IRISH SURGEONS AND SURGERY
IN THE TWENTIETH CENTURY

This book is dedicated to my wife Mary and to the wives of all the Irish surgeons of the twentieth century.

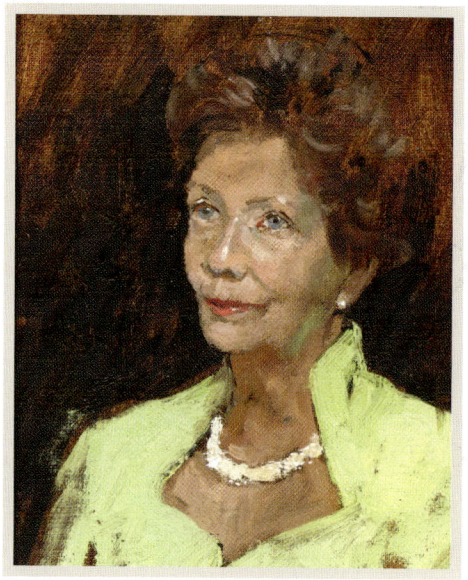

IRISH SURGEONS AND SURGERY IN THE TWENTIETH CENTURY

EDITED BY
PROFESSOR BARRY O'DONNELL

GILL & MACMILLAN

Gill & Macmillan Ltd
Hume Avenue, Park West, Dublin 12
with associated companies throughout the world
www.gillmacmillan.ie

© Barry O'Donnell
978 07171 4307 8

Index compiled by Cover to Cover
Design by Design Image, Dublin
Printed by GraphyCems Ltd, Spain

This book is typeset in 10 pt Berling Roman on 16 pt leading.

The paper used in this book comes from the wood pulp of managed forests. For every tree felled, at least one tree is planted, thereby renewing natural resources.

All rights reserved.
No part of this publication may be copied, reproduced or transmitted in any form or by any means, without permission of the publishers.

A CIP catalogue record for this book is available from the British Library.

5 4 3 2 1

CONTENTS

	Foreword *by Professor Frank Keane, President of RCSI*	vii
	Introduction	ix
	Acknowledgements	xxi
1	Chronicle of Twentieth-Century Surgery	1
2	The Development of Surgical Training in Ireland (*W. A. L. MacGowan and Barry O'Donnell*)	13
3	Surgeons' Lives	29
4	Smaller Hospitals and County Surgeons	43
5	Professors of Surgery, Queen's University Belfast	51
6	Belfast Surgeons	63
7	Surgeons in Northern Ireland by County (excepting Belfast)	97
8	Specialist Surgeons in Northern Ireland	127
9	Professors of Surgery in the Republic of Ireland	163
10	Surgeons by County in the Republic of Ireland	207
11	Dublin Surgeons, Classified by Hospital	265
12	Cork, Galway and Limerick Surgeons	333
13	Cardiac Surgery in the Republic of Ireland (*Mr Maurice Neligan*)	363
14	Neurosurgeons in the Republic of Ireland	379
15	Obstetricians and Gynaecologists (*Dr John F. Murphy and Barry O'Donnell*)	387
16	Ophthalmic Surgery (*Dr John Nolan*)	407
17	Orthopaedic Surgeons in the Republic of Ireland	451
18	Ear, Nose and Throat Surgery in the Twentieth Century (*Mr Andrew J. Maguire*)	475
19	The Evolution of Paediatric Surgery (*Prof. E. J. Guiney*)	539
20	Plastic Surgeons in the Republic of Ireland	551
21	Urologists in the Republic of Ireland	559
22	Anaesthesia (*Prof. Richard Clarke*)	577
23	Radiology (*Prof. David McInerney*)	603
	Afterwords	620
	Notes	627
	Index	629

FOREWORD

If the twentieth century can be regarded as the Golden Age of world surgery, it sprang from the well-fertilised soil laid in the previous century. In Ireland medicine and surgery evolved from the internationally renowned 'Dublin School' of which Abraham Colles was, by common consent, the outstanding Irish surgeon. The Royal College of Surgeons in Ireland, founded in 1784, represented Dublin surgery only until about fifty years ago. Even then it was seen as a body that held examinations and granted Diplomas of Fellowship but had little relevance for surgeons in training or established practitioners. This has changed completely in recent years and the College now devises and supervises training programmes, organises postgraduate education and has a wide supervisory, though not disciplinary, role in the specialty.

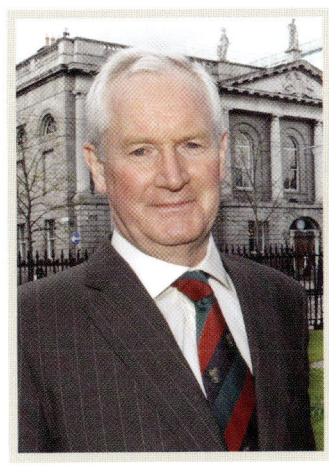

Professor Frank Keane

The history of the College has been admirably covered by J. D. H. Widdess in *The Royal College of Surgeons in Ireland and its Medical School 1784–1984* (1984), and Sir Charles Cameron's *History of the Royal College of Surgeons in Ireland and of the Irish Schools of Medicine* (1916) has a number of short biographical sketches. These are all related to doctors associated with the College. This book attempts a wider canvas and looks, all too briefly in many cases, at the lives of the great majority of those who practised surgery on the island of Ireland in the century past, whether or not they had any association with the College. Leafing through these biographical sketches will provide material for discussion on the place in our history of the varied members of this large cast. 'Who was the best?'

The editor has had a close association with the College before and after his Presidency (1998–2000). Barry O'Donnell is as Cork as the river Lee, drisheen or, perhaps tellingly, the Blarney Stone. He qualified as a doctor from University College Cork and then spent six years in England, the last fifteen months as Senior Registrar at the Hospital for Sick Children, Great Ormond Street, London. In 1955, the Ainsworth University College Cork Travelling Scholarship ('a magic carpet') took him to the Lahey Clinic, Boston, where he worked with the world famous Dr Richard B. Cattell. He also worked at the Floating Hospital for Infants and Children in Boston with Dr Orvar Swenson.

In June 1956, at the age of 29, he was appointed to the staff of Our Lady's Hospital for Sick Children in Dublin, and it was here that he worked until his retirement in 1993. One of his proudest achievements was being the driving force behind the establishment of the Children's Research Centre in 1965. He became the first Professor of Paediatric Surgery at the Royal College of Surgeons in 1986.

In 1976, after a decade of negotiations on behalf of his colleagues, he had the unique and remarkable honour of concurrently becoming President of the Irish, British and Canadian Medical Associations.

He has published extensively, including three seminal textbooks on paediatric surgery and a biography of his hero Terence Millin. He was also Chairman of the *British Medical Journal* from 1982 to 1988. He has delivered a clutch of eponymous lectures and has been a Hunterian Professor of the English College and visiting Professor to many United States universities, including twice to Harvard.

When he is relaxing, Barry's family has been his single focus, together with his charming wife Mary Leydon, whom he has crowned 'the best decision of his life', while John, Catherine, Nicholas and Michael are all admirably and diversely accomplished. At play, he has graduated from being a stocky combative rugby hooker for his university to becoming an offshore sailor who took part in the notorious Fastnet Race of 1979. Golf continues to defeat him.

Holding a conversation with Barry is to be pleasurably assailed by a verbal brew rich in wit, story telling and anecdote, and he is the most sought after medical after-dinner speaker of his generation. If one were to describe a renaissance Bob Hope, but at the same time with a sharp political nous and commitment, scientifically sound and yet devoted to his craft, then this might give you a glimpse of the rich tapestry that goes to make up the editor. It is a testament to both his energy and creativity that, in his 83rd year, he has provided us with this documentary account of surgeons and their practice in Ireland through the last century. For this we owe Barry a singular debt of gratitude.

Frank B. V. Keane
President, The Royal College of Surgeons in Ireland
October 2008

INTRODUCTION

This book is a celebration of Irish surgeons and surgery. It covers the island of Ireland and deals with a unique and unrepeatable chapter in the history of the specialty. During a period in which the total population of the island grew about 36 per cent to just over six million people, the number of surgeons grew from about 120 in all, to over 560. The group is unique in having progressed from an age when the central function of the individual surgeon was taking responsibility for the patient and the patient's welfare to the present time when care is often shared not just with colleagues in other specialties but also with other surgeons.

Surgery is one of the pinnacles of civilised activity of the twentieth century. Intervention is central to its practice and, indeed, the alternative decision not to intervene is equally important. But when in January 2007 the *British Medical Journal* published a list of medical milestones from 1840 to 2006, surgery was not one of the fourteen selected topics. Anaesthesia rightly makes the list, with its successful dentist practitioner, William Morton, demonstrating the success of ether, in Boston in 1846. Also included is imaging, with its iconic unchallenged founder, Wilhelm Conrad Röntgen, in Würzburg on 8 November 1895. Indeed, the position of the sections on anaesthesia and radiology towards the end of this book is certainly not a reflection of their importance in twentieth-century surgery. Radiology, currently called imaging, more than any other specialty showed the surgeons what needed to be seen, while the practice of anaesthesia not only provided safe conditions during operations but also, critically almost 'unconsciously' invented intensive care, which has benefited almost every specialty in medicine as well as surgery. As editor of this book, I believe that the two biggest advances in surgery in the twentieth century were not surgical at all but were anaesthesia and radiology. Surgery has developed through a gradual accretion of fresh approaches with few peaks attributable to a single person.

Seventy per cent of people who go into hospital are admitted for some form of surgery. It is now estimated that in the developed world at least 75 per cent of the population, who currently have a life expectancy of 77 to 83 years, will have a significant twentieth-century operation before they die. In 80 per cent of solid cancers the primary treatment is surgical. It is difficult to think of an activity that is more demanding with such narrow margins between success and failure, between life and death. Despite that, there is a mixed public perception of surgery and surgeons. People are happier about surgery than they are about surgeons. To adapt George Orwell in *Animal Farm*, 'surgery good: surgeons bad.' The most frequently used adjective for surgeons is 'arrogant'. How can sociopaths with varying degrees of adaptation populate a pinnacle of human achievement? Surgeons are constantly explaining themselves to the public and it is accepted that when you are explaining, you are losing. Members of the public live with the paradox, 'The surgeons are an arrogant, greedy, temperamental crowd, but I am lucky: I have one of the caring ones.' It is doctors, and particularly surgeons, who make hospitals great, though at present many hospital websites seem to be dominated by litanies of administrators. Nobody goes to hospital in the hope of meeting an outstanding and sympathetic administrator, and the home page of the domain is not the place to acknowledge their important contribution to the smooth running of the institution.

There is no identity kit for a typical surgeon. Any meeting of the specialty will confirm this. 'The long and the short and the tall' are all there. There are those with a sometimes fatal fluency and those silent by choice. In any gathering of them there will be a generally upbeat attitude, particularly about the most recent innovation. Patients like upbeat surgeons and positive predictions. Many have taken to heart the management mantra, 'Be proactive.' Sir Anthony O'Reilly, the colourful Irish industrialist, has said, 'Surgeons are an optimistic group and the truth is only a temporary embarrassment to them.' F.D. Moore of Harvard has said, 'Surgery is organised optimism.' At the turn of the millennium, a gathering of the leading surgeons of the world was invited to Scotland for a couple of days to attempt to identify the qualities that make for a first-rate surgeon. The only conclusion possible was that very few had all the qualities outlined as desirable. It was wryly commented that while these great and good were away, the quality of surgery at their home base probably did not suffer.

This all-too-brief examination of some hundreds of careers indicates little common ground. In the early part of the century, they were all individualists, and strong ones at that. As the concept of teams and a more collegiate approach takes over, these peaks of personality have tended to flatten out. One thing that requires saying is that the majority had a considerable amount of intelligence, ability and stamina. Some academics believe that medicine attracts second-class brains. Certainly we might not measure up to the particle physicists. 'In science there is only physics. The rest is stamp collecting,' said Nobellist (Chemistry) Sir Ernest Rutherford. The qualities that make for a successful surgeon are mostly the qualities that make for success in other professions. To these are added the necessary manual requirements. Perhaps nine out of ten who want to do surgery have the handicraft potential. The tenth, the odd one out, may provide end results which are comparable with the best, even if the operation is not pretty. The subject has a certain mystique and the courage displayed in other areas may come in useful in the operating theatre. On the other hand, a former Chief Medical Officer of Health for England and Wales told the editor that he had 'never put in a stitch' in his life and that, when faced with suturing a small scalp laceration, in his intern year, he realised that he never would. He had never 'scrubbed up' to assist an operation and his only knowledge of operative surgery was from screens of one kind or another. Not the sort of background that would provide a sympathetic insight into the challenges faced by operating surgeons.

Access to a medical school became competitive only about 1960. Before that, if you showed up with requisite fee or scholarship and the minimum scholastic requirements, you were admitted. Since then, medicine requires the highest academic requirements. The number of women entering the profession increases every year, though the number of women surgeons remains depressingly low and there is no woman general surgeon included in this book. But the great majority of those men who have had successful surgical careers have had honours degrees and many, a great many, have topped their class at graduation. Their interests, often rugby, sailing and subsequently golf, are to some extent markers for an energetic, strenuous life, where sustained vigour and resilience are the most needed, perhaps the central, requirements for survival.

There was a popular television programme about surgeons some years ago called *Your Life in Their Hands*. The title could be adapted for the present work as 'Your Life *was* in Their Hands'. Mostly, indeed almost all, safe hands.

It is hoped that this exercise will not deter others from doing something similar in future years. Perhaps an update will be required every thirty or forty years. Don't make the gap too long. There are some regrets. It took some time to develop the Brief Biography form which formed the basis of many of the entries, and there were still some omissions. More anecdotes would have enlivened the book. Gossip adds spice. Next time, living surgeons might be asked to nominate a trainee who might add something to the pen portrait. Even some of the deceased surgeons' trainees might be tracked down for a comment.

Population of Cities and Towns

The population of cities and towns with hospitals is given. 'That which can be measured can be understood,' said Lord Kelvin. The editor has a quirky interest in numbers of all sorts. There is probably a clinic somewhere that could help him with this addiction. The twenty-first century census of the population is used to give some sense of what happened regarding where hospitals were sited in the past. It will be seen that it sometimes had little to do with the size of the population served but much to do with political pressures. When the numbers are seen, there will the usual cries of anguish and claims that 'our place is much bigger than that and besides we drain a population at least three times that figure'. The point must be made that cities and towns have statutory boundaries and the figure given live within these boundaries. In Northern Ireland, the county boundary system has been abolished for all but football teams, but it was a powerful factor in where hospitals were sited in the past. Local government is one of the greatest legacies of British rule but hospital siting is not one of them.

The Present Surgical Workforce (2006)

The use of the word 'manpower' to describe the workforce is now more objectionable than ever as over 50 per cent of graduates are women. In 1900, there were about 120 surgeons of all disciplines, including eye surgeons and ear, nose and throat surgeons, on the island of Ireland. Sixty-one were in Dublin and twenty-two were in Belfast. At present, there are 345 surgeons in the Republic. The population in 2006 was 4.3 million, which means that there is one surgeon for every 12,463 persons. (In France, the figure is one surgeon for every 2,608 of the population — almost five times as many pro rata. France is widely regarded as having a better health service, little in the way of waiting lists and almost no international doctors.)

The following figures were provided by Royal College of Surgeons in Ireland (RCSI) Director of Surgical Affairs, Professor Arthur Tanner: general surgeons 112 (+ 25 vascular); cardiothoracic surgeons 10; neurosurgeons 10; ophthalmic surgeons 30; trauma and orthopaedic surgeons 72; ear, nose and throat and head and neck surgeons 36; paediatric surgeons 6; plastic surgeons 18; urological surgeons 26. There are perhaps 40–50 other surgeons who are in private practice only and who do not hold a public appointment.

These figures represent the lowest ratio of surgeons to population in the developed world. They are a shameful disgrace.

Though overseas graduates are in the majority in the junior posts, those who are in specialist registrar training appointments are Irish in a proportion of perhaps ten to one.

The population of Northern Ireland in 2006 was 1.75 million. There is one surgeon for every 8,064 persons The following figures were provided by Professor George Parks, Emeritus Professor of Surgery, Queen's University, Belfast: Workforce Northern Ireland: total number of surgeons 217, of whom: general surgeons 76; cardiothoracic surgeons 9; neurosurgeons 6; trauma and orthopaedic surgeons 45; plastic surgeons 7; paediatric surgeons 6; urological surgeons 14; ear, nose and throat surgeons 25; ophthalmic surgeons 29.

WRITING BRIEF BIOGRAPHIES OF SURGEONS: THE ISSUES AND DILEMMAS

The core of this work is a series of brief biographies of the surgeons who worked in Ireland in the twentieth century and either died or retired before 2005. Initially it was proposed that just one hundred of Ireland's twentieth-century surgeons should have a mini-biography. The commissioning committee later changed this and the decision was taken that *all* Irish surgeons should have an entry. This was a vastly greater task. There has been no previous effort to do this.

Sir Charles Cameron's *History of the Royal College of Surgeons in Ireland: The Irish Schools of Medicine, etc*, last edition 1916, was frequently mentioned to the editor. The College at that time was almost completely a Dublin institution and the book was about those who had held office in it.

J. B. Lyons has written *An Assembly of Irish Surgeons* (1984), which was a collection of elegant essays on the Presidents of the College from 1900 to 1986. Material from this was plundered and used with gratitude. *The Lives of The Fellows of the RCS England* has been a source of accurate facts but only a minority of Irish surgeons, perhaps less than 15 per cent of all, took this qualification in the twentieth century. But no one had attempted a wider canvas. The editor now knows why.

Biographies began with lives of the saints but later secular subjects began to be studied. It has been said that there have been fewer saints since the Middle Ages because it is easier to check up on the candidates' credentials. Biographers are certainly becoming franker and now aspire to critical secular life depiction. Plutarch's *Lives*, published about AD100, was an early example of the collective genre, while Raphael Holingshed's (died *c.*1580) *Chronicles* of over three million words are thought to have provided Shakespeare with at least twelve of his plots. Sir Walter Raleigh may have been biography's first martyr. He was beheaded on the orders of the gay King James I, for criticising princes, although none of his biographical subjects had lived after Christ, 1,500 years previously. So let biographers beware. This is slow work. It is consoling to the editor that John Aubrey's 400-page, rich in anecdote, *Brief Lives*, took almost thirty years (1669–96) to complete.

The biographical part of the book then set out to produce pen pictures of Irish surgeons who worked in Ireland during the twentieth century and had either died or retired by the end of 2005. Sadly this end point had to be rigidly imposed, which meant that some distinguished surgeons within months of retirement are excluded. Few who graduated after 1965 are included. The cut-off date was put in so that those in active practice could not complain that a modest, restrained, or even critical, entry might not reflect their real qualities and so might affect their practice.

A minimum of two letters each, with a two- or three-page 'Brief Biography' form to be filled in, was sent to each contact, either to the individual, or a relative. The Internet was used where this was feasible. Much of the information was collected when Internet use was growing rapidly but by no means universal. The editor's generation had an astonishing number who were not 'connected', and these 'unwired retired' made the task more difficult by an order of magnitude. The form collected the basic facts of birth, education, family, qualifications, training, appointments, interests and recreations. There was a personalised accompanying letter in an attempt to get away from the dreaded 'direct mail shot', and a reasonable deadline for returns. Whitehall decrees that letters unanswered in six weeks go into the 'dead letter' file, a file that is sometimes circular.

The entries in this book are called 'brief biographies' but this is a somewhat inflated description as many are only a couple of lines on professional qualifications. When the editor claims, as he does, that every effort was made to include as much information as was reasonable, it is difficult to measure this effort. There are gaps that a critic might consider could have been plugged by a little more 'digging' by the editor. More work might have produced more facts, but there is a law of diminishing returns, particularly with the earlier subjects. The editor slowly learned that half a day might be spent tracking down a single pair of dates (birth and death) and that even then one of them might be wrong.

The method employed was to scour the *Medical Directory*, using the hospital staff entries at the back of the, initially one-volume, book, and select the surgeons' names from the submitted lists. These names would then be tracked down and the directory entry extracted as a basis for further enquiries. This was done for every ten years of the century up to 1990.

To compress an active life into a word capsule is a considerable challenge. The best-known effort to do this is the (British) *Dictionary of National Biography* (DNB), which now stretches to sixty volumes and 60,000 pages. It allows up to 5,000 words for a single entry. The people to be included, all deceased, are selected by the editors, and contributors are contacted. Contributors have usually either known or written about the subject, or both. It has attracted the tag 'The Great by the Good'. A basic data sheet is completed and the facts are checked against public records, including the size of the estate. The contributor supplies an essay on the subject. Hagiography and other forms of hero worship are firmly discouraged.

In *Who's Who*, which is published annually, the subjects of entries are all alive, and the subject fills in the questionnaire. It is completely factual and there are neither comments on personality nor indeed any attempt at measuring achievements. The length of an entry is no measure of worthiness, as editorial excisions are rare.

Newspaper and journal obituaries are written soon after the subject's death and the writer, even where there is no signature, may well have an eye to surviving and grieving close relatives. These may not always have revered the deceased but may be vocal about any adjective that reflects critically on their relative's memory. This may make the obituary boring even when the subject was not. But there should be some attempt at assessment of the life and work of the deceased. The keen edge is where courtesy meets unwelcome revelations. Too much sensitivity and discretion can make a dull picture. Courtesy is a key attribute of an obituary. It's nice to be frank. It's even nicer to be nice. A phenomenon or practice has been described called 'posthumous parallax' which consists of bending life histories towards all that is light and wholesome and away from anything that might reflect unfavourably on the dead. The interpretation of obituaries is more an art than a science. The obituarist is not on oath. The trade descriptions act does not apply — which is just as well. Appreciations are written by someone who knew the deceased and who sometimes elaborates on that person's private life in the context of professional achievements. They are normally initialled, allowing easy identification by the family circle.

The eulogy is an address given by a close friend or, in H. H. Asquith's slightly more distancing words, 'a frequently encountered acquaintance'. It is usually delivered at a service of remembrance, in the presence of many who knew the deceased well, and is usually long on virtue and colour. The only criticism allowed is a humorous mention of some harmless foible. Close observers can sometimes see the eulogist's nose getting longer, as for Pinocchio, as he warms to his task.

This is not a collection of eulogies but it is not meant to be misleading. The editor has a duty not to mislead. There is an effort to produce a good patchwork, which is not always a character photograph. Posterity is too often condescending of great effort. If there were but one wish for this book it is that there might have been more anecdotes. It is teasing that they are out there and that we don't have them.

OBJECTIVES AND DILEMMAS

The format chosen for this account is an attempt to combine the facts as in *Who's Who* and an effort to encapsulate a lifetime into a few sentences or a few hundred words if the information is available. This was easier when the editor knew the subject but some remarkable portraits have been assembled by other witnesses. Many of the subjects are still alive, and this may make for a less than critical appraisal. There has been an effort to be generous, unsentimental and intelligent. It is necessarily opinionated. Any attempt to animate the few available facts involves the use of carefully chosen but sometimes sharp adjectives. Every effort is made to portray people as they were and as they would wish to be remembered. There are inevitable inbuilt conflicts in this approach. Clarity and concision can also create problems. 'Everything should be made as simple as possible but no simpler,' said Albert Einstein. It is hard to be subtle in 300 words. Of all professions few surgeons are really dull.

There is a greed for information out there. Professional and amateur biographers are writing extended essays, chapters and even books on really minor characters in the past. Biography, some say, should be bold, opinionated, admiring, critical, but above all fair, or at least it should attempt to be fair.

There is an attempt to include accomplishments and passions. Capsule biographies require concision, confronting of priorities and a comparative frame of reference, generous, unsentimental and intelligent. Should failings as well as achievements be mentioned? The achievements, accomplishments and passions should outweigh the weaknesses. Major achievements should be highlighted, as they are not always obvious from a bald recital of the facts. Norman Tanner, the iconic London surgeon of the mid-twentieth century, said to the editor, 'Few surgeons leave anything except a few thousand satisfied patients and perhaps fifty trainees who have been influenced by him.' It has become customary to mention some foibles but where do you stop? A recent brilliant medical writer got a series of gushing obituaries and it was only when they were pieced together that it was noticed that there was nothing from any of his three living wives. Three. The young tend to want to see the whole picture, 'warts and all' as Cromwell would have it, but older people usually feel that discretion is important. In Ireland, iconoclasm is a favoured spectator as well as a participatory blood sport. 'The Irish are a very truthful race: they seldom speak well of one another,' observed Samuel Johnson. But the older one gets, the less one is inclined to tick someone off for his failings. Some relationship between work and life is attempted. Generational gaps change interpretation of adjectives as well as activities. No brief biography is retributive.

Most surgeons do their best work in the operating theatre, observed by few, with even fewer able to judge the quality of the work. Indeed, surgical masterpieces may have gone un noted by the surgeon himself. It would be quite uncommon for a surgeon to have a memory of ever having said, 'That's one of the best things I have ever done.' It's not pole vaulting, where one knows all about one's best performance. Certainly no one else, not even spouses, may know the day of their beloved's greatest surgical triumph. Perhaps the patient will know least of all. Again, a surgeon's work is confidential; the more famous the patient, the greater the secrecy. There is an attempt to major on a life's achievements and perhaps secondarily look at the life and work. This is often difficult in surgeons for whom, almost more than any other activity, their life is their work. In some biographies, a brief list of some of their publications is included to give a flavour of the surgeons' areas of interest and also to highlight what was considered noteworthy at that time.

The Second World War was the most important event of the century and many surgeons, especially from Northern Ireland, played a part, but it was disappointingly difficult to get details of how these men served. All entries are inadequate and one is drawn to the entry under Belfast's Sinclair Irwin, who spent almost five years as a prisoner of war in Europe. A few lines to cover this are most unfair.

Character assessment must be made in the context of the times. It is possible to be both admiring and highly critical. Most of us are a 'package' with a sort of balance sheet of qualities and achievements, which usually leaves us slightly better off than we might deserve. Some of the short biographies might make the subjects unrecognisable to their wives, children, operating theatre staffs, the anaesthetists who worked with them, their trainees and the hospital administrators. Widows' views on their late husbands were almost all highly favourable, indeed almost rose-coloured, even when their life relationship was less cosy.

If foibles, shortcomings, imperfections or quirks appear unfamiliar to some readers, the editor can only say that most of them have had some form of corroboration, and none, that he knows of, has been invented. Some drafts when re-read resembled more a somewhat overblown brief description, such as are submitted to the 'singles' or 'contact' columns of even our most-respected periodicals, than a brief objective penetrating portrait. There is often a real problem in trying to give an accurate picture of the subject that will not upset living relatives without misleading the reader. Where does duty lie? Others may well consult the book, edited by an amateur historian, when both the subject's immediate family and the editor have long since passed away. A single adjective may alienate more than the immediate family. There is no attempt to emulate the rose-tinted spectacles and give the sort of approach that Barbara Cartland, the romantic novelist, might have adopted. The extravagant language of the estate agent is eschewed. Against all this must be balanced the biographer's curse of personal disenchantment.

Even primary sources can conflict. Every biographer knows that all evidence is suspect. Even the subject's memory of an event may be in conflict with the facts recorded at the time. Trainees' opinions can, and do, differ widely on individual trainers. Here there are many more than one opinion. This is obvious even when dealing with close associates and friends who might be expected to have the same values. One is consoled in these assessments by the diversity, often conflicting, of comments on the Internet on restaurants and hotels. Even oral testimony can be dodgy, open to distortion, often disconcerting and frequently deliciously unpredictable. Hearty laughter at the end of a supposedly illustrative anecdote is too often a contrarian marker to its veracity. Stories are condiment. They are pepper and salt, not the meat.

The inclusion of a quirk or characteristic may enhance the perception of the subject, as well as improving the writer's provenance in other areas. Pretty well every 'Brief Biography' here will illuminate the pains, perils and pitfalls of this activity. Even professional biographers will admit to occasionally making bricks with straw.

The entries differ from many professional offerings in that they are not obsessed with sex. It is hoped that the gaps are filled without resorting to fiction. Publishers believe that what sells biographies of even minor characters are intriguing details, compelling quotes and anecdotes. There will be complaints along the lines of 'not enough about X' and 'too much about Y'. The answer is that I would have liked to have had a minimum of 300 words on everyone and would have wished for colourful material to work on, but it was not to be.

This is a slow work. I envy novelists who can make up the details of their characters and cannot be contradicted about their personal qualities. A Herculean effort was made by the editor not to settle old scores (alas, there were some) and the entries have, by his standards, if anything erred on the generous side. This is not a dictionary; it is not a directory but an attempt to provide an even-handed view of those who practised surgery at that time.

Nowadays no one would write, publish or read a totally bland anodyne biography of 300 pages so why should we expect a totally bland anodyne 300-word capsule? The dead and the living have rights; so have readers. Should readers be deceived by withholding facts and opinions about individuals that were known to all around him except perhaps his immediate family? Is respecting a couple of people's feelings more important than telling the truth? It is indeed a delicate balance that has to be struck. Disclosure improves credibility, which in turn is maintained by measured assessment. The great majority of entries are benign and there is no malignancy.

The Missing

The book is an effort to portray surgery as it was and is, and in this it attempts to include all, but there will have been some lost in the trawl. There are surgeons dead and alive who are missing from this book. This is to be regretted. No omissions are deliberate. Some other entries are only a few words and are a poor reflection of a life's work. Some of the living retired have an incomplete entry, even though they had been asked to contribute. A number of retired living surgeons did not reply to our questionnaire. Most got two letters and an opportunity to fill the gaps in their entry. Some the editor knew well enough to make a phone call hoping for a return.

Surgeons are by and large not the most reticent of the species. Retired surgeons often complain that they feel cut off from the world in which they worked so hard and to which they made such a contribution. Yet a number of them, retired, alive and well, did not 'help us with our enquiries', although there was no question of an obligation to purchase. As the book is trying to cover the ground, the only entry for some is the sparse and stark *Medical Directory* entry. In the nature of things, these entries omit information on career, family, interests within and outside surgery. There is bound to be resentment, silent or expressed, from subjects or relatives about truncated entries or omissions, and in some cases the editor is indeed responsible but in most instances he is not. Doctors are well known for not responding to correspondence. A former secretary of the IMA used to say that if you offered doctors a tenner (£10), the price of a meal for two at the time, to return a stamped addressed envelope, most of them would not do it.

Widows were by far the best respondents and they all gave glowing accounts of their deceased husbands. Sadly some offspring, even surgical offspring, did not reply or promised immediate action but failed to follow through. Many of the medically qualified descendants have written thousands of words for publication in books and journals but declined to produce the few hundred words needed for some appreciation of their forebears. Some of the directory entries do not contain even dates of qualifications or training posts.

There will be some who will say that they were not given the opportunity to compile an entry for themselves or a relative. A few of these claims will be well founded but sadly the majority of omissions are the result of oversight or a decision not to participate. The editor did not enter a witness protection programme before publication. He may regret it.

ACKNOWLEDGEMENTS

This book was conceived by the editor as a series of short biographies of one hundred of Ireland's leading surgeons over the past century. The Royal College of Surgeons in Ireland, sponsor of the publication, thought that it should try to cover all the surgeons who worked on the island of Ireland during the twentieth century and had either retired or died before the end of December 2005. All those in active practice at that date are excluded. This 'stroke of the pen' change of policy has meant a much longer gestation period; from the presentation of the idea to the publication it will be six years. It must be said immediately that without the considerable financial underwriting by the College this 'loss-leader' book would never have seen the light of day.

There are many to whom I am grateful for all kinds of support.

President Frank Keane had the difficult job of writing a foreword and for this and much else over the years I am grateful.

The College was represented firstly by Kevin O'Malley, Registrar, and then by his successor in office, Michael Horgan. Between them, in one way or another, they have provided almost sixty years of service to the institution. Michael Horgan continued the initial support given by Kevin O'Malley in the face of steeply rising budgets and delivery dates trailing off into the hereafter.

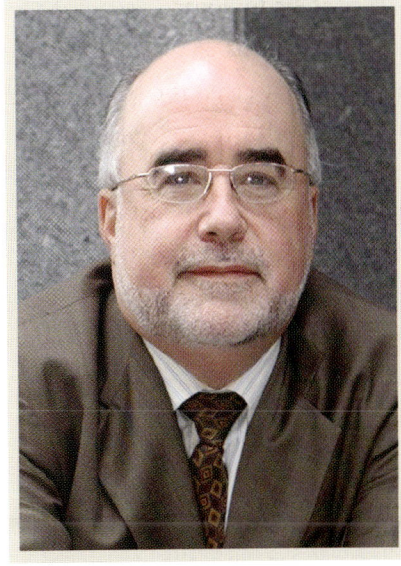

Mr Michael Horgan

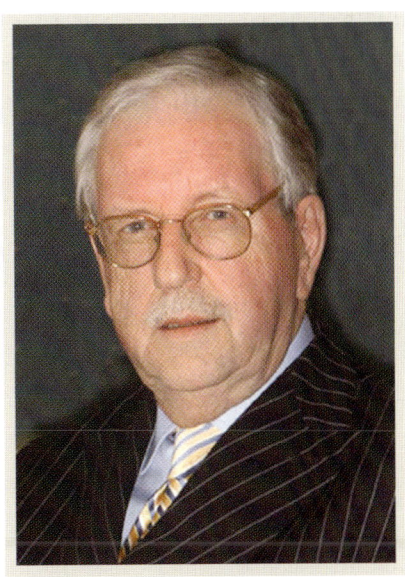

Professor Kevin O'Malley

The College owes much of its present success and prestige to the symbiosis of this pair and I have been a beneficiary at many levels but especially in the preparation of this book.

Presidents Michael Butler, Niall O'Higgins and Gerry O'Sullivan all gave support whenever I flagged. Past Presidents W. P. (Billy) Hederman, Dermot O'Flynn, Tom Hennessy and Peter McLean all weighed in with both serious and amusing material.

Beatrice Doran and Mary O'Doherty showed me what a great resource we have in the Mercer Library, and their assistance is really appreciated.

David Horgan and Christine Hamilton assisted with some tedious research and stayed close to the data at all times. Anne Gregg of the Examinations Office gallantly volunteered for secretarial assistance, for which I am grateful.

Bairbre Guilfoyle is in a special category as it was she who obtained most of the photographs and images. She was much more effective than I could possibly have been. Thank you.

The major section and chapter writers are owed a special debt of gratitude. (Sir) David Innes Williams, my old chief and friend, has said many times that 'Writing chapters for other chaps' books [was] one of the least rewarding tasks in a career'. Eddie Guiney calls it 'intellectual slavery'. This makes me more than ever grateful to those who did this work.

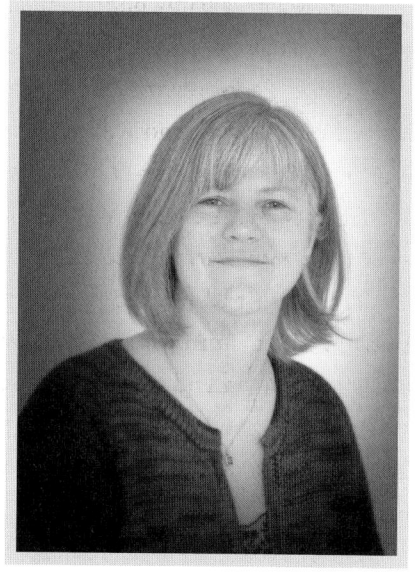

Bairbre Guilfoyle

Richard Clarke is a polished medical historian whose book, *The Royal Victoria Hospital, Belfast*, I have plundered discriminately. He brought his skills to the chapter on 'Anaesthesia' which will be quoted for a long time to come. He helped us in a great variety of ways with queries about the 'Vic' (RVH Belfast) and those who worked there.

Eddie Guiney, who has written previous chapters for books I have edited, loyally produced an account of paediatric surgery.

Bill McGowan has been associated with the College throughout his career (he qualified there sixty years ago) and is an ultimate resource on College affairs and the architect of many of the College's training programmes.

David McInerney has written the chapter on 'Radiology', as the subject was called for most of the century under review. He takes us seamlessly though the advances and those with whom they are associated in Ireland. Imaging has changed all our lives.

Andy Maguire shows his affection for and insight into his chosen specialty and casts a kindly quizzical eye over an interesting cast of ear, nose and throat surgeons, as they were then.

John Murphy has provided a graceful overview of obstetrics and gynaecology at a time when Ireland, and particularly Dublin, led the world.

Maurice Neligan's story of cardiac surgery benefits from his being so much part of it: a witness to its painful beginnings and a mainspring of its practice at its apogee.

John Nolan gallantly undertook the backwards look on the many who practised ophthalmology, this most subtle of surgical specialties, over the past century.

George Parks rewrote and substantially updated many of the Northern Ireland entries whose now flawless character and achievements has moved some into the status of 'Latter-Day Saints'.

Dermot Byrne's views on Northern Ireland's estimable neurosurgeons were expressed with warmth and clarity.

Tom Diamond worked hard to produce valuable archival material from his beloved Mater Infirmorum in Belfast. I now have a flavour of how this great hospital survived and prospered through difficult times.

Harold Browne, the ultimate sage on so much of Irish surgery, was endlessly helpful. Joe Johnson (Mayo) and Joe O'Connor (Waterford) did their counties proud.

James Nixon, Paul Osterberg and the former orthopaedic unit secretary, Betty Beavis, provided much valuable information on the 'skeleton' of Northern orthopaedic surgeons.

Gordon Loughridge made a special trip south for an enjoyable and informative session. Jack Kyle OBE, our greatest ever rugby player and the ultimate 'safe pair of hands' on the field and in the operating theatre, provided memorable insights into some of his teachers at the RVH.

David Fitzpatrick maintains his enthusiasm for Dublin medical history and I am a beneficiary.

David Lane's astute perceptions have been welcome over the past fifty years and perhaps one of the reasons I enjoy them is that they so often reflect my own views.

Stephen Lock CBE, former Editor of the *British Medical Journal*, has been my tutor in medical writing for over thirty years and it was vital to know when I took on this project that he was there to help me. He was called upon from the start to the finish — 'guide, philosopher and friend'.

Relatives and friends of deceased surgeons have given me great assistance for which I am thankful. I am in debt to all those who contributed biographies and other material about hospitals and other institutions.

There were many vital, casual, revealing conversations over tea, coffee, water (still and sparkling), and other fluids on which excise duty had to be paid.

Michael Gill represented the publishers with great calm and equanimity. He was gentle and firm as the occasion demanded and the situation did demand much of both. He was most forbearing and helpful at all times.

At an early stage in the discussions between the College and the editor, the College took legal advice about how it might indemnify, or otherwise distance itself, from what the editor might feel was appropriate to include. Readers may well feel that this was a far-sighted move by a durable institution.

Thank you all for your unselfish assistance, without which this work, so much a labour of love, would never have been published.

This book gave the editor a sense of usefulness in his declining years. Whether this is justified or not to some extent depends on how it is received.

1
CHRONICLE OF TWENTIETH-CENTURY SURGERY

CHRONICLE OF TWENTIETH-CENTURY SURGERY

1900: SURGICAL REALITIES

It has been said that it was only about 1900 that a patient had a better than even chance of benefiting from an encounter with a doctor. Diagnosis was poor and medical remedies were almost all useless, though morphine and digitalis were in common use. Smallpox was the only vaccine of any benefit. Surgical diagnosis was confined to history and physical examination. If you couldn't see it or feel it, there was no question of venturing into the unknown, and apparently unknowable, abdomen, much less the chest or brain. Fractures and joint injuries were a large part of everyday practice. The commonest non-urgent abdominal condition then, as now, was inguinal hernia. The great majority of these did not have surgery but were treated with a truss. (Winston Churchill had a truss for his hernia from 1930 to 1947.) A strangulated hernia was almost always fatal. (In 1937, at the age of 66, Sir Ernest Rutherford, the father of nuclear physics and the first man to split the atom, died in Cambridge of a strangulated umbilical hernia.) Abdominal tumours were explored only if palpable, which meant that even in skilled hands the results were dismal. The few triumphs of opening the abdomen were largely the removal of huge, largely innocent, ovarian cysts. A colostomy for malignant disease of the large bowel was a fate worse than death, due to the absence of any reliable collecting system for the constant stool. The stoma was covered with massive 'dressings'. The smell was appalling and unrelenting. And the primary tumour was rarely removed unless it was in the transverse colon. Appendicitis, which affected at least one in ten of the population, was in most cases treated expectantly in the hope that an abscess would form. This might be drained or sometimes subside on conservative management. But genuine appendicitis carried at least a 10 per cent mortality rate.

Anaesthesia was to remain unaltered for twenty-five or thirty more years, pending the invention of endotracheal intubation. Chloroform induction of unconsciousness was followed by ether inhalation or nitrous oxide. The three states of consciousness were defined by anaesthetist Zebulon Mennell (1876–1948) as 'awake, asleep and dead. You want to have them between asleep and dead'. Problems with the maintenance of an airway and lung secretions meant that any anaesthetic lasting longer than an hour was likely to prove fatal. The 'Twenty Minute School of Operative Surgery' was at its apex, and stopwatches were in frequent use for timing the, mainly extirpative, interventions. The surgeon rarely had an assistant in those early days as the house surgeon, the least experienced person in the operating theatre, was probably giving the anaesthetic, the acknowledged entry point into a position of staff surgeon. The whole concept of someone actually assisting the surgeon was late to be accepted. When it did come, there was rarely a second assistant, even in complex procedures. Much surgery took place in nursing homes, with an experienced nurse handing the surgeon the instruments and sutures, as well as assisting at the operation. As late as the 1950s, the leading gall-bladder and bile

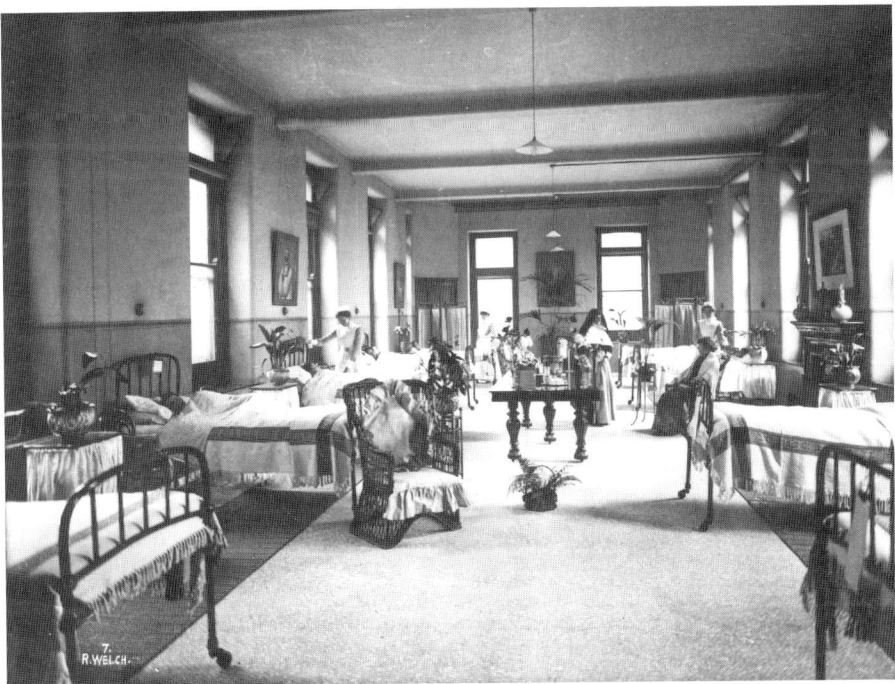

A ward in the Mater Infirmorum, Belfast, about 1900.
Spotless, polished, restful, calm and welcoming, with plants everywhere. The key figure in the right background is the overseeing nun, a Sister of Mercy, who kept it that way.

duct surgeon in the world, Dr Richard B. Cattell of Boston, told the editor that the high complication rate of such surgery in the US was largely a result of operating without adequate assistance. He said that he could not possibly make this statement in public.

A list of commonly performed procedures is a reality check. Remember that we are describing Ireland, which, because it was so poor, was then well behind the rest of the western world in medical and surgical matters. In 1900 the gross domestic product of Ireland was 68% of the rest of the UK. Most frequent were reduction of fractures and dislocation, with falls from horses causing much damage. Then drainage of abscesses and suturing of wounds, removal of superficial tumours such as cancer of the lip and breast, repair of cleft lip, amputations for infected fractures, relief of strangulated hernia, trephination for head injuries, urethral lithotomy, tapping of hydroceles and circumcision. Appendicectomy was rare, as was prostatectomy and, most surprisingly, any form of hernia repair.

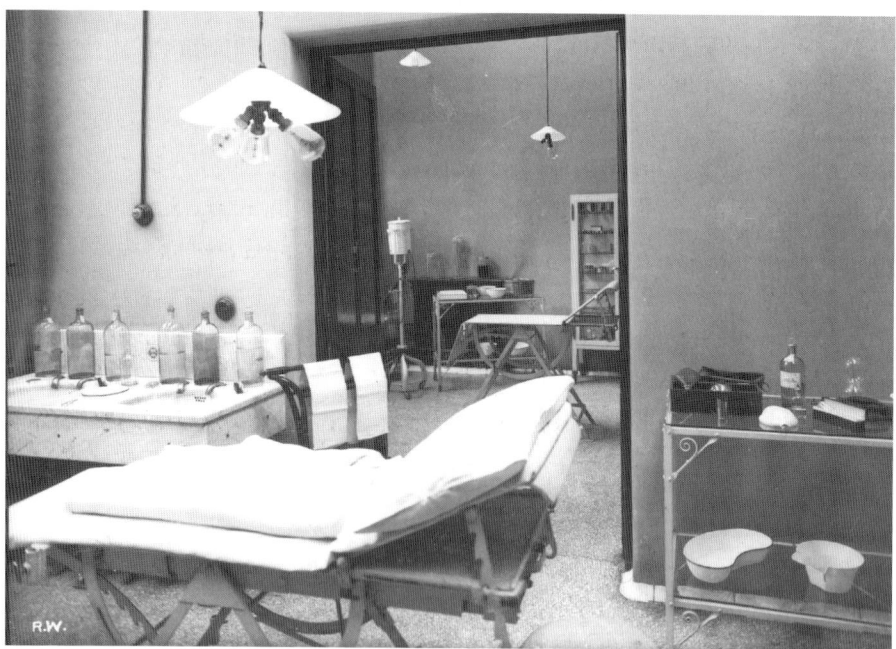

Operating Theatre, Mater Infirmorum, Belfast, about 1900.
Both operating tables are in the head up position for induction of anaesthesia. The light bulbs provided unintended heat as well as light. There was no air-changing equipment. The six jars probably contained antiseptics such as carbolic acid in various strengths. This was the antiseptic era before the change to aseptic practice. The room in the background has an irrigating apparatus. Irrigation with antiseptics was popular for a wide variety of problems at that time.

The First World War, 1914–18

The major surgical lessons of the war were: 1) no early (primary) suture of possibly infected wounds; 2) colostomy for all large bowel injuries; and 3) blood transfusion. There was little concept of any fluid replacement other than blood. All these lessons had to be relearned in the Second World War, 1939–45. Fractured shaft of femur was common and the standard treatment of a Robert Jones splint worked well in otherwise healthy young men. It worked poorly in fractured neck of femur in elderly females.

1920–1940

Anaesthesia, with the advent of endotracheal intubation, became safer, and longer operations became feasible. The biggest impact was on thoracic surgery. The cholecystogram, the test for gall-bladder function, was available in the 1930s, and chyolecystectomy (removal of the gall-bladder) became common. However, exploration of the common bile duct for gallstones remained a hazardous procedure until late in the twentieth century. Peptic ulcer was treated by gastro-enterostomy (75 per cent success rate). Colon resection for cancer was safer in some hands than others. 'Colostomy life' was still a terrible fate because of poor collecting equipment. The insertion of the Smith Peterson nail, which transfixed and stabilised the common fractured neck of femur in the elderly, was a vital *tour de force* for surgeons of that era. Breast surgery evolved from the mutilating, mandatory radical mastectomy with axillary clearance which Halsted described in 1890 to less radical surgery, simple mastectomy which was succeeded by 'lumpectomy' and then radiotherapy from the 1950s to the 1980s. Chemotherapy evolved from the 1980s onwards.

1940–1960

The really big advances were antibiotics, particularly penicillin, to combat infection, and a better understanding of the body's fluid requirements following trauma and surgery. Removal of damaged intervertebral discs for severe, persisting, low back pain became common.

Partial gastrectomy replaced gastro-enterostomy for peptic ulcer. The first kidney transplant was in 1954.

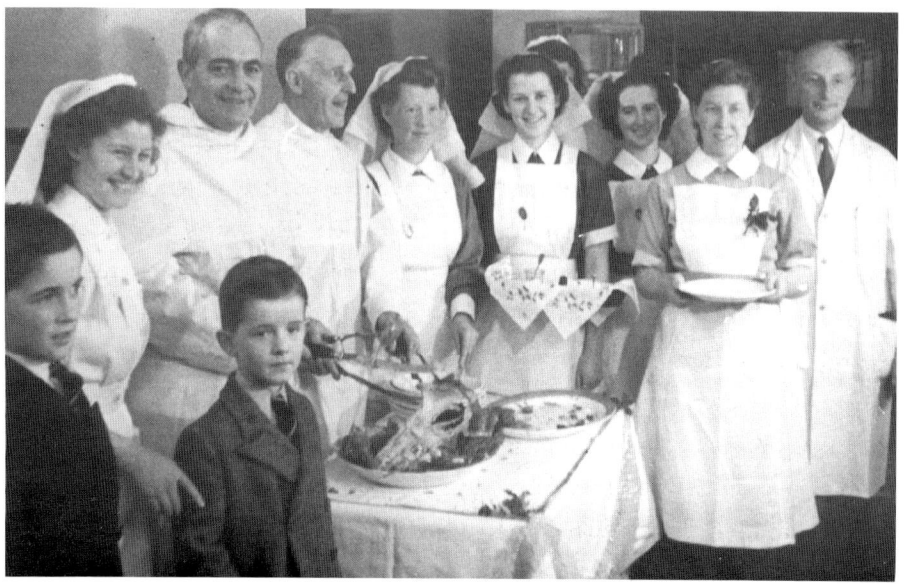

Carving the turkey
Christmas Day, Royal Victoria Hospital, Belfast, 1948.
   Surgeon James (Jamsie) Loughridge is carving the turkey assisted by Surgeon Eric McMechan on his left. All the nurses are local. Jamsie's son Gordon who was to become urologist to the RVH is on the left. In those days it was traditional for the consultant staff (called Honoraries) to visit the hospital with their children on Christmas Day. Matron would have had presents for the children.

1960–1980

The Growth of the Specialties

These two decades were dominated by spectacular growth in the specialties. Orthopaedics was completely changed by the introduction of joint replacement. The hip (John Charnley of Manchester) was first, then the knee, and later the shoulder, ankle and finger joints. Before hip replacement, osteoarthritis of the hip was treated by giving patients a walking stick if they had a limp and an osteotomy, which gave them a limp, if they had pain. At the time of writing, joint replacement is much the commonest significant elective surgical operation in the developed world. The specialty also benefited hugely from the concept of open reduction and internal fixation of fractures (the Arbeitsgemeinschaft fur Osteosynthesefragen (AO Organisation) was founded jointly by surgeons and the surgical instrument industry in Switzerland, 1958) with the introduction of a huge array of bone screws, plates and intramedullary nails. Arthroscopy was followed by arthroscopic repairs of damaged joints.

Orthopaedic surgeons gradually took over trauma in many hospitals because there was so much more that they could do, and needed to do, for limb injuries.

Lung surgery began in the 1930s with positive pressure anaesthesia, but cardiac surgery did not really prosper until the heart lung machine ('the pump') allowed prolonged intra-cardiac surgery for cardiac valve replacement and blocked coronary artery bypass using the patient's veins (1965). Coronary artery bypass was at one time (1975) the commonest major operation being carried out in the US. Perhaps the seminal operation of the century was cardiac transplant, first carried out in Cape Town in 1967 by Christiaan Barnard. Cardiac surgery created the need for intensive-care units, which in turn became one of the biggest advances in the care of the critically ill during the twentieth century.

Vascular surgery, whereby damaged vessels are replaced or, more recently, stented, awaited the gradual development of appropriate synthetic materials, and the formerly deadly rupture of an aortic aneurysm could be predicted by ultrasound, and the 'big bad bulge' replaced in time.

Urological procedures were dominated (over 70 per cent) by surgical intervention for obstructive benign prostatic hyperplasia. Newer endoscopes, particularly fibre optic lighting systems, made open prostatic surgery, even the brilliant Millin [q.v.] retropubic operation, all but obsolete. Some kidney stones could be shattered by sound waves. The biggest end-of-century controversy in urology centred on the issues of screening and surgery for prostatic cancer.

Plastic surgery grew out of the need for specialised burns management and the reconstruction of war-damaged personnel but also covered cleft lip and palate and other congenital malformations. The biggest expansion was into 'cosmetic', or as some would have it 'aesthetic', surgery for which the demand appeared limitless.

Paediatric surgery grew when it was shown that the results of newborn surgery were hugely superior in units with special teams of experts. Ultrasound imaging (1975) was more useful in paediatric surgery than in almost any other surgical specialty. Paediatric urology grew up around re-implanting the ureters as the best management for the common vesico-ureteric reflux in children. The operation is in decline having been largely replaced by endoscopic correction of the problem.

It has been said that every specialty begins to subdivide ten years after its inception. We do well what we do most often.

1980–2000

Two general innovations dominated these decades. The technological advances in imaging gave us computerised axial tomography (the CAT scan) (c.1980), which provided views of organs and body cavities, particularly the brain, chest and abdomen. Magnetic Resonance Imaging (MRI) (c.1985) further refined and defined our knowledge of the extent of disease and trauma. Neurosurgery was perhaps the biggest beneficiary of these two modalities but all specialties put them to use.

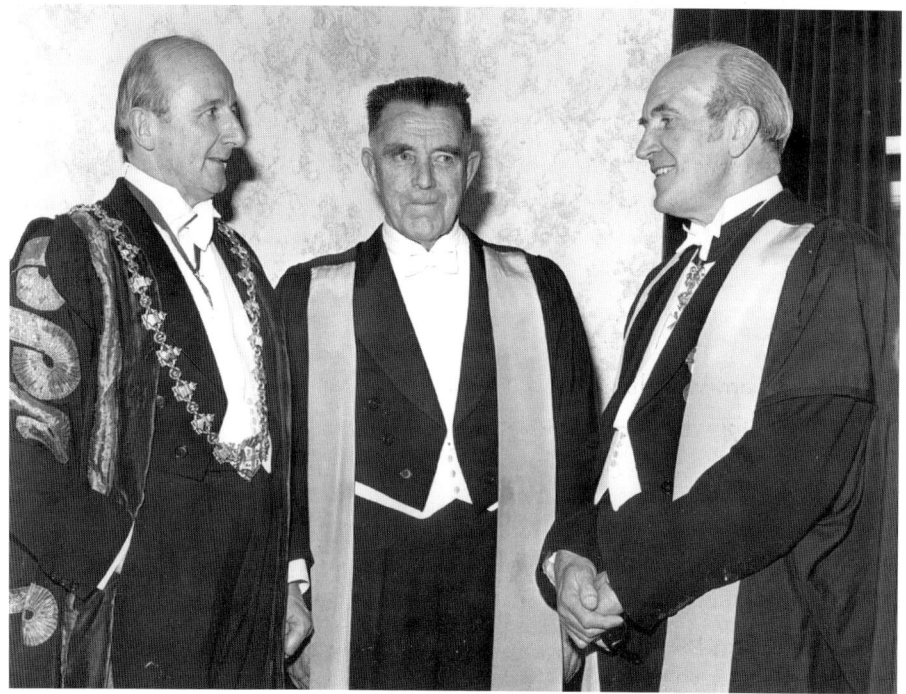

Three men in evening wear
Charter Day Dinner at the RCSI, February 1972. The dinner commemorates the granting of a Royal Charter to the College in 1784. This would have been one of the last such dinners where full evening dress was obligatory. Orders and Decorations are still worn (2008). The two surgeons with the College President were made Honorary Fellows of the College that evening.

Left: John Lanigan, Neurosurgeon, President of the College 1970–1972.

Middle: Professor Patrick Kiely, Professor of Surgery, Cork. He had taken the FRCS England. Few Cork graduates took the FRCSI until about 1965. Previous to that they went to London or Edinburgh for a Fellowship.

Right: John Corcoran, MCh, Surgeon, Mater Hospital Dublin. He belonged to a generation who were advised by UCD not to take a Fellowship at any of the Royal Colleges. They were advised that the MCh (NUI) was as good as any Fellowship. It meant, however, that he could not get a senior trainee post in the UK.

The other innovation was minimally invasive ('keyhole') surgery, which came to be used in almost every specialty. The original instrument of this genre was the transurethral prostate resectoscope but it came to encompass every intervention. Patients (and the media) loved it. Less pain and reduced bed stay were just two of the benefits.

Better treatments for cancers were emerging and with them emerged a new breed of cancer specialists: surgical oncologists. Transplant surgery continued to get the media headlines as the urgent search for organ donors intensified in some dramatic narratives.

Those with an overall responsibility for ensuring that the necessary services are available have a snowballing responsibility. The general population is getting older and has a greater potential for getting sicker with each passing year of life, and then there is so much more that can be done for each sick person. Most of the sick survive to require attention for the same or another condition later in life.

The Discards of Surgery

There were some startlingly dramatic but useless operations practised by a few surgeons. Usually the innovator had the biggest experience. The best known was the total removal of the colon as a 'septic focus', as advocated and practised by Arbuthnot Lane (1856–1943) of Guy's Hospital, London, in the first two decades of the century. This had absolutely no scientific basis of any kind. But the concept of septic foci lived on and wholesale teeth extraction, called 'dental clearance' as 'septic foci', was carried out well into the open-heart surgery era of the 1960s. (In 1942, the editor, aged 16, was advised to have all his teeth out on these grounds, but refused.) But perhaps the best paradigm is the surgical saga of King George VI (1895–1952) who was circumcised at birth by an east end of London mohel. This procedure is no longer routinely carried out, outside America, except for religious reasons. He had his tonsils removed in early childhood. Tonsillectomy has not disappeared but is in steep decline. He had an appendicectomy for recurrent abdominal pain. The concept of 'chronic appendicitis' causing abdominal pain has been abandoned. He had a gastro-enterostomy for his duodenal ulcer. Gastric operations, using either resection or drainage, are no longer employed for the treatment of uncomplicated peptic ulcer. In 1948, he had a lumbar sympathectomy for obstructive vascular disease of his legs. He nearly died during surgery as he bled profusely and the operation just made his legs warmer, without any improvement in his walking. He had a lung resection for cancer in 1951 but died, probably of coronary artery disease, six months later. The vascular insufficiency in his legs, his lung cancer and his coronary artery disease were probably all caused by tobacco (he was an heroic cigarette smoker of up to sixty a day) but this relationship was not accepted until the mid-1960s.

Perhaps the most important discard was partial gastrectomy for peptic ulcer, an operation which 'cured' perhaps 80 per cent of patients but left the remainder with serious side-effects. Better control of hyperacidity by medication and a better understanding and treatment of ulcer causation did not come on the scene until the early and late 1980s respectively. But for fifty years gastrectomy had been one of the commonest major operations in surgery and was often used as form of shorthand to assess a surgical tyro's experience. 'How many gastrectomies have you done?'

SCREENING AND GUIDELINES FOR SURGICAL PROBLEMS

Is it appropriate to say something about screening for disease in a section on discards? The public has more confidence in screening for disease than most doctors. Are we to blame for not telling people that some cancer cell types are more aggressive than others and that often the prognosis in a cancer may depend more upon the cell type than on the 'stage' of the disease? The screening test is introduced with a fanfare and its subsequent abandonment or watering down is buried in the back pages or completely overlooked.

Chest X-ray as a screening procedure for carcinoma of the lung was heavily promoted in the 1950s but was proven useless and abandoned by the American Cancer Society within twenty years. Not all 'obvious' screening procedures are of value and some are misleading. The risible campaign to get youngish men to routinely examine and compare the size of their testicles (how often, gentle reader? Once a month and the August Bank Holiday?), so that the increase in size caused by cancer would make for earlier diagnosis, was shown to be worthless when it came to results. The present big campaigns are in breast cancer where screening has been shown to be of much value though perhaps not as important as team management; testing stools for bleeding bowel cancers, which will certainly produce logistical problems; and measurement of prostatic specific antigen (PSA) for prostate cancer.

The value of screening for prostatic cancer is much debated in Europe, and the fact that half the urologists in the UK have not had their PSA measured is an important pointer. In the USA, the issue is dangerously beyond debate and any suggestion that it is less than essential and 'potentially lifesaving' is regarded as highly seditious. Solid tumour cancer seems to be settling into some sort of 80/20 rule, as in engineering, where 80 per cent of cancer patients do well on conventional treatment, and the 20 per cent with bad histology have a poorer response to treatment. Screening symptomless schoolgirls for silent bacteriuria and possible disease, particularly vesicoureteric reflux, does uncover some problems but it has been largely abandoned except as a research tool.

'Guidelines' for the management of many, indeed almost all, conditions are now in favour but there is ample evidence that many surgeons ignore them. Evidence Based Medicine (EBM) is a huge vogue with its own dedicated journals and computer databases, but some surgeons seem impervious to its dictates.

Informed Consent

Informed consent was a phrase that took root in the last quarter of the twentieth century. Up to then, perhaps from the 1950s, there *might* in some cases, if the patient were important or insistent, have been a brief discussion between patient and surgeon, but it was very much one-way. Prior to that, there was no discussion whatever. The surgeon proposed what was to be done and the only question was 'When?' Many surgeons rarely spoke to patients in public hospitals. The patient's name was put on the operating list and the procedure was carried out, frequently with the patient knowing little of what was done. The patient was grateful for the attention of the great man, who may, or, more often, may not, have done the operation himself, and if it was a success, then so much the better. If it was not a success, the surgeon had 'done his best' and there the matter ended.

One extremely distinguished London consultant, who had a slight deafness, which could be tactically increased if the occasion demanded, rarely spoke to patients at all but stood at the foot of the bed and said either 'Tuesday' or 'Thursday', which were his operating days. He then moved on. If a postoperative patient were causing anxiety, he would not visit on the grounds that 'it would be bad for morale'. It would be a mistake to believe that in Irish public hospitals behaviour was widely dissimilar. Sir James Black, the Nobel prize-winner, told the editor that the reason he gave up clinical medicine in favour of research pharmacology was that he was so upset at the way consultants spoke to and treated their patients in the wards of his medical school teaching hospital. Attitudes to the totally inarticulate were, if anything, worse. A surgical peer of the realm (that narrows it down a bit) said to the editor (c.1957) 'I would love to repair a tracheo-oesophageal fistula' (a rare and difficult chest operation in a seven pound (3.4 kg) infant). 'I hope I will be sent one.' He had never even seen the operation. The ethical wasteland and complete lack of responsible attitudes that lie behind that statement by such a leading surgeon are awesome.

The main change came when a more educated population began asking questions about the proposed intervention and its possible complications. From the surgeon's point of view, the change accelerated when there were a few well-publicised medico-legal cases in which the dissatisfied patient successfully sued for damages. The entire picture changed within a decade, perhaps the 1970s. Until then, a well-worded apology for the less-than-perfect outcome was all that was required, and the various medical insurance bodies advised that this was the correct course. As damages got bigger and bigger, the same bodies advised that any admission of liability should be carefully couched and, importantly, not made before the insurers approved the phraseology. Now pre-operative options had to be fully explored and the acronym BRAT (benefits, risks and alternative treatments) became part of the surgeon's (and patient's) lexicon.

At the turn of the twentieth century, patients began to appear with information downloaded from the Internet, and the issue became further complicated. The time-honoured 'Trust me; I'm a doctor' became changed to 'Trust me; I'm a website'. Second opinions had rarely been offered and were even more rarely asked for. 'You need an operation' 'I'd like a second opinion' 'OK; you don't need an operation' was an imaginary dialogue between doctor and patient, in America of course, but there was more than a grain of truth in it. A prominent breast surgeon told the editor that he now spends more time discussing options and management than he did on the actual surgery. In one institution, the 'consent for treatment form' for repair of an inguinal hernia is now eleven pages long.

Most surgeons can talk most patients into having the operation they propose, and a good professional will not flinch from the medico-legal issues involved, but all are now aware that consent must be fully informed.

2
THE DEVELOPMENT OF SURGICAL TRAINING IN IRELAND

W. A. L. MacGowan and Barry O'Donnell

THE DEVELOPMENT OF SURGICAL TRAINING IN IRELAND

Surgical training, from the earliest times, was essentially an apprenticeship, and in this respect surgeons were similar to the other skilled craftsmen. Indeed, the Middle Ages Guilds, which controlled the Barber/Surgeons, laid down an apprenticeship of five to seven years, followed by a period of a further three years as a journeyman or employee. Another two years were spent as a practising surgeon before being admitted to the Guild, which in Dublin was the Guild of St Mary Magdalene, which was incorporated by Henry VI in 1446.

In 1784, the surgeons separated from the Barbers and Periwig Makers to form their own College of Surgeons, by Charter of George III. It was shortly after this that surgical training education, evaluation and certification were introduced by the College. The first Letters Testimonial Examination was held in 1784. However, the credit for this profound change must go to the French, in Paris, where Louis XV in 1731 founded the forerunner of the surgical colleges, the Académie Royale de Chirurgie. It was there that Sylvester O'Halloran went to study and conceived the idea of an Irish College of Surgeons, with a motto adopted from the Collège de St-Cosme in Paris, *Consilio Manuque* (By wisdom and hands). The School of Surgery in the College was modelled on its French counterpart, and included in its curriculum Anatomy, Physiology and Pharmacy, as well as Surgery.

Surgeons need training and it is widely acknowledged that much of this training is achieved on an apprenticeship or craft model. The defining activity of a surgeon is operating and while one can read about an operation and have it carefully described to a class or smaller group, or even one on one, there is absolutely no substitute for seeing the procedure, and, better still, assisting at it, and, best of all, being assisted through it by an experienced craftsman. Films of various kinds are of increasing use. As has been said in another context, premarital courses are a good idea, and everyone should do one, but they are little preparation for the real thing.

Indeed, it could be said that surgical training in 1900 had not changed much in the previous two hundred years. It was still on a one-to-one apprenticeship basis. The hospitals had very few resident medical officers and the few who were there were general-purpose doctors, serving all members of staff. This was an advance, in that the trainee worked with a handful of people rather than a single 'master' (a term still employed in the devil/master relationship in the Irish law system). This had obvious advantages for the pupil as he (always he in those days) got to hear and see several approaches to a problem, which promoted the concept of flexibility at an early stage. The hierarchy is retained. Many surgeons employed personal assistants and paid them a small salary to carry out a variety of functions, from assisting at operations to tying up the horses to a hitching post. The concept of training as such was not in either party's mind. The object, on the one hand, was to get help and, on the other hand, to get experience. As nowadays, training involves getting experience, but experience does not necessarily mean getting training. 'Surgery is not hard to do but it is hard to get to do,' said paediatric surgeon Orvar Swenson of Boston (b. 1909). 'You spend a few years in training and the rest of your life getting experience.'

VISITING CLINICS ABROAD, 1900–1940

One of the ways of learning more about surgery in the early part of the century was to visit 'clinics', really hospitals, abroad. London and Edinburgh were nearby but the more ambitious went to the Continent, particularly Vienna (Bohler), Berlin (Sauerbruch whose patients included Mussolini, Lenin and Hindenburg) and Berne (Kocher and de Quervain). Eye surgery was particularly advanced in Vienna. After the First World War, some went to America, particularly Boston and the Mayo Clinic in Rochester, Minnesota. Travel was by boat and train. (On a travelling scholarship to Boston in 1955 the editor travelled out by boat from Cobh and sailed back to Southampton.) Flying to the US became the norm only in the late 1950s.

Few went away during their early postgraduate training years, as the favoured ones were expected to stay close to the mother hospital to give a hand. Most visits were for less than a month and some for no more than a week. A fortunate few got 'hands on' appointments, enabling them to spend more fruitful time than at the fringes of a considerable entourage. But for most it was a case of looking over the great man's shoulder and picking up useful information. The clinics were accustomed to visitors and encouraged them, for example by helping them find accommodation. Many ran structured courses of lectures and demonstrations where a fee was paid for attendance. The cost of living in post-war Europe was low, and grants or family support went a long way. Some surgeons went abroad regularly and got to know their hosts and the hosts got to know them. 'And I winked at Bohler and Bohler winked at me,' said Harry Meade, PRCSI and Professor of Surgery, UCD.

The tradition of travelling to a centre of excellence persists with the various Travelling Clubs of surgeons and 'accompanying persons' (1960) arranging visits. The custom of watching live operations in the operating theatre has been overtaken by various imaging technologies. Sub-specialisation has broken the travellers into now smaller, more international groups.

Structured Training

Structured training, as we know it today, only really got under way in these islands after the end of the Second World War. Prior to that, training was essentially an apprenticeship, on an individual basis, and largely left to the aspiring surgeon to organise himself with or without the assistance and encouragement of his mentors. The apprentice learned by assisting the surgeon. Promising trainees were given gradually more responsibility and if the chief were sufficiently influential, the trainee might be put on the staff. Competition for the solitary trainee's services at the hospital and outside was stiff, and could be acrimonious, which sometimes left him with determined enemies amongst those who felt he did not favour them. Most of the Irish surgeons up to that time confined their experience to their own alma mater, and a minority sought experience in the UK or further afield; this was usually when their career hospital appointment was confirmed.

The UK, having come through a difficult wartime period, found itself in the midst of a medical service upheaval with the introduction, in July 1948, of the National Health Service. Soon after its introduction, hospital posts were formally established for both service and training purposes. Apart from consultant posts these were:

    Senior hospital medical officers (SHMOs), a much-criticised sub-consultant grade
    Senior registrars
    Registrars
    Junior hospital medical officers
    Senior house officers (SHOs)
    House officers.

For registrars and senior registrars in surgery, the FRCS was a requirement. The plan was to have an even flow of promotion year by year from junior to more senior grades. It was also decided that the number of senior registrars should be related to consultant vacancies and that the training period at this level should be four years for all specialties. The grade of registrar was not tied to career prospects and was regarded as providing a wide range of experience. The titles of the 'trainees' caused much debate and unrest. At the beginning of the century, there were 'house surgeons' and a 'resident assistant surgeon' (RAS) who had a senior rank and would have expectations of getting on the permanent staff. Then there was the resident surgical officer (RSO) who organised the house surgeons, assisted at the biggest operations and usually had a 'list' of operations to himself. By mid-century, the terms 'house surgeon' and 'registrar' were current. To these was added the rank 'senior registrar', though this did not exist in the smaller hospitals. There was no duty roster as such. House surgeons had one half-day a week and every third weekend off, from Friday at 2 p.m. to midnight on Sunday. All house staff slept in the hospital, so the working and on-call week was 156 hours. Many teaching hospitals did not allow any annual leave. Many posts were unpaid and the trainee depended on private means or assistants' fees.

The term 'junior surgical staff' was highly unpopular in Ireland. The more senior trainees were usually in their thirties. The American term 'resident' was inappropriate where almost all of them had come to live out, even when on call. Then there were objections to the term 'trainees', on the basis that many were fully trained but did not have career appointments. Eventually the cumbersome term 'non-consultant hospital doctors (NCHD) was adopted. Our UK and US colleagues were more accepting of accurate hierarchical descriptions of posts. At the close of the century, both jurisdictions in Ireland had a higher ratio of 'trainees' to career or fully trained staff than anywhere in the developed world except Great Britain.

Electronic 'bleeps', which were carried by resident staff and went off to signify a waiting telephone call, came in about 1980, and mobile phones in the mid-1990s. Until then, most hospitals looking for a member of the surgical staff depended on a loose schedule timetable of 'Where should he be now?' The practice of wearing white coats or white jackets while in the hospital came in about mid-century, and the consultants were the last to adopt this basically hygienic measure. Name-tags on white coats came in about 1980.

It was during this post-war period that specialties of surgery started to evolve, spurred on by the wartime surgical experience, especially in trauma and orthopaedic surgery. The predominance and influence of orthopaedic surgery during this time were noteworthy.

The UK surgical colleges started in 1967 to organise surgical training and introduced courses for the FRCS and formalised recognition of senior hospital training posts. The Council of the Royal College of Surgeons of England in 1959 established a Committee on the Training of Surgeons and, through pressure of the specialty associations, Specialist Advisory Committees (SACs). To co-ordinate these SACs a Joint Committee for Higher Surgical Training, which included representatives of all four surgical colleges, was established in 1966. The SACs were established in all specialties of surgery, with representatives of all four colleges and the relevant specialty associations. Its remit was to ensure that trainees were receiving appropriate training and that there were the right number of men and women in training to fill forecasted NHS consultant vacancies. Recently (1993) the Colleges decided to amalgamate the Joint Committee with the new Intercollegiate Examinations Committee in a new body, named the Senate of Surgery of Great Britain and Ireland. The Senate has representatives from the four Royal Surgical Colleges, the Specialty Associations and the Faculty of Accident and Emergency Medicine.

Although the Royal College of Surgeons in Ireland took part in the UK committees on surgical training, the country as a whole was much slower off the mark to organise surgical training. Indeed, the earliest anecdotal records of the establishment of a surgical registrar's post were in the Mater Hospital in 1945 and in the Richmond Hospital in 1949. Before that, most aspiring surgeons started off in unpaid posts as assistant surgeons, resident surgical officers (RSOs) or resident anaesthetists, without any structured training. The favoured few were sponsored and sent abroad for training by their mentors, before being appointed to the staff of their individual hospitals. The majority had to look after themselves, with little or no assistance or, indeed, encouragement.

Surgeons on the staff of the Voluntary (teaching) Hospitals were unpaid, and usually held the title of Honorary Visiting Surgeon. Their remuneration was from their private practice. It was not until 1956–57 that a state (Department of Health) method of payment for these consultants was introduced, in the form of payment based on the number of occupied patient beds (bed days) and outpatient sessions. This method of remuneration lasted until the Consultant Common Contract was introduced in 1981.

The Council of the RCSI recognised the need for candidates to be prepared for the Fellowship Examination through an informal course in anatomy and physiology that had been in existence in the College since 1945, in preparation for the Primary Fellowship Examination. A Postgraduate Education Sub-Committee under the chairmanship of the then President, Terence Millin [q.v.], was established in 1963. A six-week full-time study course for the Final Fellowship Examination was planned with the support of the Professors of Surgery in the three Dublin medical schools. The Dublin Surgical Committee with representatives of the three medical schools was established with T. C. J. (Bob) O'Connell as its first Dean. For the first course, held in 1964, only four candidates signed on, which led to its cancellation, but it gradually gained ground. The original course for the Primary Fellowship Examination stopped in 1974. It was then reorganised, strengthened and made more relevant to surgery in the three subjects of Anatomy, Physiology and Pathology. This was very successful and continues to this day.

The four royal surgical colleges decided, in 1951, to make their respective Primary Fellowship Examinations reciprocal, but restricted entry to graduates. Up to then, the Primary Examination for the FRCSI examination could be taken by registered undergraduate medical students.

The Joint Committee for Higher Surgical Training introduced in 1966 Higher Surgical Training Programmes, initially in nine specialties, which were supervised by the SACs. Accreditation certificates were granted by the Colleges, to Fellows of the Colleges, after the satisfactory completion of training. The nine recognised specialties of Surgery were:

    General surgery

    Trauma and orthopaedics

    Otorhinolaryngology

    Urology

    Oral and maxillofacial surgery

    Cardiothoracic surgery

    Plastic surgery

    Neurosurgery

    Paediatric surgery.

The Irish College, which had been involved in the structuring of these programmes and was a member of the Joint Committee and had a representative on the SACs, decided to form a surgical training body for Ireland. This was established in 1968 and called the Irish Surgical Postgraduate Training Committee. An independent committee, meeting in the College, with the President as Chairman, it was widely representative of the College, including Fellows from Northern Ireland, the medical schools, the specialty groups, the Irish Medical Association, and the Department of Health. Its purpose was to establish and monitor the Higher Surgical Training Schemes in all specialties in Ireland. Senior Registrar posts were established for the first time in Ireland, and a rotation was set up to include the Dublin, Cork and Galway hospitals. The actual appointments had to be approved by the newly established Comhairle na nOspidéal (Hospital Council). For the first time, the formal training of a surgeon was addressed, and the quality and quantity of supervised training, with a complementary educational programme, was its objective. Operative surgery experience was, as always, a very important part of the training, but the trainee had now to be personally supervised and assessed by the consultant-in-charge. Logbooks and assessments both of the quality and quantity of training were an integral part of the evaluation of these posts and included both the trainees and the trainers. Only those hospitals that satisfied the SACs were included in the programmes. Importantly the inspection teams were drawn from the Colleges and were wholly independent.

    Trainees were encouraged to spend at least one year of their training abroad. The UK, North America and Australasia were the most popular locations. To facilitate placement of the trainees, arrangements were made with several prestigious hospitals abroad. One of the most important was an exchange programme started in 1977 between the Johns Hopkins Hospital, Baltimore, Maryland, and the Richmond Hospital, Dublin. Under this arrangement, selected Johns Hopkins surgical residents spent six months of their training in the Richmond, in general and vascular surgery. This rotation continued in Beaumont Hospital, and over fifty residents spent six months of their training in Dublin. Selected Irish trainees were placed in clinical or research posts in Johns Hopkins, for one year or more. Some twenty-five of our present-day distinguished Irish surgeons have benefited from this exchange, including five members of the present Council of the RCSI.

The first SR appointment in Ireland was in general surgery, in 1974, and the first certificate of accreditation was granted in 1976.

It became apparent that a properly structured programme was then needed at Pre-Fellowship level, which would bring together the Dublin hospitals in a joint programme. In 1973, a number of Dublin surgeons got together to devise a programme of two years, which would provide rotation between the Dublin hospitals. The programme, which started in Dublin in 1973, was modelled on a similar programme in Liverpool and provided slots in general surgery, the specialties, and accident and emergency surgery (A&E), the trainees having the benefit of exposure to many surgeons in the different hospitals where previously trainees were confined usually to one hospital and one medical school affiliation. The trainees were provided with an educational programme as well, and they usually went on to an intensive full-time course, organised in the College, by Gearóid Lynch [q.v.], prior to taking their FRCS towards the end of the two-year rotation. They then went into registrar posts in their specialty of choice, for two to three years, before applying for the highly coveted and competitive Senior Registrar posts.

A committee was set up to run the scheme, which was called the Dublin Region Pre-Fellowship Training Committee. Similar schemes followed in Cork and Galway, and the county hospitals also took part in the rotations, which were extended, in 1983, to a three-year programme. All the hospital posts involved in the rotation were subject to rigorous inspection to ensure a satisfactory level of training, along similar lines to the Senior Registrar Programmes.

An anastomosis workshop was the first of many such innovations, and operative surgery workshops were extended to other specialties, and became a very important complementary part of the practical training in surgery. Originally operative surgery was tested on cadavers in the Final Fellowship Examination but this was discontinued in the 1960s and replaced by an oral examination.

The FRCS by examination was introduced in 1843 by the English College and in the following year by the Irish College, enabled by a Supplement to the Charter of Queen Victoria. As the hallmark of the trained surgeon in past times, the Fellowship gradually retreated to the mid-training position as training expanded in length and complexity, responding to the developments in surgery itself. By the 1930s, the FRCS had become a prerequisite for appointment as a registrar or the common post of RSO (Resident Surgical Officer, who really was resident). As the specialties of surgery developed after the World Wars of 1918 and 1939, the Fellowship became out of step with North America and Australasia, where specialty board certificates and Fellowships respectively were awarded by examination on the completion of specialty training. Indeed, North American hospitals were more advanced in their surgical residency programmes, which were introduced by William Halsted in the 1880s, modelled on the German system. This was a fully structured five- to seven-year residency-training programme, followed by a Specialty Training Board Examination and Certification. It took the UK and Irish Colleges nearly 100 years to follow suit, reluctantly!

The Fellowship of the Royal Colleges, placed at the halfway mark in training, was by then an anachronism, and its status a cause of some confusion outside these islands, particularly in developing countries whose young surgeons sought the prestigious Royal Colleges Fellowship. Indeed, as early as 1959, there was a proposal to the English College to award the Fellowship only on the completion of specialty training, but this was rejected. In the meantime, to cloud the issue further, from 1966, the SACs awarded Intercollegiate Certificates of Accreditation in a specialty first, without examination, to surgeons who had completed specialty training at Senior Registrar level. Exit intercollegiate examinations, to test knowledge and competence in the specialty, were then introduced in 1989 and, in addition to the accreditation certificates, a Specialty Fellowship was awarded. A specialty suffix was added to the Fellowship, e.g. FRCS (Orth). So the successful candidates now had two Fellowships by examination, one in general surgery and one in a specialty.

In 1975, a European Directive allowed the award of a Certificate of Specialty Training by the Medical Council for the purposes of free movement in the then EEC. The certificate was granted on the recommendation of the Colleges, without further examination, to EEC citizens who had passed the Fellowship Examination and had worked for two years in a specialty, in approved registrar posts. The EU then stepped in, in 1990, and ruled that the two training certificates were incompatible. The Colleges were then forced to rethink the whole question of surgical training and evaluation in the specialties.

The British Government set up a committee to review UK specialist training, under the chairmanship of Sir Kenneth Calman, the Chief Medical Officer, and his report was issued in 1993. The Calman Report, as it is now known, changed the face of surgical training and qualifications in these islands. Surgical training was to be divided into two periods: *Basic Surgical Training* (BST), to last two years and to cover the acquisition of core knowledge and skills required by all surgeons, regardless of the specialty; and *Specialty Training* in specialty registrar posts, to last five to six years, depending on the specialty. The Fellowship was to be awarded by the Colleges, on or near the completion of specialist training, after passing the intercollegiate specialist examination.

In BST, the training posts were to be at the SHO grade, and exposed the trainees to general surgery and the specialties. A College examination at the completion of BST, replaced the Primary and Final Fellowship examinations (Parts 1 and 2). Successful candidates in this examination are awarded a Membership of the Colleges in the UK and Associate Fellowship in the Irish College. These changes started with those entering BST after July 1996. So, at long last, the Fellowship of the Colleges turned full circle and became an exit qualification, and the hallmark of the fully trained specialist surgeon.

North and South

We have seen that formal training schemes began earlier in Northern Ireland, in great measure because of the organisational improvements which were part of the National Health Service (1948). The main thrust of the various programmes was that almost all the training of surgeons took place within Northern Ireland. The Royal Victoria Hospital acted as the hub of a hub-and-spoke scheme whereby trainees spent alternating periods in Belfast and the regional hospitals until they completed the requirements. Some became fully fledged without leaving the province. This had big advantages for the consultants in the regional hospitals, as they could expect a trainee who was at a specific stage in his career, and plan accordingly. The trainee also knew years in advance where he was going to be at a given date. The disadvantage of not being exposed to a wider surgical world in England, Scotland or the USA was to some extent outweighed by the variety of the postings and, therefore, different 'chiefs' to whom one was exposed. Volumes of operations, however, did not compare with those of the big industrial cities of England. Some, 'the chosen ones', spent a year on a Fellowship in the US but this was the exception rather than the rule. Those who had served in the war were understandably anxious to settle down and begin a career post as soon as possible. The two most influential Professors of Surgery, Harold Rodgers and Douglas Roy, dominated the scene for over thirty years, and it would have to be said that neither of them was close to most of the surgeons outside Belfast.

There was a sub-group who had a somewhat different path. Catholic medical students at Queen's (about 25 per cent of the graduating classes from 1950 to 1980) would almost all have done their studentships and clerkships in the Mater Infirmorum, Belfast, rather than the Royal Victoria Hospital (RVH). This meant that when they applied for junior or senior posts at the RVH they would not be as well known to the staff and were unlikely to be successful. They went to England or possibly Scotland for further training. When they applied for consultant posts in Northern Ireland, the problem of the appointment panel 'not really knowing them', combined with an understandable loyalty to those who had given sterling service locally over the years, meant that many really well-trained surgeons were overlooked; indeed, they might not even be short-listed, and there is little question that some grave injustices occurred. A side-effect is that many able young people, though qualified to do so, did not study medicine because career prospects were so blighted. This is a somewhat sanitised version of the realities. By the 1980s, beginning with the surgical specialties, this pattern had changed radically to a 'level playing field'.

Down south, the scenario was somewhat different but it too had its failings. By and large, the Local Appointments Commission, with selection committees headed by the secretary of a government department, dispensed justice in those hospitals that they controlled. These included all the 'county' hospitals, and the Department of Health gradually took control, sometimes jointly with the local medical school, of the larger regional units.

Likely lads continued to be given advice on a path that might lead to the 'glittering prize' of a consultant appointment, but many were totally 'home-grown'. There was tremendous patronage in the hands of the professors even where independent hospital committees of management officially made the appointments. The timing of the vacancy might coincide with the end of training of a preferred candidate. Up to about 1965, many vacancies were not advertised at all. Before 1970, the major Dublin hospitals rarely appointed any to the permanent staff other than their own trainees. The category of Assistant Surgeon persisted well into the 1960s, long after it had lost its original meaning and role.

A man's regard for his institutions may, to some extent, be measured by the arrangements he makes for his succession. In business, succession planning is an early priority for all senior employees. By this criterion, some twentieth-century surgical leaders show up better than others. Some were unselfish, and likely future surgeons were sent away for experience or trained locally. Others claimed that the succession was not their business, and left their departments bereft when the predictable retirement or sudden death in office took place. Sometimes attempts were made to parachute overseas graduates into prime consultant posts, with an apparent objective of reducing private practice competition. Dysfunctional units damaged some specialties because trainees were reluctant to enter programmes where there was much internal strife. It will be remembered that for all of the twentieth century all of Ireland was a net exporter of doctors. There were many classes in which three-quarters of the graduates went abroad permanently.

Outsiders from other medical schools or hospitals found it easier to be appointed in the surgical specialties, though the growth of such specialties was not widely encouraged. Some of the Dublin teaching hospitals maintain an element of independent selection up to the time of writing and, in the past, often retained, for example, the crucial choice of extern assessor.

Trainees' Lives

As we have seen, the nature of training has changed markedly over the century. Prior to the 1960s, the trainee made his (always his) own arrangements to get experience and training. At the beginning of the twentieth century, large undergraduate teaching hospitals might have one or two house surgeons, often selected from the top performers of the undergraduate class, who might hold office for a year or two and then be expected to move on. They got free board and lodging and were expected to be on call day and night, seven days a week, fifty-two weeks a year. Since they were not paid, they depended on 'assistants' fees' from the established surgeons.

Then, a fortunate few were kept on for years and even decades, as assistants, by the 'chief', who in addition to paying fees might try to get his assistant on the staff of the institution as an 'assistant surgeon', a post which he might hold for twenty years. The assistant surgeon had no beds as of right and depended on his chief to allow him to use some of his beds. This led to massive intra-hospital rows as different chiefs espoused their own preferred assistants. Most hospitals did not appoint an assistant surgeon more often than every ten or even twenty years, and promotion to full status might take another twenty. Far from being trained in surgery, many house surgeons had anaesthesia as their principal duty, and here there was no training either.

Only those with some private means could wait for opportunities to occur. Private patients were all in private nursing homes for the first half of the century. The larger hospitals then developed a system of private wards and some few provided adjoining nursing homes.

From about 1930, the great majority of ambitious graduates went abroad, almost all to England, though those from Northern Ireland often went to Scotland, 'the mainland'. The southern Irish, like the Germans, always said 'England'. The British National Health Service (1948) changed much. The surgeons were paid and the trainees were paid. In 1949, the editor's first cheque for a month's work in The Royal Hants County Hospital, Winchester, Hampshire, was £8 (€12) after tax. For this, he was on call in the hospital for all but one half day a week, which was strictly from noon to midnight (calls after midnight were frequent), and one weekend off in every three. These conditions also applied to the intermediate training grade of registrar who was paid a bit better. Those in the top trainee grade (Senior Registrar) were allowed to live out on call. Nobody under thirty was married as there was absolutely no security and jobs were scarce. The editor unsuccessfully applied for over sixty posts when his first six months expired. The Primary Fellowship was essential for any decent jobs and there were dozens of house surgeons with the FRCS Eng waiting for registrar posts. Competition was fierce right up to the mid-1960s.

Resident Surgical Officers really were resident even at the top of the training grade of Senior Registrar. Many lived in a nearby flat provided by the hospital. In the better hospitals, there was little carousing or partying, and much on-call time was spent in the hospital library. Down the line, however, the service hospitals were staffed by itinerant trainees, including a strengthening of the stock from Commonwealth countries to include Australia, New Zealand, Canada and South Africa — people who had come for 'experience' rather than training — and the hospitals' 'messes' were much in either pre-party or post-party mode.

Despite the promise of rapid expansion of consultant surgeon numbers, the huge bulge produced by waiting ex-servicemen meant that competition for consultant posts in the period 1948 to 1960 was incredible by present standards. In 1953, a non-teaching consultant surgeon post in Kent (yes, all posts in Kent are non-teaching) attracted over a hundred applicants with FRCS Eng (no lesser breeds should apply), twelve with MS London (ditto); three of them were Hunterian Professors, and the tie-breaker was a DSO. Teaching hospitals had their own geographic 'parishes' of influence, and this was often a deciding factor.

Expansion in Numbers of Trainees

One of the issues that shows up on the most superficial study is the incredible growth in the numbers of junior, trainee or non-consultant hospital medical staff. At the beginning of the twentieth century, each major teaching hospital had perhaps two or three junior staff. Many hospitals had none. There might have been at most one hundred 'juniors' in the island of Ireland. Now every hospital has herds of NCHDs and there are perhaps 3,000 in all, about half of whom are from India or Pakistan. In the Republic, the ratio of trainees to fully trained specialists is about 2.3 to 1. It is similar in Great Britain and Northern Ireland. These ratios are unique in the world. In the US, there are five specialists to every trainee. Many large community hospitals there have only a skeleton staff of 'residents'. Most have none at all. In smaller communities, the local hospital survives by having local general practitioners, called 'family practitioners' in Canada, on emergency call and on a rota for the Emergency Department. Many large specialist units in the US are recognised for training but deliberately have no trainees. They employ sufficient staff to give constant specialist cover.

At the beginning of the twentieth century, most Irish surgeons trained at their own medical school and went abroad on educational visits only when established. Then it was realised that there were huge benefits in spending time working abroad, not necessarily in an internationally known centre, and almost all did so. At the end of the twentieth century, there was a tendency to have young surgeons completely trained at home. This has produced some first-class outcomes but it is short-sighted in the long run. All those who have worked abroad will testify to this.

ENVOI

In 1817, the Royal Colleges of Surgeons of England, Edinburgh and in Ireland held a meeting in the Boardroom of the RCSI 'to unify surgical training in the United Kingdom of Great Britain and Ireland'. As we approach the Bicentenary of that event, we can only say that, as in parliament, 'progress is reported'.

3
SURGEONS' LIVES

SURGEONS' LIVES

THE HOSPITALS

This is not a history of Irish hospitals. To begin, there were two main strands of institutions. The state ran some city hospitals and all the county hospitals, which were often not much better than workhouses. The voluntary hospitals were established mainly by the religious orders of nuns in the South and by public-spirited individuals in the North. Many were small and highly competitive rather than co-operative with their neighbours down the road.

It is worth saying that at the time of independence in 1922, there was only one hospital in the Irish Free State that was under eighty years of age. Hospitals by their nature frequently change in both structure and function. Many are worth a separate book and there have been welcome histories produced. In Dublin, the closing by amalgamation and transfer of many of the hospitals associated with the Trinity Medical School was an opportunity to record the work of these institutions. Some of the surviving Dublin hospitals have celebrated centenaries by producing histories of varying quality, in a few of which the main interest lies in the glimpse that they provide into contemporary sociology.

Dublin, Cork and many other places had voluntary hospitals that were, in the main, run by two orders of nuns, the Irish Sisters of Charity and the Sisters of Mercy. They and other women religious, such as the French Sisters of Charity who used to have huge angular bonnets based on French peasant dress at the time of their foundation, made an incalculable contribution to the Irish hospital system. They were quite unfairly classified as 'The Sisters of Mercy who have no Charity and the Sisters of Charity who have no Mercy'. These were the women who provided patient care, nurse education and the vital integrity and continuity that hospitals require. Irish medicine would be a great deal poorer were it not for the nuns.

In Cork, the closure of the Eye, Ear and Throat Hospital was celebrated by an affectionate work, *The Iron Throte*, by a staff surgeon, Denis Wilson. In Belfast, Richard Clarke's *History of the Royal Victoria Infirmary* is a model of its kind. Harold Love produced a recent history of the Royal Belfast Hospital for Sick Children, which is the sort of story that all hospitals deserve to have.

In many hospitals, there is only the slimmest or no record of those who worked there. Each institution should have a sort of 'family bible' into which entries on retiring staff might be archived. It is a sad matter of fact that two of the hardest-working Dublin surgeons of the second half of the century, Frank O'Connell and Joe McMullin, both master technicians, did not have an obituary in either the daily or medical press. To those who complain that hospitals have become impersonal places this surely is some ammunition.

Finances and Fees

There are few poor surgeons at any time but the average practitioner was much wealthier pro rata in the first half of the century than in the second. There were fewer surgeons, less than one quarter of present-day numbers. Style and really high standards of living, e.g. domestic and garden staff and grand houses, cost much less to maintain. Income tax and all other forms of taxation were low and almost optional, and fees, where they could be levied, were often large indeed and surgeons' incomes related more to highly successful present-day top bankers and stock exchange traders' fees than to other professional earnings. But the downside was serious. Few appointments paid more than a pittance, though almost all surgeons point out that they did 'insurance work' ('referees'), compiled reports on plaintiffs with personal injury claims and were available for court work.

Almost all medical fees were levied by negotiation. 'The fee should pinch but not bite,' said Harry Meade of Dublin. In the Lahey Clinic, Boston, in the 1950s, a major operation was charged as close as possible to a patient's monthly income. There the surgeon did not participate in the financial arrangements. Much work in the Irish voluntary hospitals attracted no fees at all, and even into the 1960s 'a pair of chickens' might be the reward for extensive intervention.

But elective fees could be large, though short of crippling. 'Fifty guineas for one cataract equals one housemaid for one year,' said Robert Dwyer Joyce (1938). 'One hundred guineas for a hernia repair [in 1939] and if you don't want me there are plenty of cheap fellows down (Patrick's) Hill,' said John Dundon, Cork.

P. J. Keogh was a distinguished ear, nose and throat surgeon who, in 1912, travelled by train from Dublin to Kildare to open a quinsy (abscess on the tonsil). His house surgeon asked him what was his fee for the outing and he replied, 'Seventeen pounds, four shillings and ten pence.' 'Isn't that a somewhat unusual sum? How did you arrive at that figure?' asked the house surgeon. 'Simple … it was all the money they had in the house,' replied the surgeon.

'We're from the country' was sometimes countered by, 'But you came to the city for the operation.' When a surgeon caught sight of a horse-choking bundle of twenty-pound notes, the patient explained, 'It was for the hospital.' 'You didn't plan on buying the place by any chance?' was the retort. In a largely rural country, farmers became adept at concealing their holdings, and almost all entered their occupation as 'small farmer'. It then became a battle of wits to find out the real situation. The confrontation between the educated cosmopolitan surgeon and the cunning peasant was often a sight to behold. One such 'small farmer' was advised by Professor Harry Meade to walk around the boundaries of his property every day as rehabilitation for his hernia repair. 'I couldn't do that, Surgeon. I'd be dead,' said the man. Point taken.

Some surgeons did not bring trainees with them on a ward round in which patients were about to be discharged. This was to ease any embarrassment between patient and surgeon at the request for fees. Some, indeed, insisted that all patients, howsoever poor and though fully entitled to free services, would contribute something for the intervention. Coins changed hands at times and, in the early 1950s, a dilatation and curettage might attract only five shillings. The guinea consultation fee of the 1920s, 1930s and 1940s became three guineas, and in the 1960s one secretary would keep the £1 17s change out of a £5 note ready in a white coat pocket, having been advised that 'It's the shillings of the guineas that pay your salary.' It was not unheard of for a surgeon to come into a ward in a smaller hospital and go immediately to a patient who was waving a pound note. This patient would be immediately discharged. The other patients, who did not dare to go home without the doctor's specific permission, would learn the lesson, and the following day there would be a green leafy forest of waving pound notes to greet the 'beloved physician'. Many, many patients never attended for follow-up and thus could avoid any financial negotiations. 'The time to collect the fee is when the tear is in the eye,' said John Kiely, Cork.

Two issues changed much. In 1948, the National Health Service became law and, in Northern Ireland, consultants were paid by the state for their services. Many surgeons chose full-time contracts with no private practice, although the option to engage in private practice was enshrined in all proposed contracts. The new salaries were generous by the standards of the day. 'I stuffed their mouths with gold,' boasted Aneurin Bevan (1897–1960), the Health Minister who pushed through the legislation. A critical sop to the profession's leadership was the provision of extra payments, on a tiered basis, colloquially called Merit or Distinction Awards, which were distributed by the profession itself. The top awards almost doubled salaries and almost all of these were awarded to academics and other full-time personnel. Crucially there was an indexed public service pension provided.

By 1970, inflation had eroded salaries and the NHS consultants were the worst-paid in Europe (the editor was President of the BMA from 1976 to 1977 and fielded some heavy criticism for pointing this out) but the Conservative Government of Margaret Thatcher began, in 1979, to restore differentials rapidly. Private practice in Northern Ireland had never been particularly lucrative and this influenced decisions in contractual issues, and a high proportion worked 'wholetime' in the public interest. Private Health Insurance, dominated in the UK by the British United Provident Association (BUPA), did not rise above 14 per cent participation by the population of the UK. Much of this was in south-east England where over 30 per cent were covered, while enrolment rates in Northern Ireland and Scotland were nearer to 6 per cent. Fees were agreed between the insurers and the profession. The increase in elective operations, such as joint replacement, cataracts, hernia repair and varicose veins, increased the enrolment in private insurance.

Things were very different in the Republic. Surgeons were employed in two entirely different ways. On the one hand, the government, through the largely fair and successful central Local Appointments Commission, controlled appointments in the Local Authority Hospitals which comprised all but a handful of hospitals outside Dublin, and on the other the powerful Voluntary, almost all teaching, Hospitals in Dublin were outside government control and made their own arrangements about appointments. The Local Authority appointees had a salary and limited rights to private practice, rights which were often tightly enforced by their employer's representatives. There were few private hospitals outside the three cities of Dublin, Cork and Limerick, and so for patients who wished for private treatment there was no alternative to the local hospital. Many such simply went to the nearest city for elective procedures.

For those in the Voluntary Hospitals, there was no realistic salary until the mid-1980s, and dependence on private practice continued in what was then a poor country by Western standards. There was the continuing issue of a largely public service without a serious public pension. Negotiations on a Common Contract for Consultants lasted almost two decades (1970–90), with generations of negotiators passing the 'baton' before agreement was reached whereby consultants are paid about the same salaries and pensions as High Court Judges. This was over forty years after a salaried service with the right to private practice was introduced under the British National Health Service, in 1948. There was no question of merit awards. On the other hand, private health insurance under a government-guaranteed, but not subsidised, body called the Voluntary Health Insurance Board (VHI), introduced in 1956, prospered and participation rose from 3 per cent in the early days to over 50 per cent by the turn of the millennium. Modest income tax relief on the premiums helped growth. The given reason for the growth in VHI coverage was the waiting lists for surgery but, in truth, although there was some exploitation of delays, these were no worse than in Northern Ireland.

Patients were increasingly seeking choice of an institution that would provide private rooms with en-suite bathrooms, a surgeon of their choice, or more often their general practitioner's choice, and options on the timing of any interventions. It is fair to say that the Blackrock Clinic in Dublin proved that major surgery could be as safe in private institutions as in the public hospitals of the medical schools. Rapid expansion of private facilities followed with the country's prosperity from 1993 onwards. Private fees remained at about two-thirds the insurance benefits available in Northern Ireland, but increasing frustrations with practice problems were making full-time contracts attractive to some of those outside the bigger centres. A major attraction of private practice outside the public hospital was the 'can do' attitude of all staff in the private institutions and an anxiety to get as much work as possible done in the shortest time.

Lifestyles

Surgeons' lifestyles and position in society changed and mainly declined during the twentieth century. They are still ranked near the top, just below nurses and well ahead of lawyers, in tables of public trust where politicians and journalists vie for bottom of the league, with traffic wardens, double-glazing salesmen, swimming-pool attendants and used-car vendors in between. As a group, surgeons are unpopular with the media, possibly jealous of their proven intelligence, based on the entry requirements for universities and medical schools, but probably largely because of their substantial incomes. Few surgeons are retiring by nature and the adjective most often applied to the group is 'arrogant'. Certainly most of the successful ones are self-confident, and patients like to have cheerful upbeat doctors at all times. Many groups, such as leading industrialists and job creators, sports stars, media personalities, and even prominent performers have overtaken them in public esteem. Sub-specialisation means that 'the eminent surgeon' is now the 'eminent colorectal surgeon' or 'eminent orthopaedic surgeon', which have a less glamorous ring.

They have been one of the last groups to dress formally. The long frock coat, cutaway in front, was worn into the 1920s, and some in Dublin wore the 'pepper and salt' striped trousers with black jacket, white shirt, detachable collar and grey tie into the mid-1960s. There has been a sharp decline in formality and in hospitals it is not always easy to tell if someone in jeans is the senior surgeon or someone there to fix the air conditioning. It has been said that surgeons now dress formally only for giving evidence at court. In the operating theatres, well into the 1950s, surgeons just removed their jackets and waistcoats and put on aprons for surgery. Some had shirts with detachable sleeves made. The concept of the cotton unisex theatre tunic and trousers came from the USA in the late 1950s, and the disposable paper-based suit in the 1980s.

There is a durable urban myth that surgeons die young, particularly those who continue to work after 65 years. This may well have had some substance up to about 1960. Until then, the great majority of surgeons, and the rest of the population (at least 80 per cent of males) smoked cigarettes and other forms of tobacco. The pipe, in particular, became almost a symbol of sagacity, while the big cigar, which sometimes contained as much tobacco as ten cigarettes, suggested power with phallic overtones. This was the most common cause of heart and vascular disease, and sudden fatal heart attacks were common in smokers from 40 years of age onwards. Doctors were the first group to give up smoking, and the average age of death of surgeons in the *Lives of Fellows*, published by the RCS (Eng), from 1960 onwards was over 80 years. Sudden death from heart attacks in younger men (40–60) is now much less common, and vigorous intervention in myocardial ischaemia is part of the reason, but the main reason is the recognition of the dangers of smoking. It has been shown recently (2004) that deaths in the USA from cardiovascular disease have halved since 1970. Better treatment is part of the picture, but it is a startling piece of data.

Another reason why earlier surgeons died in harness was that they could not afford to retire and they hung on to their hospital and medico-legal work long after they were past their best. Life expectancy was perhaps fifteen years shorter up to the 1970s than at the time of writing (2007). The British Civil Service stopped funding pension contributions in the mid-1920s, having discovered that most retirees lived only a couple of years after retirement. Their premature demise was thought to have been caused by the break with their work routine but it is now realised that the real cause was tobacco. Even after the Second World War, there were stories of surgeons walking up and down Harley Street hoping for a heart attack, as their practice had vanished to younger men and they had no substantive savings. There was no concept of pensions for the self-employed until the 1960s.

Marriage and Family

In the early years of the century, few surgeons married young. The future was uncertain and until, and for some time after, they got a substantive appointment they could not support a wife and children. Osler constantly reminded apprentices that 'Wives and children are hostages to fate and impedimenta to great enterprises', while the critic Cyril Connolly, under the heading 'Enemies of Promise', named 'the pram in the hall'. In those days, children followed marriage quickly and almost without pause. In 1900, only 20 per cent of married women had fewer than four children. One third of married women had seven or more children. Sir Arthur Chance married twice and had thirteen children. His successor but one as President of the RCSI, Sir John Lentaigne, had eight children. His wife Phillis, who had the eight children in eleven years, died prematurely. There was little reliable contraception in those days, and in some quarters it was thought to be morally reprehensible. 'The greatest curse of civilisation is contraception,' thundered Winston Churchill (one son, four daughters).

Divorce and separation were almost unknown amongst surgeons until the closing years of the twentieth century. It may be said that, in the first third of the century, surgeons married into 'society' and sometimes met their future brides at race meetings or black-tie dinner dances. In the middle third, they married nurses. This to some extent reflected the long hours both groups of trainees worked in the hospital and the fact that both groups 'lived in'. The massive building behind the hospital, with as many beds as the hospital itself, was the nurses' home and was almost as secure as Fort Knox from predatory male trainee surgeons. The hospital was the focal point of a self-contained active social life. In the last third of the century, many surgeons married colleagues, reflecting the increased numbers of women in the medical schools, over 55 per cent at the time of writing. No consultant surgeon in the period under review had a 'partner' — that is, lived openly with a woman who was not his wife. Gay partners were unknown. How quickly times are changing. Early on, most wives did not have negotiable skills and few were university graduates so could not afford to leave the family home even had they wished to do so. A few surgeons led chaotic and baroque lives.

The Surgeon's Day

The daily timetable of the surgeon has changed radically over the century. In the early years, the day might have started at about nine o'clock with a round of his patients in the nursing homes. Then he went to his hospital to see what patients had come in overnight. There was no concept of an operating 'list' until well into the 1930s. Operations, mainly trauma, were carried out as soon as possible but in no particular sequence. At present, most surgeons begin the day at their hospitals at eight o'clock. A full day's operating ends at about 5 p.m., when the operating theatre nurses are replaced by the 'night staff'. A round of the postoperative patients means that few surgeons' days end before 6 or 7 p.m. If not operating, the surgeon may well begin in the Outpatients Department, seeing referred new patients or following up those previously operated on. After this session, there will be letters to be dictated about the patients who attended, trainees' references to be written, and questions from management to be answered. There may be unit meetings, staff meetings, management meetings, budget meetings, research meetings, journal clubs where recent worthwhile publications are discussed, tutorials of trainees and possibly undergraduates. With the insatiable demand for doctors, almost all hospitals have undergraduate students seconded to them, and the students enjoy the experience as they are given more responsibility. But they want to be taught and shown 'how to do it'.

There is a present (2007) controversy about the appropriate number of hours a surgeon should work. It seems that 40 hours, to include on call, will be agreed. As up to the present most surgeons work, including on-call work, about a seventy-hour week it is difficult to predict how this will work out.

Honours, Awards and Distinctions

A Complex Taxonomy

No Irish doctor has won the Nobel Prize for Medicine. No one has come near. The prize is tied to innovation, and perhaps only Terence Millin's description of retropubic prostatectomy (1945) achieved worldwide recognition if not practice. Up to 1922, all Irish surgeons were theoretically eligible for Fellowship of the Royal Society (FRS). There has been no such award North or South in the twentieth century.

There were no surgical peerages, hereditary or 'life'. At the next level, in purely British 'patronage office' terms, a knighthood was offered to each president of the RCSI until 1925. (The Patronage Office (Ceremonial Secretariat) was located in number 10 Downing Street and the key figure, the Secretary, must be a practising member of the Church of England.) Outside the presidency of the RCSI a few knighthoods were awarded in the early years but none since. Sir Ian Fraser's knighthood came while he was President of the BMA (1962–63). There have been dozens of lesser political awards in Northern Ireland, particularly to those who gave so much service in the 'Troubles' (1968–98). The Republic of Ireland has no honours list of any kind.

Election to the presidency of one's home surgical college, though sometimes reflecting specialty recognition, geographic need or even diligent long service, is the top award in the eyes of most observers. The four 'home' Royal Colleges of Ireland, England, Edinburgh and Glasgow all award some variation of honorary Fellowship to worthy, well-screened recipients. There is a certain pecking order, with Edinburgh the most generous and England being somewhat more circumspect and carrying a scarcity value. ('Pinning Boy Scout proficiency badges on one another,' tartly observed the doctor wife of an Irish College President.) Abroad, the most prized is the Honorary Fellowship of the American College, which is at present limited to one hundred living surgeons, which usually means two for Ireland. Links with the South African and Australasian Colleges are sometimes strengthened by an exchange of honours. Few, indeed, are given to those under 55 years of age, and the charismatic heart-transplant surgeon Christiaan Bernard (1922–2001), who performed what was arguably the most important single operation of the twentieth century (first heart transplant, 1967) was turned down for the honour by two colleges.

The Association of Surgeons of Great Britain and Ireland is the senior society of surgeons of this region. There have been seven presidents from Ireland, Sir William Taylor 1925, Andrew Fullerton 1931, Harry Meade 1949, Sir Ian Fraser 1958, Patrick Fitzgerald 1967, Terence Kennedy 1981, and George Parks 1992. The Society of British Neurological Surgeons has had two presidents from Ireland, Adams A. McConnell and Derek Gordon. The British Association of Urological Surgeons has had two Irish presidents, Terence Millin and John Fitzpatrick. The British Association of Plastic Surgeons, now the British Association of Plastic, Reconstructive and Aesthetic Surgery, has had two Irish presidents, Norman Hughes and Michael Earley. The British Association of Paediatric Surgeons has had four Irish presidents, Barry O'Donnell, Edward Guiney, Victor Boston and Raymond Fitzgerald. Neither the British Orthopaedic Association nor the Society for Cardiothoracic Surgeons in Great Britain and Ireland has had an Irish surgeon as president.

The senior American surgical societies, of which the American Surgical Association is the most prestigious, and the one that recruits from all specialties, keep a place or two for the Irish. The common practice of making a distinguished visitor a Visiting Professor is a largely north American distinction. Perhaps only they have the funds to make the title a reality. It is certainly an area where these islands lag behind.

Eponymous addresses to learned societies, outside one's home base, in the name of a, usually deceased, distinguished doctor are another important, sensitive measure of distinction. Presidencies of international and national specialist societies are prized. Some, such as the presidency of the Surgical Section of the Royal Academy of Medicine in Ireland, are often an amiable collegiate pat on the back for solid support of the organisation over the years.

Few surgeons are honoured by non-surgical bodies. Being asked to examine at home and overseas is rightly perceived as a mark of integrity, as is the less common invitation to go on the editorial board of a reputable journal. Time-serving in the vital functions of secretary or treasurer of an organisation is often rewarded. 'Ninety per cent of life is showing up,' said Woody Allen.

Publications and Research

In the first half of the twentieth century, Irish surgeons did not write many scientific papers and there was little if any organised research. Case reports abounded. They often wrote pamphlets outlining their views on specific issues, and books were written on the basis of some limited experience. There were heated debates at the Surgical Section of the Royal Academy of Medicine of Ireland, with little in the way of factual evidence, and the level of data proof was low. Only big series of patients were seen and results published from the US and the UK. Later, the huge importance of long-term follow-up gave an advantage to smaller countries who really knew what happened to patients over the years.

The quality and relevance, rather than just the sheer volume, of research publications is becoming an increasingly important measurement of an institution's claims to be a teaching hospital. Belfast had been productive in the second half of the century but the chronic understaffing and underfunding in the Republic meant that there was little to be proud of until about 1980. The reality was that up 1990 there was not enough money to carry out the simplest of audits, let alone do basic research. It takes time and money to establish a culture of research. It didn't happen.

Surgical Travelling Clubs

Surgical travelling clubs became popular in Ireland after the Second World War. A group of surgeons would travel together to a venue to which they had an *entrée*, usually a university hospital, and spend perhaps two or three days and nights learning what was happening there, and often inviting the hosts to return the visit. Wives were brought along and the trips extended further and further afield. The clubs had all sorts of advantages because, in addition to acquiring 'local knowledge', the surgeons were told of developments nearby and of recent personnel changes, and were able to make enquiries about visits elsewhere. Admission to the clubs was by election, usually following a guest appearance on an outing. (Not all who went on 'outings' were elected to membership ... ask the editor.) Affability and 'clubability' (Dr Samuel Johnson) were crucial considerations. Members of the club got to know each other better than before. Men shared rooms all the time in those more innocent days. Many of the memories of visitations were of 'debate' lasting well into the night. There was always a shopping excursion for the ladies. Attendance was monitored and

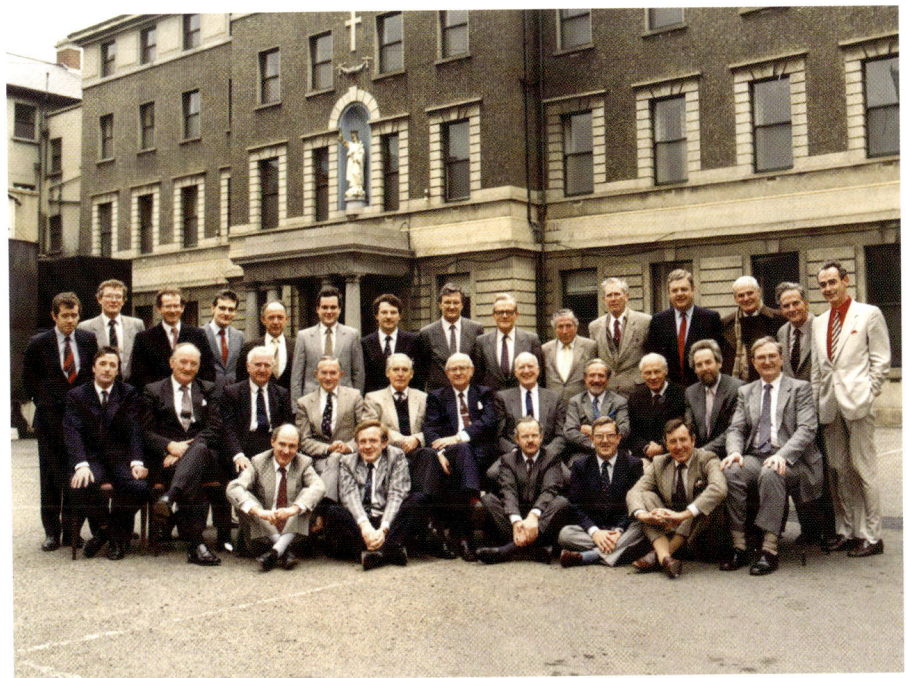

Surgical Discussion Group Meeting, Charitable Infirmary, Jervis Street, Dublin 1987.
The meeting was held to mark the closure of the hospital. The twenty-nine surgeons in the photograph represented one third of the general surgeons of the Republic at the time.

Back row, left to right: *John Kelly (Mercy Hospital, Cork), Paddy Broe (Beaumont Hospital, Dublin), Finbar Lennon (Our Lady of Lourdes Hospital, Drogheda), John Drumm (Limerick Regional Hospital), George Lyons (Bons Secours Hospital, Tralee), Ronan O'Connell (Mater Hospital, Dublin), Joe Deasy (Beaumont Hospital, Dublin), Frank Cunningham (Meath County Hospital, Navan), John O'Sullivan (County Hospital, Wexford), George Cantillon (Barrington's Hospital, Limerick), Finbar Henley (Kerry County Hospital, Tralee), John Fitzpatrick (Mater Hospital, Dublin), Frank O'Connell (Mater Hospital, Dublin), David Lane (Sir Patrick Dun's Hospital, Dublin), James 'Shay' Murphy (St Vincent's Hospital, Dublin).*

Middle row, left to right: *David Bouchier-Hayes (Beaumont Hospital, Dublin), Bernard Murphy (Regional Hospital, Galway), Sean Baker (Bantry County Hospital), Joe Hanley (Donegal County Hospital, Letterkennny), Harold Browne (Richmond Hospital, Dublin), Patrick Collins (Jervis Street Hospital, Dublin), Vincent Sheehan (Our Lady of Lourdes Hospital, Drogheda), Harry Murray (Meeting Sponsor), Thurloc Swan (County Hospital, Sligo), Eoin O'Brien (Physician and medical historian, Jervis Street Hospital), Joe Johnston (Mayo County Hospital, Castlebar).*

Front row, left to right: *Brian Lane (Jervis Street Hospital, Dublin), Gerry O'Sullivan (Mercy Hospital, Cork), Arthur Tanner (Adelaide Hospital, Dublin), Tom Hennessy (St James's Hospital, Dublin), P. E. (Paddy) Kiely (Bons Secours Hospital, Cork).*

expulsion was threatened, and sometimes carried out, for those who missed perhaps three meetings in a row.

As specialisation grew, there was pressure on the specialist surgeons to join their own specialist travelling clubs, and, in many, the club's membership went from the entire spectrum of surgery to general surgeons only. The specialist clubs took on an international and inter-continental flavour, and the 'generalist' clubs declined somewhat while understandably remaining highly popular with the true general surgeons, particularly those working outside university centres.

The Irish Surgical Travellers' Club

Harold Browne has written a fascinating account of the origin and history of this, the premier travelling club in Ireland. The account is archived in the Library of the RCSI. It began when Colman K. Byrnes and John Kiely ('K John') visited the Mayo Clinic together in 1954 and were together on the ship back. The numbers increased over the years and there were up to twenty surgeons and accompanying wives at some meetings. Over the years, they visited Bristol, Birmingham, Paris, Heidelberg, Cambridge, Russia and Richmond, Virginia, amongst other places.

The Ulster Surgical Travellers

This club was founded in 1955 with, inevitably, Ian Fraser as Life President. The first secretaries were Ronnie Loane [q.v.] and Will Hanna [q.v.]. The number was kept to twenty-five and an equal division of representation between Belfast and the rest of Northern Ireland was targeted. Ian Fraser opened doors abroad then, as always, and the Club is going strong at this time.

4
SMALLER HOSPITALS AND COUNTY SURGEONS

SMALLER HOSPITALS AND COUNTY SURGEONS

An Act of Parliament in 1765, 'for the erecting and establishing public infirmaries or hospitals in this Kingdom', brought into being the County Infirmaries or County Hospitals, one or more hospitals for each county. A surgeon was appointed as caretaker of each hospital, his salary was not to exceed £100 per annum and he was obliged to live within one mile of the infirmary. Indeed, he often lived within the usually spacious grounds. Most of these County Infirmaries were built within ten years of the passing of the Act. As the buildings crumbled, their replacements varied greatly. There was little medical or surgical activity in the infirmaries until about 1900 and they were often looked upon as places to which the poor went to die.

The Infirmary was from the beginning an object of huge local and political pressures. Aside from being a place to put the sick, it became, over time, the biggest employer in largely rural communities. Ninety per cent of the staff were female and were at the bottom end of the pay scale, but in an area without any industry, besides agriculture, it was one of the few sources of a regular income and jobs were usually for life. The political pressures resulted in some remarkable anomalies. The largest town in the county was not always selected. Cashel was less than half the size of Clonmel but was selected as being more central in County Tipperary. Worse, in Counties Cavan and Wexford there were two hospitals in completely different locations. One was for medical and maternity cases and the other was for surgery. Because of the county system of local government even towns of less than 2,000 in population might have a County Hospital. There were always extravagant claims of the population served and substantial overlaps of catchment areas, which, if added together, would give the country more than twice the number of census inhabitants. Even in the USA, in all but a handful of world-famous named institutions with highly specialised services, it is widely held that 75 per cent of surgery comes from within a 25-mile radius of the hospital.

The initial battles for location were as nothing compared with the battles when it came to closing them or reducing their services in the late twentieth century. A flavour of this may be got from the claim of a local county councillor that there would be no county football team in the future if the county were deprived of its maternity services, as there would be no native-born footballers. In Northern Ireland, the battle between, for example, Enniskillen and Omagh to keep both their hospitals open was an epic of its genre. In fairness, this was not just an Irish phenomenon as throughout the world the hardest thing a politician can face is the closure of his or her local hospital. But the argument was weakest where the population was most thinly spread.

The locals supported the hospital and there was always fund-raising and pressure for the improvement of facilities. In the 1990s visiting a town fund-raising for a CAT scanner posed a moral dilemma. If the hospital were going to continue to admit head injuries, and inevitably it would, then it was much better that it would have a CAT scanner. But anything that encouraged its self-sufficiency would make it harder to close, which every objective report had advised. If one had relatives or friends in the town or knew some of the general practitioners or even the surgeon, the dilemma became sharper. Often the strongest argument for expansion was that the deadly sporting enemy — that is, the nearest town or county — already had such equipment. This was such a political wrangle that it led the editor to suggest incautiously that a hospital should be built in the full view of every polling booth.

For much of the century, one of the major controversies within surgery in the Republic and Northern Ireland was the staffing of the smaller hospitals. In the Republic, in the year 1968, there was a seminal report drawn up at the request of the then Minister for Health, Sean Flanagan, and the medical profession. This was carried out under the chairmanship of the hugely respected Professor Patrick (Paddy) Fitzgerald. At the time, a total of forty hospitals in the state were offering full services twenty-four hours a day, seven days a week, fifty-two weeks a year. In the cities, surgeons had multiple hospital appointments and so even relatively small surgical units appeared to have adequate cover. Duty rotas for 'on call' were loosely drawn up and cover for annual holidays, sick leave and the increasing demands of study leave and attendance at meetings at home and abroad were gradually put in place.

But for much of the time under review the position in the smaller county and local hospitals was much less satisfactory. In many, the trained permanent surgical staff consisted of a single surgeon with a number of 'trainees'. These trainees might number from one to seven, and there were more as the century wore on, with a general shortening of working hours and increasing pressure from the directives of the European Union. Most of these 'junior staff' were from India and Pakistan and came to get training; latterly they were also attracted to the much higher salaries and overtime payments (which sometimes exceeded the salary) than they could get in such a post at home. A few stayed long enough to want to get career posts in the state, and perhaps got citizenship along the way, but these appointments were few and far between. It should be said that many of the Irish graduates who went to the UK and the USA as trainees often did exactly the same.

Getting the sick to hospital is always a vital issue. A patient's distance from a hospital has in the past been measured as the actual mileage rather than the time taken to get there. When infirmaries were founded, the transfer was by some form of horse-drawn vehicle, to include commercial stage and mail coaches, and these were the standard method of getting from town to town or town to city. From about 1850 onwards, the railways provided a faster link. For the next fifty years, the train seemed the future of transport, and the roads were neglected, yet according to Tommy Hogan, Chairman of CIE (the national rail company, 1970), 'If the car had been invented before the train there would be no railways in Ireland.' The motor car did not become common until after 1910 and they were not reliable until the introduction of Henry Ford's Model T (1908–27). Motor ambulances came into use after the First World War. Before that, they were horse drawn. But transport of the sick has changed radically with improved roads, many of which now are dual carriageways or motorways. This has meant that patients would be ensured good care even if they were a greater distance from a hospital. However, arguments about 'the golden hour', the first hour after a road traffic accident or a coronary thrombosis, have reignited the issue of having a hospital nearby.

In the United States, Canada and Australia, these hospitals are sometimes called rural hospitals, and the surgeons, rural surgeons, have their own organisations and societies, but this designation is not acceptable in this still quite rural country.

The County Surgeon

Whether liked or not, accurate or not, the term 'county surgeon' was part of our lexicon in the twentieth century. From the 1940s onwards, it was quite common for a newly appointed county surgeon to have spent more time in postgraduate training than many of those appointed to Irish teaching hospitals. Their training was often in busy hospitals in the non-university towns and cities in England. There are over a hundred communities of more than 100,000 in England alone, and the surgical experience to be had there was wide ranging and intense. Bolton, Oldham, Rochdale, Wigan, Stockport, Barnsley, Doncaster and Rotherham, just to take the Greater Manchester and South Yorkshire areas, each had populations of around 200,000 and were all bigger than Cork. Many of these formerly sooty cities had only one or two hospitals, the 'Royal' and the 'General', with the Royal usually outranking the General, and all the problems came through to these two. It may be said that supervision was often loosely interpreted, but the 'trainees' who spent years in such hospitals certainly knew how to operate even if they did not always generate a significant list of publications.

The Front Line

Partly because of their isolation but in part due to their self-selection, many of the county surgeons developed into full-blown 'characters'. Like other species of wildlife they are under threat from the removal of the 'hedgerows' or strict county boundaries determining where shall be the focal hospital of the area. Being on call at all times was a serious demand. Local politicians in the county council could and would and did phone the county surgeon to get a voter or a member of the voter's family a hospital bed ahead of the waiting list. This became even more of a problem where it might be proposed that an elderly person with no medical problems, but who posed a considerable social burden, be admitted to the acute hospital from whence it became almost impossible to discharge them 'home'. 'I'll try to get the Council to buy that piece of gear you wanted,' might be the inducement.

The same politicians, and indeed other staff members, would urge the surgeon to build up the hospital and its local reputation by providing a wider range of services. As the county surgeon was dependent on private practice for most of his income and the county council had much patronage, this had a certain appeal, but one man (they were almost all men) could cover only so much and some may well have overstretched their expertise. A cabinet minister sustained multiple injuries in a car crash. He was not driving, which was just as well. Bulletins on his progress in the county hospital were published daily in the national press. A specialist surgeon called the county surgeon, offering to take the patient into his unit.

'He's not fit to be moved,' said his surgical guardian.

'If you like, I'll go up and see him then.'

'Ah he's not that bad'. Analyse.

One of the issues about which they all complained was the isolation. They sorely missed the chance to discuss clinical problems with colleagues in the way they had experienced in their training. This feeling of isolation and unavailability of easy consultation with colleagues cannot be overemphasised. The professional part of this was important but there was a social element as well. The county town in the early and middle twentieth century would have had only a handful of people who had had third-level education. This meant that the surgeon's social circle was narrow. He quite inevitably became Captain and President of the local golf club and his golf partners would be a cross-section of the community, but the personnel for dinner parties were drawn from perhaps six or twelve other couples. Many towns were without a proper bookshop much less a live theatre or concert hall. A surgeon's spouse, and few spouses worked outside the home in those days, though a leader in local society also had seriously limited social outlets. For a variety of reasons, the children would often be sent to boarding school at the age of 12 if not earlier.

Then there was being in the public eye at all times so that sidling down to the local pub for a pint on a Friday evening was usually out of the question. There were other invasions of privacy. Until about 1975, a phone call to the local regional or university hospital, for help or advice, went through the local post office telephone exchange where an eavesdropper, ostensibly checking the connection, might overhear the local surgeon expressing concern about a particular patient. The post mistress (for it was always 'she') might well feel that her vow of discretion to the Department of Post and Telegraphs, as it was, was overridden by the imperative of warning the relatives and a wider audience of the surgeon's uncertainty, and worse. 'This isn't the first time that this has happened,' she might say. Automatic telephone exchanges, by making calls for advice genuinely confidential, also made them more frequent and probably saved lives.

Medico-Legal Work

One of the perks of being a solo county surgeon was the demand for medico-legal reports and court appearances. Personal injury cases were in the majority and a high percentage of these involved the outcome of road traffic accidents. The adversarial system which pertained in the Republic after partition meant that there were often two surgical witnesses, often giving different versions of the injuries and the future life of the plaintiff, and then, as true professionals do, going off to a convivial lunch together. In addition to providing income, this provided a welcome respite from the daily round or appearance at the coalface; it was an opportunity to go to where the High Court was sitting, often in Dublin, and gave the county surgeon an opportunity to meet his colleagues who might also be involved in other cases the same day.

A problem was that when the solo county surgeon was in court for the day, and one got paid twice as much for a day as for a half-day, there was no inducement to cut short the absence from the home base or encourage barristers to get the surgeon's evidence over early. The fort was held by junior 'trainees', almost none Irish born, who were sometimes under orders not to send away any patient and certainly not to pass on or pass up any problem that might have further medico-legal spin-off. So the victims of road traffic accidents were sometimes impounded, pending the return of the proleptic expert witness, or managed by an inexperienced resident. It then became important not to be involved in a damaging road traffic accident when the High Court was sitting.

At the time of writing, almost all smaller hospitals have a minimum of three consultant surgeons so that adequate cover is available at all times. There remains the issue of patients who require sub-specialty care, such as complex orthopaedic and vascular procedures. The medico-legal implications of a less than perfect outcome have now added another layer of responsibility to surgical staff.

Epilogue on County Surgeons

Looking at the lists of solo surgeons in smaller, often county, hospitals, one is struck by how a few individuals could have provided all the surgical services in that community for perhaps the first seventy years of the century. Typical of this are the counties of Fermanagh, which had only four surgeons over the entire century, and Mayo, which has a parallel story. It is a tribute to their durability and almost Darwinian 'survival of the fittest' that so many lived for so long. Many of the earlier surgeons were appointed in their middle or late twenties and stayed in office into their seventies, as pensions for many decades were either non-existent or derisory, and early retirement was never a voluntary option. They were surely a breed apart, and there may be more surgeons in each hospital now but the question is: Are they better? They could hardly be. The county surgeon made a wide general contribution to the life of his local community. He knew how to organise events and how to make them happen. He was involved in first-aid classes, the Red Cross, Civil Defence, the Hospice movement and many committees for the improvement of life in 'his' town. Above all, he was often a father figure whom the locals knew they could trust.

We salute the solo county surgeon.

5
PROFESSORS OF SURGERY, QUEEN'S UNIVERSITY BELFAST

PROFESSORS OF SURGERY, QUEEN'S UNIVERSITY BELFAST

From 1900 to 1908, the Belfast medical school was part of the Royal University of Ireland (RUI) and was called Queen's College, Belfast (QCB) RUI. With the disbanding of the Royal University of Ireland in 1908 it became Queen's University Belfast (QUB).

SINCLAIR, Thomas C. B., MP

Professor of Surgery (1886–1923) and
Belfast Surgeon

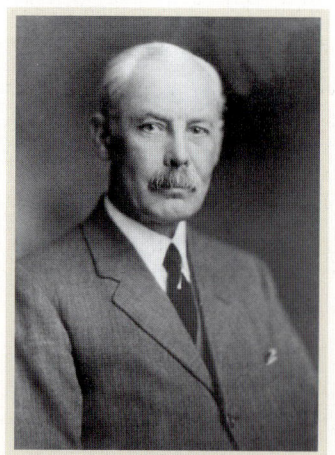

b. 17 December 1857, Belfast, third child and second son of Samuel Sinclair (flax merchant) and Isabella Sinclair (*née* McMorran)
m. Unmarried
Educ. Educated privately; Queen's College, Belfast
d. 1940

MCh, LM, 1881; MD, RUI (first class hons and gold medal); MRCS Eng, 1882; FRCS Eng, 1886; Member RCS England 1882 London Hospital, Vienna, Berlin. Malcolm Exhibition, Belfast Royal Hospital, 1880.

Surgeon, Ulster Hospital for Children and Women, Royal (subsequently Royal Victoria) Hospital (1885–1923), Forster Green Hospital, the County Antrim Infirmary and the Lisburn and Coleraine Cottage Hospitals. Appointed Professor of Surgery in 1886 at age 29, in succession to Alexander Gordon, and was in the Chair until 1923.

Colonel, Army Medical Service, 1915–18 (active service).
Registrar, Queen's University, 1919–31, Pro-chancellor 1931. Represented Queen's on the General Medical Council from 1917 onwards.
Senator, Parliament of Northern Ireland, MP from Queen's to Imperial Parliament, Westminster 1923–40.
Active in BMA; President, Ulster Medical Society, 1895–96.
Commander of the Bath (CB) 1917.

Author of Articles: 'Perinephritis', Quain's *Dictionary of Medicine*, 2nd Edition; 'Surgical Diseases of the Pleura', Encyclopaedia medical contribution; 'Jejunal Enterectomy for Artificial Anus — Recovery', *British Medical Journal*, 1888; 'Gastro-enterostomy with Senn's Plates for Pyloric Stenosis', *British Medical Journal*, 1894 (first account of gastro-enterostomy in Ireland); 'Anthrax treated by Excision', *British Medical Journal*, 1900; 'Hernia in the Foramen of Winslow', *British Medical Journal*, 1909; 'Excision of Epileptogenic Centres in Traumatic Epilepsy', *Medical Press*, c.1908.

Thomas Sinclair was the outstanding figure in Northern Ireland surgery for the first quarter of the twentieth century. He would have been unusual in Belfast at the time in having taken the FRCS Eng examination. As a Colonel in the AMS, he performed a post mortem on the great German air ace, Baron von Richthofen; the post mortem proved that the flier was shot in the air rather than after capture.

Professor for thirty-seven years in all, he had mentored almost every surgeon in the province. A born teacher, he had a fine mind, was a wise clinician, had a dextrous, meticulous technique at the operating table and was assiduous in postoperative care. He had a large private practice and charged big fees appropriate to his status, but he never let his practice interfere with his lecture schedule. He rarely visited London until 1913 and wrote little. His long tenure and somewhat isolated situation meant that he had little contact with his colleagues outside the North, which in turn meant that few of his trainees benefited from a spell elsewhere.

Never robust, he was slightly above average height, spoke with a quiet voice in a recognisably North Irish accent and was a Presbyterian. Well dressed and dignified, always with a dark pinstripe suit, he keenly attended medical meetings and was formal but friendly at close quarters. He hunted every Saturday of the season, played golf and was an expert skater.

FULLERTON, Andrew, CB, CMG (Andy) PRCSI 1926–1929

Belfast Surgeon, Professor of Surgery (1923–34) and first Belfast Surgeon to be PRCSI

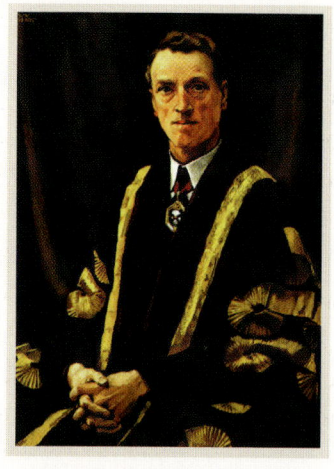

b. 1868, Cavan, third of 7 sons of a Methodist minister
Educ. Lurgan College; Queen's College, Belfast
m. Married; 3 children
d. 1934

MD, RUI, 1893; MB (first class hons and exhibitioner), 1890; MCh, QUB, 1913; FRCSI 1901 (QCB); FACS (Hon.)

Postgraduate training for two and a half years at the Miller Hospital, London, and the West Kent Hospital, Maidstone.
Surgeon, RVH, Belfast (1902–33); clinical lecturer in surgery QUB; consultant surgeon, Cripples' Home, Belfast; honorary surgeon in charge of outpatients, Belfast Hospital for Sick Children.
Temporary Colonel, Army Medical Service (precursor of the Royal Army Medical Corps); Consulting surgeon, British Expeditionary Force, France.
Scholar, QCB; examiner in surgery (Fellowship & Conjoined Board) RCSI; honorary demonstrator in anatomy, QCB.

Author of 'Colles's Fracture and Other Fractures and Disjunctions at Lower End of Radius and Ulna' and 'Case of Meningo-encephalocele Treated by Excision of the Mass', *British Medical Journal*, 1901; 'Operation for Fixing Movable Kidney', *British Medical Journal*, 1904; 'Anastomosis between Common Bile Duct and Duodenum for Obstructive Jaundice', *British Medical Journal*, 1907.

Fullerton had a glittering undergraduate career at Queen's College, Belfast. Following training in England, he set up practice in Belfast. His practice was always small as he had a difficult spiky manner, which cost him dearly. Brusque and sharp-tongued, he was the very opposite of his long-time assistant, Ian Fraser [q.v.], who remarked that he always had to have a lecture in his pocket in case the professor failed to appear. Fullerton's not particularly sympathetic character was to some extent a product of strict upbringing and modest circumstances. He was quite formal at all times, particularly regarding terms of address. He met a number of British and American surgeons at the Front in France and kept in touch with some of them. He visited the Mayo Clinic in Minnesota and was one of the first in Ireland to require white, presumably linen, trousers and shirts for the males in the operating theatre. His cold carapace collapsed with the death of his wife from inoperable cancer, leaving this almost friendless man with three young children.

He greatly cherished the presidency of the RCSI and is alleged to have said, 'In the field of surgery there should be no border'. This was misinterpreted in the North and was thought to be the reason why he was not awarded the knighthood which came with the office in those days. His difficult manner would certainly have contributed to this disappointment: knighthoods follow local soundings as well as recommendations. His mentions in the Honours Lists — a CB, Companion of the Bath — is the lowest of the three classes of that Order of Chivalry and similarly CMG, Companion of Michael and George, is the lowest of its Order. These distinctions may seem unimportant outside Whitehall where the usual recipients reside but for a touchy man with expectations of a knighthood they fuelled a resentment that was never far from the surface.

He became involved in urology and had every latest cystoscope. His peptic ulcer was not relieved by Sir Berkeley Moynihan's gastroenterostomy. He had a transurethral resection for prostatic hypertrophy in London. Shortly afterwards, he developed an unrelated malignant colon obstruction and, having refused a colostomy, he died a few hours after surgery.

CRYMBLE, Percival Templeton

Professor of Surgery (1934–45) and Belfast Surgeon

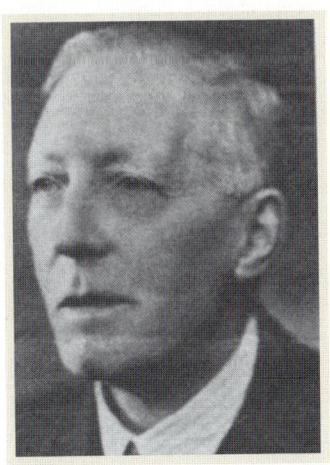

b. 1880
m son, Barry Templeton [q.v.], was an orthopaedic surgeon
d. 1970

MB, RUI, 1904; FRCS Eng, 1908 (QCB, London Hospital, Vienna). Mackay Wilson Travelling Scholarship, 1909.

Surgeon and radiographer, St John Ambulance, Brigade Hospital, France.
Lecturer in applied anatomy, QUB.
Surgeon, Royal Victoria Hospital, 1918–45. Surgeon, Hospital for Sick Children.

Author of 'The Peritoneum' Quain's Anatomy, vol. II, part ii; 'The Muscle of Treitz and the Plica Duodeno-Jejunalis', *British Medical Journal*, 1910; 'Gun-shot Wounds of Chest', *British Medical Journal*, 1918.

Crymble's main interest was in anatomy and then inevitably thyroid surgery. Many of his publications dealt with anatomical issues. He was one of the last surgeons to have been a practising anaesthetist in his earlier days.

RODGERS, Harold William, OBE

Professor of Surgery (1947–73)

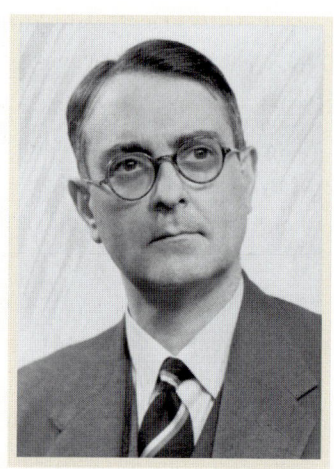

b. 1907, Bombay, son of Major R. T. Rodgers (medical officer and governor of a prison in India)
Educ. King's College School; St Bartholomew's Hospital
m. Margaret Boycott; 1 s (medical), 3 daughters (1 medical)
d. 2001

MB, St Bartholomew's Hospital 1931; FRCS 1933; MD (Hon.), Belfast, 1981.

Honorary Lieutenant Colonel, Royal Army Medical Corps.
Chairman, Court of Examinations, RCS Eng.
President, British Society of Gastroenterology; surgical section, Royal Society of Medicine.

Following training at St Bartholomew's Hospital in London, Rodgers was appointed Senior Assistant Surgeon at that hospital in 1938. At the outbreak of war in 1939, he joined the Royal Army Medical Corps and was awarded the OBE, in 1943, for forward surgery in the First Army in North Africa and subsequent courageous surgical care of an isolated Guards Regiment, which for four months held a vital crossroads outside Tunis under heavy bombardment. He went on to serve in Italy and France. When the war ended, he returned to St Bart's from where he was preferred to a highly fancied Ian Fraser [q.v.], for the Chair of Surgery at Queen's. Ian Fraser eventually did not contest the office. The result, more through complementary differences of approach than any real synergy, benefited the Medical School and Belfast by allowing both to do what they did best.

Harold Rodgers was the first full-time clinical professor at the university, and at the time Belfast was a great example of what the National Health Service did for academic surgery by allowing the creation of full-time chairs and appropriate support staff. He was, in essence, a facilitator who developed a corporate approach (though he probably would not have recognised the description) to surgical research, collaborating with the university scientific departments, in addition to NHS medical and nursing staff. A flourishing department evolved with a major interest in gastroenterology, particularly portal hypertension, peptic ulceration and, inevitably, the care of the traumatised patient. Academic activity was encouraged and papers flowed out of Belfast. He was pivotal in the development of the new Institute of Clinical Science (opened 1954), on the university site adjacent to the Royal Victoria Hospital.

Harold Rodgers was best known for the introduction of sclerotherapy in the management of bleeding oesophageal varices and, together with George Johnston [q.v.], he championed this as a vitally important mode of management. He was also a pioneer in the use of diagnostic peritonoscopy. His previous military experience helped him to shape the efficient Belfast system of rapid evacuation and treatment of casualties resulting from 'the Troubles' in Northern Ireland.

He was a good communicator who undertook a great deal of undergraduate teaching in the era of didactic lectures. Postgraduate training was greatly enhanced by developing a structured regional rotation of surgical trainees, thought to be the first in these islands. When teaching and training in the operating theatre, he sometimes proceeded in an unhurried fashion as he revelled in displaying detailed anatomy to junior staff or when assisting a trainee. However, in other circumstances, he was indeed a slick operator. The Wednesday staff ward round was notably ponderous, commencing at nine o'clock sharp, followed directly by the departmental lunch, beginning anytime from one o'clock onwards, coffee break included.

Somewhat austere, and not particularly approachable, he was, however, tolerant, fair, unselfish and extremely generous. There were those who found him remote and elitist while others who knew him best were much impressed by his undoubted integrity, unfailing dedication and immense compassion for mankind. He was totally devoid of small talk, and perhaps shy. He was an active churchman (Church of England transposed to Church of Ireland) and his beliefs pervaded his professional life.

He had a genuine interest in the developing world, culminating in many visits, not only to universities and teaching hospitals but also to remote medical missionary stations in rural Africa and India. There was some criticism that he was little seen in Northern Ireland outside the Royal Victoria Hospital. Following retirement from Queen's in 1973, he spent three years in the new University of Ife in Nigeria, as Foundation Professor of Surgery, and then worked for a time in Nepal and Nazareth. He returned to London for a period, finally settling near his family, including many grandchildren, in Birmingham. In retirement, he frequently returned to Belfast and even attended graduation ceremonies. He was understandably orientated towards the RCS Eng and was rarely seen in Dublin.

Throughout his life, he and Margaret were most hospitable, welcoming friends and strangers to their open home. He enjoyed gardening, painting, writing poetry, walking, travel and keeping in touch with colleagues and former students.

WELBOURN, Richard Burkewood (Dick)

Professor of Surgical Science (1958–63) and Belfast Surgeon

b. 1919, Rainhill, Lancashire, youngest of 5 children; his father was an engineer
Educ. Rugby School, Emmanuel College, Cambridge, Liverpool University
m. 1944: Rachel Haighton; 1 s, 4 d
d. 2005

BA, 1940, Camb; MB, BChir, Camb, 1942; FRCS Eng, 1948; MA, MD (on nutrition following gastric resection), Camb, 1953; DSc, QUB, 1985

Fellow in surgical research, Mayo Foundation; research assistant, Department of Surgery, University of Liverpool.
Senior registrar, surgical professorial unit, Liverpool Royal Infirmary.
Graded surgeon, Royal Army Medical Corps.
Professor in surgical science, QUB; surgeon, RVH, Belfast, 1953–63.
President, Surgical Research Society.
Distinguished Service Award of the International Association of Endocrine Surgeons (Stockholm 1991).

When he had finished his house jobs, Dick Welbourn was called up by the Royal Army Medical Corps. He landed in Normandy with a forward medical unit and saw unbelievable carnage. He stayed on in Hamburg after the end of the war.

In 1947, he went to Liverpool under Professor Charles Wells. He was awarded a Fulbright Scholarship to Mayo Clinic, in 1951, where he learned the techniques of surgical research. He was there to 'ride the crest of the cortisone wave' doing adrenalectomy for Cushing's syndrome under cortisone cover. He went to Queen's University Belfast in 1952 as consultant and lecturer and was subsequently appointed Professor of Surgical Science; he stayed at Queen's for eleven years.

He was invited to fill the Chair and Directorship of the Department at the Postgraduate Medical School, Hammersmith (1963–79) and Professor of Surgical Endocrinology (1979–83). He was a great believer in, and practitioner of, teamwork and collegiate attitudes. He organised many courses on surgical endocrinology. He developed close links with Dr William Longmire of the University of California, Los Angeles (UCLA) and a priceless annual exchange Fellowship followed. Welbourn lectured everywhere, wrote easily and profusely and upheld and enhanced the reputation of the Hammersmith. A devout Christian, he was an expert on medical ethics, to which he made many contributions. When he retired in 1983, he went to UCLA to write *The History of Endocrine Surgery*. He was a great fan of John Hunter and was influenced by his writings.

He was thoughtful, reserved, courteous and unflappable. His strongest expletive was 'Bother' which, with 'Oh dear', would rank at the absolute bottom of a surgeon's taxonomy. He was a brilliant analyst of surgical research methodology and was absolutely meticulous in the preparation of everything. The annual party at his home when he was in London was a wonderful affair, with his wife Rachel greeting all the guests, many of whom she had never seen, by their first name. The rumour was that their children were also prepared with names and photographs of the guest list. He had a fine sense of humour and was highly popular with colleagues, especially in the US.

ROY, Arthur Douglas (Douglas)

Professor of Surgery (1973–85) and Belfast Surgeon

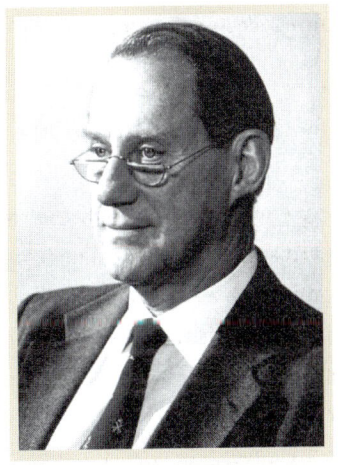

b. 1925, Paisley, Scotland, son of Arthur and Edith Mary Roy (*née* Brown)
Educ. Paisley Grammar School; Glasgow University
m. 1st in 1954: Monica Bowley; 3 d. 2nd in 1973: Patricia McColl
d. 2003

MB ChB (Commendation), Glasgow, 1947; FRCSI, 1976; FRCS Glas, 1963; FRCS Ed, 1952; FRCS Eng, 1952; FACS, Glasgow, 1979

Royal Army Medical Corps 1948–50.
Surgical registrar posts in Glasgow and Inverness; senior surgical registrar, Aylesbury and Radcliffe Infirmary, Oxford 1954–57; consultant surgeon, Western Infirmary and honorary clinical lecturer, University of Glasgow, 1957–68.
Foundation Professor of Surgery, University of Nairobi, Kenya, 1968–72; Professor of Surgery, QUB.
Consultant surgeon, RVH, Belfast, City Hospital and Royal Belfast Children's Hospitals.
Fellow, Association of Surgeons, East Africa, 1968.
Member Council RCS Ed, 1979–85.
Chief of surgical services, Ministry of Health, Oman, 1985–88.
Professor of Surgery, Sultan Qaboos University, Oman, 1986–88.

Douglas Roy was one of more than twelve surgeons trained in Glasgow by Professor Charles Illingworth who became a Professor of Surgery. This wonderful record of self-perpetuating excellence was in part due to Illingworth's plan of making sure that all his trainees did a year's research, after which many were sent to the US to complete a Fellowship and then, critically, were brought back to Glasgow to 'spread the news'. Roy headed up three university departments of surgery in three continents.

In Belfast, he stimulated, encouraged and cultivated the young, and wisely delegated responsibility. There was a productive research team, which he led in an unselfish manner. He was a fine technical surgeon, widely respected for his work on abdominal surgery as well as trauma. For eleven years, he chaired the surgical training committee of the Northern Ireland Council for Postgraduate Medical Education. He was elected to the Council of the RCS Ed from 1979 to 1985. He was a perceptive and popular examiner and as such was much in demand in university and college circles at home and abroad. He was kind, considerate, friendly and hospitable.

His relations with the strong, productive, Department of Anaesthesia at the Royal Victoria Hospital were uneven. He had been accustomed to doing much surgery in Kenya under spinal and regional anaesthesia and was sometimes impatient with the highly successful academic approach of the specialty at Queen's. There were those there who felt that he retained a slight flavour of the Colonial District Commissioner.

Roy retired to Honiton, Devon, where he put his considerable administrative skills at the disposal of the local community. He took up gliding and continued to sail and garden. He died from Parkinson's Disease, having been nursed devotedly by his wife.

PARKS, Thomas George (George) PRCSI 2000–2002

Belfast Surgeon and Professor of Surgical Science (Personal Chair) (1982–97), Professor of Surgery (1997–2000)

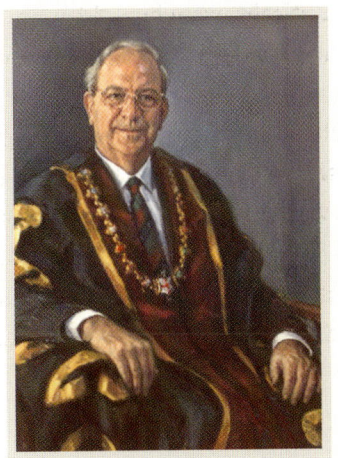

b. 1935, Lurgan, youngest son of Christopher and Evelyn Parks (*née* Turkington)
Educ. Technical School, Lurgan; Queen's University Belfast
m. 1964: Elizabeth Mahood, daughter of Robert and Lily Mahood; 1 s (Rowan academic hepatobiliary surgeon, Edinburgh), 2 d

MB (hons), QUB, 1959; MCh, QUB, 1966; FRCS Ed,1963; RCS Glas, 1981 (*ad eundem*), FRCSI, 1983 (*ad eundem*), FRCS Eng (election), 2002. Hon. Fellow, College of Surgeons, Academy of Medicine of Malaysia, 2002

Postgraduate training at RVH, Belfast; City Hospital, Belfast; St Mark's Hospital and Royal Hospital, London. Spent three months visiting leading departments in US before taking consultant appointment.

Senior lecturer in surgery, QUB (1971–73), reader in surgery (1973–82), Professor of Surgical Science (Personal Chair) (1982–97), Professor of Surgery and head of department, QUB (1997–2000).

Consultant surgeon, Belfast City Hospital and RVH, Belfast, 1971–97; RVH 1997–2000.

President, Association of Surgeons of Great Britain and Ireland, 1992; coloproctology section, Royal Society of Medicine; Irish Society of Gastroenterology; St Mark's Association and many other associations.

Greatly influenced in training by Harold Rodgers [q.v.], George W. Johnston [q.v.] and Terence Kennedy [q.v.].

His principal interests were in gastrointestinal surgery, particularly colorectal disease and trauma. His research interests were along the same lines and there were 160 publications, including thirty-seven book chapters.

George Parks was an absolutely first-rate operating surgeon. Nothing was too good for his patients. He was also in great demand for examining at the RCSI, RCS Ed, RCS Glas, Queen's University Belfast, and editorial boards including the *British Journal of Surgery*. Notably he was the only Queen's graduate to be Professor and Head of Department in the second half of the twentieth century. He was untiring in his availability for committee work on all aspects of surgery and was particularly involved with undergraduate education and curriculum development, that frustrating mirage of the ever-changing views of perfection.

His outside interests were camping and caravanning in Europe, travel, reading and DIY. No description of George would be complete without including his happy marriage to Elizabeth. His religion (The Brethren) is a central part of his life and he may be one of the few professionals who give a genuine tithe to their church. A hugely popular, totally honourable, admired, trusted and committed man who smiles easily. He is conciliatory rather than confrontational in his approach to problems, and his was a peaceful and productive presidency of the RCSI.

6
BELFAST SURGEONS

Royal Victoria Hospital (RVH)

BARROS D'SA, Aires Angelo Barnabe

Vascular Surgeon

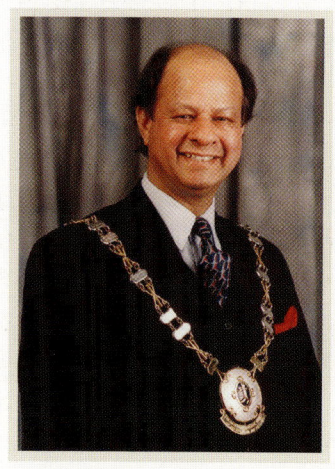

b. 1939, Nairobi, Kenya, third son of Inaçio Francisco Purificação Saúde and Maria Eslinda Inês
Educ. Duke of Gloucester School, Nairobi; Queen's University Belfast
m. 1972: Elizabeth Thompson, MB (daughter of Hugh and Mary); 4 d (Vivienne, MA, hons, Oxon, MB, MRCP; Lisa; Miranda; Angelina)
d. 2007

MB, 1965, QUB; MD (hons), 1975; FRCS, 1969; FRCS Ed, 1969

Postgraduate junior posts as house officer, RVH, Belfast; demonstrator, Department of Anatomy, QUB; registrar/senior registrar in general, cardiothoracic and vascular surgery, RVH, Belfast and other hospitals; senior tutor, Department of Surgery, QUB.
Brief attachments in the USA at Tufts New England Medical Center, Boston; Massachusetts General Hospital, Boston; Henry Ford Hospital, Detroit; and Methodist Hospital, Houston. Clinical Fellow, Reconstructive Cardiovascular Research Center International and Providence Medical Center, Seattle, Washington; principal investigator of joint research project between Seattle and Ospedali Reuniti, Bergamo, Italy.
Member, research grant-giving bodies, 1986–2003: DHSS Northern Ireland Clinical Research Awards Advisory Committee (1986–93), RVH Research Fellowship Committee (1988–94), British Vascular Foundation (1995–2003).
Regional Adviser, RCS Eng, 1988–94.
Royal College of Surgeons of Edinburgh representative on Northern Ireland Council for Postgraduate Medical and Dental Education, 1989–97.
President of the Vascular Surgical Society of Great Britain and Ireland, 2001–02. Executive and Council of the Association of Surgeons of Great Britain and Ireland.

Calvert Lecturer, RVH, Belfast, 1973; Hunterian Professor, RCS Eng, 1979; Visiting Professor to institutions in USA, Europe, Australia and South Africa (1980–2001).
77th James IV Surgical Traveller, representing British Isles, to North America, Australia and South East Asia, 1983.
Joint lectureship of the Royal College of Surgeons of Edinburgh and the Academy of Medicine of Singapore (Hon. membership), 1989.
Gore Visitor by the Royal Australasian College of Surgeons (Hon. membership), 1994
Chevalier International Knightly Order of St George (KtStG), 2001.
Deputy Lieutenant, County Borough of Belfast, 2003.

Barros D'sa participated in athletics and hockey up to university level, declining gradually thereafter to the status of spectator mainly of rugby and cricket. His other interests included reading, music (blues, jazz, classical, opera) and the arts generally. He was also involved in organisations concerned with wildlife and environmental protection and with medical relief in Africa. The following pen picture was provided by a former trainee, Paul Blair of the Regional Vascular Surgery Unit, RVH, Belfast:

'Aires was an impressive sight as his white Porsche swept into the consultants' car park at the Royal Victoria Hospital in 1970s Belfast. Apart from an old "Queen's" scarf perpetually draped round his neck he was otherwise a picture of sartorial elegance. Tall and of athletic frame, he had a definite physical presence, which could be both inspiring and intimidating. En route to wards 17 and 18, he would chat to staff irrespective of their rank and was on first name terms with porters and cleaners. In the operating theatre, a meticulous dissection technique, based on sound knowledge of anatomy, and a fearless approach to surgery, coupled with tremendous affection for his patients, made him an outstanding surgeon. Even in the middle of long and difficult procedures, Aires remained calm and quite capable of conversation on a wide variety of subjects, which is not surprising given his erudition, his extensive library and love of travelling.

'In contrast to his coolness under pressure in the operating theatre, he had a quick temper, dispensing with diplomatic skills, particularly when dealing with bureaucrats, patients who smoked, or laziness and incompetence amongst his staff. Ward rounds were never dull when Aires located cigarettes in the locker of a 'non-smoking' patient or when his nursing staff had been abused. On one such occasion, his registrar having spent all night repairing the popliteal vessels of a kneecapped individual, Aires arrived on the ward and, finding the nurses and junior medical staff being terrorised by this boorish patient, simply wheeled him out and refused to have him readmitted. The 1970s saw the worst of "the Troubles" and, along with his colleagues, Aires dealt with many horrific injuries sustained by the victims of bomb and bullet. Although his experience made him an international authority on such injuries, he despised terrorism and had no time for extremists from either side.

'A dynamic individual who believed in a direct uncompromising approach to patient care and most other problems, Aires was held in high esteem by the people of Ulster and was always remarkably tolerant of their inability to pronounce his name correctly.

'Aires was a strong supporter of the arts, and as a patron of the Ulster Orchestra had a regular seat with his wife in the front row of the balcony at Friday night concerts. A gifted artist, he would provide his own illustrations for the many chapters and books he authored and, when teaching medical students, often arrived early and covered the blackboards in the lecture theatre with detailed anatomical drawings. A lover of fine wines and good food, Aires was a generous host and would frequently entertain both senior and junior medical staff at his Belfast home.'

CAMPBELL, Robert

Belfast Surgeon

b. 1866
Educ. RUI, Queen's College, Belfast and Trinity College, Dublin
d. 1920

BA, RUI, 1887; MB (hons, first place and exhibition); MRCS Lond, 1893; FRCS Eng (by exam), 1896 (QCB and TCD)

Surgical registrar, Chester General Infirmary. Demonstrator of anatomy QCB, RUI. Surgeon, RVH, Belfast (1900–20); Belfast Hospital for Sick Children.

Robert Campbell was the pioneer of aseptic surgery in Belfast. It has been said that the biggest advance in surgery was when the surgeons began washing their hands before, instead of after, the operation. He wore rubber gloves and a face mask, originally used by French surgeons to keep their beards out of the wound, but in his case to stop the cough droplets getting to the wound. He wrote on a wide variety of subjects but his *Lancet* paper (1904) on 'The Operative Treatment of Hernia in Infants and Young Children illustrated by 114 Consecutive Cases', many of them done as outpatients, represented a huge triumph at the time. A subsequent paper in 1907 described 1,500 cases, with only one death, which he stated was caused by chloroform poisoning.

He suffered acute nephritis in childhood and this went on to become chronic glomerulonephritis, which caused his early death at 54. Though often ill, he was unremittingly conscientious in the care of his patients.

The RVH and the Ulster Medical Society established a memorial oration in his honour. The oration has been given every two to four years since 1922, and some of the most distinguished physicians and surgeons from all over the world have been so honoured.

CLARKE, Stewart Desmond (Stewart)

Belfast General and Transplant Surgeon

Educ. Queen's University Belfast

MB, QUB, 1955; MCh (hons), QUB, 1959; FRCS Ed, 1960; FRCS Eng, 1961

Postgraduate posts included lecturer, Department of Surgery, University of Sheffield; tutor and registrar, Department of Surgery, QUB.

Consultant surgeon, RVH, Belfast; Belfast City Hospital; and Musgrave Park Hospital.

Stewart Clarke began renal transplant in Northern Ireland in 1968. He resigned in 1974 to run the surgical service in Ahmadi, Kuwait, for nine years. He retired to Midhurst, Sussex.

FRASER, Ian James (Sir) 'Ian' KB, OBE DSO

Belfast Surgeon and President RCSI 1954–56

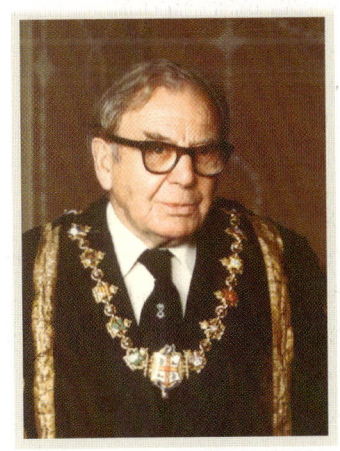

b. 1901, Belfast, son of Dr Robert Fraser and Margaret Fraser (*née* Ferguson)
Educ. Royal Belfast Academical Institution 'Inst'; Queen's University Belfast
m. 1931: Eleanor Margaret Mitchell, daughter of Marcus A. and Alice Jane (*née* Cuthbert); 2 s (John d. tuberculous meningitis 1938; Ian Marcus (Mark) is GP in Tonbridge, Kent), 1 d (Mary Alice)
d. 1999

MB (first class hons), QUB, 1923; MCh (commendation), 1927; MD, Belf, 1932; FRCS Eng, 1927; FRCSI (first place), 1926; FACS, 1945; DSc (Hon.), Oxford & New University of Ulster; FRCS Glas (Hon.), 1972; FRCS Ed (Hon.), 1976; GCStJ

Postgraduate junior posts at RVH, Belfast. Visits to Guy's Hospital and the Middlesex Hospital, London, Paris and Vienna.
Surgeon, Royal Hospital for Sick Children, 1927–66; surgeon, RVH, Belfast, 1945–66; surgeon-in-ordinary to HE The Governor of Northern Ireland.
President, Association of Surgeons of Great Britain and Ireland (1957–58), President, BMA (1962–63)

Ian Fraser was Ireland's most distinguished surgeon of the twentieth century. In his early career, as assistant to Professor Andrew Fullerton [q.v.], he showed great loyalty to this able but difficult man. His first Millin's prostatectomy (1947) was on Fullerton's chauffeur and he did it with Millin's book describing the operation open in the operating theatre, and a nurse turning the pages as for a tyro piano recital.

He volunteered for the Royal Army Medical Corps at the outbreak of war in 1939 and served in West Africa, North Africa, Italy, on the invasion beaches at Arromanches, Normandy, and ended as Brigadier in Agra, India, in 1945. He was involved in early trials of penicillin 'in the field'. Not just 'a good war' but a really great war.

A fine clinician, he was also an enthusiastic teacher, illustrating many problems with a reminiscence of a similar patient seen elsewhere, perhaps at one of the many medical schools at which he examined. He was a first-rate natural operator. Paediatric surgery had always been a particular interest and, despite all the calls on his time, he regularly attended the annual meeting of the British Association of Paediatric Surgeons, where he was feted.

He was not particularly interested in research and he had a particular aversion to animal experimentation. But he knew how to write an article that would be published and he passed this skill on to his trainees. He had a lifelong devotion to the St John Ambulance Association, in which, as usual, he reached the top rank in Northern Ireland. He served the Royal Belfast Academical Institution as a governor. It is a measure of medicine's drop down the league tables of social importance that his name is not in the Wikipedia's list of twenty-five distinguished alumni, which contains many evanescent media 'personalities'. He was on the governing body of Queen's University until he was nearly ninety.

Fraser loved surgery, was proud to be a surgeon, had great determination and ambition, a prodigious memory for faces as well as facts, and an infectious exuberance. He was constantly upbeat, had an inexhaustible fund of stories and anecdotes (all repeatable in mixed company), and was an inveterate gossip, always on the look out for tasty morsels. He was an expert at tailoring the story to the particular audience, which may account for varied versions of the core anecdote being given full provenance. His vision was for the whole Province and he was as loved by the surgeons outside Belfast as by the locals. With Ronnie Loane [q.v.] and Will Hanna [q.v.] he founded the Ulster Surgical Club, of which he was Life President. The club was set up to promote good fellowship between the Belfast surgeons and those outside, as well as visiting centres abroad where Ian's name was an 'Open Sesame'.

Something like Lewis Carroll's Cheshire cat, his trademark was the chuckle and, when he was gone from your company, the chuckle remained. He was a superb formal orator and gave many eponymous addresses. He was a great after-dinner speaker, careful in preparation and presentation, and made no secret of the fact that preparation was hard work. He was a superb chairman of a meeting, never ever losing his cool, and defusing confrontations before they had time to gain momentum. Ian did everything possible to bridge the gap between the two parts of this small island, and his integrity was unquestioned on both sides of that ravine, sometimes espousing southern candidates for honours against his own locals. He was the first agreed chairman of the Police Authority (1970–76). He was also a director of Allied Irish Banks whose headquarters is in Dublin.

His main interests were the history of surgery and everything Irish, be it silver, antiques, doctors, memorabilia or the island's rugby team. One never noticed that he was about 5' 6" because his frame was solid, broad shouldered and resilient. His legendary energy did not desert him over the decades. The massive eyebrows could be moved independently and sometimes, though this was indeed rare, could make any further comment by him unnecessary.

The BMA commissioned his modest autobiography, Blood, Sweat and Cheers, in 1989, and Professor Richard Clarke has written an elegant, painstakingly accurate but easy-to-read book, A Surgeon's Century: The Life of Sir Ian Fraser (2004). Together they provide a portrait of this warm, remarkable, endearing and wholly admirable man. There was nobody like Ian. He was a role model who was impossible to follow.

IRWIN, John Walker Sinclair (Sinclair, 'Sincy')

Belfast Surgeon

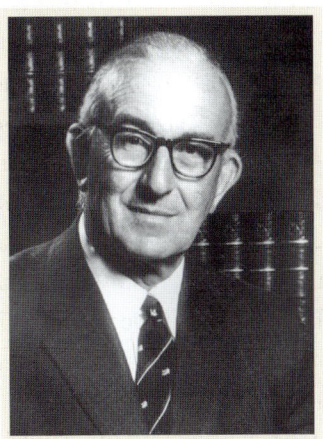

b. 1913, Belfast, son of Sir Samuel Irwin FRCS
Educ. Campbell College; Queen's University Belfast
m. 1948: Elizabeth Sherrard Fulton (Betty); 3 s, 2 d (two doctors)
d. 2004

MB (hons), QUB, 1937; FRCS Ed, 1947

Royal Army Medical Corps (Oct 1939–1945). Consultant surgeon, RVH, Belfast, 1950–78; Ulster Hospital.

Captured at the fall of France in June 1940, Sinclair Irwin, typically, stayed behind with the wounded and then spent four years as a German prisoner of war. Transported from camp to camp in cattle trucks, he was eventually incarcerated in an Oflag in Poland where, as medical officer, he compassionately cared for the plight and privations of the other prisoners of war.

Following the war, he was appointed as a general surgeon and developed an interest in vascular work. Together with Reginald Livingston [q.v.], he played a big role in the development of vascular surgery as a specialty in Northern Ireland. His clinical acumen and balanced judgment were widely recognised. In the operating theatre, those legendary hands moved with superb dexterity and great finesse. He made a big contribution to the planning and development of the hospital.

Tall, well over six foot, broad shouldered, erect and a distinguished figure, he commanded, not verbally, widespread respect in the corridors of power as well as the corridors of the hospital.

He won five Irish caps as a rugby back-row forward (partnering another legend, Blair Mayne, one of the founders of the Special Air Service, an elite fighting unit), just before the war, and scored Ireland's winning try at Twickenham in February 1939. He was fast, strong, intelligent and a very clean player with real flair. He declined an invitation to join the British Lions (rugby) tour of 1937 because it coincided with his final MB examinations. He was President of the Irish Rugby Football Union (IRFU) in 1969–70. A quiet man, with a dry sense of humour, he enjoyed his golf and his garden. He was completely admirable in every way.

Three generations of Irwins leave their indelible surgical fingerprints as master craftsmen on the Royal Victoria Hospital. His father, Sir Samuel (Sam) [q.v.] was also a rugby international at the turn of the century and was President of the IRFU in 1935–36. He is commemorated in the Irwin Postgraduate Lecture Theatre at the RVH. Sinclair's son, Terence (Terry), currently carries the surgical mantle as consultant colorectal surgeon.

IRWIN, Samuel Thompson (Sir)

Belfast Surgeon

b. 1877
Educ. Queen's College, Belfast, RUI
m. Son, Sinclair [q.v.], was consultant surgeon at the RVH, 1950–78.
d. 1961

BA, RUI, 1900; MB (hons), 1902; MCh, 1906; FRCS Ed, 1909

Coulter Exhibitioner, RVH, 1902. Assistant to Professor of Surgery, QUB.
Surgeon, RVH (1918–45), Ulster Children's & Women's Hospital, Nervous Diseases Hospital and Cripples' Institution, Belfast.

Temporary Captain, Royal Army Medical Corps.

Publications include: 'Hunger Pain & Duodenal Ulcer', *British Medical Journal*, 1909, and papers on Appendicitis.

In addition to duodenal ulcer, the disease that dominated abdominal surgery for the first ninety years of the century, Sir Samuel was also interested in orthopaedics. A quiet, expert intellectual, he was an MP at Stormont, where he held the University seat. He played rugby for Ireland (1899–1902), winning eight caps (front row of scrum), and he was President of the Irish Rugby Football Union (1935–36).

JOHNSTON, George Weir, OBE (Georgie)

Belfast Surgeon

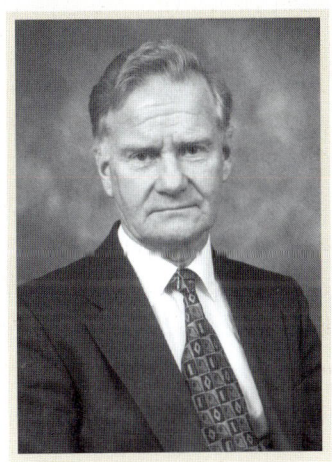

b. 1932, Ballymena, Co. Antrim, younger son of Thomas and Jane Johnston
Educ. Ballymena Academy, QUB
m. 1962: Elaine Hutton, daughter of Robert and Dorothy Hutton; 3 s (Brian is consultant gastroenterologist at RVH, Belfast, and Paul is consultant cardiologist at RVH)

MB (hons), QUB, 1956; DObst, RCOG, 1958; DCH, 1958; FRCS Eng, 1962; MCh, QUB, 1965; FRCSI ad eundem, 1977; FRCS Ed (*ad hominem*), 1995

Postgraduate posts as Senior Registrar, RVH, Belfast. Chief Surgical Assistant, St Bartholomew's Hospital, London 1965–66; Senior Lecturer, QUB and RVH, 1966–68; Consultant surgeon, NHS, 1966–95.

Hunterian Professorship, RCS Eng, 1980.
Honorary Professor of Surgery, QUB, 1990.
President Ulster Society of Gastroenterology; President Ulster Surgical Club; Board of Directors of James IV Association of Surgeons. Vice-Chairman of NI Council for Cancer Research.

As an undergraduate, George Johnston took first place in virtually every professional examination and was the recipient of a host of scholarships, prizes and medals at Queen's University. Throughout his postgraduate career, he never failed to impress. Having been senior tutor/senior registrar and subsequently senior lecturer/consultant for two years at Queen's University, Belfast and the Royal Victoria Hospital, he was headhunted for an NHS post in the RVH, to join Terence Kennedy to form one of the foremost upper gastrointestinal and hepatobiliary units in the British Isles. His NHS appointment did not deter him from taking an active role in academic surgery, and he was a prolific article writer and presenter with Professor Harold Rodgers [q.v.], Professor Douglas Roy [q.v.], Terence Kennedy [q.v.] and others. In this and so many other ways he was an answer to a professor's Santa Claus 'wish list'.

Double-blind randomised clinical trials of different forms of vagotomy and different modes of gastric drainage or non-drainage in patients with peptic ulceration received worldwide acclaim. In association with Professor Harold Rodgers, George pioneered the role of sclerotherapy in management of acute bleeding from oesophageal varices, using the rigid oesophagoscope, for many years prior to the introduction of flexible endoscopic equipment, when many centres worldwide followed their lead. For over twenty years, George was responsible for the surgical management of virtually all the cases of portal hypertension in Northern Ireland. In patients with recurrent variceal bleeding who were unsuitable for portosystemic shunt procedures, he pioneered the use of oesophageal transection using mechanical circular stapling devices. He was often called upon to deal with complex hepatobiliary problems and to treat many of the victims of civil disturbance in Northern Ireland.

George was an inspirational teacher, whether in a small group forum or as a lecturer on the international stage where he was much in demand. His great sense of humour and depth of insight are well displayed in his 'party piece' on 'How not to give a lecture'. He was a prolific author, a popular examiner and a perceptive referee of manuscripts submitted for publication.

Quick, alert, incisive with boundless energy, he was ever ready to impart his considerable knowledge and was a truly dynamic trainer with undeniable leadership qualities. Characterised by integrity, compassion and care for others, he engendered respect and loyalty in patients, nursing and medical staff alike. A devoutly committed Christian with a deep personal faith, which was an integral part of his life, he was an extremely gifted exponent of ethical values and Christian principles and was frequently invited to speak on these important topics.

Below average in height, red-haired and exuding restless energy, he was frequently at the heart of surgical meetings in Northern Ireland. In retirement, he plays golf and he gardens.

KENNEDY, Terence Leslie (TLK)

Belfast Surgeon

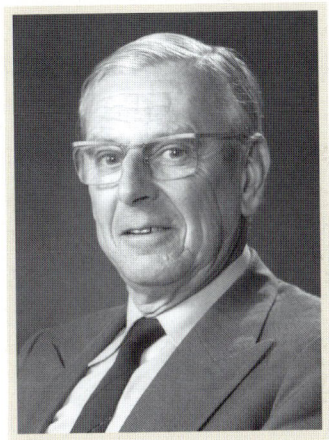

b. 1919, Plymouth, son of Matheson Kennedy (MBE, FRCS, consultant surgeon, Prince of Wales Hospital, Plymouth) and Mabel Maud Kennedy (*née* Hore); grandfather had qualified at TCD, and practised as a surgeon in British Guyana; brother, Hugh Henry Kennedy, was an orthopaedic surgeon in Epsom.
Educ. Ravenswood Preparatory School, Tiverton. Scholarship to St Edward's School, Oxford and thence to the London Hospital, where he won prizes in anatomy and physiology
m. 1949: Brigid Frances Walker; 1 s (Peter, a doctor), 2 d (Penelope is an ophthalmologist)
d. 1993

MRCS, 1942; MB, Lond, 1942; FRCS, 1946; MS, 1950; FRCSI (*ad eundem*), 1971; MD (Hon.), QUB, 1982

Royal Naval Volunteer Reserve (1942–46) in Atlantic, Pacific and Mediterranean.
Returned to London as registrar to Tudor Edwards (1890–1946); worked with Alan Perry (whom he greatly admired) and Hermon Taylor (who was pioneering gastroscopy and emergency partial gastrectomy).
First assistant to neurosurgical and thoracic firms, London Hospital (1949).
Consultant surgeon, RVH, 1950–84.
President Association of Surgeons of Great Britain and Ireland (1981); Member, Council, RCS (1981).

He published some eighty papers, a very large number for someone without academic back-up.

TLK, as he was known locally, was an excellent teacher, mentor, trainer and an extremely fine operator. He and Professor George Johnston [q.v.] established a worldwide reputation as pioneers in the development of controlled clinical trials in refining techniques in peptic ulcer surgery, with particular reference to selective and highly selective vagotomy. These seminal large studies were 'classics', leading to irrefutable publications, which helped to change the whole ethos of duodenal ulcer surgery from resectional to non-resectional methodology in the era before medicinal gastric acid inhibitors were developed.

As Chairman of the Hospital Recognition Committee, in 1984, it was said that he took no prisoners, but it was in the good cause of improving the lot of the trainees. He won awards in Denmark and Australia and was a James IV Surgical Traveller and a frequent Visiting Professor to American centres. He was essentially an NHS surgeon, albeit an Honorary Clinical Lecturer. Over the years, he maintained a close association with University Department of Surgery and supervised several postgraduates undertaking clinical or basic research for MD, MCh or PhD degrees.

He was a competitive sailor, winning, with his wife as crew, the Flying Fifteens National Championship in 1962 and again in 1966. Later he gardened, specialising in eucalyptus trees.

Tall, elegant, peppery, impatient, he did not suffer fools gladly (or at all), and he brought a breath of London dash and competitiveness to the quieter groves of the 'Vic'. In *1066 and All That* terms, he was unquestionably a 'Good Thing'.

KIRK, Thomas Sinclair ('Surgeon Kirk', 'Pa Kirk')

Belfast Surgeon

b. 1869
Educ. Queen's University Belfast
d. 1940

BA, MB RUI, 1893, QUB

Surgeon, RVH, Belfast (1897–1934); Forster Green Hospital for Consumption and Diseases of the Chest.
Surgeon, Children's Department, Tyrone Hospital; Smiley's Hospital, Larne.
Senior surgeon, Belfast Children's Hospital.
Medical Referee Workman's Compensation.
Royal Army Medical Corps, First World War.

He was known as 'Surgeon' Kirk though he had no Fellowship. He sat the exam once, failed, and then derided it. He used silkworm gut in repairing hernias (reasonable at the time), thus discarding the warning of Philip Mitchiner of St Thomas's, London: 'Use any suture you like but use catgut in your private patients.' Silk famously caused sinuses, for which the surgeon was often wrongly blamed. Wounds were loosely sutured to allow out the pus (still good practice for infected wounds). He packed his wounds with urea crystals. Patients with abdominal drains were made to lie on their faces to allow pus to drain. He used subcutaneous oxygen for chest infections, and cow's serum by mouth for infection, to raise resistance. There were other quirks.

On his retirement from the 'Royal', he was presented with a splendid, solid silver 'loving cup', and this is still passed around at staff dinners. His eccentricities were a soft target for Ian Fraser [q.v.] who always said when the loving cup was passed that he never knew a 'more unloving man'. One of his less attractive traits was that he was never, ever wrong. A life-long bachelor, it may well have been that young women looking for 'Mr Right' were not attracted to 'Mr Always Right'.

LIVINGSTON, Reginald Hamilton (Reggie)

Vascular Surgeon

b. 1923, Lurgan, Co. Armagh
Educ. Lurgan College, Queen's University Belfast
m. Sybil; 2 s, 1 d
d. 1980

MB (hons), QUB, 1946; MD (with high commendation), QUB, 1955; FRCS Eng, 1952

Postgraduate junior appointments in Belfast.
Surgical Fellow, Mayo Clinic, Rochester, Minnesota, USA.
Consultant vascular and general surgeon, RVH, Belfast, 1956–80.
Chairman NI Division BMA; Member, Council, BMA.

Reggie Hamilton and Sinclair Irwin [q.v.] formed a distinguished team in general and vascular surgery, dealing with tertiary referrals from all over Northern Ireland, with much trauma from the civil disturbances of 1968–96. He gave unstintingly of his time to many committees including the RVH Planning Committee, Eastern Health Board, St John's Ambulance, Cripples' Institute, Leprosy Mission, Belfast Bible College, Society of Friends and the YMCA.

He was a devout, unselfish, Christian gentleman whose life was focused on the welfare of others. He was a great listener who relaxed by walking in the Mountains of Mourne or along the County Down coastline. He was an accomplished silversmith with his own hallmark, symbolising a life that was genuine, authentic and exemplary.

Typically one of his last public acts was to give the Royal Victoria Annual Oration entitled 'They Comfort Me', tracing the story of nursing in the hospital and paying tribute to their loving care of the sick and dying. Ironically his terminal illness began shortly afterwards. He faced the end with great courage, serenity and absolute trust in God.

LOUGHRIDGE, James Stevenson (Jamsie)

Belfast Surgeon

b. 1901
Educ. Belfast Royal Academy, Queen's University Belfast
m. Ethel; 2 s (Gordon was a urologist in Belfast), 1 d
d. 1980

MB (hons), QUB, 1923; BSc (Physiology), 1925; MD (commendation), 1926; FRCS, 1928

Postgraduate posts in Rochdale and Manchester.
Consultant surgeon, RVH, Belfast (1945–67) and Royal Hospital for Sick Children. He stayed on as medical superintendent where his conciliatory skills were tested and not found wanting. President, Moynihan Surgical Club; Ulster Medical Society.

Jamsie was a highly popular teacher at the bedside and in the theatre and an admired colleague. He loved visits to other centres and was a much-quoted source of anecdotes and aphorisms, many culled from Holy Writ. He had a big surgical practice, based on his personal affability and his careful operative technique. He had the priceless quality of being able to create a relaxed atmosphere in the operating theatre, no matter what the problem. During the Second World War, he travelled the length and breadth of Northern Ireland and did much emergency surgery in many hospitals and even in patients' homes.

He kept very fit, though later troubled by an arthritic hip. Interests included archaeology, photography, walking and gardening. He spent his summers on Hellenic cruises. A warm, jovial, much-loved figure.

MAGEE, Reginald Arthur Edward (Reggie) PRCSI (1986–1988)

Belfast Obstetrician

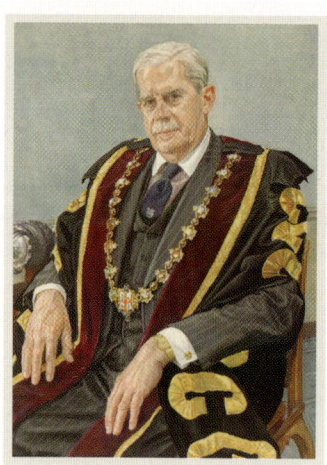

Educ. Queen's University Belfast

MB, QUB, 1937; FRCSI, 1947; FRCOG, 1967

Consultant obstetrician and gynaecologist, Royal Victoria and Royal Maternity and Ulster Hospital, Belfast.
President, RCSI, 1986–88.
Member, Council, Royal College of Obstetricians and Gynaecologists. Member, NI Hospital Authority; Senate, QUB.

Author of the clinical reports of the hospitals he served, 1963–77.

McKELVEY, Samuel Thomas Donnan

Belfast Surgeon

Educ. Queen's University Belfast

MB, QUB, 1962; MCh, QUB, 1971; FRCS Eng, 1968; FRCS Ed, 1967; DObst, RCOG, 1965.

Consultant surgeon, RVH, Belfast (1974–85); Ulster Hospital (1974–2004).
Senior lecturer in surgery, QUB.

Samuel McKelvey it was who coined the expression 'gastric incontinence' for the 'dumping syndrome' of diarrhoea, pain and bilious vomiting that sometimes occurred following vagotomy for peptic ulcer.

McMECHAN, Eric Wilson

Belfast Surgeon

b. 1910
Educ. Queen's University Belfast
d. 1980

MB (hons), QUB, 1933; FRCS Eng, 1938.

Postgraduate posts included demonstrator in anatomy, QUB; house surgeon, RVH, Belfast; registrar, St Mark's Hospital for Diseases of the Rectum etc, London.
Consultant surgeon, RVH and Belfast City Hospital 1945–68.
Lieutenant-Colonel, Royal Army Medical Corps

Eric McMechan was much admired by his colleagues and trainees including J. W. (Jack) Kyle, surgeon and Ireland's greatest ever rugby player, 'The Ultimate Safe Pair of Hands', who thought him one of the finest surgical technicians he had seen. He retired early due to ill health.

MITCHELL, Arthur Brownlow, OBE

Belfast Surgeon

b. 1865
Educ. Queen's College, Belfast
d. 1942

MB, QCB, 1890; FRCSI, 1900; Coulter Exhibitioner, Belfast Royal Hospital (later RVH), 1889.

Surgeon, RVH, Belfast (1894–1930); Ulster Hospital for Children and Women.
Lieutenant-Colonel, Royal Army Medical Corps.
Assistant Director of Orthopaedics for Ulster.

It was said that Arthur Mitchell did more between 1894 and 1928 than any other to introduce new techniques into abdominal and orthopaedic surgery. He was in on the foundation of the Association of Surgeons of Great Britain and Ireland and was Belfast's first surgical gastroenterologist. He published many papers and had a particularly low mortality in the closure of perforated peptic ulcer. In 1928, he pricked his finger during an operation and developed a crippling infection of his hand.

MORRISON, Ernest (Ernie)

Belfast Surgeon

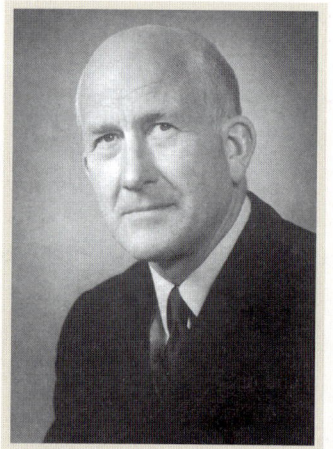

b. 1918, Coleraine, Northern Ireland, son of Samuel and Martha Morrison (farmers); brother, Ian, was a radiologist in Perth, Western Australia
Educ. Coleraine Academical Institution, QUB
m. 1st in 1945: Margaret (Peggy) (d. 1968);
2nd in 1969: Vera Loane (widow of Surgeon Ronnie Loane [q.v.])
d. 2001

MB (hons), QUB, 1942; FRCSI, 1969; FRCS Ed, 1948

Surgical registrar, house surgeon and extern surgeon, RVH, Belfast.
Consultant urologist, RVH, Belfast and Belfast City Hospital (1950–84); Consultant surgeon, Ulster Volunteer Hospital (now the Somme Nursing Home), Craigavon, and Musgrave Park Hospital, Belfast.

Ernie Morrison joined the Royal Army Medical Corps 2nd Parachute Division in 1943 and served in North Africa, Italy, France and the Middle East. He was involved in the treatment of the only chemical warfare casualties of the Second World War when the Germans launched a highly successful attack ('The Second Pearl Harbour') on Bari on the 'heel' of Italy on 2 December 1943. A secret American Liberty ship's cargo of 100 tons of mustard gas was blown into the air, causing 628 casualties and sixty-nine deaths, mostly American merchant seamen. As the mustard gas was a top secret, even the medical attendants did not know what had occurred until it was too late for some of the casualties.

A hugely popular, hard-working surgeon, he was quietly spoken and nobody ever heard him raise his voice. He initially had an interest in thyroid work and found it difficult to give this up, when he became a distinguished urologist. He was a quick and 'bloodless' surgeon, evoking the comment, 'There may have been faster surgeons than Ernie Morrison but that was before the introduction of anaesthesia.' An assistant who spent too long scrubbing up and gloving might miss half the operation.

He had a huge smile under his trademark military moustache, was 5'10", balding and burly, had been on the first rugby fifteen at Coleraine Academical Institution and never lost faith in the school's team; each year they were 'the best team in the Schools Cup', which alas they won only once in thirty years. He had great loyalties to the Coleraine Institution where he had won a King's Scholarship to study teaching, but he had second thoughts and, in one year, he completed a two-year course in science to gain entry to Queen's medical school. He taught generations of medical students and was a compassionate examiner. He regarded his membership of the staff of the RVH as being a member of the greatest club in the world.

In his declining years, he suffered a disabling stroke, affecting his left side. Fortunately like almost all surgeons he was right-handed and was well able to lift a glass with friends almost to the end. He was nursed untiringly and devotedly by his wife Vera. He was always interested in horses and was a familiar figure at Down Royal racecourse. He was also a keen huntsman and a spirited golfer. He had the priceless quality of being instantly likeable and had a sustained infectious charm.

O'NEILL, Henry

Belfast Surgeon

b. 1853
Educ. Queen's College, Belfast
d. 1914

MD, MCh, Diploma in Obstetrics, RUI (QCB), 1877; Licentiate, Apothecaries' Hall, 1877; MAO, Dublin, 1900; Barrister-at-Law, Dublin

Resident assistant surgeon, pathologist and visiting surgeon, Belfast Royal Hospital, 1879–1900.
Surgeon, Samaritan Hospital for Diseases of Women.
Health correspondent, *Belfast Evening Telegraph*; editor and proprietor, *Belfast Health Journal*.
High Sheriff, Belfast, 1905.

Something of a public-health crusader, Henry O'Neill was also much involved in wider social issues.

ODLING-SMEE, George William

Belfast Surgeon

b. 1935, eldest son of Rev. C. W. Odling-Smee and Dr Katherine Hamilton Odling-Smee.
Educ. Durham School and King's College, Newcastle upon Tyne, University of Durham
m. Anne Marie Thacker, CBE, daughter of Flight Lieutenant W. L. and Margaret Thacker;
3 s. 3 d

MB (Durham), 1959; FRCS Eng, 1968; FRCSI, 1986; BA (Classics), QUB, 2003, MA (Ancient History), QUB, 2004

Medical officer, St Raphael's Hospital, Giddalur, Andhra Pradesh, India, 1961–64.
Surgeon to Child Medical Care Unit, Enugu, Nigeria, 1969.
Research assistant, Mayo Clinic, Rochester, Minnesota, 1972.
Consultant surgeon, RVH and Mater Infirmorum Hospital, 1974–2000.
Senior lecturer in surgery, QUB, 1974. Set up first specialised Breast Clinic in NI.
Chairman, Court of Examiners, RCS Eng, 1993; examiner, FRCS, 1982–93.
Vice-President, British Association of Surgical Oncologists, 1974–78; founder chairman NI Hospice, 1979–89; chairman, Action Cancer, 1994–2000.
Ordained Auxiliary Priest, Church of Ireland, 1977; Curate at St Thomas's, 1977–90; and St George's, Belfast, 1990–2005.

Co-author with Alan Crockard (neurosurgeon) of the book *Trauma Care*.

George Odling-Smee is a tall, well-spoken gentleman, with a deep and genuine interest in his students, to countless numbers of whom he acted as counsellor and guide. For ten years, he chaired the University Medical Curriculum Committee (a position of great trust rarely given to a surgeon), and championed modernisation of undergraduate courses. A wise and sympathetic examiner who took his role in this, as in everything else, conscientiously.

PURSE, George Raphael Buick ('Barney')

Belfast Surgeon

b. 1891, Ballyclare, Co Antrim, eldest son of James Purse
Educ. Coleraine Academical Institute; Queen's University Belfast
m. Married with 2 s (elder son killed serving in RAF)
d. 1950

MB (hons), QUB, 1914; MCh, 1920; FRCS Ed, 1921.

Postgraduate posts included house surgeon, RVH; Royal Army Medical Corps 1915–18 with 8th Battalion of Royal Irish Rifles, 110th Field Ambulance Service and 48th Casualty Clearing Station. Military Cross. The Military Cross (MC) is awarded for 'Gallantry during active

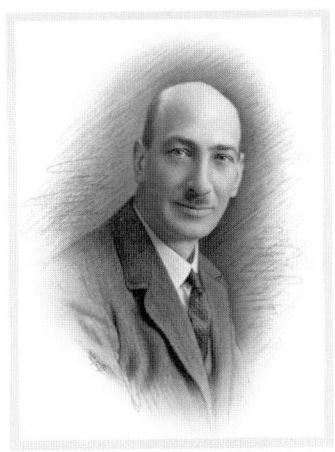

operations against the enemy'. Continued training post war in the Ulster Hospital.

Consultant staff, RVH and Ulster Hospital, 1929–50. President, Association of Thoracic Surgeons of Great Britain and Ireland; Ulster Medical Society; Ulster Tuberculosis Association.

Barney Purse had intellectual brilliance, exceptional manual dexterity and craftsmanship of the highest order. He began thoracic surgery in Foster Green Hospital and Whiteabbey Sanatorium. He carried out the first lobectomy in the RVH in 1939. He was also responsible for neurosurgery in Northern Ireland. This wide spectrum of work was carried out to the highest standards. He had exceptional stamina, talent and commitment. In character, he was quiet and unassuming. He operated with the minimum of assistance and instruments. He removed Millar Bell's [q.v.] spleen on a kitchen table and Richard Clarke's [q.v.] appendix in a similar setting. He knew the origin and modification of every surgical instrument he used and improvised further in his own workshop. He was a keen teacher, full of quiet erudition and logic, and as a skilful fast operator he was a superb teacher of technique.

He was greatly loved and admired by colleagues and patients. He was fascinated by sport and was knowledgeable on many topics outside of medicine. He had played hockey for Ireland. Later he golfed, fished, sailed and was a first-class marksman with either rifle or shotgun. He was a big man, with huge hands, slightly stooped, with a shining bald head and prominent eyes. You would certainly like to have him in your lifeboat.

STEVENSON, Howard

Belfast Surgeon

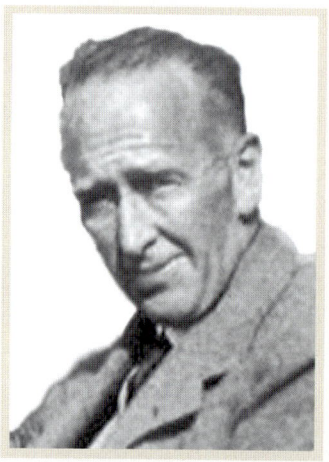

b. 1876, Lisburn; two of his brothers also became doctors, serving with the army on India (one receiving the MBE), a third serving as a chaplain with the Irish Universities Mission, a fourth receiving a Knighthood after distinguished service as Governor of Cyprus and laterally the Seychelles.
Educ. Methodist College, Belfast; RUI, Dublin, London
m. 1919: Charlotte, daughter of Sir William and Lady Liddel of Donacloney (one of the great families involved with the manufacture of linen in Ulster); son Morris became consultant thoracic surgeon, RVH.
d. 1950

BA, RUI, 1897; MB, QCB, RUI, 1900; FRCSI, 1904

Assistant resident medical officer, Royal National Hospital for Consumption, Ventnor, Isle of Wight; surgical registrar, RVH, Belfast; assistant to Professor of Surgery, Belfast.
Senior surgeon, Ulster Hospital for Children and Women, Belfast; Surgeon, RVH, 1911–41; surgeon, Throne Children's Hospital, Belfast; surgeon in charge, Limbless Branch.
Ulster Volunteer Hospital, Belfast.

Author, 'Case of Fissura Abdominalis: Oper. at age 2½ Hours', *British Medical Journal*, 1909.

Howard Stevenson was renowned for his speed and dexterity and 'the removal of a gall-bladder seemed to take seconds rather than minutes'. He was a man of few words and a story is told of a consultation that took place during an earlier time of unrest in Ulster in the 1920s. A young lad was brought into the hospital by his mother, who explained that he had swallowed one of his father's bullets! Being not too sympathetic with the cause on either side at that time, he advised the mother, 'Give him two ounces of Black Draught and don't point him at anybody for 24 hours!'

In 1938, he became MP for Queen's University. He retired in 1941 but returned from retirement to help during the war.

He was an enthusiastic golfer and every Saturday he and a group of medical colleagues went by train from Belfast to Newcastle (31 miles) to play golf at the Royal County Down Golf Club, a tradition which continued for many years.

A consummate professional and role model.

VINCENT, Samuel Anderson (Sammy)

Belfast Surgeon

b. 1909, Belfast, younger son of James Vincent (a musician).
Educ. Roseland Preparatory School; Royal Belfast Academical Institution; Queen's University Belfast
m. 1951: Lindsay Pine, Dundee
d. 1976

MB, QUB, 1933, FRCS, 1946

Training posts in Royal Berkshire Hospital, Reading, and Tyrone County Hospital, Omagh. Major, Royal Army Medical Corps. Four and a half years overseas on troopships, in the Western Desert, Sicily and Italy.
Surgeon, Ulster Hospital for Women and Children, 1947–73; Musgrave Park Hospital.

His published work includes papers on biomechanical engineering and on electrical and other aspects of enuresis in childhood. He described the characteristic sign of a child with bladder spasms as a 'curtsey' sign, where the child, usually a girl, lowers her pelvis and bends her knees in an effort to either pass or retain urine.

Shy, quietly spoken, extremely kind, considerate and conscientious, Sammy Vincent taught applied clinical anatomy to preclinical students whom he also invited to his operating lists. These were hugely popular outings even though proceedings advanced at a very modest pace. For recreation, he painted in watercolours, played the violin and fished with the fly.

WHEELER, Thomas Kennedy

Belfast Surgeon

b. 1848, son of a GP
Educ. RUI
m. married; 3 s, 1 d (all of whom became doctors)
d. 1923

MD, RUI, LM, 1879; MCh, 1880, QCB, RUI, and St Bartholomew's, London

Consultant surgeon, RVH, Belfast, 1882–1902; Ulster Hospital for Children. Medical attendant, Methodist College, Belfast.

WILSON, Willoughby, OBE

Belfast Surgeon

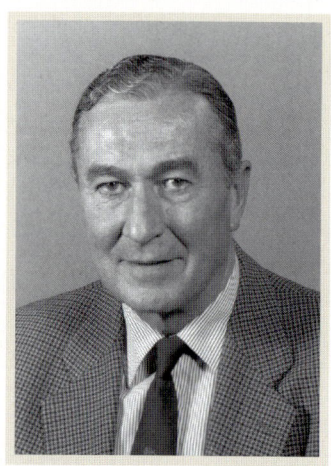

b. 1923, Straid, Co Antrim
Educ. Methodist College; Queen's University Belfast
m. Dr Kaye Browne (anaesthetist); 3 s (John, and twins David and Richard. All three started medical school on the same day and all graduated at the same time), 1 d
d. 2004

MB, QUB, 1946; FRCS Ed, 1952; FRCSI, 1969; OBE, 1982.

Training posts as house surgeon, RVH; orthopaedic house surgeon, Musgrave Park Hospital.
Surgeon, RVH, 1957–87.
President, Ulster Ileostomy Society; Vice-President, Medical Defence Union; member of numerous important hospital and Health Board committees.

At secondary school, Willoughby Wilson concentrated more on sport (rugby, cricket and tennis) than on academic studies. His first report from Methodist College read, 'A pleasant and lively member of the class. If he spent as much time at his work as he does at sport, his exam results would improve.' He went on to work harder than most.

There had been several doctors in the Wilson family tree including two older sisters, and, while a Resident House Officer, Willoughby had negotiated with a relative to go into General Practice at £750 per annum with a car provided (a very generous offer in those days). When he told his perceptive surgical mentor, Barney Purse [q.v.], what he was about to do, Barney replied, 'You will not; you are starting Anatomy on 1 October and I have arranged it with Professor Walmsley.' And so an illustrious surgical career began.

Appointed as a general surgeon with an overseeing role in the A&E Department, he was a hugely talented natural operator who could turn his hand to anything. He specialised in colorectal surgery and partnered Eric McMechan [q.v.], who had trained at St Mark's, London. Their reputation as the fastest abdominoperineal team in the field was highlighted when a group of visiting surgical dignitaries joined them in theatre after a too leisurely breakfast to witness them finalising closure of the wounds.

Willoughby was an expert endocrine surgeon. Like many other surgeons in Northern Ireland, he contributed enormously to the care of victims of 'the

Troubles'. He was the consultant surgeon on duty during three of the province's most horrific terrorist bomb blasts — The Red Lion, the Electricity Board in 1971 and The Abercorn in 1972. He was awarded the OBE in the New Year Honours in 1983. One of the most moving letters of thanks he had ever received was written on a plain piece of paper: 'Thank you for saving my life,' it read and was signed, 'A Terrorist'.

Willoughby was a superb communicator, who took a real interest in teaching and training undergraduates and postgraduates. He was a role model to which they might aspire and a charismatic figure within the hospital, much loved by his patients and widely regarded as a 'surgeons' surgeon'. In addition, he was amusing, convivial company.

Elegant, of medium build, immaculately turned out, with film-star appearance, a look-alike of the handsome, dashing cricketer Denis Compton, he had great energy and gave his all to the hospital he loved.

His interest in sport never waned. He was an enthusiastic supporter of the Irish fifteen both at home and abroad and enjoyed golf, gardening and horse riding.

WOODSIDE, Cecil John Alexander ('Cocky')

b. 1895
d. 1955

MB, Belf, 1917; FRCSI, QUB, 1925

Captain, Royal Army Medical Corps, First World War.
Assistant to Professor of Surgery, QUB.
Surgeon, RVH, Belfast, 1933–42.
Visiting surgeon, Craigavon Hospital Belfast to 1955.
Consultant surgeon, Admiralty Northern Ireland.
President, Northern Ireland Branch BMA.

'Cocky' Woodside's main interest was urology.

Belfast City Hospital

BELL, David Millar

Consultant Surgeon

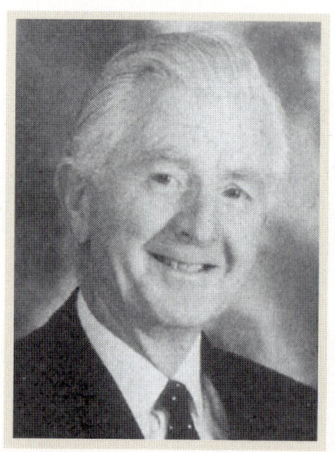

b. 1920, Cookstown, Co. Tyrone, elder son of W. G. Thompson Bell and Emma J. Bell
Educ. Rainey Endowed School, Magherafelt, Co. Tyrone; Queen's University Belfast
m. 1956: Sheila Margaret Wilson (FFARCS), daughter of Cecil and Madge Wilson; 1 s, 3 d
d. 2007

MB, QUB, 1945; FRCS Ed, 1948; FRCS Eng, 1950; FRCSI (*ad eundem*), MSc (Surgery), University of Illinois, 1957

Postgraduate junior appointments at RVH, Royal Belfast Hospital for Sick Children; Research and Educational Hospitals, Chicago, Illinois, USA.

Consultant surgeon, Belfast City Hospital, 1958–86; Musgrave Park Hospital, 1960–85. President, Ulster Medical Society; Ulster Surgical Club; Moynihan Surgical Club.

A really general surgeon with a particular interest in mouth and neck surgery, David Millar Bell did much thyroid surgery and virtually all the parathyroid surgery for Professor Mollie McGeown (1923–2004), Northern Ireland's leading nephrologist.

Bell worked in Chicago and did research under the legendary Dr Warren Cole. He produced durable papers on the importance of giving chemotherapy for liver metastases on the operating table and the superiority of half-strength normal saline to normal saline in postoperative fluid requirements. He presented papers on his work to the American College of Surgeons in San Francisco. In Chicago, the academic and teaching ward round was on Saturday morning and the research progress reports were given on Saturday afternoon. The 120-hour trainee's week was the norm. Dr Cole spoke of going to a 'ball game some Saturday' but it never actually happened.

Bell thoroughly enjoyed his time in surgery. He particularly enjoyed his travels with the various surgical clubs. He played first fifteen rugby at school, then enjoyed tennis, badminton and hunting with the North Down Hunt.

CURRY, Rodney Campbell

Belfast Surgeon

Educ. Cambridge

MB, BChir, Camb, 1952; FRCS Eng, 1961

Consultant surgeon, Belfast City Hospital.

The RCSI presented Rodney Curry with the seldom-bestowed College Medal in recognition of his service as a valued examiner at graduate level. The College has many, many examiners but Rodney's contribution was exceptional. He is also remembered as a gracious and generous host at his home.

EKIN, William Hugh

Belfast Surgeon

Educ. Cambridge

BA (Natural Sciences Tripos), Camb, 1931; MA, MB, BChir, 1937; FRCS Ed, 1947; LMSSA, Lond, 1933; DPH, Belf, 1939 (Cambridge & Westminster)

Postgraduate junior appointments as house surgeon and casualty officer, Westminster Hospital London.
Assistant medical officer, Route District Hospital, Ballymoney.
Consultant surgeon, Belfast City Hospital

HANNA, William Alexander (Will)

Consultant Surgeon

b. 1927, in Broach, near Bombay, India, elder son of William Hanna and Margaret Hanna (*née* Blair)
Educ. Campbell College, Belfast; Edinburgh University
m. 1954: Dr Patricia R. Hunter (TCD; a fourth-generation doctor), daughter of Dr Joseph and Winifred Hunter; 1 s, 2 d (Dr Winifred Hanna is a fifth-generation doctor)

MB, Edin, 1950; FRCS Ed, 1958

Postgraduate junior appointments as house surgeon, Downe Hospital, Downpatrick; Whittington Hospital, London (with Will Davey). Demonstrator in anatomy and physiology, Edinburgh University, 1951–52.
Medical officer, Irish Presbyterian Mission Hospitals, Gujarat State, India, 1953–61. Senior registrar, Banbridge Hospital, Banbridge, 1961–62; Department of Surgery, QUB/Belfast City Hospital, 1963–65.
Consultant surgeon, Belfast City Hospital, 1965–92.

A former registrar writes: 'Will Hanna was one of the first specialist colorectal surgeons in Northern Ireland. Long before any specialty associations existed, he and his colleague George Parks [q.v.] developed their practice in the City Hospital, and trainees queued up to work there. Being Will's registrar provided a number of challenges, not the least of which was interpretation, as neither he nor George ever completed a sentence. After a five-minute conversation between the two of them, one knew that something was going to happen to somebody on Wednesday, and some detective work was then required to work out exactly what was going on. Will was an enthusiastic and patient trainer. There were no cross words in theatre. If things were difficult, he would say, "Oh deary me!" and you knew that things had really taken a turn for the worse if he exclaimed, "Oh deary, dear, deary me!" He was always kind and considerate to the patients, and his practice and his enthusiasm for the subject are the reason why many of us have followed his footsteps into colorectal surgery.'

MEGAW, John McIlroy

Belfast Surgeon

Educ. Queen's University Belfast
d. 1972

MB, QUB, 1938; FRCS Ed, 1948

Major, Royal Army Medical Corps (surgical specialist).
Resident surgical officer, Walton Hospital Liverpool; Mill Road Infirmary, Liverpool.
Consultant urological surgeon, Belfast City Hospital; Musgrave Park Hospital, Belfast.

Ulster Hospital

LOGAN, Hume Charles James (Hume)

Consultant General Surgeon

b. 1931, Lisburn, Co. Antrim, only son of Isaac Logan and Margaretta Logan (*née* Charles)
Educ. Campbell College, Belfast; Queen's University Belfast
m. 1958: Eileen E. Wallace, daughter of Samuel and Anna Wallace; 1 d

MB, QUB, 1955; MCh (hons), 1966; FRCS Eng, 1960; FRCS Ed, 1960; FRCSI (*ad eundem*), 1976

Postgraduate junior appointments included rotating senior house surgeon and registrar posts in Northern Ireland, 1957–61 and again 1963–65; registrar, Leicester Royal Infirmary 1961–62. During his two-year spell as a senior registrar at Leicester Royal Infirmary he

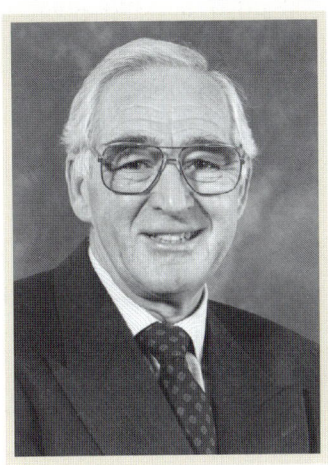

became close to his chief, J. C. (Claude) Barrett, VC, who left him some family heirlooms in his will.
Fellow, Lahey Clinic, Boston, Massachusetts, USA, 1962–63.
Research Fellow, RVH, Belfast, 1965–66.
Surgeon, Ulster Hospital, 1968–96.
President, Ulster Medical Society 1991–92.
Fellow, British Medical Association; honoured to be asked to give the inaugural Ulster Hospital Lecture and the Gary Love Memorial Lecture.

Hume Logan is a man who looked after his patients and always did his best for them. His insights into a surgeon's career are interesting: 'When you're young and learning the trade of surgery, operating seems the most important part of the job. Later, things change.' The part Hume enjoyed most was the follow-up clinic, as he felt it was there that he saw in what way, if any, he had helped his patients.

A man of beliefs and convictions, he has a tremendous loyalty to the Ulster Hospital, about which he has written an affectionate and interesting book, *The Ulster at Dundonald*. He has also taken a serious professional interest in medical representative affairs, an activity that is not particularly popular with surgeons, many of whom disdain 'medical politics' until a government or an agency threatens to alter their lives by 'stroke of the pen' legislation; it is then that they turn to experienced respected representatives like Hume.

His recreations include woodturning, golf and old car restoration. He is also interested in local and Irish history.

McCALISTER, Alexander, TD, Order St John (Alex)

Belfast Surgeon

b. 1925, Belfast
Educ. Ballymena Academy, Co. Antrim; Queen's University Belfast
m. 1st in 1956: Dr Claire Johnston (d. 1985), daughter of James and Annie Isabella Johnston; 2 s (Peter, MB, Edin, is GP in Scotland), 2 d. 2nd in 1989: Heather Hector *née* Deans, daughter of T. J. Deans and Nora McBride

MB (first class hons), QUB, 1948, with Marion Sims Medal and McGrath Scholarship; MCh, QUB, 1962; FRCSI, 1953; FRCS Eng, 1954

Postgraduate training included senior surgical registrar Northern Ireland training circuit, mainly RVH. Visiting Fellow, Lahey Clinic, Boston, Massachusetts.

Consultant surgeon, Lurgan and Portadown Hospital, Co. Armagh, 1960–68; Ulster Hospital, 1968–89.

Honorary surgeon to the Queen, 1979–81.

Royal Army Medical Corps, Territorial Army Reserve, 1953–81. Promoted Colonel. Honorary consultant in surgery to the Army, 1983–90.

Alex McCalister's family background was 'modest'. His father was Royal Irish Constabulary and then RAF during the Second World War. His mother left school at the age of 12, on the death of her father. The local church minister thought that Alex would make a good carpenter (true), but his father found the fees for the local grammar school where he was advised to become a doctor by a great headmaster, W. A. Bell MA. Continuous scholarships put him through. He was greatly influenced by Sir Ian Fraser [q.v.].

Average build, unassuming, with a very private personality. His two main interests were and are his work and his family. He had a great interest in the clinical teaching of undergraduates and postgraduates. His secretary, to whom he dictated his outpatient letters, told a colleague, 'The more difficult the patient was, the nicer he was to them.' Secretaries really know.

SHAW, Joseph (Terry)

Belfast Consultant

b. 1931, son of Joseph Shaw and Jessie Shaw (*née* Morrison)
Educ. Uppingham School, Rutland (whose great musical traditions Terry upheld); Magdalene College, Cambridge; St Bartholomew's Hospital, London
m. 1964: Patricia Lee, daughter of James and Gladys Lee; 1 s, 2 d
d. 2006

MB, BChir, Camb, 1956; FRCS Ed, 1965; FRCSI, 1983

Postgraduate training at St Bartholomew's Hospital, Norfolk and Norwich Hospital.
Consultant in charge, A&E Department, Ulster Hospital, 1972–96.
Royal Navy, Surgeon Lieutenant, 1958–61. Honorary surgeon to the Queen. Royal Naval Reserve 1961–91. Retired with rank of Principal Medical Officer, RNR.
Commander of the Order of St John, Hospitaller of the Order, Commander of Ards.

Terry Shaw was a man of wide interests, including classical piano, cooking, reading, travelling and swimming. He had been greatly in demand as a scrupulously fair and disarming examiner who put candidates at their ease while gently probing lacunae in their requirements. Large, rubicund, smiling or about to smile, he was most hospitable to all. Gregarious, gossipy in the best sense, he was somebody one would wish to have in one's lifeboat. Everybody liked Terry.

MATER INFIRMORUM HOSPITAL

GILLIGAN, Conor

Belfast Surgeon

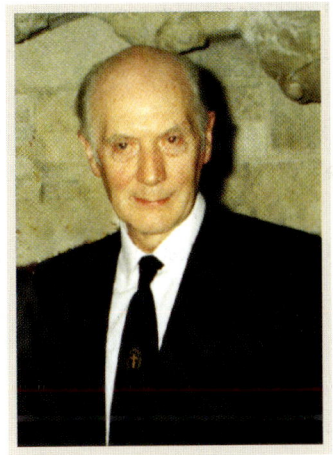

b. 1922, son of John S. Gilligan and Mary Gilligan (*née* Clarke)
Educ. St Malachy's College. Queen's University Belfast
m. 1955: Patricia Kennedy; 4 s, 2 d

MB, QUB, 1945; FRCSI 1949

Postgraduate training posts at Mater Infirmorum Hospital, Belfast; St Peter & Paul's Hospitals, and Hammersmith Postgraduate Hospital, London. Surgical registrar, Crumpsall Hospital, Manchester, 1951–52.
Assistant General Surgeon, Mater, 1952–57; Surgeon and then Senior Surgeon, 1957–87 Mater Infirmorum. Member, Faculty of Medicine, QUB, 1963–87; Clinical lecturer and examiner in surgery, QUB, 1963–87.

Member, Ulster Surgical Club, 1963–87.
Examiner in FRCSI at RCSI, 1982–87.

A very private, charitable man who was a pillar of his beloved Mater Hospital, Conor Gilligan worked long hours without any ostentation or fuss. He treated many victims of 'the Troubles' in the 1970s and 1980s, with skill and dedication. He was renowned for his commitment to bedside teaching. For decades, he was the 'Spirit of the Mater'. His pastimes include travel, history and walking.

LAVERY, Maurice Basil

Belfast Surgeon

b. 1901, Cusack Street, Belfast, second son of Daniel and Agnes Lavery (*née* Mann)
Educ. Christian Brothers School, Oxford Street, Belfast; Queen's University Belfast
m. Deborah Lee; no children
d. 1961

BSc, QUB, 1922; MB, QUB, 1925; FRCS Ed, 1931; FRCS, 1931

Postgraduate training included demonstrator in anatomy, QUB; house surgeon, St Bartholomew's Hospital, London; surgical registrar, Sheffield Royal Hospital; senior registrar, Queen's Hospital, Birmingham, 1929–32.
Surgeon, Mater Infirmorum, 1932–61; City Hospital, Belfast
Lecturer in operating surgery, QUB.

Maurice Lavery went to Queen's University Belfast, to study science but after two years he changed to medicine and finished his science degree with honours at the same time. His main interest was abdominal surgery, and he served his hospital loyally, working until a week before his death.

Shy, reserved but a really good teacher, he had a great sense of humour and shrewd judgment. He was a keen angler.

McGARRY, Philip Patrick (Phil)

Belfast Surgeon

b. 1923, Belfast
Educ. Christian Brothers School, Oxford Street, Belfast; St Malachy's, Belfast; Queen's University Belfast
d. 1991

MB, QUB, 1946; FRCSI (*ad eundem*), 1978; FRCS Eng, 1951.

Resident surgical officer, Mater Infirmorum, 1946–50.
Registrar, Royal Postgraduate Hospital, Hammersmith, London, 1950–52.
Surgeon, Mater Infirmorum, 1952–89.

Phil McGarry died in 1991 following a short illness.

MOORE, James Bernard (Barney or Brian)

Belfast Surgeon

b. 1867, Ballymena, Co. Antrim, son of a solicitor
Educ. St Malachy's College, Belfast; Queen's College, Cork; St Mungo's, Glasgow
m. Eileen McFadden of Co. Donegal. 9 children (Their distinguished novelist son, Brian Moore, 1921–99, was described by Graham Greene as 'my favourite living novelist'; Seán became Professor of Pathology at McGill University, Montreal, Canada; Seamus was a Belfast GP)
d. 1942

MB (hons), RUI (QCC), 1890; FRCSI, 1909

Surgeon, Mater Infirmorum Hospital, Belfast.
Clinical lecturer and examiner in surgery, QUB; examiner in surgery, RCP and SI.

Barney Moore's undergraduate degree was from Cork because Bishop Denvir and Bishop Tohill of Down and Conor Diocese both objected to Catholic students attending Queen's College, Belfast, a mainly Presbyterian institution. On graduation from Cork, he went to St Mungo's in Glasgow, where he studied pathology and, as at Cork, took first prize in the subject. He started in general practice but was appointed Assistant Surgeon of the Mater in 1896 and received a full staff appointment in 1900. He was Honorary Secretary to the Medical Staff Committee, 1902–20, and Chairman 1920–26, when he retired. He served as Secretary to the Surgical Division of the BMA at their annual meeting in Belfast in 1909.

An active nationalist and rigid Catholic, he talked little about himself but consistently finished the *Times* crossword before lunch. As a consultant surgeon to the British Army in the First World War, he had an armed escort to and from Victoria Barracks Hospital Wing. In the troubled 1920s, a sniper in the area meant that night visits to the Mater were a bit of a gamble. The sniper developed appendicitis and was taken to the Mater, where, despite his colourful prognostications of impending doom 'at the hands of expletive Fenians', he was operated on by Moore, and, on returning to his post, he ceased firing on him.

MORIARTY, James Joseph

Belfast Surgeon

b. 1891, Rathdrum, Co. Wicklow, son of a schoolmaster
Educ. St Mary's College, Rathmines; Blackrock College, Dublin; University College, Dublin
m. Nora Diamond; 1 s (Michael, a High Court Judge in Dublin); 1 d
d. 1975

MB, UCD, 1915

Postgraduate work as house surgeon and registrar, St Vincent's Hospital, Dublin. Bellingham Gold medal for clinical work.
Royal Army Medical Corps and served in India after First World War.
Visiting medical staff, Mater Infirmorum to 1956.

Following his service with the Royal Army Medical Corps, James Moriarty stayed on in India as doctor to the local tea-planters, returning every few years for postgraduate studies in tropical medicine in Dublin and London. He finally left India to commence general medical practice in Belfast. He had a special interest in the treatment of varicose veins. He retired to Dublin.

O'CONNELL, Sir Peter Reilly

Belfast Surgeon

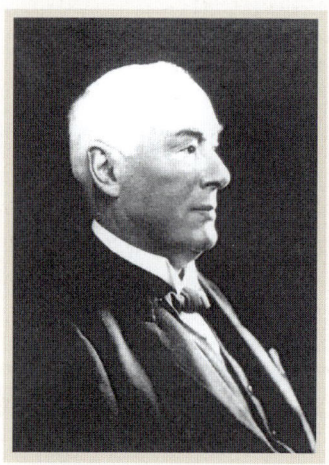

b. 1861, Maudabawn, Co. Cavan, son of Patrick O'Connell and Annie O'Connell (*née* O'Reilly)
Educ. St Patrick's College, Cavan; Queen's College, Galway
m. 1907: Jane Mary Hughes (granddaughter of the famous master baker, Bernard Hughes)
d. 1927

MD, QCG, RUI; MCh, 1885 (Catholic University, Dublin, and QCG); LM, Coombe Hospital, Dublin

In 1885, aged 24, he was appointed senior visiting surgeon to the Mater Infirmorum and remained on the staff until 1919.
Lecturer and examiner in clinical surgery, QUB.
President, Ulster Medical Society, 1910–11.
JP, Co. Antrim. Deputy Lieutenant, Belfast. High Sheriff, Belfast 1907–08.

Sir Peter became involved in politics and was the first Roman Catholic to become High Sheriff of Belfast. He was appointed to the Senate of Queen's University until his retirement. He was awarded Knight Bachelor (KB) for exceptional public service. He retired to Stillorgan, Co. Dublin, in 1919, and lived there until his death in 1927, but was buried in Milltown Cemetery, Falls Road, Belfast. After his death, Lady Jane O'Connell gave £1,000,000, to the Mater Infirmorum for a hospital bed to be named in his memory. She gave a further gift of £3,000,000 for an annual gold medal for the most outstanding Mater Hospital medical student. The hospital subsequently augmented this massive donation (£75 million in present-day terms) to provide a bursary for the winner.

O'DOHERTY, John

Belfast Surgeon

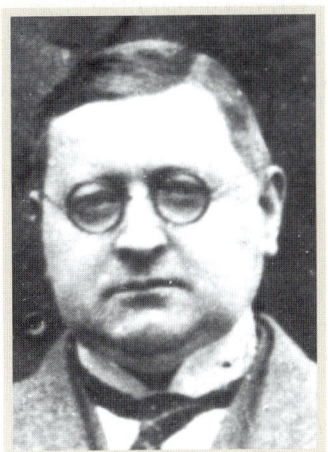

b. 1879, Magilligan, Co. Derry
Educ. St Columb's College, Derry; Catholic University School of Medicine (Cecilia Street), Dublin
m. Bridget; their daughter, Muriel, studied medicine and in later years specialised in psychiatry in England
d. 1953

LRCPI & LM, LRCSI & LM (Rotunda), Catholic University, Dublin, 1902; FRCS Ed, 1910.

Postgraduate training included house surgeon, Mater Infirmorum, 1903; assistant surgeon, 1904.
Surgeon, Mater Infirmorum Hospital.
Clinical lecturer and examiner in surgery, QUB.

Thirty years on the surgical staff of the Mater, John O'Doherty was one of the last of the truly general surgeons 'who was prepared and willing to remove the thyroid, or any expendable part from that to the uterus, and he was equally at home with the bougie or the curette'. He was a lively teacher. Some of his axioms were questionable but memorable, such as, 'What you can tie, you can cut.'

He was described as 'small, rotund, with as many waistcoats as an onion, [peering] at the world through enormous spectacles'. He published treatises on surgery. During the First World War, he was Auxiliary Surgeon at Victoria Military Barracks Medical Wing (Clifton Street, Belfast) along with his Mater Infirmorum Hospital colleague, Surgeon Brian Moore [q.v.]. They treated war casualties from the battlefields in Europe. He was interested in the clinical use of X-ray equipment. He and his wife, Bridget, contributed 50 per cent of the cost of purchasing the first X-ray operated at the Mater Infirmorum Hospital. He was a member of the British Medical Association and the Ulster Medical Society. He was a generous spirit with a great curiosity in everyone and everything.

SAVAGE, John Patrick

Belfast Surgeon

b. 1915, Downpatrick, Co. Down
Educ. De La Salle Primary School, Downpatrick; St Colman's, Violet Hill, Newry, Co. Down; Queen's University Belfast
m. Unmarried
d. 1963

MB, QUB, 1938; FRCSI, 1945

Postgraduate training as house surgeon and senior registrar, Mater Hospital.
Consultant surgeon, Mater Hospital, 1946–63. In the interim three years, he worked at Northampton General Hospital.

WRIGHT, Peter Paul

Belfast Surgeon

b. 1892, Murroe, Co. Limerick, son of a member of the Royal Irish Constabulary, who was stationed there. Parents moved to Portadown while he was an infant.
Educ. Marist College, Dundalk; Queen's University Belfast
m. Annie Brady; 1 s (Brendan, GP and Senior Community Medicine doctor for Northern Ireland)
d. 1952

MB, QUB, 1914; MD, QUB, 1919; Diploma in Public Health, Liverpool, 1919; FRCS Ed, 1921.

Worked at Mill Road Infirmary, Liverpool.
Royal Army Medical Corps, 1915–17; served at Salonika and Gallipoli.
Visiting surgeon, Mater Infirmorum, 1921–52
Clinical lecturer and examiner in surgery, QUB.

Peter Paul Wright worked at the Mater Infirmorum until his death. He had Polycythaemia Vera and a terminal sudden unexpected haemorrhage ended his life. His wife, Annie, died a few years before him.

7
SURGEONS IN NORTHERN IRELAND BY COUNTY (EXCEPTING BELFAST)

SURGEONS IN NORTHERN IRELAND BY COUNTY (EXCEPTING BELFAST)

ANTRIM

BALLYMENA (POP. 28,112)

HANNA, William Swanston (Bill)

Ballymena Surgeon

b. 1916, Belfast, son of David Hanna and Elizabeth Alison Hanna (*née* Swanston)
Educ. Royal Belfast Academical Institution; Merchiston Castle School, Edinburgh; Queen's University Belfast
m. 1951: Margaret Seale, daughter of Theophilus and Roberta Seale, Co. Kilkenny; 1 s, 2 d (one died in 1964).
d. 1988

MB (hons), QUB, 1942; FRCS Ed, 1948; FRCSI (*ad eundem*), 1979.

Postgraduate training as house officer, RVH, Belfast, 1942.
Surgeon Lieutenant-Commander, Royal Navy Volunteer Reserve: HMS *Tyrian* (Destroyer) (1,802 tons), March 1943–Dec 1944, visited Brindisi, Bari, Malta, Taranto, Palermo and Cairo. HMS *Empire Macrae* (Merchant Aircraft Carrier), Atlantic Convoys (8,250 tons) Jan–July 1945. HMS *Perseus* (Aircraft Carrier), Sept 1945–May 1946 to Sydney.
Registrar, RVH and Belfast City Hospital, 1946–50.
Surgeon, Mid-Antrim Hospital Group, Waveney Hospital, Ballymena, 1951–81.
Founder member, Northern Area Postgraduate Medical Centre, Waveney Hospital. Member, Faculty of Medicine, examiner and clinical teacher, QUB, 1973.
Distinction Award, 1969 onwards.
Founder chairman and later president, local Cancer Research campaign, 1956.
Founder member, Royal Naval Association Mid-Antrim.

Bill Hanna's three years in the Royal Navy were an important part of his life. At the Waveney Hospital, he initially worked single-handed, on call 24 hours a day and seven days a week, taking his entitled holidays only when a locum could be found.

He was a great raconteur and many have happy memories of hilarious encounters with him. He told many stories against himself, the touchstone of a true humorist. With Ronnie Loane [q.v.] of the South Tyrone Hospital, Dungannon, he was one of the founders of the Ulster Surgical Club. A Memorial Lecture to them both is given annually at the October meeting.

He was Captain and President of Castlerock Golf Club, Co. Derry and President of Ballymena RFC 1967–83, a period which saw its growth from modest beginnings to one of the major forces in Irish rugby.

Men like Bill Hanna should have been the subject of a vast Grade One Preservation order. He passed away prematurely at the age of 71, and the world around him was so much poorer for his departure.

STINSON, Robert (Roy)

Consultant Surgeon

Educ. Queen's University Belfast

MB, QUB, 1947; FRCS Ed, 1962

Postgraduate training as senior registrar, South Down Hospital Group; senior registrar and house surgeon, RVH, Belfast.
Consultant surgeon, Antrim and Ballymena District Group.

BALLYMONEY (POP. 7,818)

MARTIN, William

Ballymoney Surgeon

Educ. Queen's University Belfast

MB, QUB, 1933; FRCS Ed, 1937.

ROBB, John

Belfast and Ballymoney Surgeon

b. 1932, Downpatrick, Co. Down, elder son of John C. (Jack) Robb [q.v.] and Jessie B. Robb (*née* Wilson)

Educ. Murchison Castle School, Edinburgh (1945–50); Queen's University Belfast

m. Sylvia Sloan, daughter of William Sloan (FRCS, FRCOG), and Alexandra Shaw (MB), both of whom worked in Manchuria; 2 d, 2 s (John Daniel, MB, Newcastle-upon-Tyne, training in cardiothoracic surgery, London. William Bryson MB TCD, training in general surgery, Dublin)

MB, QUB, 1957; FRCS Eng, 1961; FRCSI (*ad eundem*); LLD, TCD, 1985; Diploma in Irish, University of Ulster (Coleraine), 2002

Postgraduate training included senior house officer, Professorial Unit, RVH, Belfast, 1958; senior house officer, Down Hospital, Downpatrick, 1959; registrar, General and Vascular Unit, RVH, 1961–62; Mid-Ulster Hospital, 1962–63; registrar, plastic surgery 1962–63. Lecturer in surgery, QUB, 1964–66. Sent by Northern Ireland Hospital Authority to study medical undergraduate teaching and postgraduate surgical training in USA and Canada, 1964–65. Surgical officer, Trauma Unit, King Edward VIII Hospital, Durban, 1966; Orthopaedic & Trauma Unit, Baragwanath Hospital, Soweto, Johannesburg, South Africa, 1967.
Senior registrar, Nuffield Unit, Musgrave Park Hospital, Belfast, 1968; Royal Hospital for Sick Children, Belfast, 1968.
Consultant/lecturer, RVH and QUB, 1968–73 (upgraded to senior lecturer).
Consultant surgeon, Route Hospital, Ballymoney 1973–92.
William Doolin Medal, Irish Medical Organisation, 1988.
Council, New University of Ulster, 1973–76; RTÉ Authority, 1973–74.
Senator, Seanad Éireann, 1982–89; QUB, 1992–2002; Founder and Chairperson, New Ireland Group, 1981–98, which was dedicated to conciliation of the warring factors on the island of Ireland.

John Robb is a sincere and totally genuine idealist who has made substantial sacrifices for his beliefs. He became fluent in the Irish language as part of his commitment to his role in the New Ireland Group.

Tall, handsome, groomed, articulate, warm and genial, he makes a wonderful first impression and continues to have the priceless quality of being instantly likable. 'Patience is the rarest of political qualities,' said HH Asquith, Prime Minister 1908–16.

Larne (pop. 17,575)

WILSON, H.

Larne Surgeon

Educ. Queen's University Belfast

MB, QUB, 1927; FRCS Ed, 1934

Postgraduate training as house surgeon and resident medical officer, Royal Hospital, Wolverhampton; house surgeon, West London Hospital.
Senior surgeon, Moyle Hospital, Larne and Smiley Hospital, Larne.
Consultant in surgery, East Antrim Hospital Management Committee.

ZAHEER, Syed Asgher

Consultant Surgeon

Educ. University of Allahabad; University of Lucknow

BSc, Allahabad, 1949; MB, Lucknow, 1954; FRCS Ed, 1961; FRCS Eng, 1962

Surgical registrar, South East Kent Group Hospitals, Wrightington Hospital Manchester.
Consultant surgeon, Merthyr and Aberdare Group Hospitals.
Consultant surgeon, Moyle Hospital, Larne; East Antrim Group Hospitals.

Syed Zaheer resigned from his post at the Moyle Hospital to work in the Middle East.

Lisburn (pop. 42,110)

GREIG, George William Vause (Bill)

General Surgeon

b. 1914

Educ. University of Leeds

MB (hons), Leeds, 1937; MRCS Eng, LRCP, Lond, 1937 (Leeds); FRCS Eng, 1949

Postgraduate training included senior surgical registrar, United Leeds Hospitals.
Lieutenant-Colonel, Royal Army Medical Corps.
Consultant surgeon, Daisy Hill Hospital Newry; Lagan Valley Hospital, Lisburn.

Bill Greig was a general surgeon with an interest in urology. When in Daisy Hill, he treated patients from South Down, including the coastal town of Kilkeel from which he had operated on so many patients with chronic peptic ulceration that one group of houses was known among the locals as 'Gastrectomy Row'.

Bill (also known as Vause) was a quintessential Englishman and when he came to Daisy Hill Hospital there was much speculation about how he would get on in an institution which was a combined local council hospital and workhouse. The locals held him in awe. His physical appearance was that of an austere and superior human being but he was invariably polite and well mannered to everyone. It was important to call him 'Mister' rather than 'Doctor', and the many in Newry who were not aware of the distinction were brought to heel. The distinction survived his demise and hospital staff got into the habit of addressing any mature doctor as 'Mister'. He had no waiting list for appointments and the clinic did not finish until all patients were seen. His notes were a model of concision.

At the end of the day, he would get into his distinctive Jaguar and, on his way home to Rostrevor, he would stop at Warrenpoint (the Crown Hotel Lounge Bar) for refuelling (gin and tonic), a cigarette and the *Times*, and woe betide any peasant who dared to interrupt him. He was a heavy smoker and when a huge mass was found on a chest X-ray, the worst was assumed. However, Bill refused intervention and went fishing in his caravan. He had the last laugh as the lesion was benign and disappeared.

YOUNG, George Ivan

Lisburn Surgeon

Educ. Queen's University Belfast

MB, QUB, 1949; FRCS Ed, 1956; FRCS Eng, 1956.

Postgraduate post as senior registrar, RVH, Belfast.
Surgical Fellow, Lahey Clinic, Boston, Massachusetts.
Consultant surgeon, Lagan Valley Hospital, Lisburn.

DICKSON, Ronald Ritchie

Lisburn Surgeon

b. 1917
Educ. Methodist College; Queen's University Belfast
d. 1962

MB, QUB, 1941; FRCS, 1949

Postgraduate work: St Helen's Hospital; RAF (posted to Rhodesia); surgical registrar, Belfast City Hospital, RVH, Lagan Valley and Banbridge Hospitals.
Consultant surgeon, Lagan Valley Hospital, 1954–62.

Calm, quiet and perceptive, Ronald Dickson was an extremely dextrous surgeon, devoted to his hospital where he spent much time planning a new surgical block. His recreations were sailing, carpentry and photography.

Newtownabbey (pop. 56,811)

LAIRD, Robert Marshall

Consultant Surgeon

Educ. Queen's University Belfast

MB (hons), QUB, 1942; FRCS Eng, 1951

Post graduation served as Flight Lieutenant, Royal Air Force Volunteer Reserve.
Demonstrator in physiology, QUB.
Surgical registrar, Preston Royal Infirmary.
Senior consultant surgeon, East Antrim Hospital Group.

KEMP, Richard Ernest (Ernie)

Surgeon

b. 1927, Bangor, Co. Down, elder son of Herbert W. Kemp and Theresa Kemp (*née* Stewart)
Educ. Bangor Grammar School, Queen's University Belfast
m. 1955: Pearl Gaston, daughter of Joseph and Margaret Gaston; 1 s, 1 d

MB, QUB, 1954; FRCS Eng, 1958

Served in Royal Navy, 1946–48.
Surgeon, Newtownabbey Hospital Group 1964–92.

Armagh

Armagh City (pop. 14,265)

DEAN, H. C. C.

Surgeon

b. 1898
Educ. Trinity College, Dublin

BA, Dub, MD, 1924; MB, 1921; DPH, 1922; FRCSI, 1924, LM (Rot), TCD

Postgraduate positions as resident medical officer, Royal Hospital for Incurables, Dublin; clinical surgical assistant and resident medical officer, Royal City Dublin Hospital.
Medical officer, Depot Royal Ulster Rifles.
Surgeon, Armagh City Hospital.
Medical officer, Armagh Royal School; Macan Asylum for the Blind; HM Prison and Post Office, Armagh.

BALMER, John Herbert (Jack)

Consultant Surgeon

LRCPI & SI & LM, 1939, RCSI; FRCS Ed, 1948; FRCSI (*ad eundem*), 1970

Postgraduate positions as house surgeon, Jervis Street Hospital, Dublin; principal registrar, RVH, Belfast.
Major, Royal Army Medical Corps.
Consultant surgeon, Armagh City Hospital; Craigavon Area hospitals.

Craigavon (includes Craigavon, Lurgan and Portadown)

GRAHAM, William John Hill (Billy)

Consultant Surgeon

b. 1928, older son of William John Graham and Charlotte Ewart Graham (*née* Hill)
Educ. Methodist College, Belfast. Queen's University Belfast
m. 1958: Florence Joyce Lindsay (d. April 2006)

MB, QUB, 1953; DObst, RCOG, FRCS Ed, 1961; FRCS Eng, 1962; FRCSI, 1981

Consultant surgeon, Craigavon Area Hospitals; North Armagh Hospital, Banbridge; Dromore Hospital Group.

Billy Graham was consultant surgeon in Banbridge Hospital and then in the new Craigavon Hospital. He was a general surgeon who later developed an abiding interest in urology and led the development of a urology unit in the Craigavon Area Hospital.

Grey-haired, moustachioed and never without his glasses, slung around his neck with a piece of nylon fishing line, he enjoyed fishing, shooting and sailing, preferably while chatting to surgical friends. He was calm and approachable and, when asked, always willing to offer advice and help. He was receptive of new ideas, supportive of his younger colleagues and perceptive enough to know when 'a word in your ear' was required.

LURGAN AND PORTADOWN (POP. 9,210 AND 21,299)

BASSETT, William Waring

Consultant Surgeon

Educ. Queen's University Belfast

MB (hons), QUB, 1928; FRCSI, 1933

Postgraduate positions as tutor in obstetrics, QUB; senior demonstrator in anatomy, QUB; house surgeon, RVH, Belfast.
Senior consultant surgeon Lurgan & Portadown Hospital.

DOWN

ARDS DISTRICT HOSPITAL

CALDER, Alexander Mackay, OBE

Surgeon

Educ. University of Edinburgh

MB, ChB, Edin, 1928; FRCS Ed, 1930

Surgeon, Ards District Hospital.

BRAIDWOOD, Walter Standish

Consultant Surgeon

b. 1905
Educ. Cambridge University; Queen's University Belfast

BA (mechanical science), Camb, 1926; MB, QUB, 1938; FRCS Ed, 1947

Consultant surgeon, Ards Hospital, North Down.
Major, Royal Army Medical Corps.

Having qualified and practised for a number of years as an engineer, Walter Braidwood studied medicine and trained in surgery. His first consultant post was at the Waveney Hospital, Ballymena. Later he moved to Ards Hospital, North Down, and while continuing as a general surgeon he developed a special interest and expertise in hand surgery. In this field, he put his engineering background to good use and acquired a well-deserved reputation.

MITCHELL, Oswald Henry Anderson

Consultant Surgeon

Educ. Queen's University Belfast

MB, QUB, 1949; FRCS Ed, 1961

Consultant surgeon, North Down Hospital Group.

BANBRIDGE (POP. 11,448)

GALLAGHER, Herbert William (Herbie)

Consultant Surgeon, North Down

b. 1917, Portadown, son of Rev. R. H. Gallagher BA (sometime President, Methodist Church in Ireland) and Helen McIlroy Gallagher
Educ. Methodist College, Belfast; Queen's University Belfast
m. 1944: Sister Dorothy Joyce Townsend (Territorial Army Nursing Service, in Madras, India; d. 1997; 1 s, 1 d

MB, QUB, 1939; FRCS Ed, 1946; FRCSI (*ad eundem*), 1977

Post graduation: Royal Army Medical Corps, 1940–45; Regimental Medical Officer for 15 months. Graded (trainee) surgeon with service in England, Egypt and India.
Registrar, City Hospital Belfast, 1946.
Consultant surgeon, Banbridge Hospital, 1946–64.
Consultant surgeon, North Down Hospitals Group, 1964–77.
President, Ulster Medical Society, 1977; honorary secretary, Ulster Surgical Club.

Formerly involved in sailing and walking, Herbie Gallagher now enjoys historical research. He is interested in the Brontë connection and lives of Ulster doctors. He is active in a wide range of community services, travels with his family and, at 89, loyally reads his BMJ. His wife taught him prize-winning embroidery and he remains the only male member of the Northern Ireland Embroidery Guild.

DOWNPATRICK (POP. 10,113)

TATE, Thomas Marshall

Surgeon, County Infirmary, Downpatrick

b. 1866

Educ. Trinity College, Dublin

BA, Dub, MD, TCD, 1890; Diploma in State Medicine, 1889; LM, Rotunda Hospital, Dublin

Surgeon, County Infirmary, Downpatrick, Co. Down, 1889.

ROBB, John C., OBE (Jack)

Consultant Surgeon, Downe Hospital

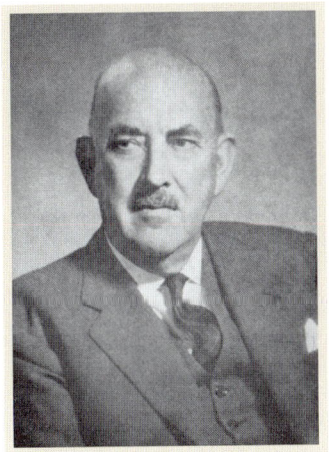

b. 1882, Dundonald, Co. Antrim, son of Alexander Robb, 1839–1909, rancher and gold miner in British Columbia, Canada, 1860–80
Educ. Campbell College, Belfast; Queen's University Belfast
m. 1928: Jessie B. Robb, eldest child of Daniel Martin Wilson (Unionist MP for West Down 1918, Solicitor General for Ireland 1918–21, junior member Lloyd George's cabinet, Westminster); 2 s (John [q.v.], is retired surgeon, Ballymoney), 2 d
d. 1968

MB, QUB, 1914; MD, MCh, QUB

Medical Officer, 108th Field Ambulance, 36th 'Ulster Division' in the Battle of the Somme.
Ulster Volunteer Force Hospital (for wounded soldiers), Belfast, 1919–22.
Medical inspector of brothels, Calais, 1919.
Assistant surgeon to Thomas Tate [q.v.] at Downe Hospital, 1922–27.
Surgeon, Downe Hospital, 1927–57
Deputy Lieutenant, Co. Down.

John Robb was captain of three golf clubs, including Royal County Down. A huge lady presented with abdominal pains. Jack thought that he felt something solid, and X-ray showed an artery forceps 8 inches long. She had previously been operated on in a London hospital. The forceps was removed, the patient was told that she had had adhesions, and the cleaned, polished and labelled instrument was returned to the London hospital theatre with a note: 'Found in Mrs X and returned with thanks'.

BOYD, John Stewart, OBE (Johnny)

County Surgeon, Downe Hospital

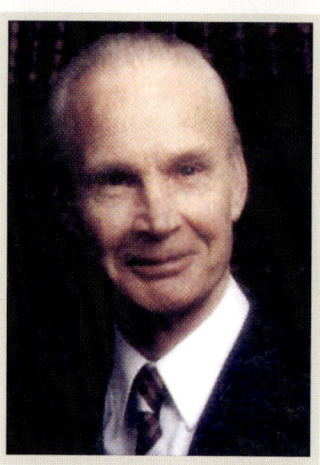

b. 1917
Educ. Queen's University Belfast
m. Kathleen; 2 d
d. 2002

MB, QUB, 1941; FRCS Ed, 1948

Flight Lieutenant Royal Air Force Volunteer Reserve, 1942–46.
618 Special Mosquito Squadron. Orthopaedic registrar, Musgrave Park Hospital, Belfast. Surgical registrar, Tyrone County Hospital, Omagh. County Surgeon, Downe Hospital.

In peacetime, Johnny Boyd co-designed and constructed an ambulance for coronary and trauma patients. He spent more than thirty years in Downpatrick. A lifetime of service compressed into so few words seems unfair.

COLE, Graham Jacob

Consultant Surgeon

b. 1933
Educ. Queen's University Belfast
d. *c.*1975

MB, QUB, 1956; FRCS Ed, 1964; MCh (hons), QUB, 1968
Postgraduate posts as lecturer and senior tutor, QUB; registrar, University Hospital, Ibadan, Nigeria.
Consultant (general surgery) Ards and Downpatrick Hospitals.

Author of a chapter in *Companion to Surgery in Africa*, 1967.

A promising surgical career was unfortunately cut exceptionally short after only a few years at consultant level due to Graham Cole's tragic death while still in his early forties.

Lurgan and Banbridge

ALLEN, Patrick John (Pat)

Consultant Surgeon

b. 1934
Educ. Queen's University Belfast
m. Amy; 1 s (deceased), 3 d
d. 1993

MB, QUB, 1957; FRCS Ed, 1962; FRCS Eng, 1963

Postgraduate positions as house surgeon, RVH, Belfast; senior registrar, St Mark's Hospital, London; research assistant, St Bartholomew's Hospital, London.
Consultant surgeon, Lurgan Hospital and Banbridge Hospital, 1969–72.
Transferred to Craigavon Area Hospital when it opened in September 1972.

Pat Allen emigrated to Chatham (pop. 105,000), in south-west Ontario, Canada, in 1973. He had a special interest in colorectal and subsequently vascular surgery, which was just becoming a serious specialty when he was at his best. He built up a progressive unit in Chatham. Two former anaesthetic colleagues speak highly of him as a pleasant, easy-going, sociable man who was easy to get along with on the crucial anaesthetist/surgeon interface. He was a really fine operator and he never, ever, lost his temper. His new life in Canada began auspiciously with a large family home and garden on the banks of the Canadian Thames. His wife did the gardening and he cooked. His only son died in a tragic accident. Subsequently Pat's life became destabilised and his own premature death was another tragedy.

Newry (pop. 21,633)

NASH, David Tyrie Llewellyn

Newry Surgeon

Educ. Trinity College, Dublin

MB, TCD, 1946; FRCSI, 1951; LMCC, 1956

Postgraduate posts as resident surgical officer, Royal Devon & Exeter Hospital; senior surgical registrar, Belfast Hospital Group.
Surgeon, Daisy Hill Hospital, Newry.

BLUNDELL, James (Jimmy)

Consultant Surgeon

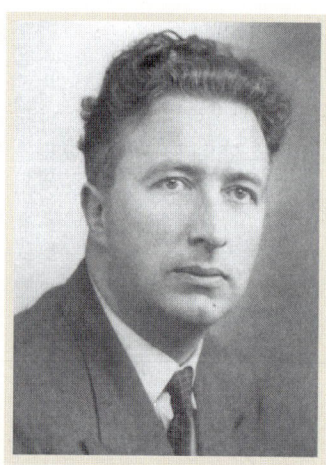

b. 1923, Newry, younger son of John and Jane (*née* Cruikshanks) Blundell
Educ. College of Technology, Belfast; Queen's University Belfast
m. Marie Ann Larkin (SRN at Belfast City Hospital); 3 d (eldest daughter a consultant haematologist), 1 s

MB, QUB, 1949; FRCS Ed, 1956; FRCSI (*ad eundem*), 1977

Postgraduate training in Leicester General Hospital; demonstrator in anatomy, QUB.
Consultant surgeon, Daisy Hill Hospital, Newry.
Captained QUB Cricket Team (fast bowler).

Jimmy Blundell is one of the great characters of Northern Ireland surgery. He left school at the age of 16 and worked as an apprentice at Harland & Wolff shipyard. He attended night classes and left to study medicine when he reached the intermediate part of the BSc in Naval Architecture. He was surgical registrar to Sir Ian Fraser [q.v.], with whom he had great rapport. He was trained at a time when competition for consultant posts was incredibly intense but then the National Health Service advised that every hospital practising acute surgery should have a minimum of two consultant general surgeons. This resulted in six time-expired registrars in Belfast being appointed consultants in Northern Ireland.

One of his favourite organisations was the Ulster Surgical Club, which was founded to encourage the peripheral surgeons to maintain social and academic connections with the centre. Membership was by invitation and only 32 active members are allowed.

Earlier, Jimmy Blundell, like many others, had signed on as a ship's surgeon because cargo ships found it economical to carry a doctor to avoid quarantine regulations and allow ships to enter port quickly for their port medical examination. He was very happy in these posts as they enabled him to see places all over the world and be paid for the privilege.

But he had a serious side and was highly regarded by his colleagues who made him one of the two Northern Ireland representatives on the Central Consultants and Hospital Specialists Committee of the British Medical Association in London. He was most anxious that the Irish Medical Association and the British Medical Association should have a closer liaison, and in 1969 there was a successful three-day meeting in Drogheda. Jimmy and his wife Marie hosted the programme arrangements in their home. Unfortunately the meeting coincided with the outbreak of terrorist activity in Northern Ireland, and further meetings were suspended. However, his gestures of goodwill, as well as his warm generous spirit, are remembered.

Always cheerful, optimistic, outgoing and highly popular, Jimmy Blundell integrated easily as the Master Surgeon in his home town. The world would have been a poorer place without him.

FERMANAGH

ENNISKILLEN (POP. 11,436)

Just four loyal, hardworking surgeons, Leonard Kidd, Horace Flemming, Jack Strahan and Alistair McKibbin, covered the surgical services in Co. Fermanagh in the twentieth century. They were a durable quartet. They had to be.

KIDD, Leonard

Surgeon

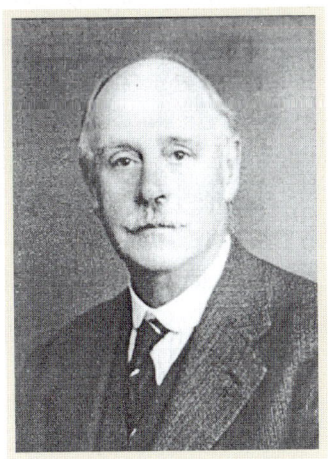

b. 1864

Educ. Trinity College, Dublin; Carmichael College, Dublin; University of Edinburgh

LRCPI & LM, 1887; LRCSI, 1887; BA, MD, 1888 (TCD, Carmichael College, Dublin, and University of Edinburgh)

Medical officer, Portora School.
Direct (elected) representative, General Medical Council, London.
Medical attendant, Royal Irish Constabulary; medical referee for many insurance companies.
President, IMA; Ulster branch, BMA.
Surgeon, Fermanagh County Infirmary, 1897–1937.

Leonard Kidd began in Enniskillen as a General Practitioner. Hospital patients then were few as patients actively avoided going into hospital in the belief that they would never leave it alive. (This belief persisted into the mid-1950s and the editor worked in a London hospital which was referred to locally as 'Feet First'.)

When Kidd arrived at the Fermanagh County Infirmary, gas lamps lighted the hospital and there were zinc basins in the wards. He was a man of immense energy and brought about changes: new wards, electric light (1925), X-rays (1928), central heating (1931), and a children's ward (1935). One of his duties was to be personally responsible for opening the infirmary gates in the morning and closing them at night. There was no state aid and the finance came from voluntary subscriptions, bazaars, hospital balls and legacies. Patients contributed what they could afford (perhaps £1 a week) and were informally assessed on the basis of how many cows they had. Dr Kidd's daughter, Miss Rita Kidd, came to the hospital from school, became the first secretary in 1925, and retired in 1961, having done all the budgeting and secretarial work for 36 years.

On his retirement (1937), Leonard Kidd received the highest commendation for his life's work. The Chairman of the Committee of Management said, 'He was pre-eminently the poor man's doctor. With him the hospital always came first.'

Just thinking about those wearying trips to London for General Medical Council meetings, by train to Belfast, ferry to Stranraer and train to London, makes one appreciate what professional representation meant in those days. Add in the trips to Dublin for the IMA, and side trips to Belfast for the Ulster Branch of the BMA, and you get a picture of a wonderfully dedicated man.

FLEMMING, Horace Townsend

Enniskillen Surgeon

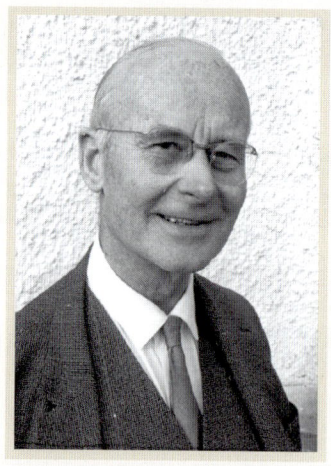

b. 1907, Timoleague, West Cork, son of Rev. Lionel and Mary Flemming
Educ. Manor Preparatory boarding school, Fermoy; Brighton College (founded 1845); Trinity College, Dublin
m. Unmarried
d. 1999

MB, TCD, 1929; FRCS; FRCSI

Postgraduate appointments in England (Cheltenham, Lincoln, Northampton and Chesterfield) as resident medical officer.
Surgeon superintendent, County Hospital, Fermanagh, 1937–72.

The Erne Hospital opened in 1964. Horace Flemming was the last of the single-handed appointments in Northern Ireland. There were no specialists and he was responsible for surgery, medicine, obstetrics and gynaecology, ENT, radiology and dispensing. Outpatients (a novel idea at the time) were seen on Monday, Wednesday and Friday, while operations were carried out on Tuesday, Thursday and Saturday. He would induce the anaesthesia himself and then supervise the house surgeon from the side of the table. If blood transfusion were needed, he had to make all the arrangements locally. Fortunately Enniskillen was an RUC training depot and the young recruits responded willingly and promptly to the call for donors, especially as a bottle of Guinness was the reward.

Patients were still afraid to come into the hospital and the wards were half-empty. An elderly patient with a strangulated hernia had his operation by Horace under local anaesthesia, in his home, by the light of an oil lamp, with a GP holding a torch.

He was an excellent clinician, which was even more important then when there were no laboratory services within 80 miles. Jack Strahan [q.v.] remembers him correctly diagnosing appendicitis in a ten-month-old baby, which was a spectacular achievement. He kept up to date through his Surgical Travelling Club. When the Smith-Peterson pin revolutionised the treatment of fractured neck of femur in the elderly, Horace went to Belfast to see the operation. He then built himself an orthopaedic operating table, which was still in use forty years later. Gradually other specialists were appointed but he remained a solo surgeon for twenty-seven years.

Part of his success was his total integration into the local community. He sailed his dinghy, Maeve (1909), and could be called ashore by lighting a flare or by loud hailer. He was a keen golfer and took his holidays in May for the 'Mayfly'. Sometimes he went to Chile to sail with his brother Lionel, a distinguished journalist. This helped to maintain his year round suntan. Bridge was an essential social skill in those days before television, and he was more than proficient. He was involved in the Amateur Dramatic Society and was a talented watercolourist. He was active in the Masonic Order. A life-long bachelor of the old school, he was strict but fair and hugely respected.

Remote areas needed remarkable men and the people of Fermanagh were fortunate that he was one of four such in the twentieth century.

STRAHAN, Jack

Consultant General Surgeon, Enniskillen, Co. Fermanagh

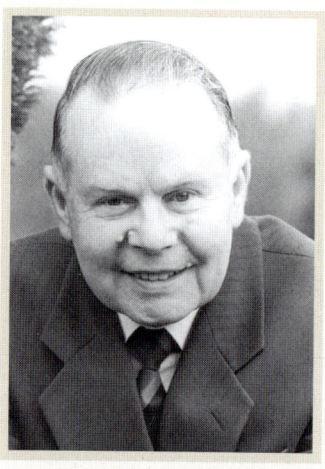

b. 1938, Broughane, Co. Antrim, fourth son of Samuel (farmer) and Elizabeth Strahan
Educ. Ballymena Academy; Queen's University Belfast
m. Unmarried

MB, QUB, 1956; DRCOG, 1958; FRCS Ed, 1962; MCh, QUB, 1971

Postgraduate appointments as house surgeon, RVH, Belfast; Royal Belfast Hospital for Sick Children; Royal Maternity Hospital, Belfast.
Senior house officer, Belfast City Hospital.
Registrar, RVH; Belfast City Hospital; Downe Hospital; registrar, Mid-Ulster; Magherafelt; Banbridge Hospital; Erne Hospital; Enniskillen; Coleraine Hospital; Royal Infirmary, Bradford.
Consultant general surgeon, Erne Hospital, Enniskillen, 1972–98.

Jack Strahan worked single-handedly at the Erne Hospital for over a year and in 1973 was joined by Andy McKibbin [q.v.] and then for most of his working life worked a one-in-two rota. He worked hard and in close co-operation with his colleague. Besides general surgery, they had a responsibility for orthopaedic trauma. Throughout the 1970s and 1980s, there was a fairly steady stream of trauma from terrorist activity. Since 1998, all orthopaedic trauma is cared for by the orthopaedic surgeons.

In addition to his interest in trauma and minor orthopaedics, Jack was interested in gastroenterology and breast surgery. His work was very demanding but rewarding, and the Fermanagh people appreciated the quality of care he gave. 'On the other hand, one had to live with one's mistakes in a closely knit community,' he remarked.

Jack Strahan is of average build and is notably conscientious and particular in his work. He set high standards for himself and others. He refers to himself as 'somewhat independent and not the best at delegating'. Patients first and always are the only true measure of a surgeon.

In retirement, his hobbies are gardening, painting and restoring an old farm cottage.

McKIBBIN, Alistair, OBE (Andy)

Consultant Surgeon, Erne Hospital Fermanagh

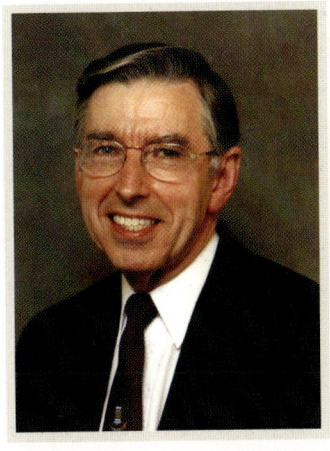

b. 1936, Portglenone, Co. Antrim, eldest son of Charles W. McKibbin and Annie McKibbin (*née* Kyle)
Educ. Ballymena Academy, Co Antrim; Queen's University Belfast
m. 1968: Lilian Dunlop, daughter of Henry and Jean Dunlop; 2 s, 1 d

MB, QUB, 1960; FRCSI, 1969

Postgraduate training entirely within Northern Ireland but with posts of increasing responsibility as senior house officer, registrar (3? years) and senior registrar (almost three years), which involved rotations into specialist units ('neuro', plastic, orthopaedic, urology and A&E), as well as a total of seven hospitals, which provided great basic training in the generality of surgery.
Consultant in General Surgery with a special interest in urology, Erne Hospital, Enniskillen, 1973–98.

Andy McKibbin worked a one-in-two rota for most of his professional life, much of the time with inexperienced junior staff. He practised 'shared care' with his close colleague, Jack Strahan. He had long outpatient clinics and operating sessions, which frequently overran, putting a premium on maintaining good relationships in the operating theatre and in his home. He loved urology and the theatre floor was sometimes awash and overflowing, as if to prove this.

The IRA outrage that was the Enniskillen Bomb on Remembrance Sunday, 8 November 1987, was etched in his memory. There were eleven deaths and fifty-four significant injuries. He and a senior registrar from Belfast, Mr Malcolm Brown, dealt with the majority of patients. Five patients were transferred to specialist units by helicopter. Five of those killed and several of the seriously injured were personal friends. Enniskillen's population is 11,436, and everyone knows the surgeons and the surgeons know everyone. Attending funeral after funeral for the next week was an emotional experience. For this and other services, he was awarded the OBE.

He enjoyed the new 'sciences', especially the wave of information technology and minimally invasive surgery.

He is serious but happy, hardworking but retiring, agreeable but a workaholic, and, above all, kind and caring. The patients often identified him as 'the wee man with the glasses'. He physically dragged his heels, alerting staff to his approach. His social life is low key and divided between family, hobbies and the church. He gardens, computes, cycles and travels. Without detracting in any way from the qualities of the surgeons in the affected institutions, it can be said that the preservation order that hangs over the Erne Hospital is in no small part due to men like Andy McKibbin.

Londonderry

Coleraine (pop. 20,721)

BAILIE, Hugh William Cochrane

Consultant Surgeon

b. 1915
Educ. Queen's University Belfast

MB, QUB, 1938; FRCS Ed, 1948

Postgraduate work as surgical registrar and house surgeon, RVH, Belfast.
Acting Major, Royal Army Medical Corps, Army blood transfusion service.
Senior surgeon, Coleraine and Portrush Hospital Group.
Consultant surgeon, Coleraine Hospital.

Hugh Bailie was sole consultant surgeon at Coleraine for many years, but was joined in later life by Ian Hardy Greer [q.v.].

GREER, Ian Hardy

Consultant Surgeon, Coleraine and Ballymoney Hospitals

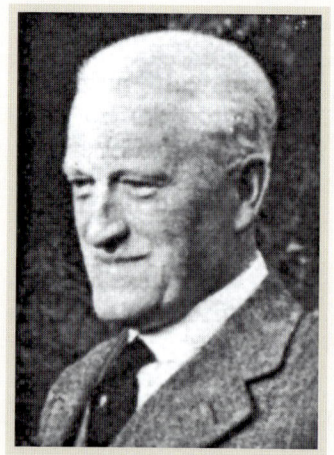

b. 1920, Belfast, only son of H. L. Hardy Greer (consultant obstetrician and gynaecologist, Royal Hospitals, Belfast) and Mamie Greer
Educ. Campbell College, Belfast; Queen's University Belfast
m. 1955: Ruth Beatty, 2 s
d. 1976

MB, QUB, 1949; FRCS Ed, 1957

Postgraduate work included demonstrator in Anatomy, University of St Andrews.
Senior surgical registrar for four years at University College Hospital, Ibadan, Nigeria (under Professor

Will Davey, a QUB graduate, a committed Christian and a fine technical surgeon who himself had been trained in London by Norman Tanner. Davey was a strict disciplinarian who put patients first at all times).
Consultant surgeon, Coleraine and Portrush and N. Antrim Hospital Groups.

Ian Greer resigned from QUB Medical School, after one year of study, to join the RAF at the outbreak of the Second World War. He trained as a navigator and was crew on the Catalina Flying Boats which flew out of Castle Archdale, Lower Lough Erne, Co. Fermanagh (the furthest west RAF station) on anti-submarine patrols. Later, when flying a Halifax bomber, he had to parachute out of his plane over Germany. He was taken to Stalag Luft 111 on the day after the 'Great Escape', a legendary break-out from a German prison camp. He cherished his membership of the Parachute Club, a club whose members had had to abandon a damaged plane by parachute. He wore with pride a silk tie presented to him by Irwins, the manufacturers of war-time parachutes.

Recreations included sailing Olympic Finn (a single-handed, fiercely competitive and physically demanding dinghy class) into his fifties; he also qualified for the world championship of the 420 class (a two-'man' dinghy). With his wife as co-driver, he competed in West African motor rallies in a Mercedes which he obtained from the Stuttgart factory.

LIMAVADY (POP. 10,350)

ROEMMELE, Peter Michael

Surgeon

Educ. University of Edinburgh

MB, ChB, Edin, 1943; FRCS Ed, 1948

Postgraduate appointments as resident surgical officer, Lewis Hospital, Stornoway; senior surgical registrar, Royal Infirmary, Edinburgh.
Surgeon, Roe Valley Hospital, Limavady.

DERRY/LONDONDERRY (POP. 72,334)
Londonderry City and County Infirmary, established 1789 (60 beds)

MILLER, W. (Sir)

Surgeon, 1900

HUNTER, W. B.

Surgeon, 1920

MILLER, Joseph Ewing

Honorary Surgeon, 1920

Educ. Trinity College, Dublin

AB, Dub, MB, 1885; LM, Rotunda, TCD

Postgraduate appointment as house surgeon, General Infirmary, Chester
Honorary surgeon, Londonderry County Infirmary.
Surgeon, HM Prison, Londonderry.

HALL, Henry Potter

Consultant Surgeon, 1920

Educ. Queen's University Belfast

MB, QUB, 1913; MCh, 1920, QUB

Captain, Royal Army Medical Corps.
Assistant to Professor of Surgery, QUB; assistant to medical superintendent, Radium Institute, London.
Surgical registrar, clinical assistant and house surgeon, RVH, Belfast.
Consultant surgeon, City and County Hospital, Londonderry; Masserene Hospital, Antrim.
Clinical lecturer and examiner in surgery QUB; lecturer and examiner, Joint Nurses' Council.
Surgeon, Belfast City Hospital; Ulster Volunteer Force Hospital, Belfast.
Honorary surgeon, Belfast Hospital for Sick Children.

Author of 'War & Surgery', *Ulster Med Journal*, 1945.

McLOUGHLIN, James Neill

Honorary Surgeon, 1920

Educ. University of Edinburgh

MD, Edin, 1910; MB, 1906.

Honorary surgeon, Londonderry County Infirmary.
Lieutenant, Reserve Royal Army Medical Corps.

1949

PYPER, John Graham (Graham)

Londonderry Surgeon, 1949

b. 1912, Bangor, Co. Down, son of John Pyper and Elizabeth Pyper (*née* Patton).
Educ. Bangor Grammar School; Queen's University Belfast
m. Patricia Brightman; 3 s, 1 d
d. 1987

MB (hons), QUB, 1935; FRCS Eng, 1946; MD with gold medal (by thesis), QUB, 1938

Postgraduate training in RVH, Belfast; demonstrator in physiology, QUB.
Consultant surgeon, Royal Navy; Captain, Royal Army Medical Corps 1939–46. Mentioned in dispatches.
Senior surgeon, Waterside, City & County and Altnagelvin Hospitals, Londonderry.
Surgeon to the Royal Navy in Northern Ireland.
Member, Court of New University of Ulster; Magistrate.
Resident surgeon, Ascension Island (two tours) after NHS retirement.

At the beginning of his career as a consultant, Graham Pyper was working virtually single-handed in this city of 70,000 souls and could seldom get out of the hospital where he was engaged in so many activities. He was Chairman of the Building Committee and lived to see Altnagelvin Hospital, in Londonderry's Waterside area, opened in 1960. It was the first hospital built in the UK after the Second World War. When his colleague, Harry Bennett [q.v.], arrived, Harry did most of the political advocacy and Graham did most of the operative surgery.

Graham Pyper's commitment to his patients and his institution was legendary. His over-riding pre-occupation and consumer of his time was always the hospital. His recreations included springboard and high-board diving (he represented British Universities in the World Student Games in Turin, 1933), photography, walking and sea bathing. Every hospital needs a Graham Pyper. Not all get one.

BENNETT, Harry Milne, OBE

Londonderry Surgeon, 1949

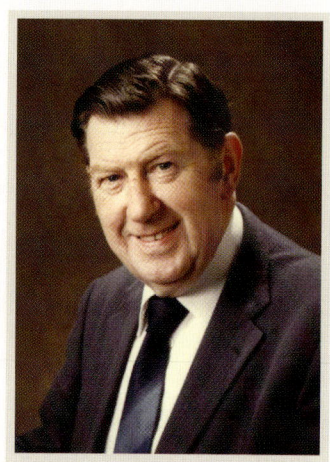

b. 1918, Bangor/Rockmount, Coleraine, son of W. Harry D. and Ida Kathleen Bennett
Educ. Coleraine Academical Institution (1930–35); Queen's University Belfast
m. 1941: Hazel Hall (d. 1990); 3 s, 1 d
d. 1990

MB, QUB, 1940; FRCS Ed, 1948

Postgraduate appointment as house surgeon, RVH, Belfast.
Captain, Royal Army Medical Corps, 1941–46; posted first to East Anglia then to India and Burma with the 14th Army (the 'Forgotten Army').
Registrar, RVH, Belfast and Musgrave Park, 1946; senior registrar, City and County Hospital, Londonderry, 1949.
Consultant surgeon, City & County and Waterside Hospitals, Londonderry, 1949–60.
Altnagelvin Hospital, Londonderry, 1960–83.
High Sheriff, City of Londonderry.

Harry Bennett was a stalwart of the BMA and long-time chairman of the Western Division, representing the NI Committee for Hospital Medical Consultants for twenty years. Journeys to London and back took a long time in the days before regular flights. (The editor can testify that Northern Ireland was never overlooked while he was there.)

He had a tough start in life as his father was killed in the trenches in 1918, before Harry was born. At Coleraine Academical Institution, he obtained every possible scholarship, and there is a plaque commemorating his unique achievements.

When he went to Londonderry, he threw himself into the design of the new hospital, which was to become Altnagelvin. He had looked after the casualties of Bloody Sunday (1973), at which twenty-six civil rights protesters were shot, fourteen of them fatally, and he was at the centre of the drama of the no-warning INLA bomb at the Droppin' Well village pub in nearby Ballykelly (1982), when eleven soldiers and five civilians were killed, and sixty-six others injured. The dead and survivors were brought to Altnagelvin. Harry became emotional even thinking about these people's lives being taken from them.

Susan Freeman, his ward sister for twenty-three years, described him thus: 'a people person, kind, caring, compassionate, generous and blunt. Always thinking of the people he worked with as well as his patients. I could not have had a better boss.'

Col. Desmond Whyte said, 'He combined physical stamina, alertness, mental agility and ready acceptance of responsibility.'

He was a keen Rotarian and was made a Paul Harris Fellow, the highest award in the organisation. He kept a meticulous diary for twenty-five years but it would have required the full resources of the cryptographers of Bletchley Park to decipher any of his writing.

In retirement, he played more golf and more bridge, while remaining active as Chairman of the Old People's Association, the local Cancer Research branch and the Friends of Altnagelvin, of which group he was probably the greatest friend. He was in every way a big man, with a full head of hair when he died in the hospital he loved and where they loved him. In his own words, he was 'still fighting the bureaucracy of the NHS'.

Every community and every hospital should have a Harry Bennett, and Derry/Londonderry, with all its misfortunes over the years, was fortunate to have had him. His death notice, written by his children, said, 'He cared more for others than he cared for himself.' A fitting tribute to an admirable man.

MAGHERAFELT (POP. 6,682)

BRENNEN, Wilfred Macaulay, OBE (Wilfie)

Surgeon, Mid-Ulster Hospital, Magherafelt

b. 1912
Educ. Queen's University Belfast
m. Muriel Earls; 3 s (Michael is a Belfast plastic surgeon), 1 d
d. 1984

MB, QUB, 1935; FRCSI 1939, C St J

Postgraduate appointments as clinical assistant, Belfast Hospital for Sick Children; surgical registrar, RVH, Belfast; tutor in surgery, QUB.
Surgeon, Mid-Ulster Hospital, 1945–77.
Chairman, Advisory Committee on Surgery, NI Hospitals Authority.
Commissioner, St John Ambulance Brigade, Northern Ireland.
Examiner, Joint Nursing & Midwifery Council; NI Royal Society of Arts.

Wilfie Brennen was a very fast, self-sufficient surgeon, who often operated with nursing assistance only. He used various modes of transport from his home to hospital, including bicycle, motorcycle, car, horse or his own two feet, either walking or running.

He had a central involvement in the Marriage Guidance Council, and was also Chief Scout for Northern Ireland.

TYRONE

Dungannon (pop. 9,190)

CREIGHTON, Patrick Urling (Paddy)

Consultant Surgeon, South Armagh and South Tyrone Hospital

b. 1919
Educ. Queen's University, Edinburgh
d. 1970

MB, QUB, 1942; FRCS Ed, 1948

Postgraduate appointments as senior surgical registrar, RVH, Belfast.
Consultant surgeon, South Armagh and South Tyrone Hospital.

Paddy Creighton was a big, kind, considerate man who retired early due to ill-health.

LOANE, Robert Cecil Ronald (Ronnie)

South Tyrone (Dungannon) Surgeon

b. 1918, eldest son of Hugh Loane and Martha Loane (*née* Coulter)
Educ. Methodist College, Belfast; Queen's University Belfast
m. 1950: Vera Harland, daughter of Henry and Helen Harland; 2 s (one a dentist), 1 d
d. 1968

MB, QUB, 1941; FRCS Eng, 1949; FRCS Ed, 1949

Postgraduate appointments as surgical registrar, RVH, Belfast; demonstrator in anatomy, QUB; rehabilitation specialist, Royal Air Force Volunteer Reserve; registrar, Omagh Hospital, 1950.
Consultant surgeon, South Tyrone Hospital, Dungannon, 1951–68.

When Ronnie Loane arrived in Dungannon, it was difficult to persuade patients to come into the hospital as 'the workhouse was a place where you went to die'. The old building was lit by gas, the mattresses and pillows were filled with straw (1951), there were two outside lavatories and one inside lavatory for 130 geriatric patients, and a ten-foot by ten-foot operating theatre. It took fifteen years to get a new hospital, which he never lived to see.

With Will Hanna [q.v.], he formed the Ulster Surgical Club, and there is a memorial lecture in the Club to commemorate the two founders.

Ronnie enjoyed golf and camping abroad with family. He skied and loved Switzerland. He enjoyed reading and the company of friends and colleagues, especially Will Hanna. When his wife Vera began to teach the children to ride, Ronnie joined the 'school' and developed a good 'seat'.

As a single-handed surgeon he was extremely hardworking and always available to help a colleague. But he sometimes had the frustration of having to cancel a holiday at the last moment through not being able to get locum cover. He loved his home, just two miles outside Dungannon, and was a devoted husband and father. He suffered a massive heart attack at the age of 50. The stress of the post was undoubtedly a factor. Sir Ian Fraser [q.v.] wrote a warm obituary in the BMJ. A great gentleman.

LOWRY, John Barbour

Consultant Surgeon, South Tyrone Hospital

Educ. Queen's University Belfast

MB, QUB, 1949; MCh, QUB, 1961; FRCS Ed, 1954

Senior registrar and Purse Research Fellow, RVH, Belfast.
Senior registrar, Postgraduate Medical School, Hammersmith Hospital, London.
Consultant surgeon, South Tyrone Hospital.

WARD, John Turner

Consultant General Surgeon, South Tyrone Hospital

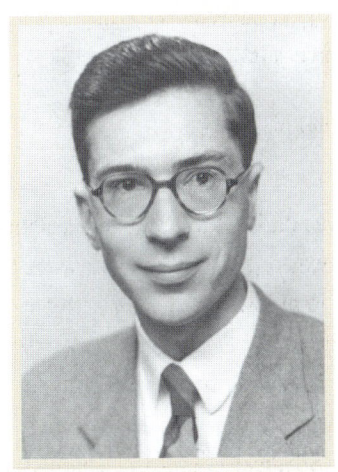

b. 1932, Ipswich, Suffolk, only son of Richard Ward (FRCSE) and Mary Ward (*née* Turner). He was the son and grandson (and to become a father of) surgeons
Educ. Epsom College; Queen's University Belfast
m. 1958: Cecilia Arnold, MB, daughter of Robert and Charlotte Arnold, MB; 3 s (one, FRCS Orthopaedics, England), 1 d
d. 1984

MB, QUB, 1958; MCh, Belf, 1962; FRCS Eng, 1964; FRCS Ed, 1964

Postgraduate appointments as senior registrar, general surgery, Belfast City Hospital; Registrar and Tutor, QUB; Senior house officer (general surgery), RVH, Belfast.

Fellow, Cleveland Clinic, USA, sixteen months.
Consultant General Surgeon, South Tyrone Hospital, Dungannon, 1969–84.
Locum Consultant surgeon, Cleveland Clinic, 1968.
Secretary, Ulster Surgical Club; High Sheriff, County Tyrone, 1983–84.

A colleague, John Watson of Armagh, writes, 'He was an outstanding surgeon with great hands, common sense and humility. An exceptional man.'

His widow, Dr Cecilia Ward, writes: 'He always said that his ambition was to practise general surgery in the country and, forgoing encouragement to train in other specialties, he stuck to his intention. The Troubles gave him the ultimate challenge. During the 1970s, Dungannon had the miserable distinction of being the most frequently bombed town in the Province. Almost daily there was an appalling incident. Working a one-in-two rota before mobile phones, he spent his captive time restoring our home. He rewired and extended a traditional cottage on Cruit Island (off west Donegal coast) and was so professional that an apprentice joiner asked him where he had served his time. He enjoyed sailing: racing in the River Class (28') on Strangford Lough or pottering round the Donegal coast in a Drascombe Lugger. He liked the faster models of cars. He became a wine expert. He was happy in his work, devoted to his family and fun to be with.'

Tall, thin (could not gain weight), active and attentive, John Ward had great compassion and integrity. A most admirable professional and a complete gentleman.

OMAGH (POP. 17,280)
Omagh County Infirmary, established 1763 (50 beds)

Surgeons, 1900–20

THOMPSON, Edward Charles

Surgeon, Tyrone County Infirmary Hospital

Educ. Trinity College, Dublin

AB, Dublin; MB, TCD, 1871; FRCSI, 1885

Surgeon, Royal Navy; medical officer, HM Prison, Omagh.
Surgeon, Tyrone County Infirmary Hospital.

Nine Publications in his entry in the *Medical Directory* in 1900, ranging from 'Hygiene' to 'The Trial of the Maguires for murder, with analysis of the medical evidence'.

EATON, Arthur Hugh McCulloch TD

Surgeon, Tyrone County Infirmary Hospital

Educ. Queen's University Belfast

MB (hons), QUB, 1922; FRCS Ed, 1927

Postgraduate appointments as house surgeon, RVH, Belfast; resident medical officer,
St Helen's Hospital; tutor in obstetrics, QUB.
Surgeon, Tyrone County Hospital; Omagh General Hospital.
Temp. Lieutenant-Colonel, Royal Army Medical Corps.

Author of 'Acute Gastro-Duodenal Perforations' (Presidential address, NI Branch of BMA, 1947)

SMYTH William Francis (Bill)

Consultant Surgeon, Tyrone County Hospital

b. 1916, Downpatrick, Co. Down
Educ. Christian Brothers School, Newry; Queen's University Belfast
m. Anne; 8 s (one a GP), 2 d
d. 1990

MB, QUB, 1938; FRCS Ed, 1948

Postgraduate appointments as surgical registrar, RVH, Belfast; Mater Infirmorum Hospital,
Belfast; Belfast City Hospital; surgical specialist, Royal Army Medical Corps.
Assistant surgeon, Belfast City Hospital.
Consultant surgeon, Tyrone County Hospital.

Bill Smyth was a devoted father and enjoyed his large family. Outside of the family his only interests were the hospital and surgery.

MALTBY, Alfred Cecil Victor (Cecil)

Tyrone Surgeon

b. 1919, Ballymoyer, Armagh, son of Rev. R. W. Maltby and Eileen Maltby
Educ. Portora Royal School, Enniskillen; Trinity College, Dublin
m. 1954: Catherine; 2 s 1 d (an ENT consultant in Halifax, Nova Scotia, Canada)
d. 1999

BA, TCD, 1940; MB, TCD, 1943; FRCSI, 1949

Postgraduate appointments as house surgeon, Southport Infirmary; registrar, RVH, Belfast; surgical registrar, Royal Berkshire Hospital, Reading.
Rotating posts in Belfast and Altnagelvin Hospital, Londonderry.
Surgeon and Lieutenant, Royal Navy Reserve, serving in the Far East.
Consultant surgeon, West Tyrone Group Hospitals.
High Sheriff of Co. Tyrone.

Cecil Maltby played competitive snooker into his eightieth year, was a single-figure handicap golfer while Captain and President of Omagh Golf Club, and sailed his large ketch to the South of England. He was a great raconteur, and Jimmy Blundell said, 'You left his company feeling that it was great to be alive.'

PINTO, Domingos Joseph Diago Teodoro, OBE (Dominic)

Tyrone Surgeon

b. 1937, Goa, India, second son of Jeromino Z. Pinto and Rosa A. Pinto (*née* Lobo)
Educ. Dr Rebeiro Goan School, Nairobi; Royal London Medical School
m. 1st in 1962: Virginia M. P. Dryden (d. 1975), daughter of Anthony and Elizabeth Dryden; 2nd: Olga Molek, daughter of Anton and Angela Molek; 2 s (one a doctor), 1 d

MRCS & LRCP, Lond, 1962; MB, Lond Hospital, 1962; FRCS Ed, 1966; FRCS Eng, 1967; MS Lond, 1970

Postgraduate appointments as senior house officer, Southend General Hospital; Addenbrooke's Hospital, Cambridge; Ipswich General Hospital.
Rotating surgical registrar and research registrar, Middlesex Hospital, London.
Senior lecturer, Makerere University, Kampala, Uganda.
Scientist and honorary consultant, MRC Northwick Park Hospital, 1973–80.
Consultant surgeon, Tyrone County Hospital.
Deputy Lieutenant, Co. Tyrone 1997; High Sheriff of Co. Tyrone, 2002.

Dominic Pinto's greatest satisfaction was to teach junior medical staff and nurses. For eighteen years, he arranged for two surgical trainees to come from Goa and Bombay, and had them incorporated into the Northern Ireland Surgical Training Programme. He continues to teach anatomy at Queen's University, Belfast.

He is an active member of many community voluntary organisations. He is also a keen Rotarian, Knight of the Order of Malta, and a member of the Ancient and Most Benevolent Order of the Friendly Brothers of St Patrick.

Having formerly played hockey and cricket, he is now a keen golfer and past Captain and President of Omagh Golf Club.

8
SPECIALIST SURGEONS IN NORTHERN IRELAND

SPECIALIST SURGEONS IN NORTHERN IRELAND

CARDIOTHORACIC SURGEONS

BINGHAM, John Alexander Walton

Belfast Cardiothoracic Surgeon

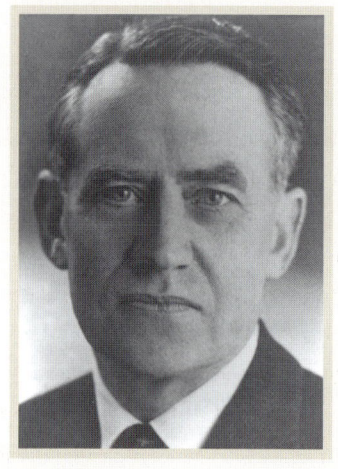

b. 1911, Belfast, son of John Alexander Bingham (chemist) and Essie Jane Bingham (*née* Carlson)
Educ. Methodist College, Belfast; Queen's University Belfast
m. Unmarried
d. 1983

MB, QUB, 1934 (many prizes); FRCS, 1938; MCh, 1946

Resident surgical officer, King Edward VII Hospital Windsor, 1934–37; Queen Mary's Hospital, Roehampton, 1938.
Major, Indian Medical Service, Sept 1939–45 (India and Malaya).
Registrar, Brompton Hospital, London, 1946–47.
Consultant thoracic surgeon, Royal Belfast Hospital for Sick Children, 1950–76; RVH, Belfast, 1950–76.

Going, as John Bingham did, immediately to England for training and experience was not usual for a Belfast graduate in those days, but his training, particularly in Roehampton (rehabilitation), stood him in good stead dealing with battle casualties, particularly amputations. His MD was on the mechanism and management of causalgia.

Quiet, careful, reserved and monosyllabic, Bingham had got a 'Blue' for cricket. However, he could explode in a torrent of staccato volubility. Given to unpunctuality, he was not a great communicator. His operative technique was quick and meticulous. If a problem arose, it was repaired before anyone outside the field knew about it. He 'whistled while he worked' and insiders could tell how the operation was going by the pitch of the rather tuneless whistle.

He was an enthusiastic golfer and played with the same medical foursome for thirty-three years. His favoured topics were golf, golf [sic], cricket and the Stock Exchange.

CLELAND, John (Jack)

Belfast Cardiac Surgeon

b. 1935

Educ. St Malachy's College, Belfast; Queen's University Belfast

MB (Hons), QUB, 1958; FRCS Ed 1962; FRCS Eng 1963

Postgraduate registrar, RVH, Belfast. Mayo Clinic, Rochester, Minnesota
Cardiac surgeon RVH, 1971–1995

PG Mayo Clinic for two years under John Kirklin and Dwight McGoon, two of the brightest stars in the world of cardiac surgery, and both of whom thought highly of Jack. From the Mayo he published useful, durable research on post-operative fluid management. He was instrumental in setting up a completely dedicated and protected cardiac surgical intensive care, high dependency and cardiac surgical ward in the Royal Victoria Hospital. It was based on the Mayo Clinic model. He had a particular interest in cardiac valve disease and surgery for congenital heart disease. He continued to write articles and contribute to meetings over the years.

He was demanding and autocratic but never wrong. Mortality of cardiac surgery was high in those early days and 'tempers became slightly frayed' on many occasions. There was a haze of smoke when he came away from the operating table. He was known as 'Black Jack', but has a high number of loyal trainees who are now consultants. He was supportive of junior staff when needs be. Jack was one of the first of his faith to be appointed to a frontline consultancy in the RVH. AE (Freddie) Wood, a trainee, said of him, 'A small, very intense man with piercing blue eyes, smoking a pipe and chewing gum.'

His hobby was art and he became even more accomplished during later years. He and his wife Pat were avid collectors of Northern Ireland artists. In retirement he went to live in Spain. He developed renal failure but came back to Dublin for a kidney transplant.

GIBBONS, John Robert Pelham, MBE, TD

Consultant Thoracic Surgeon, Belfast

b. 1928, Birmingham
Educ. Leeds University
m. Marie-Jeanne; 4 s (2 doctors), 2 d
d. 1999

MB, Leeds, 1954; FRCS Eng, 1960; FRCS Ed, 1960

Postgraduate appointments as senior registrar with Donald Ross at National Heart Hospital, London, where he assisted in Britain's first heart transplant.
Nuffield Travelling Fellow to Australasia.
Consultant thoracic surgeon, RVH, Belfast, 1977–93.
Consultant, Royal Free Hospital, London.

John Gibbons developed a unique experience in treating gunshot wounds to the chest and oesophagus and was awarded a Hunterian Professorship on the subject. At the end of the war, he enlisted in the Royal Warwickshire Regiment and saw active service in Palestine. He was President of the Northern Ireland Branch of the Parachute Regiment and kept up his links with the Royal Army Medical Corps.

He loved teaching and examined for the Edinburgh College. Self-deprecating, he had no time for arrogance. He was interested in travel, railways and good food and wine.

A popular and imposing figure, he passed away following cardiac surgery.

MOLLOY, Patrick John (Pat)

Belfast Cardiac Surgeon

b. 1928, New Zealand
Educ. University of Otago, New Zealand
m. Jewel; 9 d, 1 s (tenth child: Irish)

MB, Otago NZ, 1952; FRCS 1960

Surgical registrar, St Charles Hospital, London; senior surgical registrar and Leverhulme Research Fellow, thoracic surgery, Guy's Hospital, London.
Consultant thoracic surgeon, Broadgreen Hospital, Liverpool.
Consultant cardiac surgeon, RVH, Belfast, 1968–73.

Pat Molloy was something completely different: a New Zealander who had trained in heart surgery at Guy's in its glory days of (Lord) Russell Brock and Donald Ross. Young, with huge energy and boundless optimism, he was a superb organiser and a gifted leader who could carry the team with him no matter how hard he expected them to work. He was the major force in restarting open-heart surgery in the Royal Victoria and they were soon doing five cases a week from a standing start. He was widely admired professionally and socially, and his decision to leave Belfast for bucolic New Zealand was a widespread source of great regret — and not just because he gave great parties where some of his nine daughters helped with the entertaining.

O'KANE, Hugh Oliver Joseph

Belfast Cardiac Surgeon

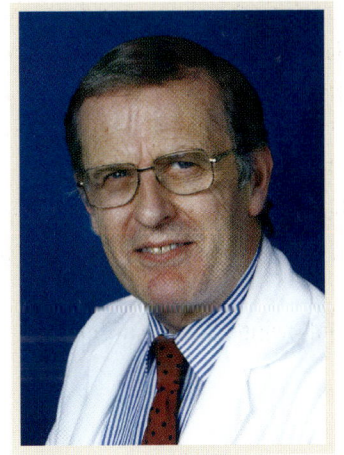

b. 1935, Belfast, fifth son of Felix Kane and Margaret Kane (*née* McKeever); one of a family of six boys one girl.

Educ. St Patrick's College, Armagh (Vincentian), 1947–53; Queen's University Belfast, 1953–60 (State Exhibition School)

m. 1973: Breige McGuckian, daughter of Gerald and Mona McGuckian; 2 s (Hugh F., MRCS), 2 d (Anna M., a doctor)

BSc (hons physiology), QUB, 1957; MB, QUB, 1960; FRCS Ed, 1963; MCh, QUB, 1969; FRCSI (*ad eundem*), 1995.

House officer, Mater Hospital, Belfast, 1960–61; demonstrator in physiology, QUB, 1961–62; surgical registrar and senior surgical registrar, NI Hospitals Authority, 1962–67.

Surgical Research Fellow and senior resident in clinical renal transplant, 1967–69, Mayo Clinic Rochester, Minnesota, USA.

Cardiothoracic Fellow, Mayo Clinic, 1969–71.

Attending staff and instructor in surgery, Jewish Hospital, Washington University, St Louis, Missouri, 1971–73.

Assistant Professor of Surgery, Washington University, St Louis, Missouri, 1971–73.

Consultant cardiac surgeon, RVH, Belfast, 1973–2000.

President, Irish Cardiac Society, 1990–92.

Founder member, European Association of Cardiothoracic Surgeons, 1987.

Intercollegiate examiner in cardiothoracic surgery.

Member, Specialist Advisory Committee (SAC) cardiothoracic surgeons, visiting professorial division cardiothoracic surgery, U. Illinois, 2000.

Hugh O'Kane returned from six years in the US as a trained, polished, technically talented surgeon, following on from the charismatic Pat Molloy. He pioneered the use of the internal mammary artery as graft of choice in these islands, and introduced the valuable bi-leaflet heart valve (St Jude). He pioneered 'Self-Managed Anticoagulation' and proved its effectiveness.

His most famous patient, by far, was Sir Ian Fraser [q.v.], who sailed through bypass surgery at the age of 88. On the trolley in the anaesthetic room, Ian, ever the joker, said to Hugh (a Catholic), 'I hope you have forgiven us... Use the internal mammary (Hugh's 'party trick') for the graft if you can.' After surgery, Hugh said, 'We had to use veins. We will use the internal mammary next time.' (This story was told to the editor by Ian. It has the ring of truth but then Ian never let the facts spoil a good story.)

Between 1953 and 1963, he played Gaelic football for Antrim and he played for Queen's between 1953 and 1959. He was a full University Blue for four years and captained the first Queen's team to win the intervarsity Sigerson Cup in 1968. He was 5'10" but played mid-field and was a renowned jumper. He also played basketball for Queen's (Half Blue in those days) in 1957. He enjoyed golf to twelve handicap at Portstewart Golf Club. (Someone has said, 'Low handicaps don't seem to go with long CVs.') Everybody, absolutely everybody, you ask about Hugh has the same answer, 'Hugh was a perfect gentleman inside and outside the operating theatre.'

SMILEY, Thomas Boyd, MC (Tom)

Consultant Surgeon

b. 1917, Castlewellan Co. Down
Educ. Methodist College, Belfast, where he was head of school and captained the 1st rugby XV; Queen's University Belfast
m. Elizabeth Mills; 3 s (2 doctors, both in New Zealand), 1 d
d. 1981

MB, QUB, 1939; FRCS, 1948

Royal Army Medical Corps, 1940–45; taken Japanese prisoner of war on the fall of Singapore, he greatly admired, as did so many others, the example set by Julian Taylor FRCS (University College Hospital, London) in the camp (Taylor operated in his bare feet, then and afterwards, with the most primitive of instruments, including a much-prized razor blade). Smiley's life was saved when the metal cigarette case in his breast pocket deflected a Japanese bayonet. He was awarded the MC and twice mentioned in dispatches.
Resident surgical officer, Brompton Hospital, London (under (Sir) Clement Price Thomas).
Consultant surgeon, RVH, Belfast, 1951–77; also at Forster Green and Whiteabbey Hospitals.

Before chemotherapy for tuberculosis, there was a great deal of operative surgery on patients with advanced disease. This surgery was physically exhausting as the lobectomies were carried out through masses of adhesions, and the thoracoplasties were prolonged and bloody. Add to that that little was known about the real blood and fluid losses of patients at that time and there is a picture of depressing intervention depleting patient and surgeon. When tuberculosis was no longer on the operating list, Tom Smiley turned to oesophageal and then cardiac surgery. He carried out the first mitral valvotomy in Ireland while still a registrar. With John Bingham [q.v.], he established the open-heart surgical programme.

A big, enthusiastic extrovert, he loved the countryside, was a keen huntsman, and farmed 60 acres in Magheragall, but on retirement he moved to Norfolk. Ironically he went back to Kuala Lumpur, Malaysia, as Visiting Professor of Surgery, in the year before his death.

With an aldermanic figure, his bluff exterior hid sensitivity within. He was wont to sing the songs of Zion while operating. His favourite was the 23rd Psalm ('The Lord's My Shepherd'). Fittingly he died following reading a lesson at church.

STEVENSON, Howard Morris (Morris)

Belfast Thoracic Surgeon

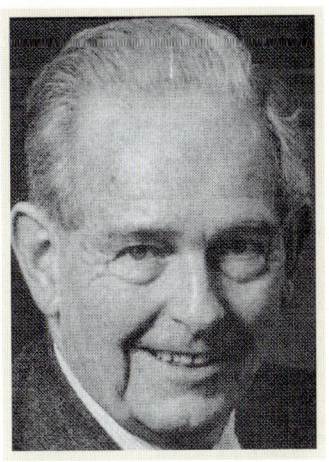

b. 1920

Educ. Queen's University Belfast

m. 1944: Phyllis Wilson, daughter of Rev. Robert J Wilson (a Presbyterian minister who became Principal of Assemblies College, Belfast); 1 s (John Howard, a plastic surgeon in Dundee), 2 d

d. 2003

MB, QUB, 1943 (Honours and many prizes); FRCS Ed, 1948

Postgraduate appointments as Surgeon Lieutenant, Royal Naval Volunteer Reserve, 1944–47. Trained as a cardiothoracic surgeon at the Brompton Hospital in London.

Surgical registrar, RVH, Belfast; resident surgical officer, Brompton Hospital, London. Consultant RVH, Belfast, and Forster Green Hospital, 1951–86.

Morris Stevenson began doing all the cardiac and thoracic work but later concentrated on the purely thoracic work. There was a big volume of chest trauma as 'the Troubles' wore on and he summarised his experience in an important article, 'A Review of 158 Gunshot Wounds to Chest' (*British Journal of Surgery*, 1978).

At the Brompton, he trained under Sir Clement Price Thomas (son of a Welsh miner), who was a great inspiration to him. Price Thomas it was who operated on King George VI for cancer of the lung in 1951. (Following the publicity surrounding the surgery, literally hundreds of patients and relatives wrote to Price Thomas asking him to do their operation. The National Health Service did not allow for choice of surgeon but Price Thomas was a prodigious worker and he did acquiesce in a number of cases.)

On his return to the RVH, he worked with John Bingham [q.v.] and Tom Smiley [q.v.], building up the cardiothoracic unit in Northern Ireland. He was an outstanding and meticulous surgeon, greatly respected by his colleagues. With them he contributed greatly to the care of the appalling number of casualties, particularly in the 1970s. He greatly enjoyed his surgery and the colleagues with whom he worked; he often mentioned in particular the late, great John Dundee, Professor of Anaesthetics, who worked with him for twenty-seven years, a period of time over which he had the great pleasure in saying that they 'never had a disagreement'.

He was a skilled and enthusiastic photographer. He also enjoyed woodworking and took particular pride in making a desk — a Davenport — which, like everything he did, was constructed with great skill and meticulous attention to detail. He often said that his greatest pleasure in life was his family to whom he devoted so much time. The July holidays in Donegal were the highlight of his year.

Shortly before he died, a former trainee wrote, 'A surgeon who worked with great speed, but without haste, a gentleman whose words I heeded, whose surgery I respected and whose manners I tried to emulate, who endeared himself to his nursing staff, his patients and his colleagues'. Trainees and secretaries really know. A most admirable professional and gentleman. A really lovely man.

NEUROSURGEONS

BAILEY, Ian Campbell

Belfast Neurosurgeon

b. 1929, Dublin, son of James Rowland Bailey and Hilda Bailey (*née* Campbell).
Educ. St Andrew's College, Dublin; Trinity College, Dublin
m. Married with 2 s, 1 d

BA, TCD, 1951; MB, TCD, 1953; FRCSI, 1959; FRCS Eng, 1963

General surgical training in Dublin; neurosurgical training in Belfast and in Guy's Maudsley Neurosurgical Department, London.
Consultant neurosurgeon in Belfast, 1967.
Spent four years in the University of East Africa (Makerere) in Kampala, Uganda, where he was instrumental in setting up the Department of Neurosurgery.

Ian Bailey returned to Belfast about 1975 and worked there until his retirement in 1995. He was interested in vascular neurosurgery, with particular concentration on the difficult condition of brain and spinal AVM (arteriovenous malformation).

Bailey's great gift was his calm and unhurried address of clinical problems. He was an indefatigable operator whose patience in the theatre and wards was legendary. Not academic by nature, he encouraged others in the Department to engage in such activity and was the leader in several multi-centre trials. He never lost his love of Africa and continues to visit that continent, even in retirement. He was the first Southerner to become a Consultant Neurosurgeon in Northern Ireland.

BYRNES, Dermot Patrick

Belfast Neurosurgeon

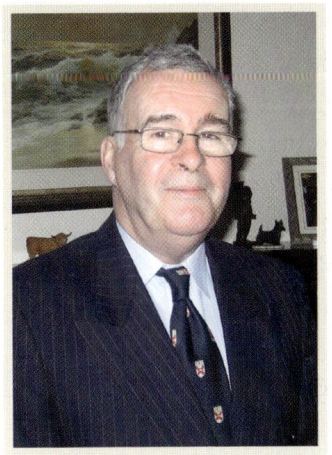

b. 1939, Dublin, son of Prof. Colman Byrnes [q.v.] and Mary Byrnes (*née* Lane)
Educ. NUI
m. 1967: Dr Toni Lawler (a classmate in UCD); 2 s (Colman K., a colorectal surgeon in Northern Ireland; Tiernan, a trainee neurosurgeon), 2 d (Sheena, a consultant in intensive care in Exeter; Aisling, a criminal defence barrister in London)

MB (prizes) NUI, 1963; FRCS Ed, 1967; FRCSI, 1969; Fellow, Academy Medical Science (Founder Fellow), 1998

Postgraduate appointment as demonstrator in anatomy, UCD, 1964–65.

Basic surgical training at Mater Hospital, Dublin; Royal Infirmary of Edinburgh; Kildare County Hospital; and Richmond Hospital, Dublin.
Tutor in surgery, senior registrar grade, Professorial Unit, Richmond Hospital, Dublin.
Neurosurgery training: senior registrar and registrar, RVH, Belfast, 1970–73; Atkinson Morley's (St George's) Hospital, London, 1973–74.
Chief resident, paediatric neurosurgery, Johns Hopkins Hospital, Baltimore, Maryland.
Assistant Professor of Neurosurgery, University of Maryland, 1975–79.
Senior lecturer in neurosurgery, 1979–95, QUB.

Consultant neurosurgeon, RVH, 1979–2004.
Lecturer in medical ethics, QUB.
Consultant neurosurgeon, King Faisal Specialist Hospital, Riyadh, Kingdom of Saudi Arabia; Ibn Al-Bitar Hospital, Baghdad, Iraq.
Member, Council, RCSI, 1993–2006; honorary librarian, RCSI.

Dermot Byrnes' main clinical interest was in head injuries and other CNS trauma. He was involved in the organisation of services and was a tireless volunteer for many committees. A prolific provider of articles, abstracts, book chapters and the spoken word from the podium, Byrnes did all that might be expected of him and much more.

He is 5'6", feisty and hugely energetic; the surgical gene of his professorial father is dominant. He had been superbly trained in the best places and his professional talents, together with his leadership skills and dedication, represented a massive loss to the Dublin unit at a time when these qualities were never more needed. He flowered in battle-scarred Belfast. A consummate, caring professional.

CALVERT, Cecil

Belfast Neurosurgeon

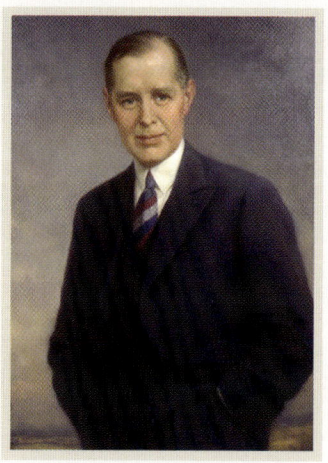

b. 1894
Educ. Queen's University Belfast
m. married; no children
d. 1956

MB (first class hons), QUB, 1922; FRCSI, 1926

Postgraduate basic surgical training, Belfast.
Assistant surgeon, RVH, 1935, as a general surgeon.
Royal Army Medical Corps, 1939–45.
Oxford Neurosurgical Unit (with Hugh Cairns).
Consultant neurosurgeon, director of Neurosurgery Department, RVH, Belfast.

Cecil Calvert was invited to join Hugh Cairns at the Oxford Neurosurgical Unit ('The Nutcrackers Suite'), specialising in head injuries. Cairns, an Australian Rhodes scholar who went to Oxford, was a driven, exacting, charismatic figure and the outstanding British neurosurgeon of the day. Calvert returned to Belfast in 1945 as the first consultant neurosurgeon, initially sharing beds and operating facilities with other specialists. In 1947, the Department of Neurosurgery was opened at the RVH and Calvert became director.

He was a meticulous surgeon to the point that his slowness in the operating theatre was legendary. This was the Harvey Cushing tradition, which he inherited from Cairns, and Cairns got from Cushing himself. His list frequently went on long after midnight, but he would appear back at eight in the morning. There were the usual stories of the wound allegedly healing as he finished sewing the scalp.

Calvert was very much part of the neurosurgical establishment in the UK and active in the Society of British Neurological Surgeons. Tall, immaculately dressed and somewhat aloof, even stern, he was perhaps too reserved to be a great teacher.

He was married but had no family. Tragically he lost his life in a road traffic accident on his way to a colleague's funeral (Ronnie Loane's) in Omagh. There is a Calvert Room in the unit, a Calvert Medal and a Calvert Lecture, all features of the admirable collegiality of the Belfast neurosurgical unit.

FANNIN, Thomas Francis

Belfast Neurosurgeon

b. 1938, Ballymoney, Co. Antrim, son of Robert Fannin and Jean Fannin (*née* Morrison)
Educ. Ballymena Academy; Queen's College, Belfast
m. 1964; Joy Black; 3 s, 1 d (a nurse)

MB, QUB, 1962; MD, QUB, 1967; FRCS Ed, 1969

Postgraduate training in pathology (three years), followed by basic surgical training in Belfast; neurosurgical training in Belfast, Edinburgh and Montreal.
Consultant neurosurgeon, Sheffield, 1977–79.
Consultant neurosurgeon, Belfast, 1979–90.

Thomas Fannin's particular surgical interests were in surgery of the pituitary and trigeminal neuralgia. He was the one of the unit who was most involved in paediatric neurosurgery. He was out of the mould of the enthusiastic surgeon: he loved operating. He was most conscientious and concerned for the welfare of his patients and, importantly, his staff alike. His use of colourful but not rancorous language in the operating theatre was well known. He was extremely popular in his hospital and was an excellent supporter of his colleagues. He seemed to know every GP in Northern Ireland personally!

Outside medicine, he walked, gardened, enjoyed his cottage in Donegal and assisted his wife in running her business in Lisburn.

GLEADHILL, Colin

Belfast and Dublin Neurosurgeon

b. 1914, Yorkshire
Educ. University of Edinburgh
m. Deirdre (a GP); 3 s (David, a physician; Ian, an A&E consultant), 1 d (Valerie, a consultant paediatrician)
d. 1991

MB, Edin, 1939; MD, 1941; FRCS Ed, 1948

Postgraduate appointments in neurosurgery in Edinburgh (with legendary Norman Dott), and in the Richmond Hospital, Dublin.
Consultant neurosurgeon, RVH, Belfast, 1957–79.

Appointed to the Richmond Hospital, Dublin, Colin Gleadhill had differences with Adams A. McConnell [q.v.], who was somewhat autocratic and whose manner was in stark contrast with Colin's egalitarian views.

His main surgical interests were in neurovascular conditions and sellar tumours such as the pituitary and craniopharyngioma. He was much loved by the junior staff whom he constantly championed.

A charming and sociable man, with strong left-wing views, Gleadhill was an expert sailor. He also had a vintage open Bentley tourer, complete with bonnet strap and running boards, in which he sat attired, 1930s-style, in a leather helmet. He was ruggedly handsome, and as an ex-amateur boxing champion, he carried considerable facial evidence of his past prowess.

GORDON, Derek Stanley, OBE, CBE

Belfast Neurosurgeon

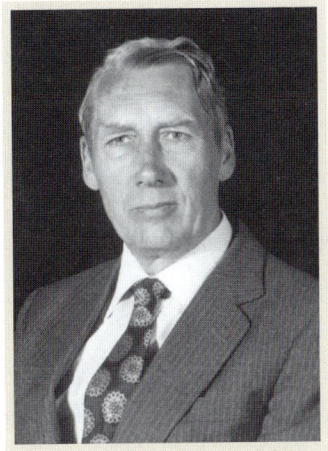

b. 1926, Belfast, son of Ernest Gordon and Ann Gordon (*née* McFarlane); two of his brothers were also doctors.

Educ. Methodist College, Belfast; Queen's University Belfast

m. 1953: Mavis Bell; 3 s (one a consultant plastic surgeon in Belfast), 3 d

MB, QUB, 1948; MCh (with commendation), 1957; FRCS Ed, FRCSI (*ad eundem*), 1979

Postgraduate training initially in pathology and later in general surgery at RVH, Belfast.
Neurosurgical training, also in Belfast, with Cecil Calvert [q.v.], and Massachusetts General Hospital and Harvard University, Boston, USA, under William Sweet; also at Massachusetts Institute of Technology.
Consultant Neurosurgeon, RVH, Belfast, 1958–89.
Examiner, Royal College of Surgeons, Edinburgh.
Member, General Medical Council, 1985–94.
President, Society of British Neurological Surgeons, 1986–88.

Derek Gordon practised as a consultant surgeon at the Royal in Belfast until his retirement in 1989. He was President of the the Society of British Neurological Surgeons. He was only the second Irishman, after McConnell [q.v.], to hold that position. As an examiner in the Royal College of Surgeons in Edinburgh, he was instrumental with others in setting up the Specialist Fellowship in Neurosurgery, which was the first college and first specialty to do so, against some opposition at the time.

As a student, he captained the QUB athletics team. An outstanding figure in a strong department, he was tall, at least six foot, calm and perfectly groomed, with a distinguished appearance. He was admired and trusted by his colleagues and seems to have been born to chair every group, large or small, with which he was ever associated. He had a brilliant analytical mind and polished surgical skills.

When the operating microscope came to neurosurgery, he embraced it with enthusiasm and was essentially self-taught, with the help of his great friend and colleague, the internationally admired Gordon Smith, of the ENT Department.

Arguably his greatest clinical achievement was his leadership by example during most of the Northern Ireland 'Troubles', between 1969 and 1990. The continuous flow of brain and spinal injuries of novel and devastating nature was unknown in a western European hospital since the Second World War. Clinical decisions and operative management had to be re-learned. Gordon calmly deployed 'the troops' such as registrars Fannin [q.v.], Crockard and Byrnes [q.v.], insisted on maintaining operative standards and principles, and at the same time did not allow patients with core neurosurgical conditions to be forgotten or neglected. Many lessons were learned, not least the reality of futile and wasteful effort. There were treatment advances including titanium cranioplasty, which Gordon developed jointly with Blair of the School of Dentistry. Under his guidance and support, a routine system of intracranial pressure monitoring was developed.

His sense of humour, cleverly concealed just under the surface, and his authoritative dignity never slipped during times of greatest pressure and tension. He was certainly the father figure of Northern Irish, indeed Irish, neurosurgery in the second half of the twentieth century. Altogether a most admirable professional and role model.

TAYLOR, Alexander Robertson (Alec)

Consultant Neurosurgeon

b. 1916, son of a Scottish manse
Educ. University of Aberdeen
m. Alice Campbell-Bannerman (a close relative, perhaps a granddaughter, of Henry Campbell-Bannerman, British Prime Minister 1905–08); several sons, none of whom entered the medical profession
d. 1978.

MA, Aberdeen, 1937; MB, Aberdeen, 1941; FRCS Ed, 1946

Trained in neurosurgery in Edinburgh (under the great pioneer, Norman Dott).
Consultant neurosurgeon, RVH, Belfast, 1952–74.

Alec Taylor had a particular interest in spinal cord surgery. He also had a flair for research and was responsible for setting up a system of measuring cerebral blood flow, using an arterially injected isotope. This system was used clinically in the management of both subarachnoid haemorrhage and head injury.

An outgoing, very learned man, he was a stickler for the English language. He could be somewhat off-hand with his patients and others. His health was not particularly robust and he resigned for health reasons in 1974. He died in Scotland.

ORTHOPAEDIC SURGEONS

ADAIR, Ian Victor

Belfast Orthopaedic Surgeon

b. 1940, Belfast, son of James and Elizabeth Adair

Educ. Bangor; Queen's University Belfast

m. 1965: Margaret, in Bangor, where both of them went to school; 2 s (Andrew Ian, an orthopaedic surgeon; Stephen Richard, an obstetrician); 1 d (a dental surgeon)

MB, QUB, 1965; FRCS Ed, 1969

Postgraduate junior appointments as senior registrar in orthopaedics, Musgrave Park Hospital, Belfast. Postgraduate Fellowship to Ottawa.
Consultant orthopaedic surgeon, RVH, Belfast, and Musgrave Park Hospital, Belfast.
President, Irish Orthopaedic Association.

Ian's main interest was in spinal conditions and particularly spinal fusion. When he got married, in 1965, he was still a houseman and people rarely got married from such a junior position. He described his time in Ottawa as 'A wonderful experience'. Toronto at the time was probably the leading orthopaedic teaching centre in the world and there were close ties between Gordon Armstrong, his boss, and the 'Silver Fox', the uncrowned king of Canadian orthopaedics, Robert Salter. Armstrong had a large research programme in spinal surgery for the Canadian National Research Council. Ian's research involved early attempts to develop spinal cord monitoring during spinal deformity surgery, and the use of photogrammetric techniques for scoliosis screening. About his time in Canada, he said, 'My time away taught me the huge value and benefit to professional and family life of learning to swim in a "big pool" and yet not forget the roots... I have tried to pass this lesson to my family and juniors.'

After university rugby, Ian went back happily to play scrum half for Bangor RFC.

BAKER, George William

Belfast Orthopaedic Surgeon

Educ. Edinburgh University

MB, ChB, Edin, 1939; FRCS Ed, 1943; MChir Orth, Liverpool, 1948

Postgraduate junior appointments as house surgeon, Edinburgh Royal Infirmary; clinical assistant, Orthopaedic Department, Royal Infirmary, Edinburgh; assistant surgeon, Princess Margaret Rose Hospital, Edinburgh.

Consultant orthopaedic surgeon, Belfast City Hospital; Royal Belfast Hospital for Sick Children; Musgrave Park Hospital, Belfast; and Orthopaedic Hospital, Greenisland.

George Baker's main interest was in paediatric orthopaedics. He quickly established an excellent rapport with his patients and could put a nervous child at ease the moment he saw them. He left Northern Ireland in the 1960s to take up a post in his native Scotland.

BAIRD, David St Clair

Londonderry Orthopaedic Surgeon

b. 1933, Belfast, son of James Baird, said to be the first qualified dental surgeon in Northern Ireland; his mother was Scottish and had been a telegraphist in the General Post Office, Edinburgh.

Educ. Royal Belfast Academical Institute, 1943–50; Queen's University Belfast

m. Married with 3 s (Ian St Clair, killed in road traffic accident, 1997; Alasdair Crawford BSc, software engineer; Stuart James PhD, population geneticist)

MB, QUB, 1956; FRCS Ed, 1961

Postgraduate junior appointments as registrar, Harlow Wood Hospital, Nottinghamshire, 1963–64; senior orthopaedic registrar, Musgrave Park Hospital, Belfast.

Consultant orthopaedic surgeon, Altnagelvin Hospital, Londonderry.

David has a great interest in the Scout movement, having been a Wolf Cub at 7, a scout at 11, and later Medical Officer, County Commissioner and now County President. His hero is a faithful 'Old Scout', a long-dead national school teacher who was a patient teacher and a really kind man.

CALDERWOOD, James William, OBE (Jimmy)

Consultant Orthopaedic Surgeon, Eastern Health and Social Services Board

b. 1936, Londonderry, son of Rev. J. W. and Kathleen Calderwood

Educ. Foyle College, Londonderry; Queen's University Belfast

m. Married to a doctor; 2 d (both doctors; Catherine is consultant obstetrician/gynaecologist)

MB, QUB, 1966; FRCS Ed, 1970

Postgraduate junior appointments as house officer and senior house officer, RVH, Belfast; senior registrar, Northern Ireland Hospitals Authority; assistant to Professor R. Tubiana, Hôpital Ambrose Paré, Paris; registrar and Fellow of Professor Harold E. Kleinert, Jewish Hospital, Louisville, Kentucky, USA.

Consultant orthopaedic surgeon, Eastern Health and Social Services Board, at Belfast City Hospital and Musgrave Park Hospital, 1975–2001; RVH, Belfast, 1980–2001.

President, Ulster Medical Society, 1997–98.

Author of 'Analysis of Fractures in Belfast — in Particular Due to Gunshot Wounds and Bomb Injuries', Injury, 1975.

Jimmy Calderwood's main interest was in surgery of the hand, and especially arthroplasty of the finger joints. Golf is a passion and earlier he enjoyed squash and skiing.

CRYMBLE, Barry Templeton

Orthopaedic Surgeon, Northern Ireland Hospitals Authority

b. 1924, son of Professor P. T. Crymble [q.v.] (Professor of Surgery, QUB)
Educ. Campbell College; Queen's University Belfast
d. 1990

MB, Belfast, 1945; FRCS, 1951

Postgraduate junior appointments at the Wrightington Hospital, Wigan, near Manchester (with Professor Sir John Charnley).
Consultant orthopaedic surgeon, Northern Ireland Hospitals Authority, 1957–84.

Barry Crymble was the first surgeon to do the Charnley hip arthroplasty in Northern Ireland. (He may also have been the last, as he continued to perform it until his retirement, although many 'improved' variants were introduced.) His other area of interest was paediatric orthopaedics, in which his practice was extensive, and he delivered an outpatient service throughout Northern Ireland.

He was a keen golfer, a member of the Royal County Down Golf Club and President of the Golfing Union of Ireland. He had been a skilful hockey player in his youth. He was great fun at parties where he entertained on the piano and told amusing stories with great timing.

DILWORTH, George Raymond (Ray)

Consultant Orthopaedic Surgeon, Belfast

b. 1943, Belfast
Educ. Royal Belfast Academical Institution; Queen's University Belfast
m. Patricia; 1 s, 1 d (physiotherapist)

MB, QUB, 1969; FRCS Ed, 1973

Postgraduate training on North of Ireland Surgical Training Scheme; AO scholarship to Graz, Austria.
Consultant orthopaedic surgeon, Musgrave Park and Ulster Hospitals, 1980–2001.

His principal interest was in adult and children's foot surgery.

For recreation, Ray Dilworth enjoyed music, playing the saxophone, dance and concert bands. He is currently a member of the band of the Northern Ireland Fire & Rescue Service. Since retirement, he has completed a BA (hons) and an MA in Music. He also enjoys walking and gardening.

FENTON, George Irwin

Londonderry-Based Orthopaedic Surgeon

b. 1914, Seskinore, outside Omagh, Co. Tyrone, son of Samuel and Margaret Fenton
Educ. The Academy, Omagh; Queen's University Belfast
m. 4 s

MB, QUB, 1938; FRCSI, 1948

Postgraduate appointments at RVH, Belfast City Hospital and Musgrave Park Hospital.
GP, 1939–41.
Regimental Medical Officer, Royal Sussex Regiment, 1941–46.
Consultant orthopaedic surgeon, NW Hospital Group, based in Londonderry with clinics in Enniskillen and Omagh.

At 93, gardening is his main pastime. His former interests were horses, dogs, fishing and shooting.

JAMES, William Victor (Jimmy)

Belfast Orthopaedic Surgeon

b. 1923, Westcliff, Essex
Educ. Beckenham Grammar School, Kent; Southfield School, Oxford; Guy's Hospital, London
m. 1954: Sheila Martha Greaves, at Southwick, Sussex

MB, BS, Lond (Guy's Hospital), 1951; MRCS, LRCP, 1951; FRCS Ed, 1959

Senior government orthopaedic surgeon, Federation Rhodesia and Nyasaland. Government surgical specialist, Ndola, North Rhodesia.
Consultant orthopaedic surgeon, Musgrave Park Hospital, Belfast, and Northern Ireland Orthopaedic Service, 1967–88.
Chairman, Northern Ireland Prosthetic and Orthotic Aids Service.
Director, Rehabilitation Engineering Unit, Musgrave Park Hospital, Belfast.
Consultant to UN, Kingdom of Saudi Arabia, Foreign Office, UK.
Lieutenant-Colonel, 204 General Hospital, Territorial Army Volunteer Reserve, 1970–88.

As the years advanced, Jimmy became an international authority on disability, particularly those caused by amputations. The proliferation of land mines in civil conflicts meant that his advice was in constant demand. He has lectured all over the world and given a number of named addresses.

LOWRY, John Henry

Belfast Orthopaedic Surgeon

b. 1929, Belfast, son of Henry and Evelyn Lowry
Educ. Royal School, Armagh; Queen's University Belfast
m. 1958; 4 d, 1 s (J. P. Lowry, consultant radiologist, Belfast City Hospital)

MB, QUB, 1954; FRCS Ed, 1959; FRCSI (*ad eundem*), 1981

Postgraduate training: house officer, RVH, Belfast, 1954–55; demonstrator in anatomy, QUB, 1955–56; senior house officer, registrar, RVH, 1957–61; registrar and senior registrar, Notley Hospital, Braintree, Essex, and the London Hospital, 1962–64.
Consultant orthopaedic surgeon, RVH, 1965–89.

John Lowry performed the first hundred total knee replacements during the 1970s in Belfast. His recreations include equestrianism of all types and golf.

MACAFEE, Alastair Lowry

Belfast Orthopaedic Surgeon

b. 1935, Belfast, son of Professor C. H. G. Macafee CBE (Professor of Obstetrics and Gynaecology) and Margaret Crymble Lowry (daughter of Professor Charles G. Lowry, FRCSI)
Educ. Rockport Preparatory School, Glenalmond, Perthshire; Trinity College; Queen's University Belfast
m. Audrey Wilson, daughter of C. S. Wilson, MCh, and Margaret Gregg, FRCSI; 2 s (David Alastair Lowry Macafee is a surgical trainee), 2 d (Barbara Elizabeth Macafee, MD, is an anaesthetist)

MB (hons), QUB, 1959; MB (pathology), 1963; FRCS, 1967; FRCSI by election, 1980

Postgraduate junior trainee posts, RVH, Belfast (three years, morbid pathology); QUB (under Professor J. H. Biggart, MD), five years, general surgery. Began training in orthopaedics in 1968, with many visits abroad, especially to Switzerland, Berne, and Davos.
Consultant trauma orthopaedic surgeon, Ulster Hospital and Musgrave Park Hospital, 1973–95.
President, Irish Orthopaedic Association.
Medical director, Musgrave Park Hospital.
President, North of Ireland Medico-Legal Society.

Alastair Macafee's major interests were in hip replacement and trauma of joints. In retirement, he enjoys gardening, golf and woodwork.

McLEOD, Norman Walker

Consultant Orthopaedic Surgeon, Belfast

b. 1924
Educ. Belfast Royal Academical Institute; Queen's University Belfast
m. 2 s (Neil McLeod Harpur is consultant anaesthetist, Ulster Hospital)

MB, 1946; FRCS Ed, 1956

Trained at Belfast City Hospital and Musgrave Park Hospital; Sanderson Children's Hospital, Newcastle upon Tyne; Hexlan Hospital, Hull; and Belfast hospitals.
Consultant orthopaedic surgeon, Musgrave Park and Belfast City Hospitals.
Chairman and secretary, Irish Orthopaedic Club.

Published 'The First 100 Knee Replacements in Belfast' with J. H. Lowry [q.v.].

Norman McLeod's recreations include golf and sailing.

MARTIN, Norman Samuel, MBE (Mil.)

Belfast Orthopaedic Surgeon

b. 1912, son of the manse
Educ. Campbell College, Belfast; Queen's University Belfast
m. Son is an orthopaedic surgeon in South Africa
d. 1992

MB, 1935; MD, QUB, 1939; FRCS, 1941

Postgraduate junior appointments as orthopaedic registrar, Wingfield Morris Hospital, Oxford (with Professor Gaythorne Girdlestone); he helped to develop an innovative technique for arthrodesis of the hip.
Surgical specialist, Major, Royal Army Medical Corps.
Surgical specialist, EMS, Belfast.
Consultant orthopaedic surgeon, RVH, Belfast, Belfast City Hospital, Musgrave Park Hospital, Belfast, and Northern Ireland Orthopaedic Service, 1948–77.

Norman Martin joined the Royal Army Medical Corps immediately after getting his FRCS in 1941. He served in Burma throughout the war and was a proud member of the Burma Star Association, never missing the annual parade past Belfast City Hall.

Although he was a general orthopaedic surgeon, his great interest was in spinal tuberculosis, and he carried out many posterior and anterior spinal fusions, as well as surgery for fractures of the cervical spine. He published on all of these subjects.

He was a keen photographer and the Department of Orthopaedics has preserved many of his films. He was also a keen fisherman and his secretary was under instruction not to book major elective operations during the month of May, at which time he 'disappeared' to catch trout with the Mayfly at Lough Sheelin. His faithful dog, Bun, accompanied him. An enthusiastic motorcyclist in his early years, he would ride his motorcycle to Enniskillen for the clinic, often with his fishing rods across his back — ready for a day on Lough Melvin.

MOLLAN, Raymond Alexander Boyce (Rab)

Belfast Orthopaedic Surgeon

b. 1943, Belfast, son of Alexander Mollan and Margaret Emma Mollan (*née* Boyce)
Educ. Belfast Royal Academy, Queen's University Belfast
m. Rev. Dr Patricia Anne Fairbanks Scott (BSc, BD, first class hons, PhD); 3 s (2 medical practitioners, Ian Alexander and Andrew John), 1 d (Susan Patricia, medical practitioner)

MB (hons), 1969; DObst, Lond, 1972; FRCS Ed, 1974; MD, QUB, 1981; FRCSI (*ad eundem*), 1985; FRCS Eng (*ad eundem*), 1992; theological diplomas and certificates, Belfast Bible College, Church of Ireland Theological College, St John's Nottingham, 1993–98; Missiology (mission science) Module, BD Level (first class hons), QUB, 1998; MTheology, QUB, 2001

Postgraduate training: nine years at the RVH, Belfast, which included training in junior posts in obstetrics and senior posts in general surgery and orthopaedic surgery; multiple training visits to Europe, South Africa and North America, 1978–79.
Consultant orthopaedic surgeon, Ulster Hospital, Musgrave Park, 1979–81.
Senior lecturer and Professor of Orthopaedic Surgery, QUB, 1981–95;
Consultant surgeon, RVH and Musgrave Park Hospital, 1979–95.
Council, British Orthopaedic Association, 1986–95.
Chairman, Continuing Education Committee of the British Orthopaedic Association; member, Senate, Royal Colleges of Surgeons; founder, British Hip Society; editorial board of *Hip International*.
Taught and examined MTheology in Missiology at QUB and Belfast Bible College. The focus is the interface between medicine and theology.
Colonel Davis Memorial Scholarship, 1977; Robert Jones gold medal and prize — British Orthopaedic Association, 1981; Johnston & Johnston Travelling Fellowship, 1982; World Health Organisation Fellowship, 1984.

A general surgeon with a special interest in trauma, particularly those following road traffic accidents, Rab Mollan also had a special orthopaedic interest in biomaterials, biomechanics, bone and joint infection and arthroplasty. He represented the best of Ireland, North and South and was a great ambassador for the island in Great Britain and further afield. He resigned to take a part-time post as Theology Deacon in the Church of Ireland.

NIXON, James

Belfast Consultant Orthopaedic Surgeon

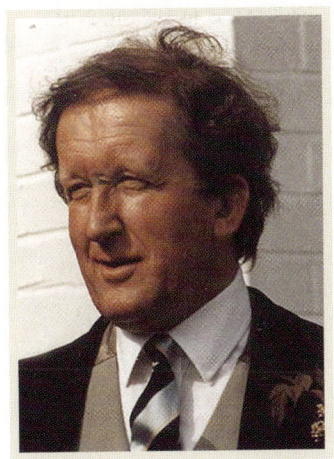

b. 1943, Belfast, son of Dr R. S. (Bob) Nixon, GP and Local MP, and Veda Nixon (*née* McKee); grew up in Bangor, Co. Down
Educ. Bangor Grammar School; Trinity College, Dublin; University of Liverpool
m. 1967: Catherine Nesbitt, daughter of Ronald and Ella Nesbitt, Dublin; 1 s (Alexander), 1 d (Holly)

Foundation scholar, 1964; BA, 1964; MA, 1968; MB, TCD, 1967; LM (Rotunda), 1969; DRCOG, 1969; FRCSI, 1971; FRCS Eng, 1972; MCh Orth, 1975

Postgraduate training in Dublin, Belfast, Londonderry, Liverpool, and Durban.
Consultant orthopaedic surgeon, Musgrave Park Hospital, Belfast City Hospital.
Honorary Professor of Orthopaedic Surgery, QUB.
President, British Hip Society; Northern Ireland Medicolegal Society.
Secretary, Irish Orthopaedic Club when it changed to Association.
Examiner in QUB, RCSI, Intercollegiate Speciality Board.
Editorial board, *Journal of Bone and Joint Surgery*.

Published papers on fat embolism, joint replacement, infection, and education.

James Nixon's special interests within surgery included adult hip surgery, bone and soft tissue tumour surgery, and education. His recreations included rugby at university, sailing (Trinity 'Pink', Irish Helmsman Champion), cruising Ireland, Scotland and the Arctic. He has served as Chairman of the Royal Yachting Association, Northern Ireland; Vice Commodore of the Irish Cruising Club; Rear Commodore of the Royal Ulster Yacht Club; and member of the Royal Cruising Club. He is the author of *Royal Ulster — a Yacht Club and its House*, 1999.

He has contributed enormously to orthopaedic and trauma surgery in Northern Ireland. Highly regarded amongst his peers he acquired a well-deserved reputation and built a valuable tertiary practice of revision hip surgery. Endowed with a determined, innovative and courageous disposition combined with distinct leadership qualities, he was willing and able to confidently face challenges and tackle complex problems whether in the clinical or administrative arena, or on the high seas.

OSTERBERG, Paul Harald

Consultant Orthopaedic Surgeon

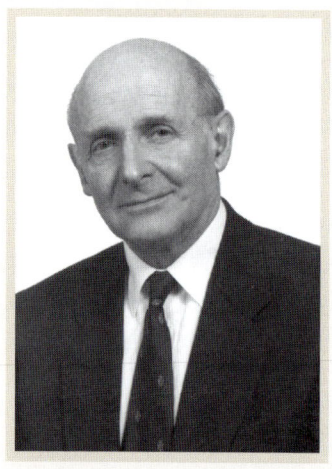

b. 1926, Copenhagen, son of Harald and Ethel Osterberg (Danish Consul General; civil engineer)
Educ. St Columba's College, Dublin; Trinity College, Dublin
m. 1952: Valerie Goodbody (d. 2006); 2 d

MA, MB, TCD, 1953 (prize-winner, anatomy and obstetrics); FRCSI, 1959; FRCS Eng, 1961

Postgraduate training: intern and registrar, Sir Patrick Dun's Hospital; registrar, RVH, Belfast; Royal National Orthopaedic Hospital, London; senior registrar, Northern Ireland Orthopaedic Service.
Consultant orthopaedic surgeon, RVH and Musgrave Park Hospital Belfast; Northern Ireland Orthopaedic Service, 1964–90.
Visiting Professor, Pahlavi University, Shiraz, Iran, 1956.
Founding surgeon in charge of spinal injuries unit, Musgrave Park Hospital, Belfast.
President, Irish Orthopaedic Club; Irish Orthopaedic Association.
Executive Committee British Orthopaedic Association, 1979–80.
Orator, Royal Victoria Hospital, 1989, on 'Lure and Lore of Surgery'.

Influenced by Professor R. I. Wilson [q.v.], Sir Herbert Seddon, Sir Ian Fraser [q.v.] and Professor Thomasen (Denmark).

Paul Osterberg was probably the last of the general orthopaedic surgeons of Northern Ireland. He covered all aspects of the specialty and perhaps increasing sub-specialising prompted his early retirement at age 63. Aged 10, in 1936, he had come to Ireland from a Danish childhood, via New York. As a Danish speaker, he had an interest in languages.

He served in the British Army from 1944 to 1947, where he was a lieutenant in the Queen's Own Royal West Kent Regiment, attached to the Royal Artillery in Palestine.

In his tranquil retirement, he kept up his interest in family life, sailing, gardening and world travel. He was part of Ian Fraser's bridge group and was a close friend of the great man. He has a real gift for friendship.

PIGGOTT, James (Jimmy)

Belfast Orthopaedic Surgeon

b. 1924, Londonderry, son of James A. Piggott (OBE, DL, JP) and Elizabeth M. Piggott (*née* Duff)
Educ. Foyle College, Londonderry; Queen's University Belfast
m. Joy Macilwaine (SRN); 3 d (including Anne, SRN SRCN), 2 s

MB, QUB, 1946; FRCSE, 1954

Postgraduate training appointments at RVH, Belfast; Princess Elizabeth Orthopaedic Hospital, Exeter; registrar and research assistant (with Norman Capener) for five years.
Consultant orthopaedic surgeon, Musgrave Park Hospital, Royal Belfast Hospital for Sick Children and Ulster Hospital for Women and Children, 1960–89.
Editorial board of *Journal of Bone and Joint Surgery*.
Examiner for FRCS orthopaedics, 1979–89.
President, Ulster Paediatric Society for ten years. Honorary member, British Children's Orthopaedic Society. Member, British Orthopaedic Travellers.

Jimmy Piggott's special interest was in children's orthopaedics. As a student, he played rugby and was Captain of QUB RFC. He played for Ulster, Irish Universities, Irish Final Trials, Exeter, and Devon County. In later life, he enjoyed golf and was winner of the Robert Jones Cup at Glasgow BOA, 1990.

PRICE, Gavin

Londonderry Orthopaedic Surgeon

b. 1943, Brighouse, son of Harold and Adelaide Price
Educ. St Edward's School, Oxford; Queen's University Belfast
m. Jennifer; 1 s, 1 d

MB, QUB, 1967; FRCS Ed, 1973

Consultant orthopaedic surgeon, Altnagelvin Area Hospital.
Principal orthopaedic surgeon, Addington Hospital, South Beach, Durban, 1975–79.

Gavin Price's pastimes include walking, sailing, swimming and tennis.

PYPER, James Bothwell (Jay)

Belfast Orthopaedic Surgeon

b. 1924, Bangor, Co. Down, son of John Pyper and Elizabeth Pyper (*née* Patton)
Educ. Bangor Grammar School; Queen's University Belfast
m. Dr Pauline Charlton; 1 s (Patrick, consultant surgeon Mid-Ulster Hospital), 1 d

MB (hons), QUB, 1946; FRCS Eng, 1951. As an undergraduate he won five scholarships, two exhibitions and a gold medal.

Postgraduate training posts of increasing responsibility at RVH, Belfast, Belfast Children's Hospital, Musgrave Park Hospital and other hospitals in Northern Ireland.
Registrar, Princess Elizabeth Orthopaedic Hospital, Exeter, 1953–55.
AO Basic Course, Davos, 1975; advanced course, Stoke-on-Trent, 1975. One month work-study with Professor B. G. Weber, Kantonsspital (St Gallen), Switzerland, 1977.
Chairman, Irish Orthopaedic Association.
North of Ireland Orthopaedic Service, Musgrave Park and Belfast City Hospital. Consultant, 1959–85.

In the past, Jay Pyper was a high-board diver. He is a lapsed angler and also dinghy sailed with a mutinous crew. He enjoyed hill-walking and skiing until he was over seventy. He now enjoys painting.

TAYLOR, Trevor Childs

Consultant Orthopaedic Surgeon, Belfast

b. 1943, Belfast, son of James Childs Taylor and Dorothy Ann Taylor (*née* Strong)
Educ. Bangor Grammar School; Queen's University Belfast
m. Dr Alice Swann; 2 s, 1 d

MB, QUB, 1968; FRCS Ed, 1972; FRCS (*ad eundem*), 1995; FRCSI (*ad eundem*), 2002

Belfast surgical rotation programme and Northern Ireland orthopaedic training programmes.
Resident and Orthopaedic Fellow, Hospital for Sick Children, Toronto, 1975–76.
Associate staff member (junior consultant), Bloorview Children's Hospital (Canada's largest children's rehabilitation hospital), Willowdale, Ontario, 1976.
Consultant orthopaedic surgeon to Mater Hospital, Belfast, Musgrave Park Hospital and Royal Belfast Hospital for Sick Children, 1977–2004.

TEMPLETON, John

Northern Ireland Orthopaedic Surgeon

b. 1937, Ballyclare, Co. Antrim, son of Alexander Templeton and Jane Templeton (*née* Barr)
Educ. Ballyclare High School; Queen's University Belfast
m. Patricia; 2 s (Peter, consultant orthopaedic surgeon, Leeds Teaching Hospitals, NHS Trust; Colin, Royal Canadian Mounted Police), 1 d (Claire, solicitor, London)

MB, QUB, 1961; FRCS (C), 1970; FRCS Eng (*ad eundem*), 1991

House surgeon, RVH, Belfast; junior resident, University of Saskatoon; senior resident, RVH, Montreal; chief resident, Shriners Hospital, Montreal; research registrar, Nuffield Orthopaedic Centre, Oxford.
Orthopaedic surgeon in chief, Queen Elizabeth Hospital, Montreal 1970–77.
Consultant orthopaedic surgeon, Altnagelvin Hospital, Londonderry, 1978–79.
Consultant orthopaedic surgeon, RVH and Musgrave Park Hospital, Belfast, 1979–88.
Professor of Traumatic Orthopaedic Surgery, Keele University, 1988–98; Dean, Faculty of Medicine & Health, Keele University, 1995–98.
President, British Trauma Society, 1994–95.
Medical director, Nuffield Orthopaedic Centre, NHS Trust, Oxford, 2001–04.

John Templeton's special interests were surgery and trauma. His recreations include golf and hill-walking.

WILSON, Robert Irvine, MBE (Mil.) (Bob)

Belfast Orthopaedic Surgeon and first Professor of Orthopaedics, QUB

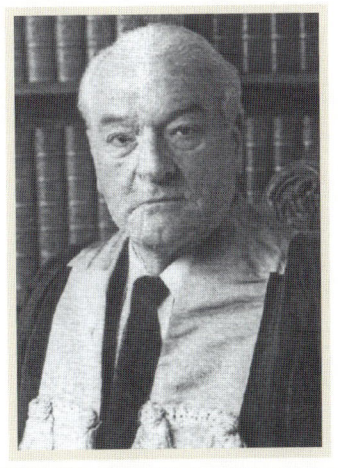

b. 1915, Belfast, son of James and Maimie Wilson
Educ. Royal Belfast Academical Institute, Queen's University Belfast
m. 1940: Kathleen Withers; 1 s (Brian, obstetrician, USA), 3 d (Patricia, physiotherapist (deceased); Maureen, retired GP in New Zealand; Oonagh, retired nursing sister)
d. 2007

MB, QUB, 1938; FRCS Ed, 1947; FRCSI (*ad eundem*), 1974

Postgraduate junior appointments as registrar, RVH, Belfast; Princess Elizabeth Orthopaedic Hospital, Exeter, with Norman Capener.
Consultant orthopaedic surgeon, Musgrave Park Hospital, Belfast; RVH, Belfast; Ulster Hospital for Children and Women, 1949–86.

Honorary Lieutenant-Colonel, Royal Army Medical Corps. Had a very active service career, particularly in Italy.

First Professor of Orthopaedic Surgery, QUB, 1979; developed undergraduate and graduate education locally and nationally.

Vice-President, British Orthopaedic Association; Chairman, Specialist Advisory Committee in Orthopaedics; editorial board, *Journal of Bone and Joint Surgery*.

President and enthusiastic supporter, Irish Orthopaedic Association.

Bob Wilson was the third consultant orthopaedic surgeon appointed, joining Jimmy Withers [q.v.] and Norman Martin [q.v.]. He quickly became the leader in expanding the service. Tuberculosis and poliomyelitis were rife at that time, and Musgrave Park Hospital had many patients for long terms. He established the Northern Ireland Orthopaedic Service with Gladys Morris, an experienced physiotherapist who had trained in Oswestry. The service created over twenty orthopaedic clinics across Northern Ireland, with surgeons, after-care nurse and secretaries travelling out from Musgrave Park. As these diseases lessened in frequency, he developed interests in hip arthroplasty, Paget's disease, fracture management and the fat embolus syndrome. He remained a well-read surgeon throughout his career. He was the long-standing Chairman of the Orthopaedic Division, which included all consultants in Northern Ireland. He was particularly effective in negotiations with government, often to the point of bluntness: 'A spade is a spade.' The steady growth of the specialty is mainly the result of his influence in those early days. (There are now forty-two consultants in post).

A big man physically, he had great charisma, which made him an excellent role model for his many trainees. The patients and staff at all levels loved him. The QUB Undergraduate Medal for Orthopaedics is named after him. He had it all and he gave his all. 'There's only one Bob Wilson.'

WITHERS, Robert James Wilson (Jimmy)

Belfast Orthopaedic Surgeon

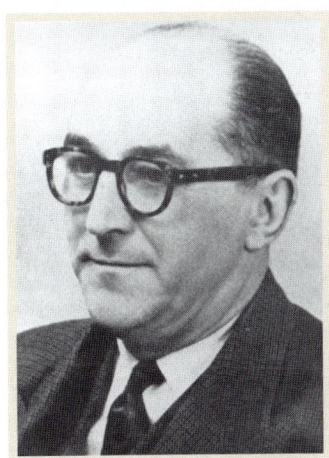

b. 1908
Educ. Queen's University Belfast
d. 1965

MB (first class hons and scholarship), 1930; MD (gold medal), 1933; FRCS Ed, 1934; MChir (commendation), 1936

Postgraduate junior appointments as house surgeon, RVH, Belfast; house surgeon, Hull Royal Infirmary, Clayton Hospital, Wakefield, and Oldham Royal Infirmaries.
Resident surgical officer, North Manchester Municipal Hospital.
Consultant orthopaedic surgeon, Ulster Hospital, Belfast, Ministry of Health Hospital, Musgrave Park Hospital, Belfast, and RVH, Belfast 1945–65.
Lecturer in orthopaedics, QUB.

Jimmy Withers was the first orthopaedic surgeon in Northern Ireland who confined his practice to the specialty. He had run a fracture clinic when he was a registrar, and built a specialty service for the whole of the province and particularly the long-stay unit at Musgrave Park.

He was a popular teacher, a fount of amusing stories, appropriate and otherwise, and an unbiased opinion in the law courts. The Orthopaedic Centre at Musgrave Park Hospital is named after him.

A dapper man, he was always well turned out, with a flower in his buttonhole; he was the epitome of the consultant surgeon of that time.

Paediatric Surgeons

SMYTH, Brian T.

Consultant Paediatric Surgeon, Belfast

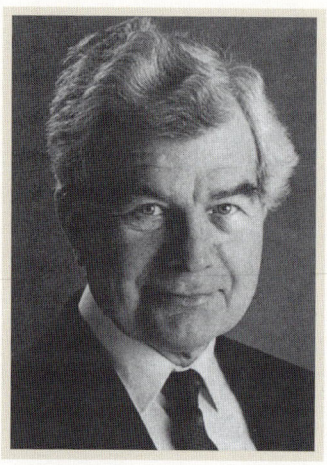

b. 1921, third son of William Smith and Flora Smith (*née* Lindsay)

Educ. Coleraine Academic Institution; Queen's University Belfast

m. 1965: Anne Disney, daughter of Frederick and Lillian Disney; 1 s, 1 d

MB, QUB, 1945; FRCS Eng, 1952

Postgraduate appointments as house surgeon and house physician, RVH, Belfast; demonstrator in Anatomy, QUB; Musgrave research student in pathology; surgical registrar, Royal Belfast Hospital for Sick Children and RVH, Belfast.

Paediatric surgical training at the Hospital for Sick Children, Great Ormond Street, London, and the Royal Liverpool Children's Hospital.

Research Fellow in Surgery, School of Medicine, Tufts University, Boston, 1957–58, with Dr Orvar Swenson, one of the giants of the specialty.

Consultant paediatric surgeon, to Royal Belfast Hospital for Sick Children and the Ulster Hospital, 1959–86.

Chairman, Ulster Paediatric Society; Medical Staff Committee, Royal Belfast Hospital for Sick Children.

Brian Smyth epitomised quiet determination. During his twenty-seven years as the first full-time paediatric surgeon in Northern Ireland, he persistently pursued the authorities to provide essential accommodation, equipment and staff necessary for a first-class service. The development of his unit had the priceless sponsorship of Sir Ian Fraser [q.v.] but progress was slow and would have daunted a lesser man. Although the major building programme came after he retired, the paediatric surgical service, which Brian pioneered, is now firmly established and recognised. He left behind a vibrant unit, which is recognised throughout the speciality. He had a special interest in the surgical management of Hirschsprung's disease and also in paediatric urology.

Brian was built like a back-row forward and his distinctive lower-register voice was never raised, except when the situation was critical. His many qualities included a ready smile, a friendly disposition and a warm sense of humour. He was popular with the entire hospital staff. When younger, he was active in rugby football, rowing and cruising under sail. He was always interested in woodwork, photography, music, Italian culture and language. In retirement, he has become an associate of the Royal Photographic Society.

BOSTON, Victor Ernest (Vic, 'Slick Vic')

Belfast Paediatric Surgeon

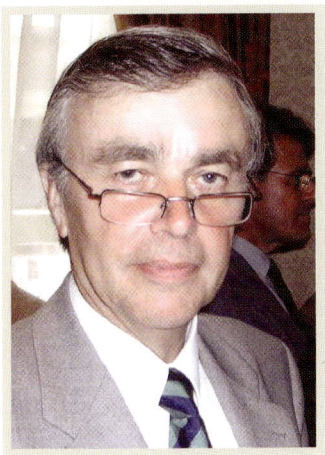

b. 1945, son of James and Joyce Boston. Maternal grandfather was a Danish missionary surgeon in Labrador.
Educ. Friends' School, Lisburn; Queen's University Belfast
m. 1968: Elaine Johnson, BA TCD; 2 adopted sons

MB, QUB, 1968; FRCS Ed, 1972; MD, Thesis, 1980; FRCSI (*ad eundem*), 1987; FRCS Eng (*ad eundem*), 1998

Commenced postgraduate training in paediatric surgery in Belfast, 1972, under Brian Smyth [q.v.], having previously been appointed General Surgeon in Edson, Alberta, Canada. Newcastle-upon-Tyne, 1973–75 under John Scott and John Wagget. Cape Town, 1976–77, under Jannie Louw, Syd Cywes and Michael Davies.
Consultant paediatric surgeon, Royal Hospital for Sick Children, Belfast; Ulster Hospital, Dundonald, 1977–2005; Belfast City Hospital, 1977–88.
Honorary senior lecturer, Department of Surgery, 1988–2005.
President, British Association of Paediatric Surgeons, 2004–06; Ulster Paediatric Society, 1989.
Member, Council, RCS Ed and RCS Eng. Editor for Great Britain & Ireland, *Journal of Paediatric Surgery*.
Chairman, Intercollegiate Board in Paediatric Surgery.

Vic Boston's research interests included Hirschsprung's disease, sepsis, nutrition and topical anaesthesia. He played an important role in the development of EMLA, the topical anaesthetic which reduces the pain of injections.

'Slick Vic' was a massively talented operating surgeon. He could complete an operation in the time it took to show a film of it — a really rare attribute. Hugely popular within the specialty, he seems to be always in good humour and was a superb colleague. His premature retirement, largely the result of a supine administrative decision, means that Belfast has lost a bright beacon surgeon and a first-rate role model.

His recreations, almost too numerous to mention, include golf: he was a Golf Blue at QUB (played down to five handicap), and represented Ireland in the Irish Universities Golf Team. He represented Ireland in 1984 in Flying Fifteen World Championship (with the 'almost' ever-loyal Elaine as the only crew). He is also a wind surfer, a paraglider, and, since the age of 52, a skier (his newest fanaticism). An exhibition-class cabinetmaker, he is also an advanced computer programmer. Even reading of his activities makes one feel lazy.

In his own words, he is 'enlarging round the middle despite all the exercise, greying, laid back. Dislikes inconsistency, injustice, dishonesty and inequality.'

Plastic Surgeons

HUGHES, Norman Campbell, OBE

Belfast Plastic Surgeon

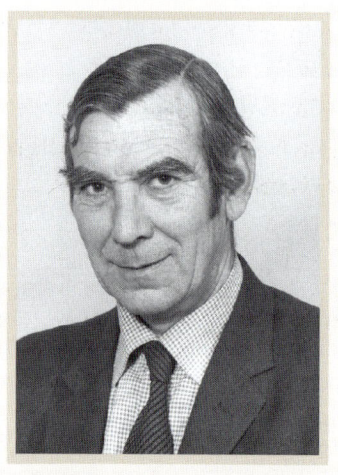

b. 1915, Bangor, Co. Down, son of William Edwin Hughes and Elizabeth Hughes (*née* Campbell)
Educ. Bangor Grammar School; Queen's University Belfast
m. 1946: Dr Rosemary Fullerton; 1 s, 2d (Mary, a GP; Anne, a geneticist)
d. 1995

MB, QUB, 1937; MRCS & LRCP, 1937; FRCS, 1947; Hon FRCSI, 1973

Royal Army Medical Corps, 1939–43.
Surgeon, Cairo, with Mortimer Shaw, from 1943.
Marks Fellowship to East Grinstead Hospital, 1947–50, under Archibald McIndoe.
Consultant plastic surgeon, Belfast, from 1950.
Chairman, Specialist Advisory Committee for Plastic Surgery.
President, British Association of Plastic Surgeons, 1977.
Hunterian Professorship, RCS, 1979.

In the Royal Army Medical Corps, Norman Hughes volunteered for the Commandos and did the full training programme of a fighting soldier, including much imposed hardship in the snow and ice of the Cairngorms. He was trained in hand-to-hand fighting with knives and pistols and was involved in the Lofoten Commando raid. He carried medical equipment in addition to personal arms and ammunition. The Lofoten islands were on the northern Norway coast, 100 miles inside the Arctic Circle, and the raid was carried out in March 1941. In 1943, the

Commandos were merged with Royal Marines and he resumed his medical career as a graded surgeon. In Cairo, he worked with Mortimer Shaw, an experienced maxillofacial surgeon, and this was to be decisive.

He returned to the RVH, Belfast, and was awarded a Marks Fellowship to East Grinstead Hospital for three years under the legendary (Sir) Archibald McIndoe, a known perfectionist and taskmaster. In 1950, he was invited to return to Belfast as a consultant to set up a Plastic Surgery and Burns Unit for Northern Ireland. He quickly built a unit of the highest quality. A most dedicated professional, he greatly enjoyed teaching and never missed an opportunity to pay tribute to the founders of his specialty. He wrote little but contributed various invited chapters to Rob and Smith's Operative Surgery.

Tall, distinguished looking, with silver hair and a permanent sailor's tan, Norman had the sort of effortless superiority which is sometimes recognisable in a school playground. An all-round sportsman, he was particularly involved in rugby, cricket, tennis and skiing, which he had learnt as a commando. He was an experienced offshore sailor and loved family cruises off the west coast of Scotland. His woodwork, as one might expect, was a model of skill and precision.

In 1992, the Regional Burns Unit was dedicated in his name, and he was there to unveil the plaque. He was the first plastic surgeon in Northern Ireland and he set the standard for that internationally known unit. Well done.

DICKIE, William Robert (Wilbert)

Plastic Surgeon, Belfast

b. 1917
m. 1st: Annabel (d.); 3 children (all doctors). 2nd: Betty
Educ. Queen's University Belfast
d. 1999

MB, QUB, 1940; FRCS Ed, 1948

Postgraduate appointments to Manchester Royal Infirmary for two and a half years.
Northern Ireland plastic and maxillofacial service. Ulster Hospital, Dundonald; Royal Hospital for Sick Children, Belfast, 1954–80; RVH, Belfast, 1958–80.
Medical Officer, British Red Cross Unit, China, the Order of St John.

Wilbert Dickie's principal interest was in hand surgery. A broken leg as a child decided his career, and an ugly scar on the back of his head decided his specialty. His hospital in China was twice evacuated because of the advancing Japanese army. He then became a relief surgeon for the Chinese government who gave him an award. He was a complete perfectionist and would scrutinise a freshly sewn wound or graft, find it wanting, open it up and do it again. This was called 'doing a Dickie'. The patients would have approved. He had a great wit and genuine humour.

He retired to gardening but also as the mainspring of a five-a-side football team called the Geriatric Dynamos. He also became a dedicated bowler.

COLVILLE, John

Belfast Plastic and Hand Surgeon

b. 1930, Belfast, elder son of James Colville and Mary Jane Colville (*née* Orr)
Educ. Royal Belfast Academical Institution; Queen's University Belfast
m. 1955: Edith Naomi Johnston, daughter of Thomas and Elizabeth Johnston; 2 s (Colin is consultant anaesthetist, Oxford)

MB, QUB, 1955; DRCOG, 1957; FRCS Ed, 1962

Postgraduate junior posts at Pittsburgh University Hospital, Pittsburgh, Pennsylvania, USA (with Willie White).
Consultant plastic and hand surgeon, RVH, Belfast; Royal Hospital for Sick Children, Belfast; Ulster Hospital, Dundonald, 1968–90.
President, British Society for Surgery of the Hand, 1988; British Association of Plastic Surgeons, 1990. Chairman, Specialist Advisory Committee on Plastic Surgery (SAC), 1987–90. Examiner in plastic surgery, FRCS.

One of the earliest to re-implant thumbs and whole hands successfully, John Colville made his own micro-surgical instruments from jeweller's tools. A 'surgical engineer' with his own well-equipped workshop in which he undertakes major metal projects up to steam engine, he now makes long-case clocks.

He was also an accomplished offshore sailor most of his life, serving as the commodore of the East Down Yacht Club, 1970, and as a member of the council of the Royal Yachting Association. He also sang with Belfast Philharmonic Choir. A warm 'late developer', who has led and is leading a full and most useful life.

SLATER, Ronald MacCollum

Belfast Plastic Surgeon

Educ. Queen's University Belfast

MB, QUB, 1955; FRCS Ed, 1964; DObst, RCOG, 1957

Plastic surgeon, Ulster Hospital; RVH, Belfast; Royal Hospital for Sick Children, 1971–91

Urologists

KENNEDY, Joseph Aloysius (Joe)

Belfast Urologist

b. 1930, eldest son of Frank Kennedy (obstetrician, Mater Hospital, Belfast) and Mary Kennedy (*née* Magee)
Educ. Queen's University Belfast
m. 1961: Claire McSparran (distinguished solicitor and sometime Chair of Belfast Port Authority), daughter of James McSparran QC (fearless Nationalist MP) and Claire McSparran; 1 s (Andrew, a surgeon), 3 d (Catriona is a GP)
d. 2006

MB, QUB, 1955; FRCS Ed, 1959; MCh, 1962

Postgraduate appointments as resident surgical officer, St Peter's Hospital, London (largely with John Fergusson); Fellow, Mayo Clinic, Rochester, Minnesota, 1961–62.
Senior registrar surgery, RVH, Belfast.
Lecturer, Institute of Urology, London.
Consultant urologist, South Belfast & Belfast Group Hospitals, mainly Belfast City Hospital.

As the first fully trained urologist to work in Belfast, Joe Kennedy set about modernising the Department with great vigour. Gentle, patient, attentive and understanding, he was popular with patients and medical staff.

Joe was tall, handsome, upright, distinguished in appearance, with sleeked hair, showing just the right amount of grey, and always well dressed — this last in part thanks to his elegant wife, Claire. He loved sailing, both cruising and racing. When racing he drove himself and his crew to distraction and was in his element in the waters round Baltimore, Co. Cork. He was also keen on gardening in their manicured home, and loved travel, food and wine. He could be impatient with the bureaucratic process, an impatience that came with a substantial price tag, but with family and friends he was a sweet-natured, kind-hearted, generous and devoted husband, parent and grandparent. Tragically he and Claire died within twenty-four hours of one another.

LOUGHRIDGE, William Gordon Galt (Gordon)

Belfast Urologist

b. son of Jamsie Loughridge [q.v.]

Educ. Harrow School, London; Queen's University Belfast

MA, MB, BChir, Camb, 1963; MD, QUB, 1966; MB, ChB, 1962, QUB; FRCS Ed, 1969; FRCS Eng, 1970

Postgraduate junior appointments as house surgeon, Hammersmith Hospital, London; University tutor in pathology, QUB; resident surgical officer, St Peter's Hospital, London. Consultant urologist, Belfast City Hospital and RVH, Belfast.
Northern Ireland Spinal Injuries Unit, Musgrave Park Hospital, Belfast, 1972–2003. Honorary consultant urologist, Musgrave Park; locum consultant urologist, Causeway Hospital, Coleraine, 2003–06.

Gordon Loughridge became one of the outstanding medical witnesses of his time. He had over thirty years' experience and unusually his work was almost evenly divided between defendants and claimants. His work ranged over clinical negligence, personal injury, road traffic accidents and industrial exposure to hazardous substances. He gave evidence in almost every major court, north and south. He holds the Cardiff University Bond Solon Expert Witness Certificate, 2005. (This hugely important development in medico-legal work means that an expert witness of the 'hired gun variety' may be questioned about their special qualifications to testify on the case under review.) A warm, generous spirit.

9
PROFESSORS OF SURGERY IN THE REPUBLIC OF IRELAND

PROFESSORS OF SURGERY IN THE REPUBLIC OF IRELAND

Departments of Surgery in the Medical Schools

Ireland began and ended the twentieth century with six medical schools. It may be the only country in the world not to have increased the number during that time. The graduating classes varied from a low of twelve at UCC in 1960 to over 250 at the RCSI at the century's end. For the first sixty or seventy years, there was a mass emigration of expensively trained doctors. Perhaps 80 per cent of each graduating class went abroad, mainly to Great Britain, and latterly, in lesser numbers, to the United States, and a trickle to Australia. By the turn of the millennium, however, there was a shortage of doctors at all levels, and overseas graduates who had spent years training in Ireland and elsewhere were filling many of the consultant posts both inside and outside the teaching centres.

There were changes in the names of four of the six medical schools during the twentieth century. They will be taken in order of foundation date.

The University of Dublin has a single college, Trinity, often referred to as Trinity College, Dublin (TCD). Trinity or TCD is used in this work. It has had a medical school since the early eighteenth century. The exact date depends somewhat on the definition of what constitutes a medical school. Catholics were prohibited from attending TCD until the early 1970s. The ban was widely ignored in later years.

The Royal College of Surgeons in Ireland has had an undergraduate medical school dating back to its foundation in 1784. It amalgamated a number of private medical schools in the late nineteenth century. Under its royal charters, it issued 'letters testimonial' and diplomas, but not a university degree until the arrangement with UCD in 1978. Together with the Royal College of Physicians of Ireland, it still awards the qualifying diploma of Licentiate of the Royal College of Physicians and Surgeons Ireland (LRCP&SI) as well as the National University of Ireland (NUI) degree. For degree-granting purposes it has become a college of the NUI.

The three Queen's Colleges, in Belfast, Cork and Galway, were founded in 1845, and quickly established medical schools. In 1879, the Royal University of Ireland (RUI) was established in Earlsfort Terrace, Dublin. It consisted of the Queen's Colleges of Belfast, Cork and Galway and the Catholic University of Ireland, forerunner of University College, Dublin. Cardinal Newman had established in Dublin what was in his eyes to be a rival to the Oxbridge universities and had called it the Catholic University of Ireland (CUI).

Catholic University Medical School was established in Cecilia Street in the Temple Bar area of the city in 1855. Its qualifications were initially not legally recognised and 'graduates' were given their 'letters testimonial' by the RCSI. This generosity of spirit was to be reciprocated a hundred years later when RCSI graduates were given their degree by UCD. The Catholic University of Ireland became a college of the Royal University of Ireland, in 1879, and then a college of the National University of Ireland in 1908.

The Royal University was dissolved in 1908 when it was divided into two, the National University of Ireland and Queen's College, Belfast. The NUI had then three constituent colleges, the University Colleges of Cork, Dublin and Galway. Queen's College, Belfast, became the independent Queen's University Belfast (QUB). In 1997, Galway became National University of Ireland, Galway (NUIG). Cork retained the name University College Cork (UCC).

Professors of Surgery at the RCSI

For the first half of the century, the professors of surgery at the RCSI were, as elsewhere, part-time appointments. The College does not allow employees to sit on the College Council. The effect of this was that those who wished to be elected to the Council, and at that time most of the Council could expect to become President in turn, had to resign their position at the College. Some then went over to Trinity and were appointed to chairs there. Trinity had two chairs, Professor of Surgery and Regius Professor of Surgery.

The Department of Surgery, Trinity College, Dublin, in the Twentieth Century

For all its academic distinction in so many fields, Trinity had no real department of surgery for the first three-quarters of the twentieth century. There are various reasons for this but the two principal ones were firstly, that there never seemed to be enough funds to employ a full-time professor, whose private practice was confined to the teaching hospital, and the appropriate back-up staff. Worldwide experience has shown that surgical academic endeavour prospers where the professor is geographically full-time — that is, where he has his entire practice on the campus of the teaching hospital. The second reason was that there were a number of, robustly competing, small hospitals under the Trinity umbrella, of which the principal, Sir Patrick Dun's, had only about 120 beds. All the professorial appointments up to 1975 were part-time and were paid at best a notional salary, on the basis that the title and associated patronage would recompense the holder. The appointment of T. P. J. (Tom) Hennessy [q.v.] in 1975 changed all that. Moving from the soon-to-be-closed Royal City of Dublin (Baggot Street) Hospital to the vast, but neglected and underdeveloped, campus of St James's Hospital on James's Street showed Trinity's centuries-old tradition of caring for the sick poor of Dublin at its altruistic best. Sir Patrick Dun's and Mercer's Hospital were closed afterwards and they too moved to the huge site, to make St James's the biggest acute hospital in the state.

Regius Chair of Surgery, University of Dublin

BALL, Sir Charles Bent, Bt

Regius Professor of Surgery, TCD, and Dublin Surgeon

b. 1851, younger son of Robert Ball, LLD
Educ. Trinity College, Dublin
m. 1874: Annie Julia Kinahan; 3 s (one was (Sir) Charles Arthur Kinahan Ball [q.v.]), 4 d
d. 1916

AB, 1871; MD, 1875; MB, MCh, 1872; FRCSI, 1879; FRCS Eng (hon.), 1900

Postgraduate appointments at TCD and Vienna; medical scholarship, TCD; senior medical exhibition and travel prize, 1872.
Regius Professor of Surgery, TCD, 1895–1916.
Surgeon, Sir Patrick Dun's & Simpson's Hospitals, Dublin.

Chancellor's consultant surgeon visitor in lunacy; consultant surgeon, Dr Steevens' Hospital, Monkstown Hospital, Orthopaedic, & Dental Hospitals, Stewart Institution & Masonic Girls' School Dublin.
Member, advisory board for Army Medical Service (precursor of Royal Army Medical Corps).
President, Dublin University Biological Association; secretary, Royal Academy of Medicine, Ireland, Dublin branch, and Surgical Section, BMA.
Member, Council RCSI. Representative of TCD on General Medical Council.
Honorary surgeon to HM the King in Ireland.
Lane Lecture, San Francisco, 1902; Erasmus Wilson Lecture, RCS, 1903.

Author of *Rectum & Anus, their Diseases & Treatment*, 2nd edition, 1894; 'Rectum' in *A System of Surgery* (edited by F. Treves, 1895); 'The Rectum: Its Diseases & Developmental Defects', 1908; 'Melanotic Sarcoma of Rectum', 'Benign Neoplasms of Rectum', 1890; 'Radical Care of Hernia by Torsion of Sac', *British Medical Journal*, 1884

Sir Charles was a hugely prominent figure in surgery in his time, rivalled nationally only by John S. McArdle (UCD) [q.v.] and Sir Thomas Myles [q.v.]. He occupied the Regius Chair of Surgery between 1895 and 1916. A man of imposing appearance, he combined a detailed knowledge of anatomy (he described a valve of the rectum which bears his name) and impressive clinical and teaching skills with a progressive and courageous approach to operative surgery. He was described as 'lavish in public work'. He was one of Dublin's pioneers in neurosurgery and successfully carried out intra-cranial operations in the late nineteenth century at Sir Patrick Dun's Hospital, but it was as a specialist in diseases of the rectum that he had an international reputation. His textbook on the subject was the standard work for many years. The title on the spine read *Ball on the Rectum*.

His family was distinguished. His eldest brother, Robert, was an FRS and Astronomer Royal in Ireland. The other, Valentine Ball, CB, was Director of the Dublin Museum.

TAYLOR, Edward Henry PRCSI 1920–1922

Regius Professor of Surgery, TCD, and Dublin Surgeon

b. 1867, eldest son of Wentworth Taylor of Tinahely, Co. Wicklow
Educ. Trinity College, Dublin
d. 1922

MD (stip. cond.), Dublin, 1896; MB, 1890; FRCSI, 1896; MCh (hon. causa) (TCD and Vienna); Surgical Travelling Prize

Lecturer in applied anatomy, TCD; assistant surgeon, Sir Patrick Dun's.
Professor of Surgery, TCD, 1906–16; surgeon, Sir Patrick Dun's Hospital.
Regius Professor of Surgery, TCD, 1916–22.
President, RCSI, 1920–22; Dublin University Biological Association.

The surgical travelling prize enabled Edward Taylor to study under Von Eiselsberg, Billroth's successor in Vienna. He returned to Dublin where he proceeded with his MD and became a Fellow of the RCSI in 1896. He produced a monograph on *Applied Anatomy* and later a textbook of operative *Surgery* (1914). His many published papers included such subjects as the treatment of peritonitis, hernia and rectal cancer, but his ability to use his anatomical knowledge in the application of new techniques is reflected in a paper on 'Researches in cerebro-cranial topography using roentgen photography', written in collaboration with W. S. ('Baldy') Haughton [q.v.].

He was assistant to Edward Hallaran Bennett [q.v.], whom he succeeded in 1906. In 1920, he was appointed PRCSI but died in office in 1922.

Taylor was cool, deliberate and resourceful in the operating theatre. He was highly respected as an upright, honourable man who, despite his many achievements, remained essentially modest. Although known as a man who could get things done, he avoided medical politics and his main interest outside his patients and his family was farming.

TAYLOR, Sir William PRCSI 1916–1918

Professor of Surgery, TCD, and Dublin Surgeon

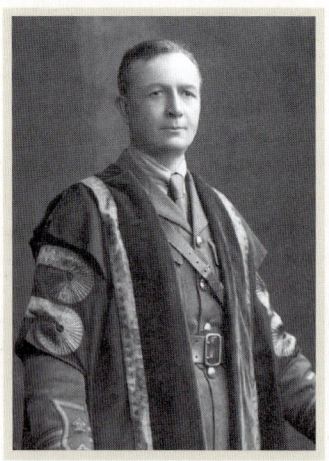

b. 1871, Castlefin, west of Lifford, Co. Donegal, son of John Taylor ('landed gentry of some generations'; they had owned the Castle of Castlefin and the townland) and Mary Jane Walker, an American doctor's daughter
Educ. Strabane Academy; Royal College of Surgeons in Ireland; Trinity College, Dublin
m. Married with 3 s, 1 d
d. 29 January 1933

RCSI (gold medal), 1893; FRCSI, 1898; MB, TCD, 1902; LLD (Hon.), McGill University; FACS (Hon.).

Assistant surgeon, Meath Hospital, Dublin, 1898–1900.
Surgeon, Meath Hospital, Dublin, 1900–22.
Member, Council, RCSI; President, 1916–18.

Colonel, Army Medical Service, 1914–18.

Regius Professor of Surgery, TCD, 1922.

Consultant surgeon, Sir Patrick Dun's, 1922. Also held appointments at the National Children's Hospital and St Ultan's Children's Hospital.

Hon. Fellow, American Surgical Association; American College of Surgeons.

President, Association of Surgeons of Great Britain and Ireland; RAMI.

As a young lad, William Taylor was not interested in either study or farming but was a fine horseman. He seemed destined to become a farmer but a local clergyman managed to stimulate in him an interest in learning, and he entered the RCSI in 1889, and graduated with a gold medal in 1893.

He earned a considerable reputation as a teacher and was an excellent clinician and operating surgeon. He initiated the change from antisepsis to surgical asepsis in the Meath Hospital. Unfortunately his interpersonal skills were less well developed and he was not on good terms with many colleagues at the Meath and at other hospitals. He frequently lamented his heavy workload with a wish that 'some other surgeon would set up in practice' to lighten his burden. In a city where there were perhaps fifty other surgeons, and which *Time* magazine subsequently called the 'backbiting capital of the world', this and many parallel remarks had wide currency. Despite his difficulties with colleagues, he was kind and considerate to his patients, and modified his fee for those who could not afford much.

In 1917, Taylor recruited and led the staff of the 83rd (Dublin) General Hospital near Boulogne, where he worked extremely hard. In 1920, the award of KBE acknowledged his service during the war.

In 1922, he was appointed Regius Professor of Surgery at TCD, an appointment that created some surprise, as he had not been much involved with Trinity in the past. He was ahead of his time in supporting the creation of one or two large hospitals instead of maintaining the numerous small hospitals in Dublin.

BALL, Sir Charles Arthur Kinehan, Bt

Professor of Surgery, TCD, and Dublin Surgeon

b. 1877, Blaenavon, son of Sir Charles Bent Ball, Bt [q.v.]

Educ. Shrewsbury College; Trinity College, Dublin

m. Elizabeth, daughter of Joseph Smythe-Wilson.

d. 1945

MB, 1900; MD, 1902; FRCSI, 1905; MCh (*Jure Officii*), 1906. Surgical Travelling Prize, 1902

Studied in Berne and Baltimore.
Assistant surgeon, Sir Patrick Dun's Hospital, Dublin; demonstrator in anatomy at TCD.
Surgeon, Sir Patrick Dun's Hospital, 1907.
Consultant surgeon, Monkstown Hospital; Drogheda Cottage Hospital.
Regius Professor of Surgery, TCD, 1934–45.

Publications included papers on perforated gastric ulcer, treatment of gonorrhoea and sterilisation of catgut.

McCONNELL, Adams Andrew (Adams A.) PRCSI 1936–1938

Professor of Surgery, TCD, and Dublin Surgeon

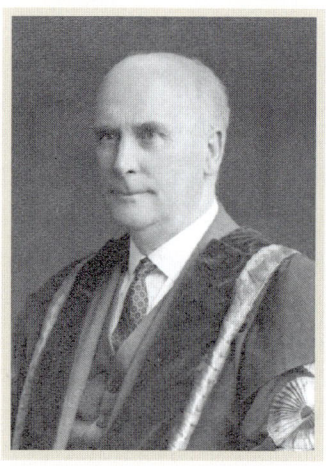

b. 1884, Lisburn, Co. Antrim, son of Dr Andrew McConnell and Margaret McConnell (*née* Adams)
Educ. Royal Belfast Academical Institute, Trinity College, Dublin
m. 1st in 1914: Nora Boyd (d. 1968);
2nd: Gladys Danesfield; no children
d. 1972

MB (first place), TCD, 1909; FRCSI, 1911, Hon. Fellow, TCD, 1956

Junior training posts at Sir Patrick Dun's Hospital.
Assistant surgeon, Richmond Hospital, 1911; surgeon, 1914.
Council member, RCSI, 1923–26; again 1930;
President, RCSI, 1936–38.

Professor of Surgery, RCSI, 1926–29.
Regius Professor of Surgery, TCD, 1946–61.

McConnell resigned from the council of RCSI when he successfully applied for the Chair of Surgery at the College in 1926. He was re-elected to the council of the College in 1930. *His principal entry is in the Neurosurgery chapter.*

PRINGLE, John Seton Michael

Professor of Surgery, RCSI and TCD, and Dublin Surgeon

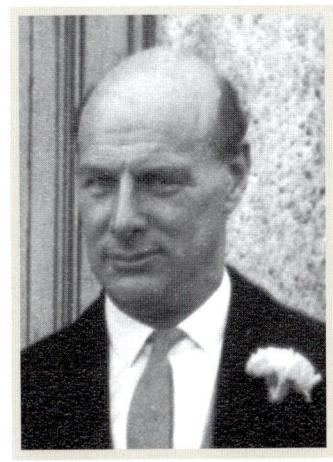

b. 1909, Belfast, youngest son of James Pringle, KC, MP of Clones, Co. Monaghan
Educ. Castle Park Preparatory School, Dalkey; Haileybury College; Caius College, Cambridge
m. 1st in 1937: Bunty Odlum (died of poliomyelitis, 1950); 1 s, 2 d (Claire, MB, TCD, 1965); 2nd in 1959: Nancy Cornwall
d. 1975

MB, TCD, 1933; MB, BChir, Camb, 1933; FRCSI, 1935; FRCS Eng, 1937

Visiting surgeon, Royal City Hospital, Dublin; Drumcondra Hospital.
Consultant surgeon, Rotunda Hospital; Stewart Hospital; Royal Hospital for Incurables.
Visiting surgeon, Mercer's Hospital, Dublin (pre war).
Major, Royal Army Medical Corps, 1939–45.
Professor of Surgery, RCSI, 1952–61.
Regius Professor of Surgery, TCD, 1961–74.

John Pringle joined the Royal Army Medical Corps in 1939, on the outbreak of war, and spent most of the duration as a medical officer on the Queen Mary, ferrying troops across the Atlantic. He was in Normandy on D Day +1 with a field surgical unit, and was actively engaged in the Arnhem campaign.

He was a cousin of Seton Pringle Snr [q.v.], PRCSI (1934–36), and like him was an expert on safe intestinal anastomosis. His career was cut short by a series of disabling strokes and he had to retire from practice, dying at the early age of 66. A quietly spoken excellent teacher, he was a highly successful professor.

KINNEAR, Nigel Alexander PRCSI 1961–1963

Professor of Surgery, TCD, and Dublin Surgeon

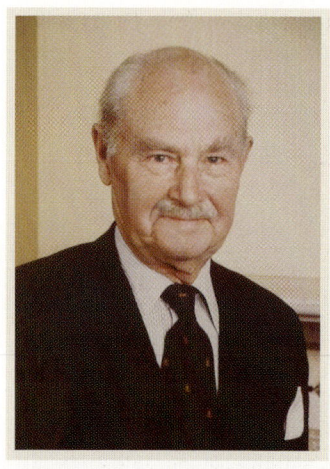

b. 1907, Dublin, son of James Kinnear and Margaret Kinnear (*née* Robinson)
Educ. Kingstown Grammar School; Mill Hill School, North London; Trinity College, Dublin
m. 1947: Frances Gardner (war widow of Flying Officer C. A. G. Thomson); 1 d
d. 2000

MB, TCD, 1930; FRCSI, 1934; FRCP&S Glas (Hon.), 1963

Postgraduate appointments as house surgeon, Sir Patrick Dun's Hospital; resident medical officer, Jersey General Hospital and in Vienna; lecturer in applied anatomy, TCD.
Assistant surgeon, Sir Patrick Dun's.
Surgeon, Adelaide Hospital, 1935–73. Surgeon, Dr Steevens' Hospital.
Member, Council, RCSI, 1946.
Regius Professor of Surgery, TCD, 1967–74.
President, RAMI, 1966–69; James IV Society of Surgeons, 1975–76.
Member, International Society of Surgeons; Irish Surgical Travellers.

Nigel Kinnear's professional career began at Sir Patrick Dun's as the solitary house surgeon. He served with the organisation Civilian Relief, under the umbrella of the British Red Cross, and had the shocking experience of being involved with the liberation of the Nazi concentration camps. He was elected to the RCSI council in 1945 while still abroad and, as he was unable to take the oath, his election was nullified. He was elected again the following year.

Like Paddy Fitzgerald [q.v.], Kinnear was a pioneer in vascular surgery in Ireland, at a time when surgical techniques and diagnostic facilities were primitive, and skill, courage and endurance were essential qualities.

He was always dressed and groomed immaculately. His precise diction and rather stern appearance belied his warm, kindly nature and his great sense of humour. His definition of borborygmi as 'the frustrated rumbles of a baffled fart', delivered with a poker face at an inaugural meeting of the TCD Biological Society, would be a typical careful use of the English language to which he was devoted. He loved to shoot and fish the Slaney with Frances.

Kinnear had enjoyed a highly successful academic career as a medical student and was equally accomplished as a sportsman, representing his university at both golf and hockey, and Leinster at hockey. He golfed into his eighties. As a surgeon, he was an inspiring role model, a great technician, a fine teacher, full of concern and compassion for all his patients and, as a crowning attribute as a professor, he was fun to work with. Few surgeons were as well and as widely loved as Nigel.

McCOLLUM, Stanley Thomas PRCSI 1976–1978

Professor of Surgery, TCD, and Dublin Surgeon

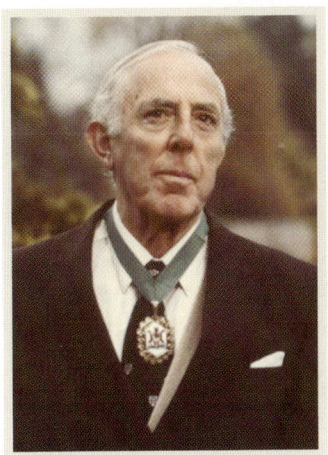

b. 1918, Athboy, Co. Meath, son of Thomas McCollum and Violet McCollum (*née* Roe)
Educ. King's Hospital School (where he took first place in Irish and was a King's Scholar); Trinity College, Dublin
m. Maeve Walker, daughter of Rev. Reginald Walker; 3 s (Peter is Professor of Vascular Surgery, University of Hull)
d. 1996

MB, TCD, 1941 (with distinction, winning Hudson scholarship and gold medal of Adelaide Hospital); FRCSI, 1944; FRCS Eng, 1947; FACS (Hon.); FRCS Ed (Hon.); FCS Australia (Hon.); FCS South Africa (Hon.)

Postgraduate surgical experience at the Adelaide and Dr Steevens' Hospitals, Dublin; Royal Northern, Hillingdon Hospital, and Rush Green Hospital, London.
Consultant surgeon, Adelaide and Rotunda Hospitals, National Children's Hospital and Our Lady's Hospital for Sick Children, Dublin.
Lecturer in surgery at TCD, and assistant to the Professor of Surgery.
Regius Professor of Surgery, TCD, 1974–81.
President, RCSI, 1976–78; International Federation of Colleges of Surgeons.
Professor of Surgery, King Faisal University, Saudi Arabia.

At Rush Green Hospital in London, he came under the influence of Henry Souttar (1875–1964), Norman Tanner, gastrectomy 'king', and J. E. Piercy, an accomplished thyroid surgeon.
His special interest subjects in surgery were thyroid and parathyroid and paediatric surgery, and he published widely in these areas.

Stanley McCollum was an absolutely first-class operating surgeon. He travelled widely in the Middle East on behalf of RCSI and, following his retirement from the Adelaide and TCD, spent some years as Professor of Surgery at King Faisal University in Saudi Arabia, and in Malaysia.

His sporting activities in college included membership of TCD's first tennis, rugby and cricket teams. In retirement, and perhaps a little before that, he golfed, gardened and did some leisure travelling. He was a devoted servant of his hospitals, Trinity and the RCSI, and had a special enthusiasm for the International Federation of Colleges of Surgeons. Precise, and perhaps austere on first meeting, he softened greatly on further acquaintance.

HENNESSY, Thomas Patrick Joseph (Tom) PRCSI 1994–1996

Professor of Surgery, TCD, and Dublin Surgeon

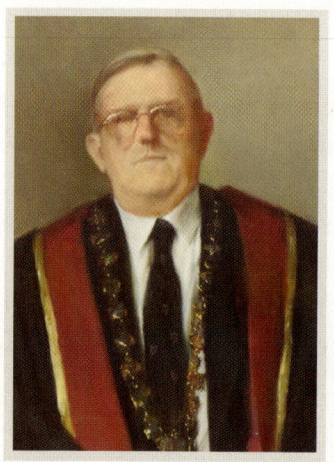

b. 1933, Kilkenny, eldest son of Martin Hennessy and Anne Kavanagh of Graiguenamanagh
Educ. Knockbeg College, Carlow; University College Dublin
m. 1st in 1959: Maura Hayden (d. 1998); 4 children (Anne is a FCARCSI). 2nd in 2001: Marta Birgitta Buckholt

MB, UCD, 1957; FRCSI, 1963; FRCS Eng, 1964; MCh, NUI, 1965; MD, 1991; FRCS Ed (Hon); FRCS Glas (Hon); FRCS Eng (Hon); FCS South Africa (Hon); FCS Pakistan (Hon).

Postgraduate appointments: internship at the Mater Hospital, Dublin; resident surgical officer, St Michael's Hospital, Dún Laoghaire; surgical registrar, Jervis Street Hospital.
Various appointments in the Liverpool region.
Surgical tutor, Mater Hospital, Dublin (with Professor Eoin O'Malley [q.v.]).
Research assistant, Minneapolis (with Dr O. H. Wangensteen).
Lecturer in surgery, TCD. Surgeon, Sir Patrick Dun's Hospital.
Honorary Fellow, American Surgical Association.
Consultant surgeon/statutory lecturer in surgery, St Finbarr's Hospital, Cork, and UCC, 1970–75.
Professor of Clinical Surgery and head of department at TCD.
Regius Professor of Surgery, TCD, 1984–98.
Foundation Dean and Professor of Surgery, Penang Medical College, Penang, Malaysia, 1998–2004.
President, Surgical Research Society of Great Britain and Ireland; Irish Society of Gastroenterology; surgical section, RAMI.

During his time as surgical tutor at the Mater, with Professor Eoin O'Malley, Tom Hennessy was exposed for the first time to surgery of the oesophagus, which became a lifelong interest. After a priceless year of laboratory research with the iconic Dr O. H. Wangensteen, in Minneapolis, with side trips to the Mayo Clinic just up the road, he was appointed lecturer in surgery at TCD and worked at Sir Patrick Dun's Hospital with Professor George Fegan.

In 1970, Hennessy was appointed to St Finbarr's Hospital and University College Cork. He was hugely popular there, which is not an easy achievement for any outsider but might be even harder for a Kilkenny man. (As has been said, 'In Cork the edge of criticism is sharpened every morning.') In 1975 he was appointed Professor of Clinical Surgery and head of department at TCD, and was appointed Regius Professor of Surgery in 1984.

Professor Hennessy continued his commitment to upper gastrointestinal surgery, with a particular interest in oesophageal surgery. He focused mainly on the pathophysiology of Barrett's oesophagus and multi-modality treatment of oesophageal carcinoma. He and his colleagues published 140 peer-reviewed papers, mainly related to upper GI and oesophageal pathology and he co-authored five books and was author of several book chapters.

He was awarded the travelling Fellowship of the James the IV Surgical Society in 1977 and was subsequently a Vice-President of the Society. He delivered several named lectures in Ireland, UK, Sweden and Japan.

Of middle height, and bespectacled, Hennessy has an aldermanic figure and measured manner of speaking which partly conceal an acute intelligence. He was well trained in the craft of surgery and the methodology of research, and patients, Trinity and the RCSI benefited. For years, before he was made President, he headed the annual election poll for the College Council. This was in appreciation of his complete integrity, legendary discretion and achievements. He never made the slightest effort to curry favour with the electorate but greatly enjoyed resuming his position at the top of the annual Council poll after his two years of presidency.

At the unprepossessing St James's Hospital he built up a world-class oesophageal unit, and his team's paper was the first from Ireland to be published in the New England Journal of Medicine. He had a great belief in the separation of Academic Chairs from private practice, and this inevitably caused some tensions in other departments where his views were not shared.

Warm, cuddly, much loved by his trainees and all who know him well, he travels widely during retirement. He made a big difference to academic surgery in Ireland.

The Chair of Surgery, TCD, in the Twentieth Century

BENNETT, Edward Hallaran PRCSI 1884–1886

Professor of Surgery, TCD, and Dublin Surgeon

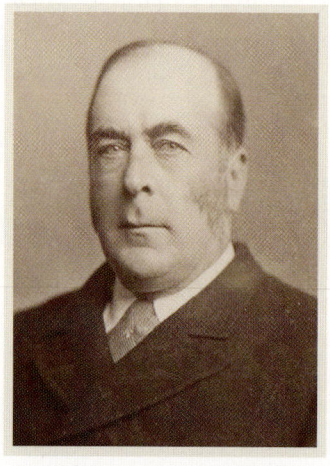

b. 1837, fifth son of Robert Bennett (barrister and Recorder of Cork, and Jane Hallaran (a doctor's daughter and a doctor's granddaughter)
Educ. Hamblin's School, Cork; Academic Institute, Harcourt Street, Dublin; Trinity College, Dublin
m. Frances Connolly Norman of Fahan, Co. Donegal; 2 d
d. 1907

MCh, 1859; FRCSI, 1863; MD, 1864; FRCS Eng (Hon.), 1900

Postgraduate appointment as demonstrator in anatomy, TCD, 1864–73.
Surgeon, Sir Patrick Dun's Hospital, 1866. His other hospital appointments were at Dr Steevens', St Mark's, the Eye and Ear Hospital and the Dental Hospital, Dublin.
Professor of Surgery, TCD, 1874–1906.
Member, Council, RCSI; president, 1884–86.

Edward Bennett entered TCD in 1854 as a medical student and attended the Meath, Dr Steevens', Sir Patrick Dun's and the Richmond Hospitals. Early in his career, he came under the influence of Robert Smith, Professor of Surgery at TCD, and developed a lifelong interest in diseases of bone. (Smith is remembered for Smith's Fracture, a fracture of the lower end of the radius in which the lower fragment is displaced forwards, unlike in the much more common Colles's fracture, where it is displaced backwards.) He eventually succeeded Smith as Professor of Surgery.

Bennett was the first graduate to be awarded the new degree of MCh. As University anatomist, he established an important collection of specimens of bone disease, fractures and dislocations. His interest in bone pathology continued and, in 1881, he described, for the first time, the fracture dislocation of the base of the first metacarpal, which bears his name.

Despite his blunt exterior, Bennett endeared himself to all who knew him. His students revered him as a teacher and a diagnostician. His sympathy and kindness towards his patients, particularly children, evoked a remarkable trust and confidence. When his health began to fail in 1904, his students and colleagues determined to recognise his immense contributions by suitable memorials. A surgical travelling prize was established. In addition, a large bronze medallion was commissioned, showing Bennett's profile. A bronze medal was also struck, showing Bennett's profile and, on the reverse side, a representation of the thumb fracture which bears his name.

Edward Hallaran Bennett was succeeded as Professor of Surgery by Edward Taylor [q.v.] who later (1916) became Regius Professor of Surgery at TCD.

GORDON, Thomas Eagleston PRCSI 1928–1929

Professor of Surgery, TCD, and Dublin Surgeon

> b. 1867
> Educ. Trinity College, Dublin
> m. married; 5 d
> d. 1929

Thomas Eagleston Gordon graduated from TCD in 1890, winning a gold medal and the Hudson Scholarship at the Adelaide Hospital. Shortly afterwards, he joined the Adelaide staff as assistant to Mr Kendal Franks. In contrast to his mentor, Franks, Gordon was a conservative and methodical surgeon.

Despite a quiet and reserved manner, he was a very accomplished teacher. His surgical interests were wide ranging and he published papers on abdominal surgery, orthopaedics and prostatic hypertrophy. When Sir Edward Taylor [q.v.] became Regius Professor of Surgery in 1916, Gordon was appointed Professor of Surgery.

Professor Gordon lived quietly at 8 Fitzwilliam Square with his wife and daughters. He was elected president of RCSI in 1928. Partial blindness in one eye forced him to withdraw from active surgery that same year.

PEARSON, William PRCSI 1950–1952

Professor of Surgery, TCD, and Dublin Surgeon

> b. 1882, Cork, son of Prof. Charles Yelverton Pearson [q.v.] (Queen's College, Cork) and grandson of Dr William Pearson (dispensary doctor in Carrigaline, Co. Cork)
> m. 1st in 1918: Monica Henty Dodd of Manchester (His family was unaware of this first marriage); 2nd in 1927: Esther Hurford, an Adelaide Hospital, Dublin, theatre sister; 1 s (John, an anaesthetist)
> Educ. Trinity College, Dublin; Johns Hopkins, Baltimore; Mayo Clinic
> d. 1976

MB, TCD, 1907 (many honours); FRCSI, 1910; MD, MCh

Assistant to Professor of Surgery, T. E. Gordon [q.v.], Adelaide Hospital.
Royal Army Medical Corps, First World War; served in France; later chief surgeon at Graylingwell Hospital, Chichester; demobilised in 1919 with rank of Lieutenant-Colonel.
Surgeon Adelaide Hospital; Ministry of Pensions Special Surgical Hospital, Blackrock.
Member, Council, RCSI, 1924.

William Pearson seems to have got first place in every examination he ever sat. This would not have surprised him. An effective and competent teacher, he was not averse to mentioning his diagnostic and therapeutic successes as illustrative anecdotes. He was supremely confident of his knowledge and was quoted as saying, 'The only time I was wrong was when I thought I was wrong, but I was proved right in the end.'

Like his successor, Jack Henry [q.v.], he was an avid fisherman. He was also a strong supporter of TCD's rugby club and faithfully attended the College Races each year. In his declining years, he admitted himself to Sir Patrick Dun's Hospital, having parked and locked his car in the parking place of surgeon Tom O'Neill [q.v.], an avowed antagonist, where it gradually rusted and disintegrated as he stayed on in the hospital, month after month, dictating his own treatment. He spent his final years in Honolulu with his doctor son.

FEGAN, George William

Professor of Surgery, TCD, and Dublin Surgeon

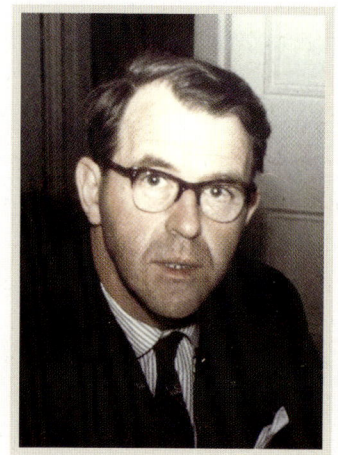

b. 1921, Cavan
Educ. Trinity College, Dublin
m. Pamela (deceased); 1 s, 5 d
d. 2007

MB, TCD, 1946; MCh, Dub, 1952; FRCSI, 1949

Postgraduate appointments at Sir Patrick Dun's and the Royal Northern Hospital, Holloway Road, London.
Assistant surgeon, Royal City of Dublin Hospital, Baggot Street, Dublin.
Visiting surgeon, Rotunda Hospital.
Clinical Professor of Surgery, TCD, 1967–73.
Member, Council, Surgical Research Society of Great Britain and Ireland.
Member, Council, RCSI, 1966–73.

George Fegan was much influenced by the story of his mother almost dying of a pulmonary embolus, following on deep-vein thrombosis after delivering herself of George. It was while he was at the Rotunda that he developed his technique of compression sclerotherapy for varicose veins. Because it was an ambulatory treatment, and because it seemed to work, compression sclerotherapy became increasingly popular, and special outpatient clinics were established at many hospitals in Ireland and in the UK. Fegan realised that if his technique were to gain wide acceptance among surgical colleagues, he would have to produce evidence as to how and why it worked. So he established a laboratory in the basement in Sir Patrick Dun's, in which the anatomy and physiology of the venous system and the pathophysiology of varicose veins were studied exhaustively. The results were communicated to the Surgical Research Society and published in peer-reviewed journals, including the *Lancet* (where the first article was not peer reviewed at all but published following an imperious phone call to the editor from Sir George Godber, Chief Medical Officer of Health in the British Department of Health and Social Services).

Fame followed and George Fegan became an internationally recognised expert on the venous pathology of the lower limb. The variegated population of patients treated and the regressive nature of the condition in the biggest cohort, the post-partum group, combined with comparatively low numbers of long-term follow-up, meant that the breakthrough did not get the credit it deserved outside Ireland. His publications were few. Innovators publish and republish and republish to get their point across but George said that his dearth of publication was a result of his dyslexia. Follow-up or lack of it, always a problem with private patients, was a real issue in the acceptance of the method.

George had many interests outside surgery. He kept a herd of Charolais cattle on his estate near Maynooth. He had a valuable collection of paintings, and he also collected antiques, with a particular interest in Irish silver. He was a man of restless energy who was constantly rushing from meetings of the Federated Dublin Voluntary Hospitals, in whose successful amalgamation he played a leading part, to academic meetings, to his operating list, to his extensive private practice, and travelling to speak at meetings. It was hardly surprising that he began to develop symptoms of angina in the late 1960s and resigned his chair in 1973.

On his resignation, in recognition of his research work, TCD appointed him Honorary Professor of Surgical Research, for the duration of his life. He retired to Zanzibar and Lamu in Kenya. He was afflicted in later life by macular degeneration but retained much of his volcanic energy.

Above middle height (just), with a head of semi-kempt hair, and always, but always, talking, he was a constant source of gossipy quotes. A bright comet that lit up our lives.

Professors of Surgery at the Royal College of Surgeons in Ireland from 1900

DWYER, Frederick Conway (Sir) PRCSI 1914–1916

Professor of Surgery, RCSI, and Dublin Surgeon

b. 1860, Dublin, son of Michael F. Dwyer (Registrar of Deeds)
Educ. Trinity College, Dublin
m. Unmarried
d. 1935

MB, TCD, 1883; FRCSI, 1898

Resident surgeon, Mater Hospital, Dublin
Visiting surgeon, Charitable Infirmary; Meath Hospital; Richmond Hospital; Mercer's Hospital.
Professor of Surgery, RCSI, 1901–19.
President, RCSI, 1914–16.
Lieutenant-Colonel, Royal Army Medical Corps, 1914 –18; knighted, 1924 for wartime services.
Chairman, Board of Governors, Richmond Hospital.

Sir Frederick Conway Dwyer's forte was abdominal surgery. He published a treatise, 'Cases Simulating Gastric Ulcer', in the RAMI Transactions. He was one of the 'Big Three' (including Sir Thomas Myles [q.v.] and Prof. Joseph O'Carroll) who provided strong leadership of the Richmond Hospital in the post-war years.

He died in 1935, unmarried, with no surviving relatives.

JOHNSTON, George Jameson

Professor of Surgery, RCSI, and Dublin Surgeon

b. 1866, Dungannon, Co. Tyrone, son of Ronald and Sarah Emily Johnston
Educ. Royal School, Dungannon; Trinity College, Dublin; and the Royal University of Ireland
m. Noreen Norman
d. 1926

BA (hons), TCD; MA, RUI, 1891; MB, BCh (hons), RUI, 1894; FRCSI, 1898, TCD (first in class and first class hons (bis.) and first class exhibitioner in biology and physiology)

Postgraduate appointments as demonstrator in anatomy, TCD; assistant surgeon, Richmond Hospital, Dublin.
Visiting surgeon, Royal City of Dublin Hospital, 1896–1926.

Professor of Surgery, RCSI, 1912–26.

Lieutenant-Colonel, Royal Army Medical Corps, 1914–18; posted as senior surgeon to the Dublin Hospital near Bologna.

Surgeon and lecturer on clinical surgery, Royal City of Dublin Hospital, Baggot Street, Dublin.

Honorary surgeon, Masonic Boys' School; honorary consultant surgeon, Royal Hospital for Incurables, Dublin.

Member, Council, RCSI.

University examiner in clinical surgery, TCD; lecturer in clinical surgery, Royal Medical Service School.

Author of 'The Superficial Mapping of the Fissure of Rolando, with Description of a Simple form of Rolandometer', Medical Press, c.1896; 'Necessity for Municipal Ambulances for Removing Cases of Accidents and of Sudden Illness from the Streets', Congr. Royal Institution Publications, Health, 1898; 'Swallowing of a Metallic Denture successfully treated by the Internal Administration of Cotton Wool', Transactions of the Royal Academy of Medicine, Ireland, 1902.

George Johnston was an excellent teacher and held in high regard by his students in the College and in the Richmond Hospital. He married Noreen Norman less than one year before his death.

CHANCE, Arthur

Professor of Surgery and Dublin Surgeon

b. 1889, third son of Sir Arthur Chance [q.v.] (PRCSI, 1904–05)
Educ. Clongowes Wood College; Trinity College, Dublin
m. 1941: Harriet McBurney
d. 1980

MA, MD, Dublin, 1912 (first place in surgery — Bennet Medal); MRCS, LRCP 1914; FRCS, FRCSI, 1915

Postgraduate appointments to Charing Cross Hospital and St Bartholomew's Hospital, London; Bohler Clinic, Vienna; Mayo Clinic, USA.

Royal Army Medical Corps 1915–18; served in France and Italy.

Surgeon, Dr Steevens' Hospital, 1916–66; Jervis Street Hospital, 1930–61; St Michael's, Dún Laoghaire; the Orthopaedic Hospital.

First Professor of Orthopaedic Surgery, TCD.

Professor of Surgery, RCSI, 1926–46.

Vice-President, British Orthopaedic Association 1954–55.

Arthur Chance was first chairman of the Federated Dublin Voluntary Hospitals, a tribute to his well-honed conciliatory skills. He was appointed to Dr Steevens' Hospital in absentia because he was on active service in France (field dressing station).

As a teacher, he was first class, attracting to his clinics scores of students from all three medical schools. He was a formidable but scrupulously fair examiner. He could be demanding as a 'chief'. He was one of the first in Ireland to specialise in orthopaedics. In later life, he became a full-time legendary medical witness. His prop was a monocle, which he carefully polished before adverting to his notes and giving his expert opinion to a, now riveted, court. The monocle could then be let drop from his eye, with exquisite timing, if he felt that some of the opposition evidence lacked credibility.

He was a keen golfer but his later passion was horse racing: he was honorary surgeon to the Curragh, Leopardstown and Baldoyle racecourses. He developed a stroke hemiplegia at 83 and was nursed devotedly by his wife, Harriet, who had been his secretary before they married in 1941. He was a warm, chuckling, rounded figure with a great love of life and surgery.

HENRY, Robert F. J. (Jack)

Professor of Surgery, RCSI and TCD, and Dublin Surgeon

b. 1901, West Dublin, son of a clerk in Guinness's.
Educ. St Stephen's Green School; Trinity College, Dublin
m. Stella Ross (also a medical student at TCD when they met, later a well-known medical illustrator (SCR), d. 1975); 2 s (George, former Master of the Rotunda Hospital; Adrian, an orthopaedic surgeon in Guy's Hospital London)
d. 1970

MB, BCh (with distinctions), 1924; FRCSI, 1927

Postgraduate surgical training, Ancoats Hospital, Manchester, with Sir Harry Platt.
Awarded Surgical Travelling Prize in TCD and gained further experience in Paris.
Surgeon, Royal City of Dublin Hospital, 1926–70.
Surgeon, National Children's Hospital, Harcourt Street; Newcastle Sanatorium; the Rotunda Hospital.
Professor of Surgery, RCSI, 1938–52.
Royal Army Medical Corps, 1939–45.
Professor of Surgery, TCD, 1952–67.
Founder member, Society of Thoracic Surgeons of Great Britain and Ireland.

At the start of the Second World War, Jack Henry joined the Royal Army Medical Corps, and was in France for the German breakthrough in 1940. His unit made its way with great difficulty to the coast and was part of the general evacuation of the British Expeditionary Force in 1940. After the war, he returned to his surgical duties in Baggot Street Hospital. The reorganisation of clinical teaching in the Dublin teaching hospitals in the 1950s resulted in the alignment of the Royal City of Dublin Hospital with TCD. As a result, Jack Henry left the staff at RSCI and joined the staff of TCD in 1952.

He was a pioneer in the field of thoracic surgery and particularly in the surgical treatment of pulmonary tuberculosis, in which he published several papers. He was a dramatic and outstanding lecturer and clinical teacher. He always had a full attendance at his clinics in Baggot Street Hospital, and those fortunate enough to attend his lectures will never forget his ringing tones and dramatic gestures, attributed to earlier acting experience. Flame-haired and energetic, Henry was a terrifying but compassionate examiner.

He was an expert fisherman and yachtsman, and had a great interest in rugby football. He died at the age of 69, whilst fishing on his beloved Lough Derg.

BYRNES, Colman Kevin (Coley)

Professor of Surgery, RCSI, and Dublin Surgeon

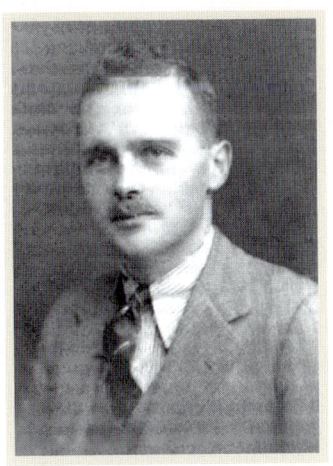

b. 1909, Bruree, Co. Limerick, son of Dr and Mrs Byrnes, one of eleven children of whom four sons became doctors
Educ. Salesian College, Pallaskenry, Co. Limerick; RCSI on a scholarship
m. 1937: Mary Lane; 4 s (Dermot Byrnes was Belfast neurosurgeon [q.v.]), 1 d
d. 1965

LRCP & SI, 1934, with many honours, prizes and distinctions during his undergraduate career; FRCSI, 1940; FACS, 1953

Postgraduate appointment as house officer, Richmond Hospital, for one year.
Captain, Indian Medical Service, 1935–37; served in the Lansdowne United Provinces of Agra and Oudh. Captain, Army Medical Service (reserve), 1939–45.
Surgical registrar, Richmond Hospital, 1938–42.
Assistant surgeon, Richmond Hospital, 1942. Surgeon, Richmond Hospital, 1956–65.
Vice-Chairman, Board of Governors, Richmond Hospital, 1964.
Professor of Surgery, RCSI, 1961–65.
Early member, Society of Thoracic Surgeons of Great Britain and Ireland.

During his time as surgical registrar at the Richmond, Coley Byrnes spent a period with Adams McConnell [q.v.] in the Neurosurgical Department. As a professor, Byrnes was an inspired teacher of the art of surgery on the wards and in the operating theatre. He led by example, as a surgeon dedicated to his patients and always available. He was a hard taskmaster ('I wear the badge with pride') but he imbued in his many trainees this dedication to duty. He was particularly fortunate to have W. A. L. MacGowan [q.v.] as a brilliant, loyal, second in command. He regarded himself as a true general surgeon, equally at home in the abdomen, thorax, cranium and limbs. His particular field of interest was in the surgery of the oesophagus and he was a pioneer in this difficult area.

He was the driving force behind the setting up of a research centre and the surgical research laboratory at the Richmond Hospital, which opened in 1970 as the Colman K. Byrnes Research Centre.

Short (certainly below average height), stocky, with bristling military-style moustache, he exuded waves of energy. His regional accent was much imitated but he always made himself clear. He was a great example of a man who, with little or no academic training, brought the RCSI Department of Surgery into the modern era by sheer sustained drive and vigour, allied to a warm, forceful personality. He was greatly loved in the profession.

MacGOWAN, William Arthur Lysaght (Bill)

Professor of Surgery and Registrar, RCSI

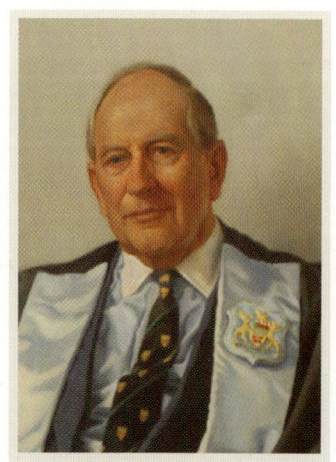

b. 1925, third child of Maurice (BL) and Eileen MacGowan
Educ. Belvedere College, Dublin; Royal College of Surgeons in Ireland
m. Joan, 4 children (son, Simon, a consultant cardiovascular surgeon in Belfast)

LRCP & SI (first class hons and Council medal for special merit), 1948; FRCSI, 1952; FACS, 1959; DSc (Hon.), University of Khartoum, 1994; FRCSI (Hon.), 2002

Postgraduate appointments as surgical registrar, Richmond Hospital, 1949–54; registrar, cardiothoracic surgeon, Frenchay Hospital, Bristol (Ronald Belsey), 1954–55; registrar, cardiothoracic surgeon, Newcastle Upon Tyne (George Mason), 1955–56. Senior lecturer in surgery, University of Khartoum (under Prof. Julian Taylor of University College Hospital, London), 1956–59.

Consultant surgeon, Richmond Hospital, Dublin, 1959–81.
Professor of Surgery, RCSI, 1967–80. Dean, Medical Faculty, RCSI, 1974–78.
Seconded from RCSI to King Faisal University, Amman, Saudi Arabia, as Charter Chairman, Department of Surgery, 1979–80.
Registrar and chief executive officer, RCSI, 1980–90; overseas contract director, RCSI, for North West Armed Forces Hospital Contract, Tabuk, Saudi Arabia, 1990–98.
Member, Medical Council; Medical Research Council.
Secretary, Irish Surgical Postgraduate Training Commission, 1980–90.
Honorary secretary, International Federation of Surgical Colleges, 1984–92.
External examiner in surgery at many universities.
Visiting Professor of Surgery, Johns Hopkins Hospital, Baltimore, USA, 1969.
Order of the White and Blue Niles (1st Class), Democratic Republic of the Sudan, 1993.

Bill MacGowan's special interests were surgical training and education, medical manpower, selection processes for undergraduates and surgical trainees, surgical problems of the developing world.

He was one of the most influential figures in Irish surgery in the second half of the twentieth century. Early signs of brilliance were rapidly translated into a huge body of achievement. Following his UK training, his post in Khartoum gave him a chance to acquire wide operative experience quickly, and he greatly admired his chief there, Professor Julian Taylor. On his return to Dublin, he loyally helped Professor Colman Byrnes [q.v.], and when he took over as Professor he made the RCSI Department of Surgery into a modern, progressive scientific unit.

His scientific talks always separated undergraduate from postgraduate surgery according to the audience; this was the exception rather than the rule up to about 1970. He promoted the concept of data-based presentations at the few surgical meetings there were. The unit prospered. When he was appointed Registrar at the RCSI, the worst of the crisis, when the Medical School was threatened with closure, had almost passed, but there was much to be done. During his decade in office, the College underwent a vital transformation from an examining body into a training institution. But the Medical School was losing money at a torrential rate and he then entered a third and vital phase on the College's behalf, when he initiated discussions with the Ministry of Health in the Kingdom of Saudi Arabia, and secured a contract to administer and staff a hospital in Tabuk in the North West Province. This institution was rapidly transformed into one of the best hospitals in the Middle East, and the College benefited financially.

Together with Dr Harry O'Flanagan, registrar 1957–80, Bill MacGowan brought the RCSI from the brink of disaster to becoming the leading international medical school in the world and secured its role as the arbiter of training standards for aspiring surgeons in Ireland. Both were graduates of the College.

Bill MacGowan, at almost 6 foot, and well over 15 stone was, and is, a formidable figure. He had the right ideas almost all the time and brooked little interference with their implementation. His symbiotic partnership with various Presidents was punctuated by a few upheavals, but the College had no better servant and he generated strong loyalties amongst his trainees. The College made him an Honorary Fellow, the highest distinction in its gift. Few deserved it more. For recreation, he enjoys tennis.

BOUCHIER-HAYES, David John (DBH)

Professor of Surgery, RCSI, and Dublin Surgeon

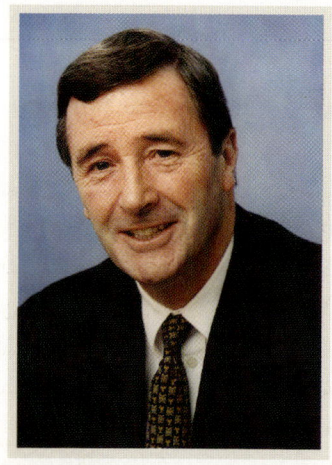

b. 1940, Dublin, son of Thomas [q.v.] (a prominent Dublin surgeon) and Mona Bouchier-Hayes (both of Limerick)

Educ. St Conleth's College (school captain); University College Dublin

m. 1966: Dr Margaret Hogarty; 2 s (David Jnr is urologist in Galway), 1 d

MB (hons), UCD, 1965 (first place, paediatrics, Coombe Hospital silver medal, obstetrics); FRCSI, 1969; FRCS Eng, 1969; MCh, NUI, 1974; Certificate Higher Surgical Training, 1975

Postgraduate junior posts in St Vincent's Hospital Dublin; Our Lady's Hospital, Navan; registrar, Western Infirmary, Glasgow, 1968–71; senior registrar, St Vincent's Hospital.
Fogarty Fellow, Massachusetts General Hospital, Boston, 1977–78.
Consultant surgeon, St Laurence's Hospital and Beaumont Hospital, 1979–2005.
Professor of Surgery, RCSI, 1981–2005. Dean, Medical School, RCSI, 1988–93. Regional director, Cancer Services, North Dublin, 1997–2005.
Millin Lecturer, RCSI, 1979.
Visiting Professor, Johns Hopkins Hospital, Baltimore, October 1980.
Chairman, Board of Examiners, RCSI. External examiner, University of Glasgow and University of Leicester.
Member, Beaumont Hospital Board.
President, surgical section, RAMI.
Chairman, Irish Association of Vascular Surgeons.
Member, Council, RCSI, since 2006.

Over two hundred publications in peer-reviewed journals, four books (joint authorship) and dozens of invited presentations.

David Bouchier-Hayes was appointed consultant at 39 and Professor at 41. His Department of Surgery was arguably the most productive in Ireland in the years 1985–2000. There was a huge output of high-quality research papers. Members of the Department, uniquely, won the top award, the Patey Prize, at the Surgical Research Society, in two consecutive years. Many, many doctoral and other theses were monitored and completed. Two Chairs of Surgery, at Cork and at Limerick, went to 'graduates'.

He excelled at predicting trends and he was the first in these islands to run courses for consultants on laparoscopic (keyhole) surgery, which drew people from all parts of the UK and Europe. He pressed ahead with minimally invasive methods in his own specialty of vascular surgery. He was a fine, thoughtful, operating surgeon.

David took an active part in the surgical and management programme at the North West Military Hospital in Tabuk in Saudi Arabia in the 1990s. This development was vital for the RCSI at the time. He was also active in the founding of the RCSI/UCD Medical School in Penang, Malaysia. Recognising the importance of management in medicine, he, with Austin Leahy, put together a Diploma of Management in Medicine and, with a neat twist, a programme of Medicine for Managers. He combined the gifts of focus and seeing the big picture, agitating, unsuccessfully, for a liberal arts semester in the middle of the medical undergraduate course. He has a long, close, personal relationship with Professor Kevin O'Malley, who was Registrar at the College for much of his tenure as Professor of Surgery, and who was a shrewd adviser.

His family had been doctors for over a century and he was arguably the fifth generation in the profession. It shows, particularly in his humanity. Above medium height, he is lean, sharp-featured, dark, good-looking and energetic. He reads widely and has a vast compendium of erudition outside medicine. Margaret is a loyal supporter and many feel that he could not have got there without her. Perilously convivial, he enjoys the company of his Fellows and they enjoy him. 'Nobody's Perfect,' is an important mantra. David is a 'package', acknowledged and gratefully accepted as such by those who know him best. He did a superb job for the RCSI and Irish surgery.

University College Cork

Queen's College, Cork (later to become University College Cork) was officially inaugurated on 7 November 1849.

Professors of Surgery, 1849–2002

Denis B. Bullen	1849–1864
William K. Tanner	1864–1880
Stephen Sullivan	1880–1899
Charles Yelverton Pearson	1899–1928
John Dundon	1828–1940
Patrick Kiely	1941–1967
Michael P. Brady	1968–1997
Paul Redmond	1998–

PEARSON, Charles Yelverton

Professor of Surgery, Cork

> b. 1857, Kilworth, Co. Cork, fourth son of William Pearson MD (GP)
> m. 1st in 1881: Christiana Dorothea Tuckey of Bantry; 2 s (William Pearson [q.v.] became Professor of Surgery, TCD and PRCSI; Charles Broderick Pearson, MCH, succeeded to his father's practice), 1 d. 2nd in 1924: Dr May Clemence Ferguson of Co. Wicklow; 2 d (Veronica, MB; Anne, BArch)
> d. 1947
>
> MD, MCh, FRCS Eng
>
> Demonstrator in anatomy; Professor of Materia Medica; lecturer in jurisprudence.
> Surgeon, the North Infirmary, Victoria Hospital, Lying-in-Hospital and Eye, Ear and Throat Hospital, Cork.
> Professor of Surgery, Cork 1899–1928.
> Examined for the Indian Medical Service, which so many Irish graduates joined at that time. Senator, NUI, 1908. Hon. surgeon to the King in Ireland, 1916.
>
> Author of *Modern Surgical Technique in its relation to Operations and Wound Treatment* (1st Edition, 1907; 2nd Edition 1911), published in London.

As Professor of Materia Medica, Charles Yelverton Pearson gave crucial evidence in a case which excited wide national interest and which led to the conviction of a medical poisoner, Surgeon-Major Phillip Henry Eustace Cross, LRCSI, of Dripsey, Co. Cork (*The Coachford Poisoning Case*, Transactions of the RAMI, 1888).

Small, sharp-featured, 'patrician', with superb elocution, which he retained all his life, he was a fine craftsman, particularly in bone surgery and skin grafting. He visited clinics in England, the Continent and the United States. He was highly regarded by patients, students and colleagues. For recreation, he sailed, fished and shot.

He resigned as Professor of Surgery after he married May Ferguson, but continued with private practice. Sight failed him around 1929 and he gave up general practice. He gave anatomy grinds to his daughter and other medical students right up to his late eighties. Though almost completely blind, he could distinguish all the carpal bones by feel alone and then assign them to their correct side.

Genes in surgery exist. Pearson's granddaughter, Patricia Eadie, is a gifted plastic surgeon who works in Dublin. This proud man would have been even prouder.

DUNDON, John

Professor of Surgery, Cork, and Cork Surgeon

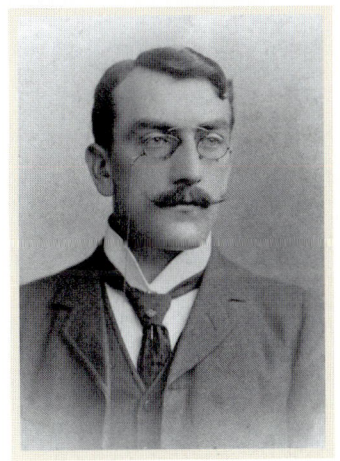

b. 1868, eldest son of Edmond and Eileen Dundon
Educ. Christian Brothers College, Cork; Queen's College, Cork
m. 1910: Mary McDonnell. 2 s (John Conor, a surgeon in Cork [q.v.]; Charles, a urologist in Canada), 3 d (one, Eileen, qualified as a doctor)
d. 1952

MB, QCC, 1894; FRCSI, 1898; FRCS Eng, 1905; MD (Hon.), NUI, 1940

Professor of Therapeutics and Materia Medica, 1900–27. His letter of appointment was signed by Queen Victoria in 1901.
Professor of Surgery, Cork, 1928–40
Examiner in surgery at RCSI.
Surgeon, North City and County Hospital, Mercy Hospital and Bon Secours Hospital.
Member, General Medical Registration Council.

His major interest was in the surgery of trauma, and he was author of an article on 'Injuries around the Shoulder Joint'.

Dundon attended the survivors of the torpedoed *Lusitania*, in 1916, and was one of six Cork citizens who had a 'pass' when the city was under martial law and had a strict dawn-to-dusk curfew, in 1920. He witnessed the burning of Cork City (11 December 1920), the most extensive single act of vandalism committed in the whole War of Independence. Later, the then Prime Minister, David Lloyd George, wrote to him as an Irish representative on the GMC, asking his opinion on how the medical profession in the South would react to an autonomous Irish Free State. We have no record of his reply.

His MD from UCC on retirement from the Chair was, as far as can be traced, a rare honorary degree conferred by the College on one of its medical graduates. In 1940, he retired for a time to Jersey, Channel Islands, partly as a result of a difference with the Revenue Commissioners, but he later returned to his beloved house in Patrick's Place, Cork, opposite Christian College, where he lived, consulted and died aged 85.

Dark, handsome, strong-willed, immaculate, extrovert, unafraid of any situation, dextrous, confident, pricey (100 guineas for a hernia in 1939), with a great sense of humour, he stressed in his teaching the basics of history taking, and the interpretation of clinical signs.

KIELY, Patrick (PK, Paddy)

Professor of Surgery, Cork, and Cork Surgeon

b. 1897, Moonakirka, Dungarvan, Co. Waterford, eldest son of John Kiely and Maryanne Kiely (*née* Moloney)
Educ. St Augustine's, Dungarvan; University College Cork
m. 1923: Mary; 3 s (two became surgeons: John [FRCS Eng. 1925–1960]; and Patrick Bartholomew [q.v.]), 4 d
d. 1998

BSc, 1918; MB (hons), UCC, 1920; MD, NUI, 1922; MCh, NUI, 1923; FRCS Eng, 1926; FRCSI (Hon.), 1972

Postgraduate appointment as demonstrator in anatomy, UCC.
Surgeon, Bon Secours Hospital, 1923; Mercy Hospital and South Infirmary, 1927.
Dispensary Medical Officer, Cork Rural District No. 2 Dispensary District, 1923–29.
Professor of Surgery, UCC, 1941–68. Dean of the Faculty of Medicine 1964–67.
Member, governing body, UCC, and Senate NUI 1934–40.

PK was by any standards a singular man. He had a brilliant undergraduate career, interrupted by three major illnesses, including tuberculosis and five months of incapacity from typhoid fever. He then got both parts of the FRCS Eng, first time, without leaving Cork except for the examinations. He had studied while conducting a general dispensing practice, on foot, in Blackpool, one of the poorer parts of the city. Getting the English Fellowship was such an event in those days that friends in

London gave a formal dinner, complete with signed menus and documented speeches, to celebrate the occasion. He had for many years demonstrated anatomy and his knowledge of structural variations was a great strength. He had enormous energy and a photographic memory, knowing all the students by name within a few days, a welcome but intimidating facility. He was a well-organised teacher: almost every clinical issue seemed to have five features, one for each of his powerful fingers, and he rarely went on to the other hand.

He was of the no-nonsense school of operating and the editor, as a student (1948), assisted him in removing a gallbladder under ether anaesthesia ('rag and bottle'), with a single nurse scrubbed. The teaching clinics on Saturday mornings, nine to twelve (unless there was a race meeting, in which case it was nine to eleven) were peppered with anecdotes of previous patients and the lessons learnt from them. He self-published a remarkable *Textbook of Surgery*, based almost entirely on his personal experience. Clinical professors of the day were paid a pittance, on the basis that the title would enhance their practice, but PK did all that could be asked of him when the medical school was under a lot of pressure and its survival was at stake. Lectures were rarely missed.

He had a huge practice from all over Munster. The GPs really trusted him. There were discarded crutches and sticks (no wooden legs!) in the hallway of his consulting rooms at the bottom of St Patrick's Hill. He had an engaging manner and a gift for enduring friendship. He had a hearty laugh but perhaps a limited sense of humour.

PK had been on the Republican side in the Civil War and was somewhat anti-British, which partly accounted for his not travelling abroad to keep up with the times. He proudly spoke, read and wrote Irish. Formidable when he felt he was under attack, he generated fierce loyalties and significant antipathies, particularly regarding his attempted 'ring fencing' of hospital appointments. He was hugely popular with the plain people of Cork who warmed to him. He was perhaps less popular with the medical profession where there had been tales of physical intimidation. He personified will power and determination.

His sporting activities were part of the legend. He played really competitive golf for high stakes and frequently walked the seven miles out and back to the golf course. He twice threw his clubs into the river Lee only to have them rescued at low tide. He loved horse racing, and perhaps his happiest moment was when his horse 'Dominick's Bar' won the Irish Grand National.

Middle height, ruddy complexioned, broad shouldered, well tailored and barbered, with a mane of black hair into his hundred and first year, he retained his volcanic energy almost to the end. A man of huge ability, imprisoned to some extent by his prejudices. Perhaps he properly belonged to an earlier generation. Iconic.

(Conflict of interest. When the editor passed the FRCS Eng in 1953 'PK' walked from his consulting rooms to our family's public house in Cork city centre to congratulate the candidate's father. Would any other professor of surgery anywhere else have done that?)

BRADY, Michael Patrick (Michael P.)

Professor of Surgery, Cork, and Cork Surgeon

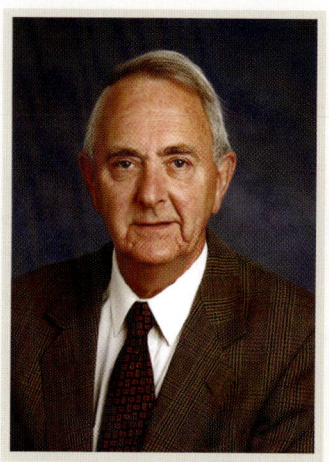

b. 1931, Accrington, Lancashire, eldest of 6 children of Michael J. (UCC graduate and Dublin radiotherapist) and Mary Rose Brady

Educ. Belvedere College, Dublin; University College Dublin

m. 1962: Leta Sue Brann of Leesburg, Virginia, USA; 5 children

MB, UCD, 1955 (McArdle prize in surgery); FRCSI, 1960; MCh, NUI, 1964; FACS, 1964

Resident surgical officer, St Luke's Hospital, Dublin; surgical registrar, Liverpool; Our Lady's Hospital for Sick Children, Crumlin, Dublin.

Two and a half years at the Peter Bent Brigham Hospital and Harvard University, Boston (under Prof. Francis D. Moore, the leading surgical scientist of his day).

Tutor/lecturer, St Vincent's Hospital, Dublin, 1962–67. Consultant staff, 1967.

Professor of Surgery, UCC, 1968–98.

Surgeon, St Finbarr's Hospital, 1968–78; Cork University Hospital, 1978–98.

Member, Medical Council; Postgraduate Medical and Dental Board; Council RCSI.

Dean of Medical Faculty, UCC.

William Doolin Lecture, 1977; Robert Adams Lecture, 1996.

Published papers on surgical metabolism and the sympathetic nervous system.

Michael Brady won every undergraduate prize while qualifying and his academic record was immaculate. When he came to Cork in 1968, he faced a different challenge. The medical school had just survived the biggest crisis of its 110-year history. An inspection by the (British) General Medical Council plainly stated that recognition of the school would be withdrawn unless full-time chairs in front-line specialties were established. From the start, he gave absolute priority to undergraduate teaching, and the students appreciated this and held him in great respect and affection. They valued his total integrity. He was a gifted organiser and was one of the first in Ireland to introduce a weekly audit meeting at the hospital. He was regarded by some as a quirky postgraduate examiner.

Throughout his thirty years as Professor, he was fortunate to be influenced by his Boston experience. The priceless link with Harvard and UCC's Ainsworth Scholarship were used to send 'likely lads' (there were no likely lassies in those days), for the incomparable stimulation and mind-broadening experience of working in the capital of the medical world. When they returned, they strengthened the stock. There was a certain inevitability that during these early days of rescuing the medical school there was little time for thoughtful research. While working, his availability for patients, few of whom were private, was legendary.

He built up the first purpose-built A&E Department in Cork at St Finbarr's, and then the first Grade I trauma centre in the country. He also founded the Southern Tumour Registry, now the National Tumour Registry.

He is interested in all kinds of sport and the theatre. Perennially youthful in appearance, of average height with brown hair, quiff intact after retirement, Michael P. is one of those who really changed things for the better. Perhaps most importantly he changed attitudes to academic surgery in Cork. He would be in everybody's list of Ireland's Top Twenty Surgeons of the Twentieth Century.

University College, Galway

O'MALLEY, Michael George (Michael, Mike O)

Professor of Surgery, Galway, and Galway Surgeon

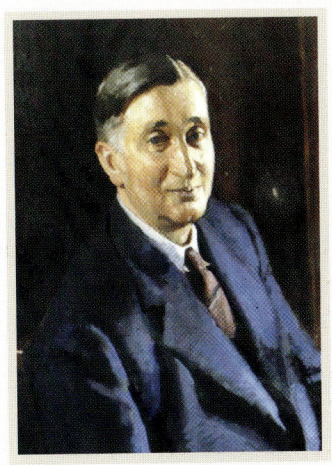

b. 1887, Maam, west of Galway; five siblings became doctors, including J. F. O'Malley, ENT surgeon to St John and St Elizabeth's Hospital, London
Educ. Rockwell College; Queen's College, Galway
m. 1916: Christina Ryan, BA; 7 children (one was Prof. Eoin O'Malley [q.v.] of UCD, and another a radiologist in Canada)
d. 1961

MB, Galway (NUI), 1910, with many distinctions; FRCS, 1915; MCh, 1919

Residency at Mater Hospital, Dublin; demonstrator in anatomy, Middlesex Hospital; house surgeon (to Sir Peter Freyer, another Galway man and the distinguished urologist who invented a 'better'

prostatectomy, at St Peter's Hospital, London). Returned to Galway, 1915.
Professor of Surgery, UCC, 1924–56.
Surgeon, Galway Central Hospital; and subsequently Galway Regional Hospital.

Widely travelled and deeply interested in medical education, Michael O'Malley raised money locally for research. Visiting examiners (and the students) also benefited from his lavish hospitality. A warm, kindly figure, slightly above average height, he looked every inch a professor, and was greatly loved at all levels.

He was a popular golfer and was President of the Golfing Union in Ireland. An expert bridge player, he was President of an International Bridge Congress in Galway, in 1954. There is a wonderful portrait by Sean O'Sullivan in the family archives.

O'BEIRN, Seán Fahy (Seánie)

Professor of Surgery, Galway, and Galway Surgeon

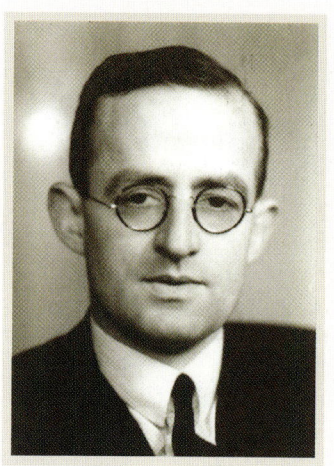

b. 1914, Galway, son of Dr Seamus O'Beirn (GP) and Sabine O'Beirn (*née* O'Malley); nephew of Prof. Michael O'Malley [q.v.] of UCG and a first cousin of Prof. Eoin O'Malley [q.v.] of UCD
Educ. St Mary's, College, Galway; Blackrock College, Dublin; University College Galway
m. Rita Sheil (d. 1992); 3 d (Ann d. 1951, aged 4 years; Geraldine, an anaesthetist; Mary Pat, a psychiatrist), 2 s (Peter d. 1992)
d. 2002

MB, UCG, NUI, 1937; FRCSI, 1940; MCh, 1945

Graded surgical specialist: Commandant, Irish Army Medical Corps, 1940–45.

Lahey Clinic, Boston, US; surgical appointment in Sligo and St Patrick's Chest Hospital, Castlerea. Assistant to Professorial Surgical Unit, Galway Central Hospital.
Professor of Surgery, UCG; consultant surgeon, Galway Regional Hospital, 1958–81 (first full-time consultant surgeon at the hospital).

A safe, careful surgeon, Seánie O'Beirn's availability and dedication to his patients were legendary. It was said that he slept with the telephone receiver cradled in his arms. He was a first-rate clinical teacher, happiest at the bedside demonstrating, with great regard for the patient's sensibilities, some clinical signs. He was immensely proud of the medical school and took particular joy in the judgment of the General Medical Council inspectors in the 1960s that Galway, with its close integration of the university and the teaching hospital, was, from their point of view, the most satisfactory of the Irish medical schools.

In 1978, he instituted an annual meeting in honour of Sir Peter Freyer, the nineteenth-century innovative urologist and UCG's most distinguished graduate, which attracts speakers from all over the world. He had a particular interest in skin cancer and through a collaborative effort with Boston colleagues was able to show that the Irish, wherever they were, had a genetic predisposition to melanoma.

A man of deep faith, he has been described as earnest, humble, sincere, honest and loyal. He was a keen sailor, racing as well as pottering in his locally built boat, a gleoiteog; it is still used by the family. He hunted with the Galway Blazers, swam all year round, and kept his figure spare by jogging. He loved opportunities to use the Irish language with his Aran Island patients. Galway and its graduates have much reason to be grateful to Seánie. His final decade was saddened by his decline into Alzheimer's disease. He was hugely popular with all.

GIVEN, Frederick (Fred)

Professor of Surgery, Galway, and Galway Surgeon

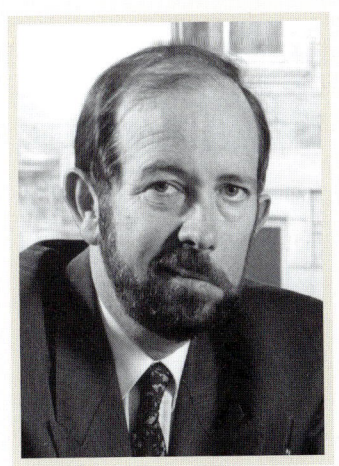

b. 1944, youngest child of Patrick and Nora Given (*née* Feehan)
Educ. Roscommon Christian Brothers School; University College Galway
m. 1968: Kathryn Deacy; 2 s (Mark, a radiologist; John, a pharmacist), 1 d (Elaine, a solicitor)

MB, NUIG, 1967; FRCSI, 1974; MSc (experimental surgery), 1980–81; FACS, 1987

Postgraduate posts in general, thoracic, urological and orthopaedic surgery rotations in Galway, 1968–74.
Surgical tutor 1974–75, Galway.
Registrar, paediatric surgery, Our Lady's Hospital for Sick Children, Crumlin, Dublin, 1975–76; senior surgical registrar, St Vincent's Hospital, Dublin 1977–78; Mater Hospital, Dublin, 1978–79.
Research Fellow, University of Alberta, Edmonton, Canada, 1979–80.
Lecturer in surgery, UCD, 1980–81.
Professor of Surgery and surgeon, University Hospital, Galway, 1981–2003.
Director, National Breast Cancer Research Institute 1991–2003.

Emeritus Professor of Surgery, 2003.
Member, Council, RCSI, 1987–93; Medical Research Council.
President, Irish Society of Surgical Oncology.
Chairman, Sir Peter Freyer Symposium (the largest surgical meeting in Ireland) for 21 years.
NUIG Alumni Award, 2004. People of the Year award, 1992.

Fred Given established the first breast unit in Galway in 1982. His research included work on angiogenesis and tumour markers. As a researcher in Edmonton his experimental animals survived when all his predecessor's animals had died. Fred put a camp bed in the animal laboratory and gave them all 'intensive care' for the vital first 48 hours. How practical.

He took early retirement partly in protest against the failure of the health service to deliver on its promises. At that time, he was one of the nation's leading experts on breast cancer. He had had a near-death experience when a silent acoustic tumour caused him to go unconscious in the operating theatre, where the quick-thinking anaesthetist, Professor Padraig Keane, intubated him and saved his life.

A gifted, bloodless operator, Fred is one of the most retiring of men. He has a caring, uncomplicated personality. A keen gardener and skier, he likes messing around in boats, and is an almost-failed golfer. Totally reliable and totally trusted by the profession, he is a tribune for Galway and for his patients.

UNIVERSITY COLLEGE, DUBLIN

HAYES, Patrick Joseph

Professor of Surgery, Dublin, and Dublin Surgeon

b. 1838, Waterford, son of Thomas Hayes and Maria Hayes (*née* Fleming)
Educ. Dr Quinn's School, Waterford; Carmichael School and House of Industry Hospitals (Richmond)
m. Elisa Hayes; 4 s, 4 d
d. 1904

LRCSI, 1859; FRCS Ed, 1879; MD & MCh, RUI (*hon. causa*), 1885

Surgeon, Mater Hospital, 1869–1903; St Michael's Hospital, Kingstown; St Joseph's Hospital for Sick Children, Temple Street; St Patrick's College, Maynooth.
Professor of Surgery, Catholic University Medical School, 1879–1903.

Many publications on colectomy, hernia, lithotomy, ovariotomy (then one of the commonest intra-abdominal operations because the swelling was palpable), aneurysm, excision of shoulder joints and particularly knee joints.

There is no record of any interaction with the RCSI.

McARDLE, John Stephen (Johnny)

Professor of Surgery, Dublin, and Dublin Surgeon

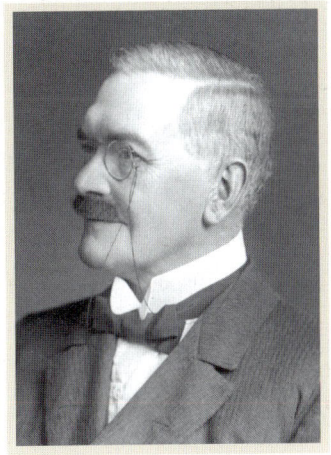

b. 1859, second son of Robert McArdle
Educ. Christian Brothers School; St Mary's College, Dundalk; Royal University of Ireland
m. 1st in 1882: Madeline King Forrest; 4 children.
2nd in 1909: Eileen Nugent; 2 d
d. 1928

MB, Catholic University, Dublin, 1880; LRCP&SI, RCSI, 1880; FRCSI, 1884; MCh, RUI *(hon. causa)*

Surgeon, St Vincent's Hospital Dublin, 1882–1928.
Consulting surgeon, Temple Street Children's Hospital
Professor of Surgery, Catholic University School of Medicine; Royal University of Ireland; University College Dublin, 1900–28.

Member, Council, RCSI.
President, Irish Medical Association, 1906–08.

Author of *Abdominal Surgery*, 1889; *Hydrocele and its Treatment*, 1888; *Students' Note-book of Operative Surgery*, 1894; *Operative Surgery for Students*, 1894; *Renal and Intestinal Surgery*, 1895; *Intestinal Obstruction and its Treatment*, 1896; *Oesophagotomy with Provisional Ligature of Carotid*; *Stricture of Pylorus Treated by Murphy's Button*, 1897; *New Method of Nephrectomy*, 1898; *Radical Cure of Hernia*, 1898; *Gastroenterostomy*, 1906. Contributor to 'Stricture of the Rectum', 'Pylorus Resection', 'Bone Tuberculosis and its Treatment' and other papers, Transactions of the Academy of Medicine, Ireland, 1884–93; 'Causation & Treatment of Arthritis Neurotica', *Dublin Journal of Medical Science*, 1885; Enterectomy & Enterorraphy', Ibid. 1888; 'Treatment of Traumatic Tetanus by Urea', *British Medical Journal*, 1885. (This partial list of publications gives a flavour of surgery at the end of the nineteenth century.)

A vigorous, fiery legend in his lifetime, Johnny, or Surgeon, McArdle was an outstanding figure in Dublin surgery for over forty years. He was a brilliant student and graduated MB with honours on the eve of his twenty-first birthday. He was on the full staff of St Vincent's Hospital at the age of 25. In his early days, he played lacrosse for Ireland, and he was passionately devoted to horses and country pursuits all his life. He was a colourful teacher and attracted the largest classes in the city. In 1889, he went to the USA, where he met the great J. B. Murphy of Chicago and was much impressed with his methods. The two men were of similar temperament.

He would operate from eight o'clock to lunchtime, have lunch at the Dolphin Hotel in Essex Street, which was owned by his in-laws, with his assistants and perhaps a visiting doctor at the table, and then consult at his home, 7 Upper Merrion Street, from two to after six. He would fit in an undergraduate lecture and would then visit the various nursing homes to see his patients. He rarely retired before 1 a.m. and by this time he would have got through five or more large cigars. He was constantly cheerful and optimistic and gave patients great confidence. He was one of the first Irish surgeons to carry out a hysterectomy. He was well versed in the surgical literature and he contributed over forty articles and handbooks covering a huge range of topics.

He had a powerful physique and was a tireless worker.

The monocle and the huge moustache completed his formidable appearance. He was an avowed nationalist and, although he believed that doctors should not get involved in politics, it was said that he flew a black flag over his house when Queen Victoria visited Dublin in April 1900. He loved horseracing and was the jockey's surgeon of choice. Oliver St John Gogarty mocked Johnny's 'miraculous' powers in a poem:

> Let Surgeon McArdle confirm you in Hope
> A jockey fell off and his neck it was broke
> He lifted him up like a fine honest man
> And he said 'He is dead but I'll do what I can'.

The nuns loved him and the legend goes that when he was acquitted in a messy marital court case, they awaited his return to St Vincent's Hospital, then a series of interlinked Georgian houses on the south-east corner of St Stephen's Green. The front door was closed but when it opened there were garlands of flowers and his much-loved champagne.

He gave part of a nationwide subscription in his honour to fund a surgical prize in his beloved St Vincent's, which is competed for to this day. The government sent a plane to circle over Glasnevin cemetery while he was being buried in 1928.

With Thomas Myles [q.v.], his main rival, Johnny McArdle in his heyday dominated the Irish surgical scene. He was the first Catholic of whom this could be said.

BARNIVILLE, Henry Leo (Barney)

Professor of Surgery, Dublin, and Dublin Surgeon

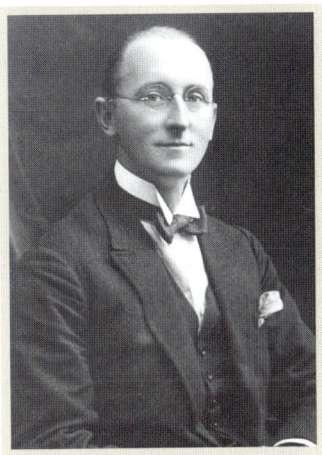

b. 1887, Belfast
Educ. Rockwell College, Co. Tipperary; University College Dublin; Frankfurt-am-Main, Germany
m. 1919: Brigid 'Bee' Weymes; 2 s (Harry was a brilliant physician at the Mater Hospital), 1 d
d. 23 September 1960

MB, UCD, 1910; MCh

Surgeon, Mater Hospital, Dublin, 1915–60.
Professor of Surgery, UCD, 1925–57.
Member, Seanad Éireann, 1922–60

Barney was very much a man of his time, and his career was mirrored by many, but few were as widely liked and successful. He was a warm, gracious, generous spirit, who gave great confidence to his patients. He lived and practised from 9 Merrion Square, a house to which he was devoted and where he entertained and hosted musical soirées. He lived in great style, with an indoor staff of five. Holidays to London or on cruises were on a grand scale: 'Nothing but the best.' His wife, 'Bee', was a central figure in Dublin medical society.

He played rugby as full back for Bective Rangers, and golf at Portmarnock and the Royal Dublin. He was an enthusiastic race-goer and punter and numbered Joe McGrath, of Sweepstake fame, amongst his close friends. He loved the Senate and loved being a Senator but contributed little to the debates and was called 'The Silent Senator'.

A busy hard-working surgeon, with a huge operative load, he was a complete generalist and dealt with many of the fractures and joint injuries of the day. All trainees had a great affection for Barney even though many felt they had learnt little. He never took the FRCSI, as this was the time of a nationalistic backlash against the College, particularly by the youthful UCD. As a surgeon, he had the priceless reputation of being lucky, and the costly one of not always sending a bill. He it was who, with Harry Meade, attended Kevin O'Higgins (Minister of Justice) when he was fatally shot in Blackrock in 1927.

He worked at a time when there was no hospital salary, patients had no medical insurance and crucially he had no pension. He was still on the staff of the Mater, with severe smoker's emphysema, at 73 years of age, when he died. Like so many of his time, he had not found it possible to provide a comfortable nest egg, but his family rallied round and he finished his life at ease and contentment in his beloved 'Number 9'.

MEADE, Henry Sords (Harry)

Professor of Surgery, Dublin, and Dublin Surgeon

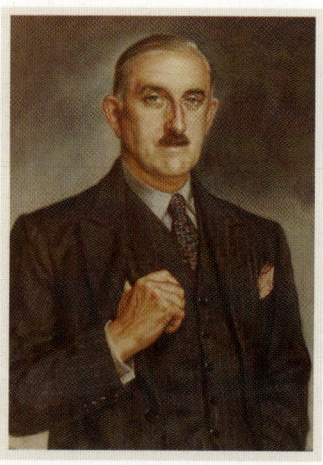

b. 1884, Amoy, South China, son of Henry John and Mary Josephine Meade. Father was in the Imperial Civil Service.

m. Avice Rooney; 2 s; 1 d (Sheila married Seamus Dundon, much-loved Professor of Paediatrics, RCSI)

Educ. Carmelite School and Catholic University Medical School

d. 1952

LRCP & SI 1909; FRCSI 1910

Dublin surgeon PRCSI 1948–50.

Professor of Surgery, UCD, 1928–52.

Became Assistant Surgeon at St Vincent's Hospital in 1913 and remained on the staff until his death. Spent a year with the 17th region French Army and went on to become a Captain in the RAMC, treating some of the casualties of the Battle of the Somme (July to September 1916).

He was a superb tutor at the bedside. He taught the importance of an unhurried history and careful physical examination. He was an absolutely first-rate technical surgeon. His brisk manner with students meant mixed but overall favourable memories of the Professor.

He lived at and practised from 9 Fitzwilliam Place, a splendid, gracious house in the longest row of Georgian architecture then existing. The family subsequently moved to 'Runnymede', a rambling Edwardian mansion on Shrewsbury Road, Ireland's most exclusive thoroughfare. It was there in 1949 that he and Avice threw a huge garden party for the Dublin meeting of the Association of Surgeons of Great Britain and Ireland. Harry was one of seven Irish Presidents during the century.

Very much an international figure, he travelled regularly to foreign clinics and was well known in Vienna.

Tall, lean, somewhat austere, and lantern-jawed, Harry had great style and gave justifiable confidence to his patients. He died of a brain tumour, which manifested itself in dramatic fashion.

FITZGERALD, Patrick Alexis (Paddy Fitz, P. Fitz)

Professor of Surgery, Dublin, and Dublin Surgeon

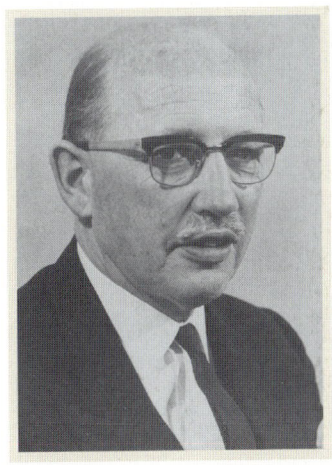

b. 1911, Waterford, second son of Alexis Fitzgerald and Elizabeth Fitzgerald (*née* O'Halloran)
Educ. Waterpark College, Waterford; Clongowes Wood College, Kildare; University College Dublin; Johns Hopkins Hospital, Baltimore
m. 1944: Dr Helen Nolan, daughter of Prof. Thomas and Florence Nolan, BA; 6 s, 2 d
d. 1978

MB (first place), UCD, 1935; MSc, MCh, MD (both in 1940); FRCSI (Hon.), 1962; FACS

Postgraduate appointments, 1937 to 1939, at Johns Hopkins University and hospitals in Baltimore, Maryland (Medical Resident Council of Ireland Fellowship); surgical laboratories of RCS Eng, London. Surgeon, St Vincent's Hospital, 1940–78, and numerous other hospital appointments.

Professor of Surgery, UCD, 1954–76.

Paddy Fitzgerald probably had more influence on the development of Irish surgery than anyone else between 1950 and 1970. He was the first of a new breed who had an extended postgraduate training, as distinct from visits, abroad, and saw what the application of scientific principles could do for the craft. He had a brilliant mind and showed early signs of excellence. He won every available award and scholarship, including a travelling scholarship from UCD.

A broadly general surgeon, he was known for his meticulous technique, which was very much in the wary, careful, exact school of William Stewart Halsted (1852–1922), and which he had learned at Johns Hopkins. At Johns Hopkins he also learned the value of the residency programmes and the importance of incorporating research into a young surgeon's training, even if he were not going on into academic life. He set up research laboratories in the grounds of UCD at Woodview, but was not particularly imaginative in designing projects. He was one of the first professors of surgery to wear a white coat in the hospital, signifying his commitment to hospital life rather than moving round to the various private hospitals and nursing homes.

His main interest was in vascular surgery, for which his technical skills were well suited. The specialty was developing slowly at the time, and myths were slow to be dispelled. King George VI of England had the now-discredited lumbar sympathectomy, in 1948, for obstructive vascular disease, and extensive thoracolumbar sympathectomies were carried out for all forms of hypertension.

Paddy Fitz was early to recognise the importance of publications in the life of the surgeon and co-authored over 100 papers, with the assistance of junior colleagues being fully acknowledged. Although eschewing medical politics as such, he was always active when professional standards were in peril and was the chairman of a government-commissioned report on hospital services (1968). This became known as the 'Fitzgerald' report, which advocated far-reaching changes in the way services were to be delivered. The report was welcomed by the then Minister of Health, Seán Flanagan, but there was little political will to implement its carefully considered findings.

He was good rather than expert at selecting young people from within the hospital for advancement and this meant that succession in various areas was 'sewn up', and the opening up of new surgical subspecialties was encouraged in a highly practical fashion.

He never took the FRCSI and thus the College missed a superb President. His avowed ambition was 'to help in the scientific development of surgery in Dublin and elsewhere, more particularly by improving the educational and research opportunities'. He certainly did everything he could to achieve these ends.

He was of medium height, balding, moustachioed (apparently a family tradition), convivial, slow speaking, wryly humorous, much imitated and greatly loved by the young who worked with him. The broader profession rewarded him with many honours, and perhaps the most appreciated was the presidency of the Association of Surgeons of Great Britain and Ireland when its meeting was held in Dublin in 1967.

He had had rheumatic fever as a child and he developed a resistant infective endocarditis, which precluded heart-valve replacement at the time and from which he died in 1978.

An Irish icon.

O'MALLEY, Eoin PRCSI 1982–1984

Professor of Surgery, Dublin, and Dublin Surgeon

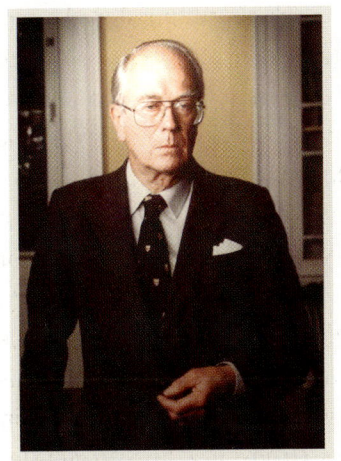

b. 1919, Galway, second son of Prof. Michael George O'Malley [q.v.] (Professor of Surgery, Galway) and Christine O'Malley (*née* Ryan). (The O'Malley family is descended from ancient Irish royalty, with lands centred in Connemara.) Four of his uncles were doctors, of whom three practised in London; Prof. Charles Conor O'Malley [q.v.] practised in Galway. **Educ.** St Ignatius' College, Galway; Clongowes Wood College (where he got first place in the country in at least two subjects in his school Leaving Certificate); University College Galway and University College Dublin
m. Una O'Higgins (1927–2006), daughter of Kevin O'Higgins (Cabinet Minister, murdered in 1927); 6 children (Kevin is a vascular surgeon at the Mater Hospital)
d. 2007

MB, UCD, 1942 (first place, first class honours and gold medal); MCh, NUI, 1947; FRCSI, 1947; FRCS Eng (Hon.), 1984; FACS (Hon.), 1984

Postgraduate appointments at HS Southend General Hospital (where London luminaries came down to operate, some of them all day on a Saturday), and various other, smaller London hospitals, including Mitcham (where he assisted Terence Millin [q.v.], who was developing his retropubic prostatectomy at the time), and the Royal National Orthopaedic Hospital for a year. Lahey Clinic, Boston (with Dr R. B. Cattell and Dr Frank Lahey). Resident surgical officer, Mater Hospital, where he lived in seven nights a week.
Consultant surgeon, Mater Hospital, 1952–85; Peamount Hospital, Our Lady of Lourdes Sanatorium, St Luke's; National Maternity Hospital.
Professor of Surgery, UCD, 1958–85.
President, RCSI, 1982–84.

Eoin O'Malley was the most influential surgeon in the Republic between 1970 and 1990. He was on every local and national healthcare committee of consequence and was the first port of call when the Department of Health needed advice on almost anything. He had been at Clongowes with Cyril Joyce, then Chief Medical Officer, who greatly admired him. Trained as an old-style general surgeon, including orthopaedics, he decided that the chest and particularly cardiac surgery was the most important area for his generation. Heart surgery had started at the rival St Vincent's Hospital, but it was not carried through, and, in the Mater, O'Malley patiently built up the team and the expertise for open-heart operations. It was one of the first hospitals on the island to report a successful series of such procedures.

He published little and most of what he did publish was in local journals, on a wide range of subjects. Although a member of a number of travelling clubs, including the James IV Association of Surgeons, he did not travel a great deal by modern standards; when he did, it was with a specific mission in mind rather than the surgical social round.

A man of great intellect and ability, tenacious, hard working, determined, and seemingly tireless, he never gave up. He had great vigour, surgical skills, intellectual depths, and honesty. He was a talented strategic thinker. Essentially modest, he was easy to work with. It is a formidable list and he was a formidable man.

He was a slow, deliberate operator, who insisted on getting it right first time. His most imitated characteristic was that of never using one word where none would do. This sometimes made lectures and informal tutorials somewhat pithy. It also meant that there were some people with whom he did not establish a warm relationship and easy rapport. His interest in tobacco was legendary but did not always stretch to purchase. Hospital Christmas pantomimes sometimes had 'him' patting the trainees' white coats in search of a packet of cigarettes. He quit, 'out of shame', at 75.

Teak tough, and just above average height, he had played rugby (wing forward in those days) for Clongowes, UCG, UCD and Connaught. He was that surgical rarity, a true intellectual, and had perhaps the highest IQ of any Dublin surgeon of the twentieth century. Some of his considered musings are still quoted. Impervious as he was to the accepted complex taxonomy of awards and honours, he lived a life of huge service to his hospital and Irish surgery. The Mater has a 'Prof Eoin O'Malley National Centre for Cardiothoracic Surgery' and it is a well-deserved honour.

O'HIGGINS, Niall John PRCSI 2004–2006

Professor of Surgery, Dublin, and Dublin Surgeon

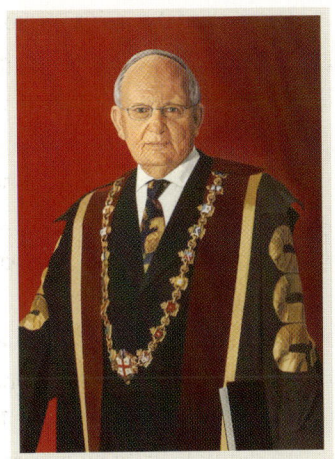

b. 1942, Dublin, son of Dr Niall B. O'Higgins (consultant psychiatrist) and Dr Joan O'Higgins (*née* O'Shea); spent most of his childhood and adolescence in Limerick

Educ. Crescent College, Limerick; Clongowes Wood College, Kildare

m. 1979: Dr Rosaleen Elizabeth Healy, emergency medicine consultant and campaigner (retired); 2 s (Eoin and Conor), 2 d (Amy, a medical student, and Lisa)

MB, UCD, 1965 (first place, first class hons); BSc in anatomy (hons), 1967; FRCS Ed, 1970; FRCS Eng, 1970; FRCSI 1970; MCh (by thesis), 1974; FRCPS Glas (Hon.); FRCPI (Hon.), 2004; FCS South Africa (Hon.), 2005; FACS (Hon.), 2006; FRCS Eng (Hon.), 2000

Postgraduate junior posts at St Vincent's Hospital, Dublin; General Hospital, Portlaoise; Farnborough General Hospital; Croydon General Hospital; Royal Cornwall Hospital, Truro; Hammersmith Hospital, London.
Registrar in surgery and cancer research, Luton and Dunstable Hospital; registrar and senior registrar in surgery, Hammersmith Hospital, and tutor in surgery, Royal Postgraduate Medical School, London; tutor in surgery, UCD, St Vincent's Hospital, Dublin.
Senior lecturer in surgery/honorary consultant surgeon, University College Hospital Medical School, London. Teacher and examiner in surgery, University of London.
Chair of Surgery, UCD and consultant surgeon, St Vincent's University Hospital, Dublin, 1978–2007.
Honorary consultant surgeon, National Maternity Hospital, Holles Street, Dublin.
Consultant and Member, Scientific Committee, European Institute of Oncology, Milan, Italy.
President, RCSI, 2004–06; chairman, Clinical Guidelines Committee.
Consultant, National Cancer Screening Service.
Professor of Surgery Emeritus, UCD.
Chairman, editorial board, European Journal of Surgical Oncology, 2001 to date; European Society of Surgical Oncology (President, 1994–98); Federation of European Cancer Societies (President, 1997–99).
Examiner in surgery in seven medical schools.
Visiting professor in United States, Canada, France, Italy, United Kingdom, Greece, Malaysia, Singapore, Bahrain, New Zealand, Denmark, Kuwait, Indonesia. James IV Surgical Traveller, United States and Canada (1982).
Honorary Fellow, Bangladesh College of Physicians and Surgeons (2004); President's Medal, RCS Ed (2006).

Niall O'Higgins had a brilliant undergraduate career and worked in eight different hospitals, two in Ireland and six in England, before his appointment as Professor of Surgery at his alma mater, St Vincent's Hospital. His ascent up the surgical ladder owed nothing to chance but much to his remarkable ability, industry and determination. He has a bibliography of 287 papers, almost all peer reviewed, and twenty-four books and chapters. His special interest is in breast disease and it was he, more than anyone else, who was responsible for the rollout of the national screening programme for breast cancer. His expertise included thyroidectomy, parathyroid surgery and the parotid, all demanding areas.

He was influenced particularly by his father, by R. B. Welbourn, Patrick FitzGerald, Selwyn Taylor, A. G. Cox and J. Ian Burn. He has not been afraid to take difficult and controversial decisions when it came to concentrating care in centres that were fully staffed and equipped to cope with the work. His twenty-nine-year tenure of the chair of surgery was the longest of any in Ireland in the twentieth century. He is a genuinely modest, highly articulate man with much idealism. He was a particularly sound clinical opinion and a highly competent operator. His heavy schedule of international, mainly European, meetings and conferences inevitably reduced his Irish appearances outside the capital. A few trainees have complained that he rarely assisted them. But in his years as President of the RCSI, he consulted widely and his was a progressive, proactive and productive term of office.

He describes himself thus: 'a serious, occasionally amusing, fastidious, concerned clinician, appreciative of students, advocate for patients, insistent that surgical technique should be anatomically-based, lacking in understanding of hospital managers, not good at compromise, sense of surgical history and heritage, analytical of surgical literature, promoter of interdisciplinary cancer care, dedicated to professionalism and improvement in standards, delighting in surgery and surgeons, respectful of scholarship.'

Niall is 5'5", with a stocky, youthful appearance that hasn't changed in thirty years. He smiles easily, and is always, always, always concerned. He has massive reserves of stamina and has frequently cycled over 100 miles in a day, has a genuine sense of humour, composes light verse apparently easily, and is interested in his children's development, reading and formerly rugby.

(Conflict of interest. Niall has been the O'Donnell family surgeon for more than twenty years. He has been wonderfully kind in this role.)

10
SURGEONS BY COUNTY IN THE REPUBLIC OF IRELAND

SURGEONS BY COUNTY IN THE REPUBLIC OF IRELAND

Hospital Surgeons by County

Carlow

Carlow (pop. 18,487)

Carlow County Infirmary established 1836 (28 beds)

BROOMFIELD, Humphrey John

Carlow Surgeon

FRCSI, 1885, RCSI (gold medallist and senior scholarship) & Vienna

Surgeon, Carlow County Infirmary, 1900.
Member, Council, RCSI.

O'MEARA, William Hy

Carlow County Surgeon, 1910–1920

LRCP & SI, LM, 1877; LM, Rotunda, 1881, TCD

Surgeon, Carlow County Infirmary, 1910–20.
Consultant medical officer of health, Carlow.
Certified factory surgeon.
Physician, St Patrick's College, Carlow; St Mary's College, Knockbeg.
JP, Co. Carlow.

QUILL, Denis

Carlow Surgeon

Educ. Trinity College, Dublin

MB, TCD, 1935; FRCSI, 1936; MCh, TCD, 1950

Postgraduate appointments as house surgeon, Richmond Hospital; orthopaedic registrar, Ancoats Hospital and Manchester Royal Infirmary.
Surgeon, Ministry of Pensions Hospital, Cosham, Portsmouth.
Consultant surgeon, Eastern Health Board; Midland Health Board; St Brigid's Hospital, Carlow.

CAVAN

Cavan (pop. 6,098)

Cavan County Hospital established 1767 (52 beds)

ACHESON, Howard William.

Cavan Surgeon

LRCPI, LRCSI, RCSI, 1881

Medical attendant, Royal Irish Constabulary.

Surgeon, Cavan County Infirmary, 1900, 1910, 1920.

McMULLIN, Joseph Columba

Cavan and Ballyshannon Surgeon

b. 1886, Donegal town, son of Timothy McMullin (Postmaster) and Bridget McMullin (teacher)
Educ. Donegal town; Blackrock College, Dublin.
m. 1913: Frances Byrne (d. 1969); 3 s (eldest, Joe McMullin FRCSI, FRCS, was surgeon at St Vincent's Hospital, Dublin [q.v.]), 8 d
d. 1963

LRCP & SI, Catholic University, Dublin, 1907; FRCSI, 1919

Postgraduate work in various English hospitals.
Burtonport, Donegal, 1912–16.
Rock and Sheil Hospitals, Ballyshannon, 1916–22.
County Surgeon, Cavan, 1922–52.

While in Ballyshannon, McMullin built his own operating table with head and foot pieces. It was there that he performed a life-saving emergency leg amputation on a train crash victim. His DIY wood saw had to be shortened to fit into the pot for sterilising. He became a local hero and the saw a family heirloom.

Working in the Surgical Hospital in Cavan, he was also physician, but was known as 'The Surgeon'. On retirement at 66, he did surgical locums in London and went as a ship's surgeon on the P&O line to South America. He loved 'the boats'.

He had no hobbies and ignored the horse and the fishing rods which his wife purchased more in hope than expectation. Radiation burns of a hand from a leaking X-ray machine required plastic surgery and forced him to drop the scalpel. He died at home of cancer of the prostate. A warm family man.

MOLONEY, Patrick Dermot (Paddy or 'PD')

County Surgeon, Cavan

b. 1904, Rineen, Skibbereen, Co. Cork, eldest son of Martin Moloney (Royal Irish Constabulary) and Eileen Collins
Educ. Royal College of Surgeons in Ireland
m. 1945: Dr Celia O'Regan (MB, UCC, d. 1973); 3 s, 6 d (none in medicine)
d. 1975

LRCP & SI, RCSI 1941; LM Rotunda, 1942, FRCSI, 1944

Resident surgical officer, Lurgan & Portadown District Hospitals.
Visiting surgeon, Portsmouth Corporation Hospitals.
County Surgeon, Cavan Surgical Hospital, 1952–69.

Paddy was a brilliant diagnostician and operator, loved and respected by his patients. He was particularly adept at dealing with young patients. He was a late vocation to medicine, having qualified aged 37. Prior to that, he had worked in an office job at Ford Motor Works of Dagenham, Essex (probably between 1920 and 1935), to where thousands of his fellow Cork men emigrated before and during the Second World War. He did a lot of tutorial work to help pay his way through RCSI.

Lean, 5'6", expressionless, neat and dapper, he wore a morning suit to work for many years. He was really formal in all ways, particularly at ward rounds, through which he smoked. No matter what the emergency, he never swore or used bad language. From over twenty years' residence he had adopted many English cultural habits and expressions and sometimes found it difficult to communicate with his Cavan patients. He never disguised his West Cork accent.

He was a skilled and devoted bridge player, and the Surgeon's Residence on Cavan's Main Street was within a few hundred yards of the bridge club and his local pub. These were almost his only interests outside his family and surgery.

HANNA, Boulos Kamel (Boulus, Paul in English)

b. 1934
Educ. Ain Shams, Egypt
m. Mary, an English nurse
d. 1992

MB, Ain Shams, Egypt, 1958; FRCSI, 1967; FRCS Eng, 1969; LMSSA, Lond, 1966, Demerdashe Hospital Medical School, Cairo.

Postgraduate work included surgical registrar, Letterkenny Hospital.
Consultant surgeon, Cavan County Surgical Hospital. 1974–92.

Pleasant, caring and sincere with his patients, Boulus came from a wealthy Egyptian family with extensive sugar plantations. He attended a private English school in Cairo where his school run was in a Rolls Royce and one of his classmates was the actor and bridge player Omar Sharif.

He had a striking presence, 6'2", broad shouldered and powerfully built; he had been a powerful swimmer of international standard, a 'good Othello'. He had no real interests outside surgery and his beautiful home at Crossdoney. Mary was seriously overweight (about 25 stone) which was a factor in keeping the couple out of local society. He and his wife died prematurely, and generously left their estate to the RCSI.

CLARE
Ennis (pop. 22,051)
Ennis County Infirmary established 1860 (60 beds)

FARIS, George

Clare Surgeon

Educ. Trinity College, Dublin
MD, Dublin, 1893; MB, 1886; LAH Dublin 1886, TCD.

Surgeon, County Infirmary, Ennis, 1900–10.

MacCLANCY, John Boetius

Ennis County Surgeon

b. 1883, Miltown-Malbay, Co. Clare
Educ. Clongowes Wood College; Royal College of Surgeons in Ireland; Catholic University School of Medicine (Cecilia Street)
m. Married with 3 s, 5 d (3 doctors and a dentist: Patrick, a consultant paediatrician at the Rotunda Hospital; Aileen, an anaesthetist, m. Harold Browne [q.v.]. All five daughters married doctors.)
d. 1964

LRCP & SI, 1907

Postgraduate training at St Vincent's Hospital, Dublin, under Surgeon Tobin [q.v.] and Dr Michael Cox.
County Surgeon, Ennis, Co. Clare.
President, IMA, 1944 and 1945.

MacClancy served as County Surgeon in Ennis for forty-five years. He did all kinds of surgery but was a particular expert on the acute abdomen. He kept up to date by reading a great deal and visiting other surgeons.

A great burly man, with a personality to match, he was a popular and fair chairman of many meetings. He was an amusing after-dinner speaker. A keen race-goer, a successful golfer and an occasional fisherman, he was a mine of information on all kinds of sporting lore.

STAUNTON, Edward G. (Eddie)

County Surgeon, Clare

b. 1917
Educ. University College Dublin
m. Joan

MB, UCD, 1939; MCh, NUI, 1945; FRCSI, 1945

Postgraduate work as house surgeon and senior house officer, St Vincent's Hospital, Dublin; senior house officer, County Hospital, Lincoln.
Registrar for three years at Becket Hospital, Barnsley (where he was taught general surgery, gynaecology and orthopaedics).
Locum county surgeon, St Mary's Hospital, Cashel, Co. Tipperary, 1947–50.
Surgeon, Ennis General Hospital, Ennis, Co. Clare, 1950–82.

As County Surgeon, Eddie Staunton was involved in such diverse problems as long bone osteomyelitis, empyema, Millin's prostatectomy, tonsil dissection and caesarean section. He was particularly adept at pinning and plating the fractured femur. Initially without a full-time anaesthetic service, he was a master of local, regional, and spinal anaesthesia. The ambulance service was developed under his guidance and this saved many lives.

Tall, handsome and rugged, with a mane of white hair, he looked every inch a surgeon, and he was every inch a surgeon. He had enormous energy and is loved by the patients and the profession. He is a keen golfer and fly fisherman.

CORK
Bantry (pop. 3,150)

BAKER, Seán

County Surgeon, Bantry, Co. Cork

b. 1923, Ennis, Co. Clare, second son of Michael J. Baker and Bridget Baker (*née* O'Dwyer)
Educ. St Flannan's College, Ennis; University College Dublin
m. 1954: Dr Marie Courtney, FFARCSI, daughter of Letty and T. C. Courtney; 2 d
d. 2008

MB (hons), UCD, 1949 (gold medal in surgery, UCD; McArdle gold medal in surgery, Mater Hospital); FRCSI, 1953; MCh, NUI, 1953; FRCS Eng, 1954

Surgical registrar, Mater Hospital, 1951–53.
Consultant surgeon, Archway Group Hospitals, London, 1955–57.
County Surgeon, Monaghan General Hospital, 1957–59.
Consultant surgeon, Cork County Council at Bantry, 1959–89
Member, Comhairle na nOspidéal for nine years.
Vice-President, Medical Council, 1989–94.
Chairman, Southern Health Board; Irish Consultants Discussion Group; Cork Board of Fisheries.
President, Medical Union; Trustee, Irish Hospital Consultants Association.

A man of prodigious energy, Seán Baker had a glittering undergraduate career, but an occasional impatience led to a falling out with some of the Establishment, and Bantry benefited. At a time when hospitals were under threat of closure, Seán, by sheer force of will and personality, made Bantry's future safe. An activist in community activities, he promoted Bantry in many other ways, too, such as developing the splendid town square, where he had a statue erected to his hero,

Theobald Wolfe Tone. He worked tirelessly for the independence of the profession and it responded by electing him to many high offices.

An expert (international standard) salmon fisherman, he bred wild pheasants and peacocks. Average height, broad shouldered, with dark wavy hair above a craggy visage, he was a voluble, amusing companion.

Mallow (pop. 8,737)

GAFFNEY, Peter Richard ('The Gaf')

Mallow Surgeon

b. 1940, son of Michael Gaffney, FRCS Eng, and Molly Gaffney (*née* Halkett)
Educ. Castleknock College, Dublin; University College Cork
m. Anne Kiely (PhD, lecturer in paediatrics, UCC), daughter of Prof. Patrick Kiely [q.v.]; 4 s (incl. Robert, Director of Clinical Skills Unit, UCC; John a solicitor; Benjamin, an engineer), 2 d (Ruth, an electrical engineer; Rachael, a legal executive)

MB (surgery), UCC, 1965 (first class hons and O'Donovan prize in medicine); Dip Trop Med and Health, London, 1967; FRCSI, 1971; MCh, UCC, NUI, 1982

Postgraduate appointments at Bantry General Hospital; Sheffield Royal Hospital; Bristol Royal Infirmary; Exeter Royal Infirmary; Mount Sinai Hospital, Toronto; Sick Children's Hospital, Toronto; Cork University Hospital, 1976–79.
Consultant general surgeon, Mallow General Hospital, 1979–2005; Shanakiel Hospital 2005 to date.
Medical officer, St Joseph's Hospital, Masaka, Uganda, 1967–69.
Reviewer of original articles for *Lancet* and *Irish Journal of Medical Science*, 1990–2001.
Captain, UCC RFC, 1963–64. London-Irish 1st Team, 1967, East Africa Team 1967–68.
First place, National Marathon Championships, Over 50, 1990; First place, Dublin City Marathon, Over 65, 2005

Author of a widely quoted article on the effective prophylaxis of wound infection in appendicitis.

Peter Gaffney is 6'3" and, according to himself, a 'fit, thin, academic, aggressive, Holy Joe'. Hospitals survive for many reasons but part of Mallow's success is the perception that the energetic Peter Gaffney/Aengus Twomey team gives the locals what they want. Mallow was recently voted the cleanest hospital in the state but the crown has become tilted in 2007.

DONEGAL
Lifford *(pop. 1,395)*
Donegal County Infirmary established 1775 (50 beds)

BOYD, John Craig

Donegal Surgeon

Educ. Trinity College, Dublin

MB, MCh, TCD, 1869

Surgeon, County Donegal Infirmary, Lifford.

BANNIGAN Charles, MC

Donegal Surgeon

Educ. National University of Ireland (Cecilia Street, Dublin)

MB, NUI, 1913

Senior house surgeon, Borough Hospital, Birkenhead.
Surgeon, County Donegal Infirmary, Lifford.

Ballyshannon *(pop. 2,715)*
Sheil Hospital established 1898

1920	Consultant surgeons	E. C. Thompson
		H. T. Warnock
		J. D. Condon, also F. W. Condon (1910)
	Visiting surgeons	J. Gordon
		J. McMullin (see under Cavan)

Letterkenny (pop. 15,231)

McGINLEY, J. P. ('JP')

Donegal Surgeon

b. 1894, Letterkenny

Educ. St Eunan's College, Letterkenny; Queen's University Belfast

MB, QUB, 1916 (first class hons; first place in surgery; gold medal in paediatrics); MCh, QUB, 1945 (dissertation on intestinal obstruction)

Dispensary doctor, Letterkenny, 1918–68.
Surgeon, Letterkenny District Hospital, 1922–60.

JP was one of the last of a breed of surgical pioneers who embraced all other specialties and offered a unique service in a remote area. In the USA and Australia, they are called rural surgeons. Co. Donegal was unique in having four of this species in various locations in the county — Ballyshannon, Donegal Town, Lifford and Letterkenny. Of the four, two had higher surgical qualifications, but JP was also obstetrician, gynaecologist and physician, and dealt with all conditions presenting to him. A surgeon to whom he referred a patient could expect insightful enquiries about the patient's progress.

On his way home from Fairyhouse Races at Easter 1916, he heard of the Easter Rising and became politically involved. He was elected TD to the first Dáil in 1918, having spent some months in Derry Gaol as a Nationalist sympathiser.

He was constantly available for his wide range of responsibilities, and had the strength and energy required. At 6'4" and built in proportion, he managed to continue his political career as well. He was a warm, generous, humorous personality, and the brilliant portrait by Seán O'Sullivan RHA, which hangs in Letterkenny Hospital, shows well the witty geniality which was so much part of this remarkable man.

HANLEY, Joseph Augustine (Joe)

Consultant County Surgeon, Letterkenny, Co. Donegal

b. 1923, Castletownbere, Co. Cork, fifth son of Michael and Hannah Hanley
Educ. Mungret College, Limerick; University College Cork
m. 1955: Dorothy Challans; 3 s, 3 d (two doctors in general practice)

MB (hons), UCC, 1948; FRCS Eng, 1953; MCh, NUI, 1954; FRCSI (*ad eundem*)

House surgeon, Mercy Hospital, Cork; General Hospital, Halifax, Yorkshire; North Middlesex Hospital, London.
Surgical registrar, County Hospital, Lincoln; North Middlesex Hospital (general surgery and orthopaedics); Royal Infirmary, Bradford, Yorkshire; Regional Hospital, Limerick. Senior surgical specialist, Royal Army Medical Corps, 1955–58, stationed in Germany.
Consultant surgeon, Sheil Hospital, Ballyshannon, Co. Donegal.
County Surgeon, General Hospital, Letterkenny, 1960–91.

Joe Hanley's professional life offers an accurate career microcosm of many of his time. An honours graduate, he went to England and changed addresses (involuntarily) eleven times during his twelve years of training. Appointed consultant at 35 years of age (younger than average), he worked single-handedly in Co. Donegal for fifteen years before being joined by J. P. Golden [q.v.]. On call, he could not go to the river or lake to fish because this was before mobile phones and he had to be available. It was entirely the surgeon's responsibility to provide a locum when he was on leave, and, if he couldn't get one, he could not leave his hospital. Joe frequently could not take entitled holidays because there were no available locums, though a sometimes locum surgeon was the legendary Dr J. P. McGinley, MCh. Joe was active in medical affairs, especially the Medical Union. In his retirement, he was interested in medico-legal work.

He described himself as 'short, wide shouldered, cheerful but could be short tempered when stressed, clubbable, gregarious, optimistic'. His recreations included rugby (Schools Munster Junior Cup Medal, 1941), golf, gardening and painting.

'Despite sleepless nights, the constant on-call and the sheer hard physical labour, the practice of medicine fascinates me with its clinical conundrums and humanitarian rewards. I would do it again,' he said. He developed motor neurone disease in his eighties. He deserved better. Much better.

GOLDEN, James P. (Jim)

Letterkenny Surgeon

b. 1941, Cork
Educ. University College Cork
d. 1998

MB, UCC, 1964; FRCS, 1973; FRCSI, 1968

House posts in North and South Infirmaries, Cork; Lourdes Hospital, Drogheda. Registrar, Regional Hospital, Limerick, 1974–75; anatomy demonstrator, UCG. Consultant surgeon, Letterkenny General Hospital, 1975–98.

A keen golfer, Jim Golden was a skilful exponent of the harmonica.

GALWAY (COUNTY)
Ballinasloe (pop. 6,129)

McCORMACK, Michael Joseph

Consultant Surgeon, Ballinasloe, Co. Galway

b. 1916, eldest son of Tom McCormack (County Physician, Laois) and Alice McCormack; three doctor brothers.
Educ. Portlaoise; Castleknock College, Dublin; Royal College of Surgeons in Ireland
m. 1951: Erina Healy; 2 s (elder son, Tom, is consultant surgeon, Kerry General Hospital, Tralee), 2 d
d. 2004

LRCP&SI, RCSI 1940; FRCSI, 1951

Postgraduate training posts in Dublin and UK (Bristol, London, Coventry and Manchester). Consultant surgeon, Portiuncula Hospital, Ballinasloe, Co. Galway. 1956–82.
Surgeon prosector, RCSI, 1982–2000.

Michael was one of the last of the old-style general surgeons who was as skilled in orthopaedics as in gastrointestinal surgery. He was a fully trained surgeon when he took up his consultant post. He loved anatomy, and the RCSI benefited from his late vocation. He played golf into his eighties at Ballinasloe and Rosses Point, Co. Sligo.

KERRY

Tralee (pop. 21,987)

Tralee County Infirmary established 1763 (36 beds)

HAYES, W. B.

Surgeon, Tralee County Infirmary

SHANAHAN, Michael

Surgeon, Kerry County Infirmary

MB, 1913

House surgeon, St Vincent's Hospital, Dublin.
Assistant surgeon, South Infirmary, Cork.
Surgeon, Kerry County Infirmary, 1920.

It was a cruel, and unrelated, coincidence that early in his tenure as county surgeon a second graveyard was opened in Tralee. Perhaps the most oft-told tale of him was the one in which he opened an empyema in the patient's bed in a remote farmhouse, which was approached by a narrow boreen. The patient died when he put the knife in. He and his assistant ran for the car, which unfortunately had been left turned the wrong way around, thus delaying his hasty exit. The relatives surrounded the surgeon and his assistant in the car and they were lucky to get away unscathed. On the way back to Tralee, the surgical apprentice asked, 'Well, what did we learn from that?' Shanahan replied 'Next time, I'll park the car heading for home, not as I did today.'

LYONS, George

Kerry Surgeon

b. 1934, Tuam, Co. Galway, second son of Jimmy Lyons and Delia Lyons (*née* Lavelle)
Educ. St Jarlath's, Tuam; University College Galway
m. 1962: Dr Fin Comer; 2 s (Jimmy a consultant in anaesthesia), 3 d (Fionnuala a consultant in anaesthesia)

MB, UCG, 1957; FRCSI, 1964; FRCS Eng, 1964

Postgraduate training as orthopaedic and surgical senior house officer posts in Kent and Sussex Hospital, Tunbridge Wells, Kent.
Registrar, Galway Regional Hospital (under Mr Bernard Murphy); St Catherine's Hospital, Birkenhead; Broadgreen Hospital, Liverpool.
Consultant general surgeon, Bon Secours Hospital, Tralee, 1965–97.

For thirty-two years, as part of a double act, with his wife Fin as anaesthetist, George Lyons provided care and attention to the people of Kerry in the 'The Bons' in Tralee. He was the most general of general surgeons, performing orthopaedic, obstetric and gynaecological surgery, as well as general surgery. He kept abreast of all innovations, mastering laparoscopic surgery late in his career.

'Small but perfectly formed', he has a great sense of fun and a mischievous but never unkind sense of humour. He is a complete gentleman. Proof of his attractive character is that he has been given the status of honorary Kerryman by that most discerning electorate.

He swam competitively in his youth and is now applying his delicate touch and decision making to the Kerry 'Seniors' Golf Tour. Many of the health service's problems would be solved if every town in Ireland had a George Lyons.

GALVIN, Colm

County Surgeon, 1957–69

See entry under Galway.

Tralee General Hospital opened 1984 (374 beds)

HENLEY, Andrew Finbarr (Finbarr)

Surgeon, Tralee General Hospital

b. 1921, Cork, eldest son of Andrew T. Henley and Agnes Henley (*née* Talbot)
Educ. Christian Brothers College, Cork; University College Cork
m. 1950: Audrey Briggs, daughter of Bertrand and Maud Briggs (d. 1981); 3 s, 3 d

MB, UCC, 1945; FRCS Eng, 1952

Registrar, Royal Berkshire Hospital, Reading.
Surgeon, Government Hospital, Georgetown, British Guiana, 1957–60; Mallow Hospital, 1960–71; Tralee General Hospital, 1971–86.

Very tall (6'3"), thin and quietly spoken, Finbarr Henley was an excellent clinician and operator who never, ever, took on more than he should. A great colleague. Some patients may initially have been daunted by the occasional Zen-like silences but quickly realised that they were getting top-class care. He retired to fish and keep bees near Macroom, Co. Cork.

SPILLANE, Dermot Francis

Surgeon, Tralee General Hospital

MB, 1963; FRCSI, 1969; FRCS Eng, 1970

KILDARE
Kildare, 1930 (pop. 5,694)

COADY, Edward Thomas

Kildare Surgeon

LRCSI & LM, 1893; FRCSI, 1901

Surgeon, Kerry County Infirmary,
Surgeon, County Infirmary, Kildare.

CANNON, Dominick John (Dom)

County Surgeon, Kildare

b. 1884, Glenties, Co. Donegal, eldest son of Cormac Cannon (hotelier) and Ann Cannon (*née* Moore)
Educ. St Eunan's College, Letterkenny; Maynooth College (where he came within one year of ordination to the priesthood); University College Dublin
m. 1920: Ellen O'Connor (d. 1987); 1 s (Paul, Professor of Pharmacology, UCD), 1 d
d. 1967

MA, UCD, 1911; MB, UCD, 1913; MAO, NUI, 1924; LM, Coombe Hospital 1925; MD (published work); MA (Philosophy), UCD, 1944

Captain, Royal Army Medical Corps, 1914–19; transferred to Royal Flying Corps (renamed Royal Air Force), 1918.
House surgeon, Royal Sussex County Hospital, Brighton.

Assistant medical officer, St Mary's Infirmary, London.
House surgeon, North Staffordshire Infirmary, Stoke-on-Trent.
Assistant visiting surgeon, Children's Hospital, Temple Street.
Assistant master, Coombe Hospital, 1922–25.
County Surgeon, Co. Kildare & Drogheda Memorial Hospital, The Curragh (which also acted as a hospital for Co. Carlow).

Dom Cannon did a significant amount of gynaecology and was an extern examiner for obstetrics and gynaecology at UCC, with Professor J. J. Kearney. He continued to contribute articles to medical journals until late in his career. The students made him President of the UCD Medical Society, which is a notable mark of their affection.

Not many other county surgeons would have read Kant for relaxation. Near retirement, he followed in his wife's footsteps and went back to college to do his MA. He was a keen trout and salmon angler and golf was an abiding interest at the Curragh. Dark-haired, 5'7", lithe, kind, humane and a good mixer, he was devoted to his work and intellectual pursuits.

MOONEY, Robert Albert Henry

Kildare Surgeon

Educ. Trinity College, Dublin

MA, Dub, 1968; MB, TCD, 1960; FRCSI, 1969; FRCS Ed, 1965.

Postgraduate training included senior surgical registrar, Royal Hospital, Wolverhampton; surgical registrar, Dr Steevens' Hospital, Dublin; Western General Hospital, Edinburgh.
Tutor in surgery, Dublin University and Meath Hospital, Dublin.
Surgeon, Curragh Military Hospital.

GIBSON, Jack

County Surgeon, Naas, Co. Kildare

b. 1909, Ranelagh, Dublin, youngest of 7 children of Henry Gibson and Millie Gibson (*née* Bailey)
m. 1937: Elizabeth James (d. 1991), youngest daughter of Robert and Ethel James, kinswoman of William James (philosopher) and Henry James (novelist); 1 d
Educ. Wesley College; Royal College of Surgeons in Ireland
d. 2005

LRCP & SI & LM, 1933 (gold medal in surgery); Dip Trop Med and Hygiene, 1934; FRCSI, 1934 (youngest ever Fellow)

Postgraduate posts in Aden and Malawi, 1935–37; McCord Zulu Hospital, 1938.
Dean of Medical Aids School, precursor of Durban Medical School, 1939.
Appointments in Emergency Medical Service, Newcastle, Liverpool and Weymouth.
GP, South Africa, 1946–49.
Surgeon, Queen Elizabeth Hospital, Guernsey, Channel Islands, 1950–58; Haile Selassie Hospital, Ethiopia, 1959.
Resident surgical officer, Dr Steevens' Hospital, Dublin, 1959.
County Surgeon, Kildare, at Naas, 1960–1974.

In Naas, Jack Gibson ran the busiest casualty department in Ireland. However, he will probably be best remembered as a hypnotist who performed 4,000 operations, including amputations and eye surgery, under hypnosis, both in Africa and Ireland. He produced cassette tapes, CDs and videos on such issues as 'The Power of the Subconscious' and 'How to Stop Smoking'. Through self-hypnosis, he cured himself of a basal-cell carcinoma and varicose veins. He was a gift to late-night chat-show hosts.

Jack Gibson lived in Naas in an eleventh-century Norman castle and was interested in camping, rugby, gardening, antiques and renovation of old buildings. He held a trump card as a medical witness, in that he feared no one. He was a short (5'5") balding dynamo, hugely colourful, and, in spite of his height, was described as looking 'a bit like Nelson Mandela' (a big influence on him, as was Mahatma Gandhi). At 95, Jack was still dapper. A legend.

KILKENNY

Kilkenny, 1900 (pop. 20,735)
Kilkenny County Infirmary established 1767 (50 beds)

JAMES, Charles Edward

Kilkenny Surgeon, 1920

Educ. Trinity College, Dublin

BA, MB, Dublin, 1874; LRCSI, 1874; LM, Dublin Lying-in Hospital, 1874 (TCD)

Senior surgeon, Kilkenny County Infirmary.
Consultant medical officer of Health Urban and Rural Districts.
Medical attendant, Kilkenny College & Switzer Charity, Kilkenny.
Medical referee, Kilkenny War Pensions Committee; Alliance and other assurance companies.
Medical officer, HM Prison, Kilkenny.

STEVENSON, Alex. Berchmans

Kilkenny Surgeon

Educ. Catholic University School of Medicine (Cecilia Street), Dublin

LRCPI & LM, LRCSI & LM, Catholic University, Dublin, 1900

House surgeon and house physician, St Vincent's Hospital, Dublin.
Medical officer, Kilkenny No. 1 Dispensary District & Union Hospital.
Surgeon, County Infirmary, Kilkenny.

PHELAN, William Joseph (Willie)

Kilkenny County Surgeon

b. 1897, third son of William Phelan and Ellen Phelan (*née* Shelly) of Cashel, Co. Tipperary

Educ. Castleknock College; University College Dublin
m. 1924: Margaret ('Daisy') Duggan; 1 s, 4 d (Peggy, MB, m. Prof. Frank Muldowney, UCD academic; Ellen is a psychiatrist in Mullingar; Dr Hendy was in Public Health in Arklow)
d. 1963

MB, UCD, 1921

Surgeon, Central Hospital, Kilkenny, 1922–42.
Surgeon, County Hospital, Kilkenny.

At the age of 25, Willie Phelan was appointed in sole charge of the Central Hospital, Kilkenny, which comprised a workhouse, an infirmary and a fever hospital. In 1942, the new County Hospital opened and he confined his practice to surgery. His patients claimed that 'his hands had been blessed by the Pope' though he had never been to Rome and the Pope had not been to Kilkenny!

He and his wife were keen archaeologists, and he was President of Kilkenny Archaeological Society in 1947 and 1963, assisting in the preservation of the beautiful, attractive mediaeval city. His other great interest was horses, which he bred, trained and raced. A model of loyalty, integrity and consideration, he had a strong sense of humour.

SCARISBRICK, Joseph Brendan Pancratius

County Surgeon, Kilkenny

Educ. University College Dublin

MB, UCD, 1946; FRCSI, 1952; FACS, 1962; Dip American Board of Surgery, 1959

Postgraduate appointments as senior resident surgeon, Roswell Park Memorial Hospital, Buffalo, New York; chief surgical resident, Baptist Hospital, Nashville, Tennessee; resident surgical officer, St Mary's Chest Hospital, Dublin.
County Surgeon, Kilkenny.

O'GRADY, Seán Francis (Sean)

County Surgeon, Kilkenny

b. 1935, son of Gerald O'Grady (pharmacist, Irish Army) and Sheila O'Grady (*née* Cassidy)
Educ. Belvedere College, Dublin; University College Dublin
m. Angela Brennan; 2 s (Paul is an orthopaedic surgeon), 2 d
d. 1986

MB, UCD, 1960; FRCSI, 1964; MCh, 1966; American Boards in colorectal surgery, 1970

Postgraduate travelling Fellowship in surgery with Harry E. Bacon, Temple University, Philadelphia, 1970–71.
County Surgeon, Kilkenny, 1971–86
University tutor in surgery, UCD; examiner in FRCSI.
Physicians' recognition award, AMA, 1971.

Seán O'Grady was an active member of, and often hosted, the 'Surgical Discussion Group'. He came from a remarkably talented musical family, played the violin and sang with a clear tenor voice. Geraldine O'Grady, Ireland's foremost violinist, is a sister. He was a founder of the Kilkenny School of Music, played first-class rugby, got a UCD rowing 'Blue' and was coach and team doctor to Kilkenny RFC. He was a warm, generous spirit, a devoted husband and proud father. He gave great service to the people of Kilkenny and was a valued part of the fabric of the city.

King's County/Offaly
Tullamore (pop. 11,098)
Tullamore County Infirmary established 1783 (50 beds)

MEAGHER, Timothy M. C.

Surgeon, 1920

Educ. Royal University of Ireland

MB, RUI, 1906

Temporary Captain, Royal Army Medical Corps (Croix de Guerre).
Medical officer, Post Office.
Surgeon, King's County Infirmary.

HUGHES, Joseph (Joe)

County Surgeon, Tullamore, Co. Offaly, 1965

b. 1926, Donegal, son of Michael and Anne Hughes
Educ. St Munchin's College, Limerick; Clongowes Wood College; University College Dublin
m. 1956: Carmel Fallon; 3 s (Kieran a GP; Joseph FRCS (otorhinolaryngology); John P. a solicitor)

MB, UCD, 1950; FRCSI, 1959; FACS, 1967

Postgraduate training in Birmingham Accident Hospital (Peter S. London), 1951–52. Registrar, Dr Steevens' Hospital, 1958; St Laurence's Hospital (Richmond) (under Prof. C. K. Byrnes and P. C. Carey), 1956–60; Salford Royal Hospital, Genitourinary Unit (Denis Poole Wilson), 1961–62. Senior registrar, City Hospital, Stoke on Trent, 1962–64.
Consultant surgeon, Midland Health Board, General Hospital, Tullamore, Co. Offaly, 1965–92.

Above average height, dark, concerned and deeply conscientious, Joe Hughes returned to Ireland fully trained. He is one of the shrinking garrison of county surgeons who soldiered on his own for many years. A tireless, neat, operator, he sometimes had difficulties getting a few days' cover for attendance at UK meetings, even for his beloved British Association of Urological Surgeons, but he kept right up to date and was held in great affection by the local population, whom he served so well. In retirement, he pursues golf and angling, as well as music and history.

DURKIN, Francis Anthony (Frank)

General Surgeon, Tullamore

b. 1945, Dublin, third son of John Durkin (labourer) and Kathleen Durkin (*née* Devaney)
Educ. Synge Street Christian Brothers Schools, Dublin; University College Dublin
m. Dr Jean Kelly from Tipperary

MB, UCD, 1969; FRCS Eng, 1978

Postgraduate training included surgical teams, St Finbarr's Hospital, Cork, 1971–72; demonstrator in anatomy, UCD; surgical registrar, Basingstoke, 1977–79 (with R. J. Heald, famous colorectal surgeon).
Tutor in surgery, UCD, 1979–80 (worked with and greatly admired Prof. Eoin O'Malley [q.v.]).
General surgeon, Tullamore.

As a student at UCD, Frank Durkin was vice-president of the Students' Union (1967). He was also Irish champion and international oarsman, and later an international rowing coach. He was a founder of Offaly Rowing Club and has been president of the Irish Amateur Rowing Union since 2002.

LEITRIM
Carrick-on-Shannon (pop. 2237)
Carrick-on-Shannon County Infirmary (52 beds)
1900

BRADSHAW, R.

Surgeon, Carrick-on-Shannon County Infirmary

BRADSHAW, R. Jnr

Assistant Surgeon, Carrick-on-Shannon County Infirmary

McDERMOTT, Patrick

Surgeon, County Leitrim Infirmary, 1920

LRCPI, LM, LRCSI & LM, 1903

House surgeon, Mater Misericordiae Hospital, Dublin; St Michael's Hospital, Kingstown.
Surgeon, County Leitrim Infirmary.

Limerick
Croom (pop. 1,056)
Limerick County Hospital

O'CONNOR, John (The Surgeon O'Connor)

Limerick County Surgeon, 1926–55

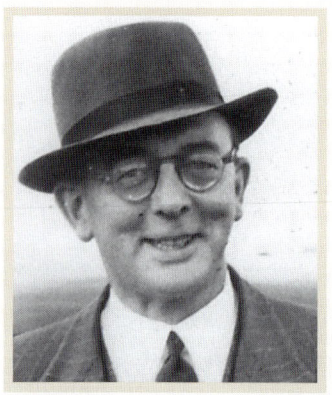

b. 1899, Limerick, third of 4 sons of Edmund O'Connor and Catherine O'Connor (*née* O'Sullivan) (both national school principals), Tervoe, Co Limerick; brothers all doctors
Educ. Mungret College, Limerick; Royal College of Surgeons in Ireland
m. 1st in 1932: Molly Dwyer-Joyce (d. 1946), daughter of Prof. Robert Dwyer Joyce (distinguished Dublin ophthalmologist); 1 s, 1 d. 2nd in 1949: Nan Heaphy (d. 1991)
d. 1959

LRCP & SI, RCSI, 1922; FRCSI, 1925

Limerick County Surgeon 1926–55, St Nessan's Hospital, Croom, Co. Limerick.
Regional orthopaedic surgeon, 1955–59.
Career visits to the Mayo Clinic. WHO Fellowship to the USA, 1958.
Freedom of the City of Boston, USA.

Appointed County Surgeon at age 28, to a general hospital of 100 beds, John O'Connor and the matron ran the entire institution with firm hands. His patients were the most important people in the hospital and they got nothing but the best, and his inspections included the kitchens. He was in the operating theatre most days until early afternoon and then he did ward rounds of the type seen in movies of the time. He was a good correspondent and read voraciously, mainly on surgical, particularly orthopaedic, topics.

John O'Connor had high intelligence, class and style. Measuring 6'1¼" in his socks, he had a splendid appearance and confident manner. He was always beautifully dressed with horn-rimmed spectacles, and trademark cigar at a jaunty angle. People really did notice when he came into a room. He was a demanding, domineering, sometimes irascible 'chief', but it was all on behalf of his patients. He took no nonsense and this style also extended to his operations and his interpersonal relationships. He prospered as a surgeon and delighted in driving his huge American car to the Dublin hospitals, to overawe his struggling contemporaries. He was an impatient fisherman.

He was dead at 59, one of that generation of surgeons who died prematurely from hard work and tobacco.

Longford

Longford Town (pop. 7,757)

Longford County Infirmary established 1767 (39 beds)
1900–1920

MAYNE, Nathaniel

Surgeon, County Infirmary

LRCPI & LM, 1872; LRCSI, 1871

LAVERTY, Thomas

Surgeon, County Infirmary

MB, RUI, 1905

STANLEY, Anthony Joseph

Honorary Surgeon, Westmeath Infirmary

BA, NUI (first class hons), 1919; MB, 1926, UCD

O'SHEA, JOHN ('John O')

County Surgeon, Longford, 1937–64

b. 1898, Cahirciveen, Co. Kerry
Educ. CBS Cahirciveen; Blackrock College, Dublin; University College Dublin
m. 1936: Agnes Patterson of Edenderry; 1 d
d. 1976

MB, UCD, 1921; MD, 1927; MCh, 1934; FRCSI, 1934

Postgraduate appointments as house surgeon, Mater Hospital, Dublin; in Nottingham, general practice; in Cahirciveen for two years; Middlesex Hospital, London.
Resident surgical officer, Children's Hospital, Manchester.
County Surgeon, Longford, 1937–64.

John O'Shea had a brilliant scholastic and sports career at Blackrock College, winning prizes and exhibition scholarships. He was an inter-provincial schools rugby player. While house surgeon at the Mater, he had a confrontation with the 'Black and Tans', when he refused to let them see a patient with gangrene, even when they threatened to shoot him.

He came to Longford well trained by the standards of the day, and, through hard work, determination and boundless energy, he established himself as one whose skill and judgment were widely known and respected.

A handsome man with impressive features, he was always neatly dressed. He sometimes gave the impression of being brusque, but underneath he was a kindly family man. He was a keen golfer and race-goer. On retirement in 1964, he qualified as a solicitor through Trinity College. He was one of the last of a durable breed of single-handed surgeons who provided high-quality services for a wide range of problems.

BARRETT, Connor

County Surgeon, Longford, 1975–92

Educ. University College Dublin

LAH, 1949; MB, UCD, 1952; FRCSI, 1958; LMC (Canada), 1965; FRCS (Canada), 1972

Postgraduate work included house surgeon, Orthopaedic Professorial Unit, Royal Southern Hospital, Liverpool; registrar, General and Genitourinary Unit, Oldchurch Hospital, Essex. Surgeon, General Hospital, Vancouver.
County Surgeon, Longford County Hospital, 1975–92.

LOUTH
Dundalk (pop. 32,505)
Louth County Hospital, Dundalk, established 1750 (42 beds)

McDONNELL, H.

Surgeon, Louth County Hospital, 1900

O'HAGAN, J. V.

Surgeon, Louth County Hospital, 1920

LRCPI & LM, LRCSI & LM, 1908 (RCSI & Catholic University, Dublin)

CLARKE, James Joseph

Surgeon, Louth County Hospital, 1950

LRCPI & LM, LRCSI & LM, Catholic University, 1907

Surgeon, Louth County Hospital.

MULCAHY, Ursula Mary

Surgeon, Louth County Hospital, 1978–2004

MB, BS, Newcastle, 1965; FRCS Ed, 1970

Postgraduate work included registrar in surgery, Sunderland General Hospital; surgical registrar, Royal Infirmary, Hull.
Surgeon, Louth County Hospital, Dundalk, 1978–2004.

Drogheda (pop. 31,020)
International Missionary Training Hospital

SHEEHAN, Michael Vincent (Vincent)

Drogheda Surgeon

b. 1912, Carnew, Co. Wexford, son of two schoolteachers
Educ. Scholarships to Castleknock College (became head prefect and got first place in the national Leaving Certificate examination); University College Dublin
m. Dr Marie de Vere from Ballina (became his consultant anaesthetist); 2 s, 3 d
d. 2000

MB, UCD (first place, first class hons) 1935; MCh, NUI, 1942; FRCS Ed, 1941; FRCS Eng, 1942; FRCSI, 1969; FICS, 1955; PhD (by thesis at age 76), UCD

Postgraduate posts in Middlesex, Hammersmith and Guy's Hospitals; Surgical Emergency Medical Service in London Hospital and St Olave's Hospital, Rotherhithe, Surrey, where he looked after many injured fliers and civilians.
Fellow in Surgery, Lahey Clinic, Boston.
Surgeon, Our Lady of Lourdes International Missionary Training Hospital, Drogheda, for 39 years.

A legend in his lifetime, Vincent Sheehan, having failed to get a post in Dublin, despite his outstanding academic and training credentials, determined to make Drogheda a centre of excellence, and he did. He rarely sent patients on the 30-mile journey to the capital. He was a really good, fast operating surgeon, who could, and did, turn his hand to anything.

His great interest was teaching and he had a staccato style of reeling off the core issues of a problem in such a fashion that examiners would sometimes ask a candidate if they had been at Vincent Sheehan's 'grind'. It didn't always help to say 'yes', but his tutorials on a Saturday morning were thronged with students from abroad as well as the locals. He had myriad slides and a binder of 'Notes on Surgery', which he subsequently published as a book. He showed the schoolmaster's genes in his didactic teaching.

Always demanding the best for the patients, he was right up to date with the surgical literature. He had applied for the Chair of Surgery at UCD, at St Vincent's Hospital, his alma mater, and felt that his rebuff was unfair. He ran the whole Drogheda hospital as a personal fiefdom and as a 'tight ship'. He preserved the highest standards and was very critical of anyone guilty of a breach. He would not have been considered an easy colleague but he loved surgery and surgical discussions and was a warm, entertaining, polymath and interesting travelling companion. He was awarded the Knighthood of St Gregory for his work in Nigeria on behalf of the Medical Missionaries of Mary. He was a great traveller and not only visited Germany, France and Spain but was fluent in each language.

Tall (5'11"), with a constant, engaging smile, he had volcanic energy. Typically, when he had to retire on grounds of age, he took a Master's degree in the then fledgling science of computers at TCD. An unforgettable character and an icon.

Mayo
Castlebar (pop. 11,371)
Castlebar County Infirmary established 1790 (58 beds)

KNOTT, Middleton O'Malley

Mayo Surgeon

> b. 1838, son of William Knott (1807–71, GP/surgeon, County Infirmary, Castlebar and Physician to County Gaol for 40 years) and Mrs O'Malley Knott (a descendant of Grace O'Malley [Granuaile]); an uncle, George O'Malley, commanded a battalion at Waterloo
> d. 1920
>
> LRCSI & LRCP Ed, 1864.
>
> Postgraduate appointments as medical officer to Militia in Castlebar; GP in England.
> GP/surgeon, County Infirmary, Castlebar, 1871–1907.
> Anaesthetist/assistant surgeon, County Infirmary, Castlebar, 1907–1927.
> Medical officer to Castlebar Gaol and the RIC.

Middleton O'Malley Knott succeeded his father as surgeon/GP in Castlebar. Until 1910, there was no operating theatre, and all surgery was done on the ward. A skilful surgeon, he was held in high esteem locally. He was replaced as surgeon by

Anthony McBride but stayed on as anaesthetist/assistant until his eightieth year. In 1919, he carried out two successful appendicectomies in one day.

A most charitable and tolerant man at a time of vicious Catholic/Protestant animosity, he contributed to the building of the local Catholic church and was the subject of a warm, appreciative obituary in the *Connaught Telegraph*. He had been an excellent horseman and successful amateur jockey.

His nephew, Lieutenant General Knott, was Director General of the Royal Army Medical Corps, 1964–66. A brother, John Knott, FRCSI, lived in York Street, Dublin. In 1916, heading for the College library, he was followed in the front door by Countess Markievicz (1868–1927), Frank Robbins and members of the Citizen Army who occupied the building for a week.

McBRIDE, Anthony ('Daddy')

Mayo Surgeon

b. 1869, son of Captain Patrick McBride (a merchant seaman from Cushendall, Co. Derry) and Hanoria (*née* Gill) of Westport
Educ. Catholic University School of Medicine (Cecilia Street), Dublin
m. Lelia Mooney; 2 s (Patrick, MB, UCD)
d. 1942

MB, RUI, 1889 (Catholic University, Dublin)

Spent a year as a ship's surgeon (did one tracheotomy) before appointment to Castlebar. County Surgeon, Castlebar, Co. Mayo. 1907–40.

When 'Daddy' McBride was appointed to Castlebar, the salary for the position was £100 a year, with house, fire, lighting and land surrounding the Infirmary; in 1923, it was £500, with no private practice allowed; and in 1940, it was £800, the starting salary for all county surgeons at that time. In 1907, he had no operating theatre, no outpatients' department, and sixty beds with straw mattresses. Each mattress had an oval hole in the tick (cover), so that the nurse could take out a bundle of straw and change it, or often just shake it. There was no WC, only an earthen closet, and two baths. There were two nurses, one for the male and one for the female ward. Domestic help did night duty.

McBride set up a Guild of Ladies and began fundraising for an operating theatre, beds and equipment, pawning his life insurance policy to finish the work. He set up a nursing school and involved the local GPs as assistants. The matron either assisted or gave the anaesthetics of open-drop ether and chloroform. He spent thirty-three dedicated years bringing the hospital up to the best possible standards, setting a headline for his successors.

McBride took the Free State side during the Civil War (1921–23). He was on the Central Council of the IMA. About 5'10", erect, with a military moustache, stiff collar and bow tie, he was most energetic and enterprising and did rounds at 7.30 a.m.

BRESNIHAN, Patrick Cornelius (Paddy)

Mayo Surgeon

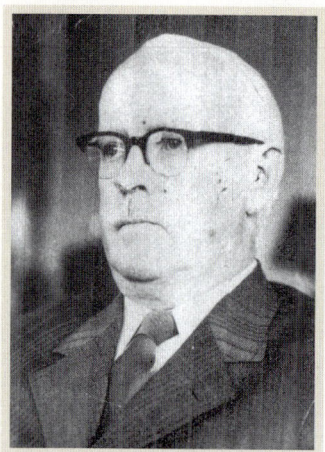

b. 1912, Castletown, Co. Limerick, first child of John and Elizabeth Bresnihan
Educ. Limerick (first place in Ireland in Intermediate Certificate, 1928); University College Dublin
m. Nora Murphy; 2 s (Eoin is consultant radiologist, Western Health Board), 3 d
d. 1987

MB (first class hons), UCD, 1936; FRCSI, 1940; MCh, 1942; MD (published work), 1843

House physician, Mater Hospital, Dublin 1937.
Travelling scholarship in pathology to Freiburg, Germany, 1937–38.
Assistant surgeon, Woolaston Infirmary, Newport, Monmouthshire, Wales; and surgical registrar, Mater Hospital, 1939–42.
County Surgeon, Mayo, 1942–76.

Paddy Bresnihan began his time in Castlebar in 1942 when the hospital had 124 beds, twenty-six nurses and two house doctors. Chronic osteomyelitis, tuberculous bones and joints, caesarean sections, gynaecology, tonsillectomies, prostatectomies and gastrectomies (the great general surgical operation of that time) were all the responsibility of one surgeon. Anaesthetics of open-drop ether were administered by the house staff. Paddy's salary was £800 a year, and private practice was tightly controlled.

Twenty years later, the hospital had a qualified anaesthetist (Dr Aubrey Bourke), a shared radiologist, and two assistant surgeons (K. Jones and Gerry Leahy). The grind of having to be always available, always in the public eye in the town, sometimes through lack of a locum unable to take his leave entitlements, and the 168-hour week was exhausting and draining. He was an ideal choice to represent the county surgeons on the committee that produced the ground-breaking Fitzgerald Report (1968), which proposed a reduced number of properly staffed hospitals.

Paddy Bresnihan was a very big man (6'2"), with imposing appearance, and was full of ideas and energy. He had been Irish High Jump Champion at 16 and became a popular golfer, inevitably captaining Castlebar Golf Club. He also shot, fished and read widely. His health suffered in later years but he lived happily in Castlebar and Spain for ten years after his retirement. An iconic county surgeon.

LEAHY, Edward Gerard (Gerry)

Mayo Surgeon

b. 1922, Miltown-Malbay, Co. Clare, eighth in a family of 12, seven of whom were doctors, including three GPs, two psychiatrists, one physician and Gerry, a surgeon.
Educ. La Sante Union, Bath; St Mary's, Rathmines, Dublin and Clongowes Wood College; University College Dublin.
m. 1959: Anne Brickley of Clonakilty; 4 d (Helen, a nurse; Yvonne, a dentist; twins Elizabeth, occupational therapist, and Barbara, marketing)
d. 2008

BComm (first class hons), 1942; LRCP&SI, 1948; FRCSI, 1953

Surgical registrar, Mercer's Hospital and Urological Unit at the Meath Hospital with Tom Lane [q.v.].
Senior registrar and first assistant (to chest surgeon Maurice Hickey [q.v.]), St Finbarr's Hospital, Cork; Sarsfield's Court Regional Sanatorium, Cork.
County Surgeon, Mayo County Hospital, Castlebar, Co. Mayo, 1963–87.

Gerry Leahy was that great surgical rarity — a fully trained competent surgeon who was happy to be second in command rather than leader. Having studied commerce in UCD from 1939 to 1942, he had begun an apprenticeship to a chartered accountant. However, after six weeks, he switched to medicine at the RCSI. He was a hardworking loyal colleague everywhere he went. He retired to Dublin in 1988.

JOHNSTON, Joseph G. (Joe)

Mayo Surgeon

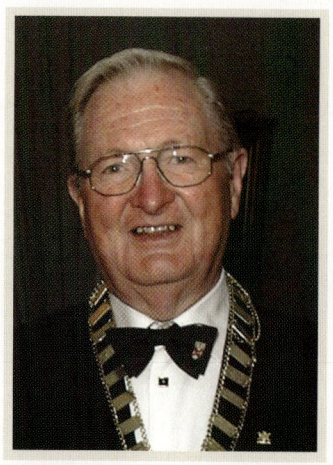

b. 1933, only child of Michael J. Johnston and Mary Johnston (*née* Golding; d. 1938); stepson of Peg Johnston (*née* Sharkey)
Educ. CBC Monkstown, Dublin; University College Dublin (Commerce); Royal College of Surgeons in Ireland
m. 1964: Siovan A. Murphy, third daughter of Seán Murphy and K. C. ('Jimmy') Murphy (*née* James); 2 s (Sean is consultant surgeon, Tullamore General Hospital), 2 d (Orla is a GP in Dublin)

LRCP & SI, LM, 1962; FRCS Ed, 1969; FRCSI (*ad eundem*), 1987

House surgeon and house physician, Jervis Street, Dublin, 1962–63.
Lecturer in anatomy, RCSI, 1963–64.
Royal Army Medical Corps, 1964–74 (served in Germany and Millbank London; saw action in Oman during Rebellion; mentioned in Dispatches).
First senior registrar in Irish Scheme/lecturer, St Laurence's Hospital, 1974–77.
Consultant surgeon and chairman, Surgical Division, Mayo General Hospital, 1977–99.
Member, Council RCSI, 1988–99; Chairman, Finance Committee, 1996–99; President, Association of Graduates, 2004–06; Examiner in FRCSI & FRCS Ed.

Joe Johnston was responsible for many, many 'firsts' at Mayo General, including 'screening' clinics and laparoscopic surgery. He was also the first 'County' surgeon to put together a three-man team of surgeons. Some wanted to do this but he made it happen. He began close co-operation with UCG Medical School.

He is a loyal graduate of RCSI who put his honed administrative skills to work in his hospital and the College. He also did a huge job for the entire community of Mayo. He was a shrewd, prolix medical politician with sound values and principles.

Joe played rugby for Greystones 1st fifteen in 1952–56, and later took up shooting, golf, gardening and hill walking. A big, rampaging six-foot, rugby forward, he became a genial chief and a great travelling companion.

MEATH
Navan (pop. 19,417)
Navan County Infirmary established 1756 (41 beds)

FINNEGAN, Laurence Patrick Joseph

Surgeon, Navan Union Infirmary, 1900

Educ. Royal College of Surgeons in Ireland

LRVP&I, 1877; LRCSI, RCSI, 1876

Medical attendant, St Finian's Diocesan Seminary.
Civilian surgeon, 5th Battalion Leinster Regiment.
Surgeon, Royal Irish Constabulary.
Surgeon, County Meath Infirmary; Navan Union Infirmary.

TIMMON, W. P.

Honorary Surgeon, 1920

LRCP, LRCS Ed, LRFPS Glas, 1905 (Ed & Dublin)

ROSS, Charles Homan Givan

Honorary Surgeon, 1920

MB, RUI, 1906; LRCPI, Catholic University Dublin, 1910.

House surgeon, Meath Hospital; County Dublin Infirmary (two years).
Temporary Lieutenant, Royal Army Medical Corps, 1915–17.
Certified factory surgeon.
Honorary surgeon, County Infirmary, Meath.

MOORE, Hy. Francis

Honorary Surgeon, 1920

MB, NUI, 1912

SHANAHAN, Edward Francis (Ted)

County Surgeon, Meath, 1955–1962

MB (hons), UCD, 1944; MCh, NUI, 1949; FRCSI, 1948; FRCS Eng, 1953

Postgraduate studies included travelling studentship in anatomy, NUI, 1945; lecturer in anatomy, UCD.
Surgical registrar, Liverpool Royal Infirmary; senior surgical registrar, Birkenhead General Hospital.
Surgeon, Meath County Council, 1955–62.

Ted Shanahan was a brilliant student. However, his postgraduate career was cut short by mental illness.

LAVELLE, James Stephen Richard Mary ('Ruaire')

County Surgeon, Meath, 1962–1984

b. 1924, eldest son of Dr Richard Lavelle of Castleknock, Co Dublin, and Mrs Lavelle (*née* O'Meara; one of five O'Meara sisters who married into the Dublin medical establishment); His uncle Edward (Eddie) Lavelle, who died prematurely, had been assistant surgeon at the Mater Hospital
Educ. Ballinasloe, Co. Galway; Belvedere College, Dublin; University College Dublin
m. Dr Ena Kenny (anaesthetist; d. 1999); 1 s (John, a urologist in North Carolina), 2 d (Ena is a psychiatrist in Portrane, Co. Dublin)
d. 2006

MB, UCD, 1949; MCH, NUI, 1957; FRCSI, 1955

Postgraduate work included junior posts at the Mater Hospital, St Michael's Hospital and St Laurence's Hospital (Richmond); two years at the Gastroenterology Unit, St James's Hospital Balham London (under Norman Tanner, the most distinguished and admired English upper abdominal surgeon of his generation).
Senior surgical registrar, St Laurence's Hospital, Dublin.
Tutor in surgery, UCD, at Mater Hospital, Dublin.
County Surgeon, Meath, at Our Lady's Hospital, Navan, 1962–84.
Visiting surgeon, James Connolly Memorial Hospital, Blanchardstown.
Surgeon, Bahrain, Arabian Gulf.
Member, Council RCSI.

A really well-trained surgeon who brought new standards to his post, Ruaire Lavelle was a highly skilled gastrectomist when that was the central operation in upper abdominal surgery. He was a dedicated teacher of surgery, both to medical students and postgraduates, and was one of the first county surgeons to be involved in training programmes organised by the RCSI. Appointed by government to Comhairle na nOspidéal (Hospital Council) from 1972 to 1985, he was trusted completely by his colleagues who elected him to the Council of the RCSI where, in time, he would probably have become president, were it not for his economic decision to go work in Bahrain, where his skills were appreciated.

Formal and dedicated, he put his patients first, last and always. He was quietly spoken, a deep thinker and held conservative, traditional views on the ethical issues of the day. Of medium height, stocky, terse and shrewd, he was seldom without his pipe.

In retirement, he returned to his O'Meara roots in Connemara and a retirement cottage in Cashel, Co. Galway, where he made life hell for the sea trout in the local lakes. He integrated into the community and became a sort of 'village explainer' for those with all kinds of problems. His twilight years were blighted by a prolonged and painful descent into Alzheimer's disease, throughout which he had wonderful family support.

HYLAND, Gabriel (Gay)

County Surgeon, Navan, Co. Meath

Educ. University College Dublin

MB, UCD, 1960; FRCSI, 1963; FRCS Eng, 1966; MCh, NUI, 1968

County Surgeon, Our Lady's Hospital, Cashel, Co. Tipperary.
County Surgeon, Meath County Council at Navan.

Monaghan
Monaghan (pop. 5,946)

Monaghan County Infirmary established 1768 (60 beds)

HALL, James Campbell

Surgeon, Monaghan County Infirmary, 1900–1930

Educ. Trinity College, Dublin

AB, Dublin, MB BCh, 1878; Diploma in State Medicine, TCD, 1878; LM RCPI, 1878

Assistant physician, Highfield & Hampstead Private Lunatic Asylums, London.
Surgeon, Monaghan County Infirmary, 1900–30.

MOLONEY, Michael

Consultant General Surgeon, Monaghan County Hospital, 1963–96

b. 1931, son of Michael Moloney and Margaret Moloney (*née* Quinliven)
Educ. O'Connell Schools, Dublin; University College Dublin
m. 1961: Eileen O'Brien, daughter of John and Mary O'Brien; 3 s, 1 d

MB, UCD, 1955; MCh, 1962; FRCSI, 1962; FRCS, 1963

Surgical tutor, UCG, 1959–62.
Consultant general surgeon, Monaghan County Hospital, 1963–96.

Influenced by Professor Neil McDermott [q.v.], PRCSI, and Anthony Walsh [q.v.], urologist, Jervis Street Hospital, Dublin.

An interesting and amusing teacher, Michael Moloney had a very well-run unit with long series of difficult operations with the minimum of complications. His recreations include tennis, golf and chess.

Queen's County/Laois

Portlaoise (pop. 15,037)

Maryborough, Portlaoise Queen's County Infirmary founded 1766 (90 beds)

JACOB, William Gardiner

Consulting Surgeon, Queen's County Infirmary, 1900

LRCP, 1881; LRCSI, 1880 (RCSI)

Surgeon, Queen's County Infirmary.

BLAYNEY, John

Surgeon, Queen's County Infirmary, 1920

Brother of Alex Blayney [q.v.], of the Mater Hospital, Dublin

O'CONNELL, Michael John ('The Boss')

County Surgeon, Laois, 1918–1952

b. 1884, Templemore, Co. Tipperary, third son of William O'Connell and Brigid O'Connell (*née* Coffey)
Educ. Rockwell College (scholarship); Catholic University School of Medicine (Cecilia Street)
m. Agnes Barry of Gort, Co. Galway (a nurse who took first place in her finals at the Richmond Hospital, Dublin, and subsequently did private nursing at the Mater Hospital, Dublin); 3 s (Liam, Dublin haematologist; Francis Xavier [q.v.], surgeon, Mater Hospital, Dublin; J. M. Brian, nephrologist Washington, DC); 3 d
d. 1954

MB, Royal University of Ireland, 1908 (first place in all subjects, Chancellor's gold medal for outstanding student of the year)

Postgraduate studies included visits to London twice a year to visit various major hospitals. Kept in close touch with the Rotunda Hospital, Dublin, where he had probably been a clinical clerk.
Dispensary doctor, Borris-in-Ossory, 1908–12; Maryborough/Portlaoise, 1912.
County Surgeon, Laois, at Portlaoise 1918–52.

Michael O'Connell's story is typical of the time. A talented, brainy man, his first post was as a general practitioner and he went into surgery without further training, as was the custom of the time, because that was what he wanted to do and he did it well. He was appointed county surgeon in 1918, initially to the County Infirmary and, in 1939, to the County Hospital. He was proud of his position as medical adviser to the Jesuit community at Emo, Co. Laois. He also had a big medico-legal and workman's compensation practice. If necessary, consultants were brought down from Dublin (a guinea a mile to Portlaoise, so the round trip was 100 guineas, exclusive of the fee).

In his early practice days, he made rounds on one of his two horses and subsequently had two cars. He had a driver who also had to be a mechanic, as cars broke down frequently. There was no heating in the early cars and he carried rugs, a hot water bottle and a flask of hot tea. There were frequent night calls. The flu epidemic of 1918 was a time of great stress. It was said that for three months he never undressed and he slept in a chair. There were few telephones but the hospital and the Garda station had one each. His work was his life but his other interest was his highly successful family. He was genial, smiling.

His funeral was one of the largest ever seen in Portlaoise. The description of the event in the newspaper the *Leinster Express* (published Portlaoise, price two pence) the issue of 25 December 1954 (sic) is a cultural capsule of another age. There were

96 Catholic clergy present and each is given his rank in that complex taxonomy, as well as whence he came to the funeral. The Minister for Health and many local politicians, as well as representatives of other churches and other professions are all listed. Last in the list is his extended family.

An epic occasion for a great man.

McCORMACK, Charles J. (Charlie)

County Surgeon, Portlaoise

b. 1923, youngest of nine children of Dr William and Germaine McCormack of Wicklow
Educ. Dominican Primary School, Wicklow; Clongowes Wood College, 1934–40; University College Dublin
m. 1955: Monica; 7 s, 4 d
d. 2003

MB, UCD, 1946; FRCSI, 1952; MCh, NUI, 1958

Postgraduate training posts in St Vincent's Hospital, Dublin; Lancashire; Sheffield; London; St Kevin's Hospital, Dublin.
Locum consultant in county hospitals in Tralee, Roscommon, Longford, Ennis and Cashel.
Tutor, St Vincent's Hospital, Dublin, 1958–59.
County Surgeon, Portlaoise, Laois, 1959–88.

At school, Charlie McCormack had been a popular all-rounder, distinguished in studies and games. As a student, his summer job was playing the piano for guests at the Butler Arms Hotel, Waterville, Co. Kerry, and his great skill enlivened hundreds of parties throughout his life. His training as detailed above shows not just how varied it was but also the appalling dislocations which were part of the wonky professional ladder of the time.

An inspiring and knowledgeable teacher, he was a thoroughly reliable surgeon and a most supportive colleague. He worked as a solo county surgeon for many years. Eventually a jovial Harvard-trained colleague joined him and put a board on his clinic door which said simply, 'County Surgeon'. Charlie reposted with his own board, which said 'Senior County Surgeon' — a designation that does not exist.

He played competitive golf off about 12 handicap and was president of the local club. He played and holidayed at Dooks in Kerry. He was a founding member of the Rugby Club in Portlaoise and was the driving force in bringing it from simple beginnings to winning the Towns Cup, which was a source of great joy to him.

Charlie was exactly what a county surgeon needed to be, with all the professional and social skills required, and an eagerness to immerse himself in the local community in a productive manner. He was loved and missed.

ROSCOMMON

Roscommon Town (pop. 4,489)

Roscommon County Infirmary established 1783 (60 beds)

1900–1920

BLAKENEY, Edward Thomas

Surgeon, Roscommon County Infirmary

Educ. Royal College of Surgeons in Ireland

LRCPI 1869; LRCSI 1869, RCSI

O'HANRAHAN, John Tobin ('Jock')

County Surgeon, Roscommon

LRCP & SI 1933; FRCSI 1937

County Surgeon, Co. Roscommon

RELIHAN, Michael

Consultant Surgeon, Roscommon County Hospital, 1977

b. 1938, Listowel Co. Kerry, eldest son of Thomas Relihan and Brigid Relihan (*née* Horan)
Educ. Presentation Brothers College, Cork; St Ita's College, Abbeyfeale, Co. Limerick; Trinity College Dublin
m. 1977: Geraldine Kennealy, daughter of Niall and Joan Kennealy; 1 d

MA, MB, TCD, 1962; FRCSI

Postgraduate posts as house officer, Richmond Hospital, Dublin; casualty officer, Central Middlesex Hospital; house surgeon, Hammersmith Hospital, London; registrar, St Finbarr's Hospital, Cork.
Research Fellow, Tulane University, New Orleans; First Assistant Surgical Fellow, Lahey Clinic, Boston (with Ken Warren, 'pancreas king'), resident in cardiothoracic surgery, Albany New York.
Surgical registrar and tutor, Royal City of Dublin Hospital, Baggot Street, Dublin.
Locum surgeon, North Eastern Health Board and South Eastern Health Board, 1974–76.
Consultant surgeon, Western Health Board, Roscommon, 1977–2003.
Examiner and demonstrator, RCSI.

bove average height with a distinguished appearance, Michael Relihan was very well trained in many sub-specialties. Diffident (by surgical standards), he paid tribute to colleagues, especially in Portiuncula Hospital, Ballinasloe, who helped him as a single-handed county surgeon. His interests include horse racing, golf, opera and gardening.

SLIGO

Sligo Town (pop. 19,735)

Sligo County Infirmary established 1760 (54 beds)

MacDOWELL, Effingham Caroll

Sligo County Surgeon, 1900–1920

Educ. Trinity College, Dublin; Radcliffe Medical School, Oxford

AB, MD, MB, MCh, 1875; FRCPI, 1883 (senior modern exhibitor and gold medallist, TCD; Radcliffe Medical School, Oxford)

Surgeon, Sligo County Infirmary, 1900–1920.
Visiting and consultant physician, Sligo District Lunatic Asylum.
JP for Sligo.

McCARTHY, Charles J. (Charlie)

Sligo County Surgeon, 1924–1958

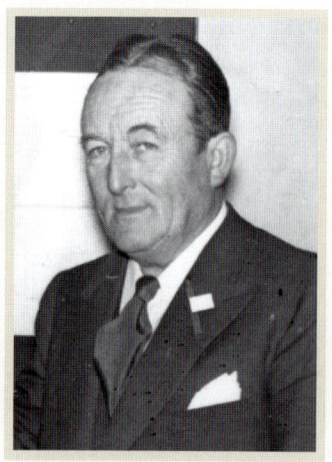

b. 1892, Tralee, eldest of 7 sons of Thomas and Margaret McCarthy (*née* Walsh)
Educ. Rockwell College, Co. Tipperary; University College Dublin
m. 1917: Mae O'Sullivan, BA (Music), daughter of Donal and Hanna O'Sullivan, Killarney; 1 s (Donal, iconic county physician, Laois)
d. 1975

MB (first class hons), UCD, 1914

Surgical training, Mater Hospital, Dublin, largely under Alec Blayney [q.v.].
Sligo County Surgeon, 1924–58.

A keen sportsman, he was on the Rockwell Senior Rugby Cup Team but it was as a golfer that he excelled. He played to scratch and once beat the International and Close Irish Champion, Dr James Mahon. He was an active member of three clubs: Rosses Point (golf); the 'Constitution', Sligo ('Social and Business'; Protestants not admitted…tit for tat of course… and that in WB Yeats' home town); and in the twilight zone, 'Beatrix's' or the 'Glue Pot' whose raison d'etre is self-explanatory. A true bon vivant, he was a competitive snooker and poker player. He regularly had champagne breakfasts in the Hibernian Hotel on his visits to Dublin, and he attended race meetings and all the big game finals.

A larger-than-life character, he was a brilliant raconteur, and stories of doubtful provenance were often attributed to him. At 5'10" in height, he was broad and strong, with great stamina, and was the solo county surgeon for thirty-four years. Deeply religious, he attributed his recovery from earlier TB to divine intervention, and perhaps there was intervention again when he survived, for eight years, a pneumonectomy (Sir Thomas Holmes Sellors in London) for carcinoma of the lung. Memorable.

BOLAND, Denis

Sligo Surgeon

Educ. University College Dublin

MB, UCD, 1936; FRCSI, 1947
Postgraduate appointments as resident surgical officer, Roscommon County Hospital; Derbyshire Royal Infirmary; Salford Royal Infirmary.
Assistant surgeon, North Western Health Board at Sligo General Hospital.
Proprietor of Garden Hill, Nursing Home, Sligo.

A large, cheerful, bucolic character, Denis Boland ran the only private nursing home in Sligo, where he did almost everything, including obstetrics and gynaecology.

SWAN, Thurloc

General Surgeon, Sligo, 1961–1986

b. 1922, London, younger son of William Swan (a GP graduate of RCSI) and Ann Swan
Educ. St George's College, Weybridge, Surrey; University College Dublin
m. 1952: Veronica Donnelly, daughter of Michael and Sheila Donnelly; 1 s, 2 d
d. 2006

MB, UCD, 1945; MCh, NUI, 1951; FRCSI, 1951

Postgraduate appointments as house officer, St Vincent's Hospital, 1946; senior house officer, Crumpstall Hospital, Manchester, 1946; senior house officer, Chase Farm Hospital, Enfield, Middlesex, 1947; surgical registrar, Leigh Infirmary, Lancashire, 1947–48.
Royal Army Medical Corps, 1949–50; served in Middle East.
Surgical registrar, St Kevin's Hospital, Dublin, 1950–52.
Assistant surgical specialist, Civil Hospital, Aden, South West Arabia, 1952–56.
Surgical specialist, Civil Hospital, Ibadan, Nigeria, 1956–60.
Consultant surgeon, Sligo General Hospital, 1961–86.

A general surgeon in the best sense of the word, Swan had an immaculate surgical technique. In retirement, he had wide interests in rugby, tennis, golf, walking, reading and classical music. Of average height, he was always well groomed, dapper and ready for inspection.

McDEVITT, Joseph Brendan (Brendan)

Sligo Surgeon, 1972–98

b. 1934, Sligo, son of Joseph McDevitt and Kathleen McDevitt (*née* McCauley)
Educ. St Macartan's College. Monaghan; University College Galway
m. Anne Marie O'Sullivan, daughter of Stephen and Molly O'Sullivan; 3 s

MB, UCG, 1958; MCh, NUI, 1967; FRCSI, 1967

Postgraduate work at UCG Hospital; Bantry General Hospital; Tralee General Hospital; Jervis Street Hospital; Our Lady's Hospital for Sick Children, Crumlin, Dublin.
Surgeon, Sligo General Hospital, 1972–98.

Brendan McDevitt really enjoyed the work and the interaction with patients, students and nurses. He was a completely reliable operating surgeon, with great judgment. In retirement, he fishes but misses the hospital buzz.

Tipperary

Cashel (pop. 2,270)

Tipperary County Infirmary established 1768 (54 beds)

RUSSELL, George Hy

Surgeon, Tipperary County Infirmary, 1900

LRCP, LRCSI, 1892 (RCSI & TCD)

HOGAN, Patrick, TD ('Surgeon Hogan')

Surgeon, Our Lady's Hospital, Cashel, Co. Tipperary, 1940

b. 1907, Rearcross, Newport, Co. Tipperary
Educ. Doon CBS; University College Dublin
m. Unmarried
d. 1972

MB, UCD, 1929; MCh, UCD; FRCS Ed

Postgraduate training in Dublin, London, Edinburgh and Vienna.
County Surgeon, Roscommon.
Surgeon, Our Lady's Hospital, Cashel, Co. Tipperary, 1940.

Initially appointed county surgeon in Roscommon, Patrick Hogan moved to Cashel when the opportunity arose. He had a 'lifestyle' disagreement with the nuns who ran Our Lady's Hospital and moved his surgical practice to his residence in John Street, Cashel, where he had an operating theatre on the top floor of a four-storey building. It is reputed that four strong men were often summoned from local hostelries to carry patients up and down the stairs to the operating theatre.

He never married and his second love after surgery was politics. In 1945, he was elected to Tipperary County Council, and subsequently became chairman. He was elected to the Dáil in 1961, 1965 and 1969. He was Fine Gael spokesman on Local Government and Health and was appointed Chairman of the Dáil Public Accounts Committee. As a sitting member of the Dáil, he tended to operate in the evenings when the House had risen. A legend even in his time, he often consulted at midnight with his jacket, stiff collar and tie discarded. He was feared but trusted by patients, many of whom saw him as a figure from a bygone age.

NOONAN, Timothy Joseph (Tim)

County Surgeon, Our Lady's Hospital, Cashel, 1957

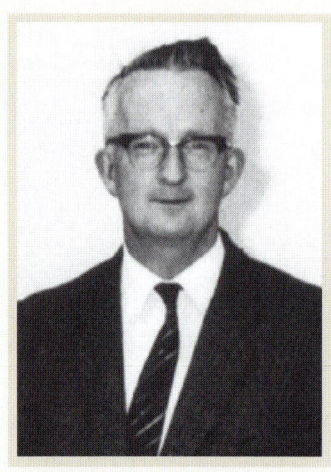

b. 1920, Ballineen, Co. Cork, first son of James N. Noonan and Elizabeth Kearney Noonan
Educ. Mount Mellary School, Co. Waterford; University College Cork
m. 1951: Eileen Cronin; 1 s, 6 d (one, Carmel, an ophthalmic surgeon in Warrington, England)
d. 1975

MB, UCC, 1944; MCh, FRCS, Ed, FACS, FICS & FRSM, Lond

Volunteered as a medical officer with the Medical Missionaries of Mary and worked in St Luke's Hospital, Anua, Oyo, Southern Nigeria, 1946–49. Ainsworth travelling scholarship from UCC to Minneapolis, Minnesota (under Prof. Owen Harding Wangensteen, with whom he established great rapport. Wangensteen was one of the world's leading surgeons at that time).
Surgical registrar, Wigan, Chepstow and Salford in England, and with John Kelly [q.v.] (whose protégé he was) at St Finbarr's Hospital, Cork.
County Surgeon, Our Lady's Hospital, Cashel, 1957.

Hugely popular and held in great respect at all levels, Tim Noonan was the ultimate iconic county surgeon. He often said that he would 'follow general surgery to the ends of the earth', though his main interest was gastroenterology. He was seldom happier than when discussing minute (but vital) details of operating technique, late in the evening, surrounded always by admiring colleagues. He was the initiator of the Surgical Discussion Group where the practical problems of patient management were dissected in depth and there were no holds barred in the debates, which excluded almost all aspects of molecular biology. There is a Noonan Medal awarded to a surgeon 'approved' by the group.

On the small side, bespectacled, slope-shouldered and prematurely grey-haired, he looked like a care-worn under-promoted civil servant, but few in the country were listened to with more respect and none was better loved. In his later years, he suffered from generalised vascular disease, survived a severe stroke in 1974, and had a subsequent lower limb amputation. The UCC medical students commemorate him by the Surgeon Noonan Society, a charity which funds students for elective work in developing countries.

Nenagh

O'DOMHNAILL, Seamus

Consultant Surgeon, Nenagh and Limerick

b. 1922
Educ. University College Cork
m. Married with 5 children (daughter, Nuala Ní Dhomhnaill, is one of Ireland's best-known poets)
d. 2006

MB (hons), UCC, 1946; FRCS Eng, 1951; MCh, NUI, 1953; Fellow, International College of Surgeons, 1966; FRCSI (*ad eundem*), 1966

Postgraduate work included demonstrator in anatomy, UCC, 1948; surgical registrar, General Hospital, Burnley, Lancashire, 1951–52; St Helen's Hospital, 1952–57.
County Surgeon, Nenagh, 1957–72.
Consultant surgeon, Limerick Regional Hospital, 1972–86.

Seamus O'Domhnaill was an archetypal county surgeon with a great love of Ireland and the Irish language, which he spoke on all possible occasions. His relaxed manner, sharp mind and ease of vaulting over examination hurdles would have ensured him a post in England's provinces but he desperately wanted to be near his roots. He built up trust and admiration wherever he went.

A keen ballroom dancer, and also a former university featherweight boxing champion, he was 5'5" in height, with curly ginger coloured hair and a boxer's nose. He was always either smiling or about to smile. A dedicated countryman, he was an international authority on gun dogs and their training. Ironically he died of a heart attack when trampled on by cattle while out with his dog.

HICKEY, John F. (Jack)

County Surgeon, Nenagh

LRCP & SI, 1948. FRCS Ed, 1959

Sometime medical missionary doctor.
County Surgeon, Nenagh.

249

Waterford

Waterford (pop. 46,736)

Waterford County and City Infirmary established 1897 (62 beds)

MAKESY, George Ivie

Waterford County Surgeon, 1900

Educ. Trinity College, Dublin

AB, TCD, 1866; MA, 1869; MB, 1868; LRCSI, 1868 (RCSI and TCD)

Surgeon, Waterford Lying-in Hospital.
Surgeon, County and City Infirmary, Waterford.
President, Irish Medical Association.

All doctors gave their services free to county infirmaries at that time, and no private patient, or anyone who could afford anything better, ever crossed the threshold. There was a bust of him in the entrance hall of the Infirmary.

MORRIS, William Richard

Surgeon, Waterford County and City Infirmary, 1900

MB, RUI, 1888 (Carmichael College and TCD)

FRIEL, Robert

Surgeon, Waterford County and City Infirmary, 1900

Educ. Trinity College, Dublin

MB, 1895; MD, 1897; FRCSI, 1898, Dublin, Cork, Vienna

Surgical traveller prize-winner, TCD, 1896.
Surgeon, Extern Department, County Infirmary, Waterford.

STAUNTON, Frederick William

Surgeon, Waterford County and City Infirmary, 1900

Educ. Trinity College, Dublin

BA, MB, TCD, 1892

House surgeon, Adelaide Hospital, Dublin.
Surgeon, HM Prison Waterford.
Surgeon, Waterford County and City Infirmary.

MORISSEY, Joseph M.

Surgeon, Waterford County and City Infirmary, 1920

FRCSI, 1901; L & LM 1895; LRCPI & LM, 1895, LM, Rotunda Hospital, 1897 (Cecilia Street & TCD)

House surgeon, Mater Hospital; St Michael's Hospital, Kingstown.
Medical officer, Cork Street Fever Hospital.
Surgeon, Waterford County and City Infirmary.

JELLETT, James William Hy

Ophthalmologist and External Surgeon, Waterford County and City Infirmary, 1920

Educ. Trinity College, Dublin

MD, TCD, 1890; MB, 1888; DPH RCPSI (hons), 1900, TCD

House surgeon, Peterborough Infirmary.
House officer, St Mark's Ophthalmic Hospital, Dublin.
Surgeon, Waterford County and City Infirmary.

HOGAN, John Joseph

Resident Surgeon, Waterford County and City Infirmary, 1920

Educ. Catholic University School of Medicine (Cecilia Street), Dublin

LRCSI & LM, Catholic University, Dublin, 1906

Resident surgeon, Waterford County and City Infirmary.

SHIPSEY, Maurice

Waterford Physician and Surgeon

b. 1891, Dunmore East, Waterford, twin son of Isaac Shipsey and Elizabeth Shipsey (*née* Walsh)
Educ. Castleknock College, Dublin; Royal College of Surgeons in Ireland
m. 1921: Edith Marguerite Kearney, daughter of William and Mary Kearney; 3 d
d. 1959

LRCSP & LM, LRCSI & LM, RCSI, 1924 (gold medal in operative surgery; senior clinical medal, Meath Hospital and many other top prizes); DPH, RCSI, 1920

Captain, Royal Army Medical Corps, 1915–18; served in Mesopotamia.
Physician and surgeon, Waterford County and City Infirmary, and County Physician (served in this post to his death).

This hugely talented man was part of a medical dynasty. He kept up his contacts with his beloved Meath Hospital, particularly with Mr Tom Lane [q.v.]. He founded the Waterford branch of the Knights of Malta Ambulance Corps, and was President of the Waterford Golf Club, an expert shot with a love of gun dogs, and physician to the Waterford Football Club.

A sheaf of twelve testimonials of Maurice Shipsey was preserved by the family. Many of the letters are 150 or more words long but some of the phrases give a flavour of the man and the time, *c.*1914: 'If Dr Shipsey remained in town he would attain one of the highest positions in the Profession' — William Taylor, Vice President, RCSI. (You have to come from any other Irish city to realise how much the word 'town' for Dublin is disliked.) 'Earnest, remarkably brilliant, industrious, talented' — Conway Dwyer, PRCSI. 'Very distinguished answering' — John W. Moore, Prof Medical, RCSI. 'Zeal and attention…kind and attentive to the sick poor…steady and gentlemanly conduct.' — Sir Lambert H. Ormsby, Past President, RCSI (and not a man to get carried away about anybody). 'Far beyond the average in his general intelligence and aptitude…the goodwill of all who knew him…by far the best man in his year…ever been popular…good sense and tact.' 'Brilliant and industrious…glad to record my admiration of his sterling worth' — Oliver St John Gogarty, MD FRCS, nationalist, poet, and ear, nose and throat surgeon. It was also said of him: 'He was a striking figure with a most amiable disposition and was loved by one and all.'

COFFEY, William Stanislaus (Bill)

Surgeon and Physician, Waterford, 1925–1964

b. 1886, Fethard, Co. Tipperary, second eldest son of Michael Coffey (miller) and Ellen Coffey (*née* Lonergan)

Educ. Newbridge College, Co. Kildare; Royal College of Surgeons in Ireland

m. 1912: Dorothy Mary Begley (d. 1958; her brother, Joe Begley, was private secretary to Éamon de Valera during the War of Independence, 1918–22, and was gaoled, while another brother was in the Palestine Police in 1918 and was killed in action); 3 s (one, Richard, a doctor).

d. 1964

MRCSI, (LRCSI), RUI, 1910

Postgraduate position in Leeds (as assistant to Berkeley George Andrew Moynihan [subsequently Lord Moynihan], with whom he met King George V several times).
Captain, Royal Army Medical Corps, Malaya (Penang and Malocca), 1913–22; Free State Army, 1922–25.
Surgeon and physician, Waterford, 1925–64.
Proprietor of a highly successful nursing home in Catherine Street, Waterford.
Medical officer, Royal British Legion, Waterford.

Bill Coffey was a general surgeon with a particular skill in skin grafting. He had a big 'carriage trade', including Lord and Lady Waterford of Congreve, but he had equal time for poor people, and in his early days some of them were without shoes. ('Treating duchesses like charladies and charladies like duchesses' was a traditional recipe for success in Harley Street.) He spoke Malay (well after nine years...), knew and disliked W. Somerset Maugham (he was certainly on the side of the majority in that one), was interested in Buddhism although a devout Catholic, and had a massive library. He farmed, collected antiques and stamps, told stories and was immersed in the history of Co. Tipperary. All in all, he was a most colourful personality and was supposed to be the 'doctor' in Molly Keane's novels. He was most highly regarded as a surgeon.

Union Hospital (St Patrick's)

WHITE, Vincent, TD

Waterford Surgeon

Vincent White worked in St Patrick's in the early 1920s. He was a Sinn Féin TD, and was one of a few surgeons to have been a member of the Dáil. As the late Jack Lynch (Taoiseach, 1967–73 and 1977–79) remarked to the editor, 'Doctors make good candidates but bad TDs because they are always rushing back to their patients.'

d'ABREAU, Abundius Joseph Grian Bhrugh

Waterford Surgeon

b. 1889
Educ. Grant Medical College, Bombay
m. 1913: Lucy Victoria d'Souza (d. 2006, in Scotland, aged 113 years; at the time of her death, she was the oldest person in Great Britain); 1 s (died aged 4), 5 d (2 medically qualified)
d. 1971

MB, BS, University of Bombay, 1912; FRCS Ed, 1922

Postgraduate work included Dr Muller's Hospital and private practice, Mangalore, India, 1912–17; Captain, Indian Army Medical Service, 1914–18 (wounded at the front in Mesopotamia [Iraq]).
Trained in radiology and radiotherapy in Germany and London, as well as urology (with Terence Millin [q.v.]).
Outpatient surgeon, Waterford County and City Infirmary.
Visiting surgeon, Maypark, John of God's Hospital, Waterford.

D'Abreu was an avid reader of medical and classical literature. Kindly to all, particularly those in trouble, socially or professionally, he prevailed upon the St John of God order to open the Maypark Nursing Home in Waterford in the late 1920s.

He was a keen cricketer, tennis and bridge player. He also greatly enjoyed the 'musical evenings' of his era, both in his home and with friends, and was co-founder, with William Watt, of the Waterford Festival Choral Society. He did not suffer fools gladly, if at all, and in his declining years he was renowned locally for his motoring 'idiosyncrasies'. Always immaculately turned out, he was the epitome of a westernised Indian gentleman.

O'REILLY, John Thomas (Jack)

County Surgeon, Waterford, 1953–1980

b. 1916, Dublin, older son of John O'Reilly and Ann O'Reilly (*née* Moran)
Educ. O'Connell's Schools, Dublin; University College Dublin
m. 1942: Dr Josephine Heffernan (d. 2001), daughter of William and Frances Heffernan;
5 d (1 nurse, 4 doctors)
d. 1980

MB, UCD, 1939; FRCSI, 1941

Postgraduate work at Brompton Hospital, London; St James's Hospital, Balham, London (with Norman Tanner, the leading abdominal surgeon of his time).
Major, Royal Army Medical Corps.
Surgeon, County and City Infirmary, Waterford, 1949–53.
County Surgeon, Waterford, 1953–80.

Jack O'Reilly's upbringing was modest but he excelled scholastically and won academic scholarships, which took him through medical school. He had a great belief in meritocracy, a love of athletics and of things Irish, and an admiration for James Connolly and his tenets. He disliked incompetence and laziness (once remarking that the only good thing he could say about a particular trainee was that he had a great appetite). He assembled a team of people completely loyal to him and he was particularly proud that some of 'his' nursing staff remained with him for most of his career. He had a strong sense of humour, and the theatre tearoom ('with tea strong enough to trot a mouse on') rang with laughter.

He never used electrocautery. His great interest was peptic ulcer, and he refused to believe that stress was a factor in ulcer, as most of his patients were phlegmatic farmers. How right he was.

A huge man with a booming voice, military bearing and moustache to match, he loved his all-female family, he frequently said, 'Blessed am I amongst women'. For over twenty-five years, he was the solo county surgeon for a population of over 50,000. Few could have done it up to Jack's standards.

POWER, William Henry (Liam)

Waterford Surgeon

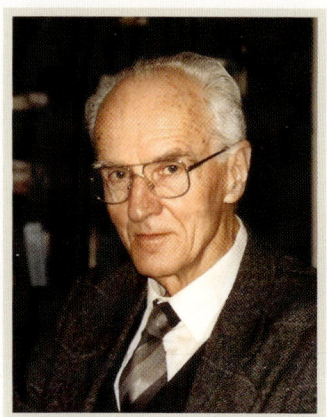

b. 1919, Cork, eldest son of John Power (Headmaster of Cork School of Art, an artist and sculptor) and Eleanor (Ellen) Power (*née* Riordan)
Educ. Presentation College, Cork; University College Cork
m. 1949: Marion Freda Milburn (d. 1987), daughter of Fred and Teresa Milburn, York, England; 4 s (2 doctors: Anthony, Dublin; Aidan, Connecticut). 2 d (Juliana, a clinical psychologist, Elgin, Scotland)
d. 2001

MB (first class hons), UCC, 1941; MCh, 1952

Postgraduate work at Winwick Emergency Hospital, Warrington, England, 1945; orthopaedic registrar, Royal Northern Hospital, London; registrar, Southern Hospital, Dartford; surgical registrar, Croom, Co. Limerick, 1951–53.
Consultant surgeon, St Patrick's Hospital, Fermoy, Co. Cork, 1953–55.
Consultant surgeon, Maypark Private Hospital, Waterford; Ardkeen Hospital, Waterford; Airmount Maternity Hospital, Waterford, from 1955.
Consultant surgeon, Waterford, County and City Infirmary, 1956–85.
Secretary, Waterford Clinical Society (an active body that brought speakers from far and near for educational and convivial meetings).

Tall and energetic, Liam Power was a true gentleman in every sense of the word and was the embodiment of courtesy. A devout Catholic who took his faith seriously, he was a careful, meticulous surgeon, who never ever took on anything outside his wide range of expertise.

A cultured family man of wide interests and great energy, Liam Power enjoyed classical music as well as opera and was an expert on Beethoven. He spoke French and German, and took pleasure in writing his referring letters in italic script. He hill-walked, swam, fished, gardened (including vine growing) and kept bees. Later, he took up painting. He was a keen dinghy sailor in a '420', which was considered a young man's boat.

The people of Waterford had a great affection for Liam Power and appreciated his care and dedication.

WESTMEATH
Mullingar (pop. 15,621)
Westmeath County Infirmary (20 beds)

MIDDLETON, William Henry

Surgeon, Westmeath County Infirmary, 1900

Educ. Ledwich (Medical) School, Dublin

LRCPI, LRCSI, 1872

KEARNEY, Anthony Joseph

Surgeon, Westmeath County Infirmary, 1900

LRCPI & LM, LRCSI & LM, 1894

1920	Honorary surgeons	J. D. Kelly
		T. J. Daly
		G. J. Gibbon

KEELAN, Patrick

County Surgeon, Mullingar, Co. Westmeath

b. 1887, Mullingar, one of 4 sons and 2 daughters of Patrick Keelan and Annie Keelan (*née* Sherrin); brother John died in First World War; Edward was Master of Coombe Hospital for Women
m. 1918: Helen Kelleher (d. 1974); 2 s, 1 d (Dr Maeve Keelan)
d. 1963.

MB, Royal University of Ireland, Dublin, 1909; LM, Rotunda Hospital

Postgraduate work included resident physician and surgeon, Mater Hospital; subsequently house physician and assistant anaesthetist.
Ship's surgeon to the Far East.
External maternity assistant, Rotunda Hospital.
Surgeon, Westmeath County Hospital, 1917–52.
Medical officer, Post Office.

Patrick Keelan was one of the pioneers of collapse therapy (pneumothorax) in tuberculosis, visiting the Brompton Hospital and Finley Sanatorium. His annual vacation was spent visiting continental clinics and keeping up to date. Much influenced by Lorenz Bohler (1885–1973) of Vienna, who had himself done some training at the Mayo Clinic, USA, he was considered an expert on trauma and was one of the first in the country to use the Smith Petersen Nail for fractured neck of femur. This was a key skill from the 1930s onwards as, if the fracture were not 'pinned', the patient would almost certainly die, usually of hypostatic pneumonia. He did the obstetrics, some medicine and radiology, with a practice throughout the midlands.

Mullingar was the first hospital to be built with funds from the Hospital Sweeps. Keelan supervised everything in the planning and construction, and the new hospital, costing £60,000, was opened in May 1936. He retired as county surgeon in 1952 but continued in practice until his death. His successor as county surgeon was Mr James O'Connell, who became a close friend.

Keelan held deep Christian values and attended Mass daily. For forty consecutive years, he also attended the doctors' retreat by the Jesuits at Milltown Park, Dublin. He went to Lourdes regularly and was given a Papal Medal by Pope Pius XII.

He was a keen deep-sea angler at Ballycotton and Port-na-Blagh. He was a fine shot and, as a keen golfer, he was Life President of Mullingar Golf Club.

Patrick Keelan was of the old school, admirable and committed to the service of others, a gentleman who had time for everyone. An avid reader and traveller in pursuit of up-to-date medical advances, he was also tender and kind, and any request for advice or assistance was answered with 'Certainly'. What a wonderful epitaph.

STANLEY, Anthony Joseph

Honorary Surgeon, Westmeath Infirmary

BA (first class hons), NUI, 1919; MB, 1926, UCD

LAVERTY, Thomas

Westmeath Surgeon

MB, BCh, BAO, RUI, 1905

O'CONNELL, James Alphonsus (Jimmy) PRCSI 1980–1982

Mullingar Surgeon

b. 1914, Belfast, son of John O'Connell (wine merchant) and Gertrude O'Connell (*née* McIvor)
Educ. Rosario Primary School; CBS, Belfast; St Malachy's College, Belfast; Queen's University Belfast
m. 1944: Dr Olivia (Bunny) Clarke, daughter of Dr D. F. R. Clarke of Co. Sligo; 6 d (Brigid is a physician), 1 s
d. 2000

MB, QUB, 1937; DPH; FRCSI; FRCS Eng

Training posts in Nottingham and Hillingdon Hospital, London.
Surgeon, Daisy Hill Hospital, Newry.
County Surgeon, Mullingar.
Council, RCSI, 1963–84; President, 1980–82.
President, IMA.

Principal interests were gastric surgery and orthopaedics.

Jimmy O'Connell was an absolutely first-class operating surgeon. Quiet, determined, with the silver hair of a surgeon from Central Casting, he never lost his clear Belfast cadence, and was highly popular, both as a surgeon and as a person.

During his term as President, the RCSI ran its first Primary Fellowship course and examination in Dammam, Saudi Arabia. Perhaps the highlight of his presidency was the conferring of the honorary Fellowship on Dr Loyal Davis of Chicago. Dr Davis was one of the most distinguished American surgeons, and he was also father of Nancy Reagan, wife of the then President of the US, Ronald Reagan. The conferring and dinner at the Irish Embassy in Washington were splendid, memorable affairs, enjoyed by President Reagan.

Jimmy excelled at billiards and was a canny golfer with a magic putter. In 1985, he suffered a debilitating stroke but was devotedly nursed back to health, and to golf, and to his winning ways.

MINA, Amal ('Mike')

Regional Surgeon, Mullingar

b. 1933, Cairo, Egypt, younger son of Girgis and Amina Mina
Educ. French Christian Brothers, Cairo; Cairo University
m. 1967: Ann Mucklow, MB, daughter of John and Hilda Mucklow; 1 d.

MB (hons), Cairo University, Kasr-El-Aini Medical School, 1957; LMSSA, Lond, 1968; FRCS Ed, 1967; FRCSI (*ad eundem*), 1989

Postgraduate training posts in Cairo University Hospital, American Baptist Hospital, Garden City Hospital, Cairo.
In UK, worked at Taunton, Bournemouth and Central Middlesex Hospital, London.
Tutor and registrar, University College Hospital, Galway.
Tutor and senior registrar, paediatric surgery, Children's Hospital, Temple Street, Dublin.
Lecturer, St Vincent's University Hospital.
Microsurgery training in UCD labs.
Consultant general surgeon, Midland Regional Hospital, Mullingar, 1979–96.

Mina continued his interest in microsurgery into practice. A highly skilled meticulous craftsman, he taught basic surgical techniques at the RCSI, and was a trusted, experienced and completely fair examiner for the RCSI at all levels. He retained an interest in medical affairs through the Irish Hospital Consultants Association (IHCA).

A great traveller, he has a deep interest in ancient sites and cultures. He is an expert on food and wine, a long-distance swimmer, and a skilled gardener. He is also an enthusiastic concert-goer and musicologist. In height 5'5", and with an engaging smile, he is a genial figure encountered at myriad medical occasions.

WEXFORD

Wexford (pop. 17,235)
Wexford County Infirmary established 1769 (56 beds)

HADDEN, David

Surgeon, Wexford County Infirmary, 1900

LRCPI, LRCSI, 1898.

HADDEN, David Jnr

Honorary Assistant Surgeon, Wexford County Infirmary, 1900

LRCP Ed, 1869; FRCSI 1882 (RCSI)

FURLONG, Stanislaus Andrew

Surgeon, Wexford County Infirmary, 1900

LRCP & LM, LRCSI & LM, Catholic University, Dublin, 1907

Postgraduate work as house surgeon, Jervis Street Hospital, Dublin; Wrexham Infirmary.
Captain, Royal Army Medical Corps.
Surgeon, Wexford County Infirmary.

SHIGGINS, Richard (Dick)

Wexford Surgeon, 1946–1957

b. 1913, youngest son of Richard and Margaret Shiggins
Educ. St Peter's College, Wexford; Royal College of Surgeons in Ireland
m. 1953: Peggy Cunan, daughter of Jim and Brigid Cunan; 2 s (Richard is in the American Hospital, Paris)
d. 2003

LRCP & SI, 1940 (Stoney memorial gold medal); FRCSI, 1943

General surgeon, Omagh Hospital, 1943–45.
Temporary surgeon, County Hospital, Wexford, 1946–57.
Consultant surgeon, Ely Hospital, Wexford, to retirement.

Influenced by Terence Millin [q.v.], Michael O'Brien and Arthur Chance. He was the first surgeon to put in a Smith Peterson femoral head pin in Wexford.

Dick Shiggins has been described thus: 'Short but commanding. Spoke clearly and concisely with a droll humour and dry wit. He shook hands with everyone. Followed the Wexford hurling teams. Enjoyed chess and his farm at Castlebridge. A man of deep faith, he was greatly loved and respected by all.'

LEE, George Angus McLean (Angus)

Wexford Surgeon

b. 1918, Dublin, son of George Angus McLean Lee and Roberta Pearson
Educ. Lindsay Road National School, Glasnevin; St Andrew's College, Dublin; Trinity College, Dublin
m. Dr Isobel Ross; 2 s; 1 d (died as an infant)
d. 1996

MB (Hudson Scholarship and Adelaide Hospital gold medal), TCD, 1942; FRCSI, 1949; FRCS Eng, 1952

Postgraduate appointments as house surgeon, Adelaide Hospital.
Surgeon-Lieutenant, Royal Navy, serving in the UK and Far East.
General surgical training: National Temperance Hospital, London; Royal Postgraduate Medical School, Hammersmith; Rush Green Hospital, Romford; St Peter's Hospital (urology).
Senior surgical registrar, at Hillingdon Hospital, Uxbridge, 1953–56.
County Surgeon, Wexford, 1957–83.
Member, South Eastern Health Board; Comhairle na nOspidéal; Colles Travelling Club.

Angus Lee was involved in the evacuation of the wounded from the Normandy beaches shortly after D-Day. He subsequently spent ten years (1947–57) in general surgical training in England, which was not uncommon at that time.

When he arrived in Wexford, the hospital was an old 'poor house' building and it required a huge amount of work and enthusiasm to bring it up to teaching hospital standard. He was particularly effective in getting modern medical and nursing record systems installed. He worked for years without a secretary. He had a huge range of expertise, 'tonsils to colons to hips and in between', and he sometimes brought a textbook of operative surgery (Rob and Smith) into the theatre suite. He was on call most of the time and worked very hard. From 1975, he was fortunate to have Johnny O'Sullivan [q.v.] as a colleague.

He enjoyed a joke but, if needs be, he would stand firm and get things done. When the *Fitzgerald Report* (1968) advised that Wexford Hospital be closed, it was Angus, more than anyone else, who ensured its survival; he lived to see a splendid new hospital opened in 1992 and it now has three surgeons.

He suffered from asthma throughout his life and then developed arthritis, but he had a happy family life and enjoyed sailing and angling He was a man of high principle, generosity, integrity and wisdom. Like his parents, he was a faithful member of the Presbyterian-Methodist Church and he was ordained to an Eldership of the congregation in recognition of his commitment. Angus Lee made a huge difference to his institution. He was greatly admired and, although it would embarrass him to hear it, loved.

O'SULLIVAN, John Phillip Brennan (Johnny)

Wexford Surgeon

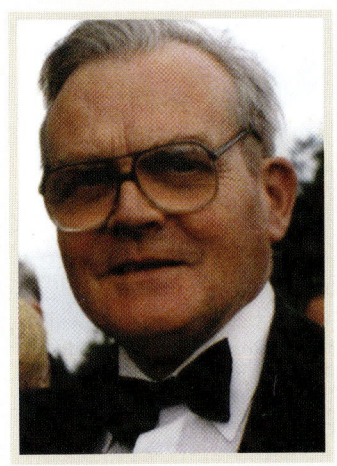

b. 1933, eldest son of Dr and Mrs M. O'Sullivan of Herbert Park, Dublin
Educ. Marlborough National School; Belvedere College, 1946–51; University College Dublin
m. 1962: Eileen Taylor (SRN); 2 d (Frances, a radiographer; Annaliese, a GP)
d. 2000

MB, UCD, 1957 (Tobin medal in medicine); FRCSI, 1964; FRCS Eng, 1967; MCh, 1969

Postgraduate appointments as senior house officer, St Vincent's Hospital; Liverpool Surgical Training Rotation Scheme, to include Walton Hospital, Broadgreen and the Liverpool Royal Infirmary. Senior registrar and tutor, St Vincent's Hospital, 1967 (under Prof. Paddy Fitzgerald [q.v.]).

County Surgeon, Tralee, Co. Kerry, 1972–75.
County Surgeon, Wexford, 1975–98.
President, surgical section, RAMI, 1996–98.
RCSI College Medal.

Johnny O'Sullivan was one of the most popular surgeons in Ireland. He was always involved, whether it was the Society of St Vincent de Paul, the school opera, captaining the successful St Vincent's Hospital's rugby hospitals cup team, or subsequently with his patients, his trainees and his colleagues. He was an active member of the Surgical Discussion Group, the Colles Travelling Club and much in demand as a sensible examiner at all levels.

He had a deep sense of professionalism and was devoted to his patients, visiting them at all hours. For twenty-five years, he was on a one-in-two on-call rota, with all the onerous implications that carried.

Johnny had a wonderful sense of humour and was a raconteur of professional standard, greatly sought after as a speaker at all kinds of functions. His imitation of a ranting Hitler made that monster human and risible. He had a great love of music and was an active member of his church choir and the Wexford Festival Singers. He had a deep faith and went on one or two pilgrimages each year. He was self-deprecating, humble and genuinely startled by any form of recognition by colleagues. His home life was exceptionally happy, and Eileen was a gracious hostess.

Tragically he developed a brain tumour within months of retirement. His funeral was a huge, inspiring event, when many whose lives he had brightened came to pay a final tribute. He was the iconic county surgeon of his time.

Wicklow

Newcastle National Hospital for Consumption for Ireland established 1896 (24 beds)

No Surgeon

Wicklow County Infirmary established 1776 (23 beds)

LYNDON, Thomas

Surgeon, Wicklow County Infirmary, 1900

MB, Dublin, 1884; MD, 1886

Surgeon, Wicklow County Infirmary, 1900.
Medical attendant, Lighthouse Keepers.
Medical referee, Workman's Compensation Act.

11
DUBLIN SURGEONS, CLASSIFIED BY HOSPITAL

DUBLIN SURGEONS, CLASSIFIED BY HOSPITAL

ADELAIDE HOSPITAL

BEESLEY, William Harold (Bill)

Dublin Surgeon

b. 1935, Birmingham
Educ. Trinity College, Dublin
m. Married with 4 children

BA, TCD, 1959; MB, TCD, 1961; MD, 1964; MCh, 1973; FRCSI, 1966

Lecturer in surgery, TCD.
Senior surgical registrar, Sir Patrick Dun's, Dublin. Senior Surgical Research Fellow, University Mt Sinai Hospital, Minneapolis, Minnesota.
Consultant surgeon, Adelaide and Meath Hospitals, Dublin; Stewart's Hospital, Palmerstown and Rotunda Hospital

Dark, bronzed, diligent and highly organised, he managed to keep a low profile even when he won the national lottery (Lotto) … twice!

BRENAN, Richard Brownell (Dick)

Dublin Surgeon

b. 1919
Educ. Trinity College, Dublin
d. 1987

MB, TCD, 1942; MCh, TCD, 1960; FRCSI, 1947; FRCS, 1956

Surgeon-Lieutenant, Royal Naval Volunteer Reserve.
Surgical registrar, Royal Northern Hospital, Holloway Road, London.
Surgeon, Nairobi General Hospital; Adelaide Hospital, Dublin, Mercer's Hospital, Dublin; Royal City of Dublin Hospital; Royal Victoria Eye and Ear Hospital, Dublin; and the Royal Hospital, Donnybrook.

Dick Brenan was a careful, courteous, considerate, quiet, hard-working surgeon. When he worked at the Royal Northern, the hospital had about 130 beds and thirty-four consultants. The resident surgical officer (surgical registrar) had the impossible job of finding beds for the patients of a hugely distinguished staff, which included R. J. (Bobbie) McNeill Love (of Bailey and Love textbook fame) and William Bashall Gabriel, the leading rectal surgeon in England, inevitably referred to as the 'arse angel Gabriel'. The private wing was visited by many of London's most distinguished surgeons, some of whom worked there when they were retired from their teaching hospitals, and some of who were well past their 'sell-by date'. The resident surgical officer became accustomed to taking detailed instructions on the telephone, as postoperative visits for complications were uncommon. 'Bad for morale.'

HEUSTON, Francis Thomas

Dublin Surgeon

b. 1857, Tipperary, son of Robert and Elizabeth Heuston (*née* Tydd)
Educ. Privately at the Manse, Tipperary; Tipperary Grammar School; Rathmines School; apprenticed to Dr Stoney and studied in the College School before becoming a resident pupil at the City of Dublin Hospital
m. 1888: Frances, daughter of Gibson and Cecilia Black; 2 s, 1 d
d. 1915

MD, MCh, Queen's University Galway, 1878; FRCSI, 1883. He gained numerous prizes and honours.

Lecturer and then Professor of Anatomy, RCSI.
Surgeon, Adelaide Hospital, 1885–1915.
Consulting surgeon, Coombe Hospital; Cripple's Home, Bray; Children's Hospital, Delgany.

Francis Heuston was an active educationalist and prepared large numbers of candidates for the Army and Navy medical departments. He died a few days after he got the news of his son's death in the First World War.

PUREFOY, Robert Dancer PRCSI 1912–1914

Dublin Obstetrician

b. 1847, Cloughjordan, Co. Tipperary, fourth son of Dr Thomas Purefoy and Alla Maria Purefoy (*née* Dancer)
Educ. Bective College, Rutland Square; Raphoe Royal School; Trinity College, Dublin
m. Unmarried
d. 1919

MB, TCD, 1872 (also won a musical exhibition prize for his singing); LRCP & SI, 1885; FRCSI, 1879; MD, TCD, 1892

Assistant Master, Coombe Hospital; Rotunda Hospital.
Master, Rotunda Hospital, 1896–1903.
Gynaecologist, Adelaide Hospital.
Examiner, TCD.

Gynaecological surgery greatly increased in volume while Purefoy was Master of the Rotunda, and the Hospital District Service had 12,811 deliveries over the seven-year period. As examiner at TCD, he examined Oliver St John Gogarty and gave him a generous mark, apparently based on Gogarty's affability and family connections. In *Ulysses*, Joyce mentions the name Mina Purefoy in connection with Holles Street Hospital.

His presidency coincided with the bicentenary of the School of Physic (TCD) and he was given an honorary LLD. His professional papers were all on complications of pregnancy and labour. He was a good judge of a horse and collected objets d'art. He also had a fine baritone voice. He may have been one of the last to wear a top hat while operating.

CHARITABLE INFIRMARY, JERVIS STREET

BYRNE, Louis Aloysius

Dublin Surgeon

Educ. Ledwich School, Dublin
LRCPI, Ledwich School, Dublin, 1886; FRCSI, 1889; L. 1885; LM, Coombe Hospital, Dublin, 1884

Surgeon, Jervis Street Hospital, 1903.
Lecturer and examiner, St John Ambulance Association.
Coroner for Dublin City.

COLLINS, Patrick Gerard (Paddy)

Dublin Surgeon and Associate Professor of Surgery, RCSI

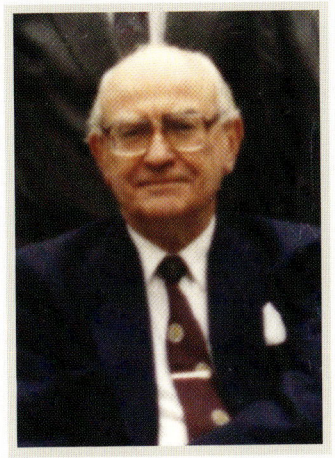

b. 1922, Cobh, Co. Cork, eldest son of Archie and Mary Anne Collins, both school teachers and staunch republicans

Educ. Presentation Brothers College, Cobh; University College Cork

m. 1st in 1952: Pauline M. Higgins (consultant anaesthetist, who predeceased him); 2nd: Catherine McGovern (former theatre sister at Jervis Street Hospital)

d. 2000

MB (first class hons), UCC, 1947; FRCS Eng, 1951; MCh, NUI, 1951; FACS, FRCSI *ad eundem*; Henry Hutchinson Stewart Scholarship in Physiology (open to all the Irish medical schools)

Postgraduate appointments in Southend General Hospital (where many London surgeons, including the master upper-abdominal surgeon, Rodney Maingot, came to operate at weekends); Derby Royal Infirmary.

Senior registrar, Sheffield Royal Hospital (with Mr James Lytle from Derry).

UCC Ainsworth scholarship to Lahey Clinic, Boston, Massachusetts (with Dr R. B. Cattell, Dr Samuel F. Marshall, Dr Herb Adams, Dr Ben Colcock and Dr Ken Warren). Consultant surgeon, Jervis Street Hospital and subsequently Beaumont Hospital, 1960–89; St Luke's Hospital

Associate and then Clinical Professor of Surgery, RCSI. Examiner in surgery, Edinburgh. Member, Council RCSI, 1991–95.

Governor and Founder Member, Irish Chapter of the American College of Surgeons.

President, section of surgery, RAMI; Pancreatic Society of Great Britain and Ireland.

Special interest was the surgery of the biliary tract, liver and pancreas. His *tour de force* was the repair of the common bile duct.

When Paddy Collins returned to Ireland, he had been training abroad for eleven years. It was a long time for an outstanding surgeon but that was what happened in those times. While he was at the Lahey Clinic in Boston (June 1953), Anthony Eden, British Foreign Secretary and Prime Minister designate, had his damaged bile duct repaired by Dr Cattell and Dr Frank Lahey (founder of the Clinic). Dr Lahey died the day Eden was discharged.

Paddy was a master surgeon with a superb brain, allied to a naturally talented technique. He enjoyed teaching and his ward round on a Sunday morning always had an overflow attendance. An intimidating but scrupulously fair examiner, he was the despair of examination chairmen as he wanted to pass everybody. He was always protective of, and kind to, the underdog, be he or she a patient or an examinee, though he could be turbulent and declamatory at times. Popular with nurses, anaesthetists and trainees — the people who really know — he was tireless in the theatre.

Paddy had a brilliant undergraduate career and was an iconic figure in the UCC medical school. He played for UCC Rugby XV (second row of the scrum) and got an inter-provincial cap for his beloved Munster. A fearless tackler and line-out jumper, he might have gone further but he had a severe distance vision problem and this was before contact lenses were widely available.

He had a sad family life. His father died when he was young, and his wife Pauline, two younger sisters, Emer (Rehill) and Fionn (Harrington), as well as his younger brother Oscar, all predeceased him. But he found happiness with Catherine. He had no children.

Tall, 6'1", burly, with an unruly mop of jet-black hair and trademark horn-rimmed spectacles — a cartoonist's portrayal would certainly include a massive cigar and his polished Mercedes. His contribution to the Cuban economy was significant. He loved stories and was an accomplished raconteur. Hugely popular and highly convivial, he was happiest discussing surgery late in the evening at an out-of-Dublin meeting.

FLOOD, John Charles, Dom Peter, Order of Saint Benedict (JC)

Surgeon, Jervis Street Hospital

b. 1898, Bristol
Educ. St Brendan's School, Bristol; University College Dublin
m. Unmarried
d. 1978

MB (first class hons), UCD; MD, MCh, BA, BComm, Barrister-at-Law

Surgeon, Jervis Street Hospital, 1935–49.
Gynaecologist, St Michael's Hospital, Dún Laoghaire.
Member, Court, Apothecaries Hall of Ireland (Dub); Governing Body, UCD; Senate, National University of Ireland.
Assistant editor, *Journal of the Irish Medical Association.*

JC Flood was a superb public speaker, having been auditor of the Literary and Historical Society at UCD. He had a remarkable voice and an intimate knowledge of criminal law and court procedure, which made him a fearsome expert medical witness. He was outspoken on all issues and did not spare colleagues or other professionals. While in surgical practice, he had a reputation for caustic wit. 'Flood has more degrees than a thermometer without the same capacity for registering warmth,' said Professor Leonard Abrahamson of RCSI. It was sometimes felt that his initials, 'J. C.', were not entirely accidental.

In 1948, he joined the Benedictine monks at Downside and was ordained a priest in 1951. He lectured in canon law and medical ethics in Rome and became a professor of moral theology for fourteen years. He continued to publish extensively.

The Reverend Mother of the community of the Mercy Order of Nuns who administered the Charitable Infirmary died. The blinds were drawn and Requiem Mass was about to be celebrated. The Reverend Mother had been a sworn enemy of JC and he went round the hospital letting up the blinds. A senior nun asked why he was not attending the Mass for the deceased, 'Waste of time, Sister. She is in hell.'

HAYDEN, Patrick Edward

Dublin Surgeon

LRCPI & LM, 1905; DPH, RCPSI, 1906; FRCSI, 1907 (UCD)

Postgraduate appointments as senior resident surgeon, Mater Misericordiae Hospital, Dublin.
Surgeon, Jervis Street Hospital, 1905–30.
Surgeon, Dublin Castle Hospitals. During the First World War, part of Dublin Castle was used as a Red Cross hospital for wounded soldiers. When James Connolly was wounded while in the General Post Office in 1916, he was taken to Dublin Castle hospital when the Post Office garrison surrendered.
Demonstrator in UCD.
Examiner in surgery, Apothecaries Hall, Dublin; RCSI.

KEEGAN, John Francis Leo

Dublin Surgeon

b. 1878, Dublin
Educ. Belvedere College; Royal College of Surgeons in Ireland
m. Rose Warren, daughter of Henry Warren Darley of Pembroke Road, Dublin

LRCPI & LM, 1901; L & LM, 1901; FRCSI, 1904

Postgraduate appointments as resident surgeon, St Vincent's Hospital, Dublin; resident physician, Cork Street Fever Hospital, Dublin; demonstrator in anatomy and examiner in surgery for Fellowship and dental finals, RCSI.

Visiting surgeon, Jervis Street Hospital, from 1930.
Consultant surgeon, London Midland Region, British Railways.
Examiner in Anatomy & Surgery Conjoint Board, RCPSI; Member, Council, RCSI.

A colleague described Keegan thus: 'A not too tall, dapper figure, quintessentially a man of Dublin; uncomplicated of mind, he typified the extroverted surgeon-figure. He gave example to all in punctuality, loyalty and moderation.'

LANE, Brian Edmond

Dublin Surgeon

b. 1937, son of Cornelius and Dr Edith Lane
Educ. Clongowes Wood College; Royal College of Surgeons in Ireland
m. 1982: Jean Dunn, FRCPI consultant in mental handicap; 1 s (Brian); 1 d (Louise)

LRCP & SI, 1961; FRCSI, 1965; FRCS Ed, 1966; FRCS, 1966; FACS, 1976

Postgraduate training in Leicester Royal Infirmary (with E. Frizelle); Luton and Dunstable Hospital, Charing Cross Group of Hospitals, London (with Prof. A. J. Harding Rains); Jefferson Medical College, Philadelphia (with Prof. Tom Nealon); Jervis Street Hospital, Dublin (with P. G. Collins [q.v.])

Consultant surgeon, Jervis Street/Beaumont Hospital, 1971–2002; Blanchardstown Hospital, St Luke's Hospital, 1972–2002.
Lecturer in anatomy, primary FRCSI course at RCSI, 1970–97.

Surgical interests included surgical critical care and inflammatory bowel disease. His best-known contribution to the literature is his continuing chapter on 'Fluid and Electrolyte Balance' in *A Short Textbook of Surgery*, originally by Hamilton Bailey and R. J. McNeill Love, but he has been a steady contributor of carefully worded articles at home and abroad.

At Jervis Street, Brian Lane was the surgeon most involved in setting up the Intensive Care Unit. The quietest of men, above average height, with dark hair thinning on top, he is the antithesis of the caricature surgeon, in that he is retiring and reserved. In his time, he was a first-rate opinion and operator, hugely admired and popular within the circle who knew him. He is now a prosector in the RCSI Anatomy Department.

MURRAY, Desmond Patrick (Des)

Dublin Surgeon

b. 1914, Dublin
m. Unmarried
d. 1984

LRCP &SI, LM, RCSI, 1937 (many medals); FRCSI, 1940

Postgraduate posts in Mercer's Hospital, Dublin.
Visiting surgeon, Jervis Street Hospital.
Consultant surgeon, Dublin Health Authority.
Member, Council RCSI.

A quiet, charming, congenial, courteous, gentleman with a good knowledge of the literature but one who was at best 'unlucky' in many of his operations. Des Murray's most frequent request at the operating table was for a 'pack' to hold firmly on whatever was bleeding at the time. His trademark phrase in the theatre was 'God knows what damage I have done now.' He was a chainsmoker and could smoke a cigarette down to the very end without taking it out of his mouth or indeed touching it in any way. This enabled him to do a sigmoidoscopy while surrounded by clouds of smoke. He had no interest in teaching. Although he was a member of the Council of the RCSI for twelve years, there is no record of his ever having spoken at a meeting.

He was interested in classical music, art, and literature. He liked to go abroad on short visits; he would just go to the airport and pick a destination based on the time of the next flight. He was born with bilateral congenital dislocation of the hips which was treated poorly, if at all, and this made his progress across a room slow and apparently ponderous. He was a lifelong bachelor of the old school, never known to have lady friends, who lived and died in the house in which he was born, in the Dublin suburb of Dundrum.

RYAN, Daniel Alphonsus (Dan)

Dublin Surgeon, Jervis Street Hospital

b. 1912, Waterford
Educ. Royal College of Surgeons in Ireland
m. Unmarried
d. 1984

LRCSI 1938, FRCSI 1941

Dan Ryan's early training at the Richmond Hospital was in anaesthesia, sometimes for neurosurgery by Adams A. McConnell [q.v.]. Many of the operations were prolonged and, from time to time, he would have to tell the surgeon that the patient was dead on the table. This never perturbed McConnell, who always responded, 'Shouldn't be long now, Ryan' and finished the operation at his normal pace. Ryan trained in surgery at Jervis Street Hospital and is remembered for writing all his letters to the referring doctors by hand and posting them himself that evening. Thus there was no record of what the letter said, but he built up a significant practice.

Cautious and conservative, he was a very neat technical surgeon. A good clinical teacher (he had been a primary school teacher before going to medical school), he used a blackboard to illustrate a point. He was vehemently opposed to all forms of change and opposed the vital kidney transplant programme which transformed the entire hospital. As a long-time member of the Council of the RCSI, he was never known to make any contribution to the debates. He had a particular antipathy to Professor P. G. Collins [q.v.] who had come to the hospital as one of the best-trained surgeons ever to return to Ireland and it was said that Dan Ryan would sit in the operating theatre, reading the paper, even if he had no operations pending, rather than let Collins in to operate. But it was Collins who eventually sorted out most of Ryan's complications.

A bachelor of the old school, he was a seriously religious man, beloved of the nuns who ran the hospital at the time.

VELLA, Leonardo Antonio (Leo)

Dublin Accident and Emergency Consultant

b. 1935, Malta, second son of Paul and Salvina Vella (*née* Balbi)
Educ. St Aloysius' College, Malta; Royal College of Surgeons in Ireland
m. 1st in 1964: Claire Crowley (d. 1982), daughter of Senator Patrick and Eileen Crowley.
2nd in 1986: Anne Marie, daughter of Bob and Joan Murphy (both BDs); 2 s (John is a nephrologist in Maine, USA)

LRCP & SI, RCSI, 1962; FRCSI, 1971; FRCPI, 1971; FFAEM, 1993

Postgraduate posts at Meath Hospital (with David Lane [q.v.], Victor Lane [q.v.] and Dermot O'Flynn [q.v.]).
Research Fellow, Our Lady's Hospital for Sick Children, Crumlin (with Barry O'Donnell [q.v.]).
Other training posts at Royal Free Hospital, London; Royal Infirmary, Leicester; Charitable Infirmary, Jervis Street (with Gerry Brady [q.v.]).
A&E surgeon, Jervis Street Hospital and subsequently Beaumont Hospital, 1972–97.
Co-founder and first President, Irish Accident & Emergency Association.

Leo Vella invented the role of A&E consultant in Ireland. A problem solver, who loves challenges, he was superb at management and organised triage. Early morning teaching sessions were held. He devised a disaster plan for Dublin, which was activated for two bombings and the Stardust nightclub fire. He also did a really good job as Research Fellow with several publications in a short time.

Leo spent the Second World War in Malta, surviving multiple close-quarters aerial attacks. Undeniably of Mediterranean origin, with the largest eyebrows in Ireland, he made his department a particularly agreeable place to work.

In retirement, he is a more than competent fly fisherman. Subspecialties often take their character from the first practitioners. Accident & Emergency (now Emergency Medicine) was lucky to have Leo Vella.

City of Dublin Hospital, Baggot Street (subsequently Royal City of Dublin Hospital)

'Baggot Street' was established in 1832 by a group of six surgeons, and for 120 years had close links with the Royal College of Surgeons in Ireland. The most famous of the founders was Arthur Jacob (1790–1874), PRCSI 1837 and 1864–65, surgeon and ophthalmologist. Another was John Houston (1802–45), who is remembered for describing the 'valves' or permanent folds in the wall of the rectum. Abraham Colles was appointed as surgeon. The 'Royal' came with Queen Victoria's visit to Dublin in 1900. During the First World War (1914–18), the hospital allocated more than thirty beds, including a soldiers' ward, for the exclusive use of wounded men from the Expeditionary Force. Some 200 casualties were treated during the Easter Week 1916 'Sinn Féin Rebellion'.

One of the features of the hospital was the huge amount of voluntary work carried out by successive ladies' committees, who raised money for all sorts of necessities. There was a highly regarded school of nursing. In the 1950s, Baggot Street lost its connection with the RCSI and became exclusively associated with TCD. At this time, it had about 200 beds.

The Cardiothoracic Centre

Open-heart surgery began with Keith Mears Shaw [q.v.], PRCSI 1980–82, in 1960. In 1971, Shaw was appointed to the Mater Hospital, and then the actual surgery was carried out there. The unit was closed in 1987, when the staff and patients transferred to St James's Hospital. At time of writing, the building serves as a community hospital with special facilities for the elderly.

CROLY, Henry Gray PRCSI 1891–1893

Dublin Surgeon

b. 1836, Mountmellick, Queen's County, eldest son of Dr Henry Gray and Isabel Gray
Educ. Nutgrove School, Rathfarnham; Royal College of Surgeons in Ireland; Royal City of Dublin Hospital
m. 1861: Anna Mary Chapman (d. 1901); 6 s (two surgeons in Royal Army Medical Corps, First World War), 6 d
d. 1903

FRCSI, 1863

Naval surgeon in the Crimean War (1853–56).
Surgeon to HM Prison on Spike Island, Co. Cork.
Surgeon, Monkstown Hospital. Examiner at RCSI.
Senior surgeon, City of Dublin Hospital.

Henry Croly served in Baggot Street for forty-six years and had exceptional energy, ability and courage, with great skill in diagnosis. He famously and uniquely ligated the second part of the subclavian artery in 1896, for which he received a congratulatory letter from Lord Lister. He was a huge, imposing man whose massive portrait is in the boardroom of the RCSI. He died of brain haemorrhage.

FITZGIBBON, Henry PRCSI 1888–1889

Dublin Surgeon

b. 1841, son of Gerald Fitzgibbon QC and Ellen Fitzgibbon (*née* Patterson)
Educ. Tutors at home; Trinity College, Dublin (arts and medicine); City of Dublin Hospital; Paris
m. Adeline Meta Foot; 4s (one, Gibbon, was consultant gynaecologist to the Royal City of Dublin Hospital)
d. 1911

MD, TCD, 1870; MB, 1866; MCh, 1867; FRCSI, 1881

Following qualification, he spent a year as a ship's surgeon, then practised in Howth, Baldoyle and Clondalkin.
House surgeon, City of Dublin Hospital.
Surgeon, City of Dublin Hospital; Mercer's/St John's Home and House of Rest, Merrion.
Surgeon, various provident societies.

MOORE, Henry MC DSO

Dublin Surgeon

b. 1867

d. 1918

LRCSI and LM, LRCPI and LM, 1892; LM, Rotunda Hospital, Dublin, RCSI

Surgeon, Royal City of Dublin Hospital, 1900–18.
Demonstrator of anatomy, RCSI.
Surgeon, Mercer's Hospital, Dublin.
Civil surgeon, South African Field Force, Boer War (1899–1902).
Medical officer, Basutoland.
Lieutenant-Colonel, Royal Army Medical Corps.

In 1918, Moore was killed on the front in France, following an explosion. (Seventy-five per cent of Great War deaths were due to heavy artillery.) He had been a civil surgeon with the South African Field Force during the Boer War and volunteered his services in 1914. His awards were for conspicuous gallantry in the field. He was 'gassed' in the autumn of 1915 but repeatedly volunteered for front-line action when he was over 50 years of age. He had often operated on badly wounded men while an assistant held a torch as operating light.

STONEY, Richard Atkinson (Stoney) PRCSI 1930–1932

Dublin Surgeon

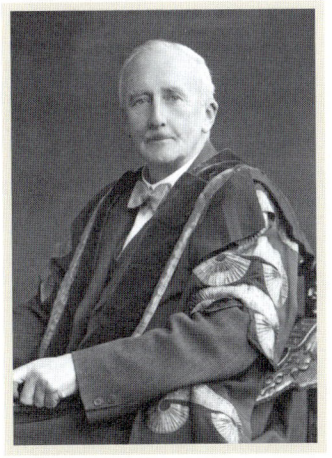

b. 1877, Dublin, son of Rev. Robert Bader Stoney, Rector of Holy Trinity Killiney, and Katherine Mabel Atkinson of Dundrum, Co. Dublin
Educ. St Helen's; Trinity College, Dublin
m. 1915: Gladys Enid, daughter of Arthur Leonard Figgis; 2 d
d. 1966

MB, 1901, TCD; FRCSI, 1906

Surgeon, Baggot Street Hospital, 1903–60.
Surgeon to the Ministry of Pensions; honorary surgeon, Masonic Boys' School.
Major, French Army, 1915–19 (Legion of Honour).
Member, Council, RCSI, 1924–66. RCSI representative on Medical Registration Council of Ireland (President 1945–63).
Member, GMC; President, RAMI, 1933–36.

A really fine technical surgeon, Stoney was also an irascible operator who once threw a stainless steel kidney dish (he used only round bowls, and kidney-shaped bowls were prohibited) out of the window of Baggot Street Hospital operating theatre, bringing the trams outside to a standstill. He did all his own wound dressings, often using BIPP (bismuth iodoform paraffin paste) and had a reputation for early uninfected wound healing, though he did not wear a surgical mask. (Surgical masks originated with French surgeons. The purpose then was to keep their beards out of the wound.) He served as surgeon in Baggot Street for fifty-seven years and was undoubtedly the surgeon of choice for most of the hospital staff; this is a touchstone everywhere. He drank a brandy egg flip at the end of the operating list.

Kind, wise and a master of procedure and committee work, he was on the Council of the RCSI for thirty-five years, and was aged 82 when, in 1959, the Council presented him with his portrait as a hint that he might retire. He responded, 'Now that the College has been so generous to me, the least I might do is continue to serve it for my declining years.' And he did. While he was President of RCSI, the sports ground at Bird Avenue, Clonskeagh was purchased, and it proved a superb investment for the College.

A rigid disciplinarian in his youth, Stoney mellowed with age about most issues except the religious divide. He was an active Freemason to the end. Tall, dignified, he had a splendid appearance in both youth and old age and had been one of the best dancers in Dublin.

DR STEEVENS' HOSPITAL

CHERRY, John Edward Cooper (Jack)

Dublin Orthopaedic Surgeon

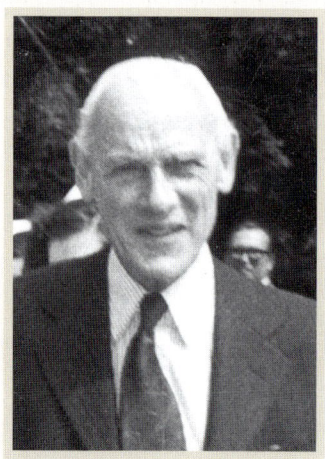

b. 1905, 92 St Stephen's Green, Dublin, son of Richard Robert Cherry (Lord Chief Justice of Ireland) and Mary (Minna) Cooper; great grandson of William Henry Porter FRCSI (surgeon, the Meath Hospital, 1819–61)
Educ. St Stephen's Green School; Trinity College, Dublin
m. Helen; 2 s, 1 d
d. 1995

MB, TCD, 1929; MA, MD, TCD, 1943; FRCSI, 1933

Postgraduate training appointments at Leicester Royal Infirmary and St Mary's Hospital, London, for some years.

Consultant surgeon, Dr Steevens' Hospital; the Incorporated Orthopaedic Hospital, c.1937 to 1980s.
Member, British Surgical Travellers Club

As an undergraduate, Jack was an outstanding rugby wing three-quarters on the invincible TCD team of the time. Terence Millin [q.v.] was captain for two years and said, 'Jack was quick as the wind, had a great pair of hands and was just a few tackles short of international honours'. He was secretary of the TCD Athletic Club and a founder member of the Knights of the Campanile. He was athletic all his life and was still riding into his eighties. It would have been most unusual for an Irish graduate in the 1930s to work at a London teaching hospital but the fact that Jack was a distinguished rugby player would have counted for much at St Mary's. The Dean of the Medical School at the time, the devious Charles ('Corkscrew Charlie') Moran, later Lord Moran, Churchill's physician, was said to meet the Cardiff trains at nearby Paddington Station to pick up rising Welsh rugby stars and enrol them in Mary's. It paid off.

Jack never took the consultants' (common) contract with the government and was able to stay on the staff at Dr Steevens' well beyond retirement date. Throughout his long professional career, he was retained by a number of large insurance companies for medico-legal work, and his evidence in court was always clear and convincing.

Slightly above middle height, with a fine upright stature to the end, he was always immaculately turned out as for a Court appearance. He had a figure which was a tailor's joy, and there was never a hair out of place. He talked all the time and his long career straddled huge changes to which he adapted with a certain impatience. 'When I was young, patients were happy to get out of hospital alive…now they want to be cured as well,' was a saying of his, oft delivered in a high pitched, crystal-clear voice to the younger generation, which eventually meant everybody. A complete professional.

Mater Misericordiae Hospital

BLAYNEY, Alex Joseph McAuley

Dublin Surgeon

b. 1870, Cushendall, son of Alexander Blayney of Cushendall, Co. Antrim; brother John Blayney [q.v.] was surgeon to the County Infirmary, Maryborough (Portlaoise)
Educ. St Malachy's College; Catholic University School of Medicine (Cecilia Street), Dublin
m. 2nd in 1920: Mary (Molly) Stanton; 2 s (John was Supreme Court Judge; Alex was anaesthetist at the Mater Hospital), 2 d (Alice is married to iconic former Chief Justice Tom Finlay)
d. 1925

MA, RUI, 1891; MB, 1893; FRCSI, Catholic University, Dublin, 1898; Stud. in Biology, RUI

Postgraduate appointments as house physician, Mater Misericordiae Hospital, Dublin; assistant demonstrator in anatomy.
Surgeon, Mater Hospital.
Professor of Biology, UCD, Catholic University, Dublin; examiner in biology, RUI.
Assistant Professor of Surgery, Catholic University, Dublin; examiner in surgery, RCSI.
Member, Council, RCSI.

Author of 'On Removal of Great Lengths of Intestine', *British Medical Journal*, 1902; 'On Two Cases of Perforated Gastric Ulcer', *Medical Press*, 1902.

'A florid athletic looking, balding man with striped trousers and expensive, highly-polished shoes' was how James Joyce described him when he saw him at Cecilia Street Medical School in 1902, when Joyce was considering a career in medicine.

He died while strolling on his beloved Portmarnock Golf Links with his wife and young children. He was President of the club at the time. He had played football for Bohemians FC, an amateur club in the semi-professional league of those days.

BUTLER, Andrew Lazarian (Andy)

Dublin Surgeon

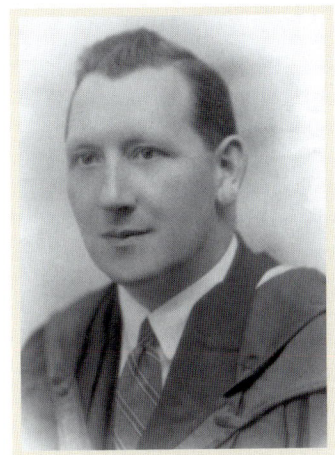

b. 1900, Myshall, Carlow, youngest of three boys
Educ. Myshall National School; scholarship to Rockwell College (1913–19); scholarship to Catholic University School of Medicine (Cecilia Street)
m. 1st wife (*née* Coughlan) from South Africa died after six months' marriage; 2nd in 1937: Eithne Doyle, Shamrock, Carlow; 3 s (Michael [q.v.], Dublin urologist and PRCSI, 2002–04), 5 d
d. 1955

MCh, NUI, 1936.

Postgraduate work at St Thomas's London and visited Mayo Clinic in 1937.
Consultant surgeon, Mater Hospital and St Anne's Hospital, 1928–55

Andy Butler's main interest was urology but he also did abdominoperineal resections and block dissections of the neck. Remembered as a sound opinion and no-nonsense operator, he was a first-class 'inspiring' teacher of undergraduates and surgical trainees. His system involved a history from the patient, a careful physical examination and then retiring out to the corridor (foot up on Mater Hospital windowsill), for an in-depth discussion of diagnostic and therapeutic options. He was excellent at drawing out trainees' opinions and gently letting them down if in error. These mini-tutorials were memorable exercises for the young. He built up a massive practice and began operating at 8.30 on the dot although 'nineish' was the usual starting time in those days.

Golf was his passion. He 'took it up late but with a vengeance' (Eoin O'Malley [q.v.]), played at Championship level (0–2 handicap) under 'A L Driver', won many prizes and became Captain of his beloved Portmarnock Golf Club. He had succeeded Alex Blayney [q.v.] on the Mater Staff when he, Blayney, died on the same course while he was club President.

A huge man, well over six foot and weighing about eighteen stone, he was highly popular right through his life at school, university and as a surgeon. He died aged 55, on board a ship, returning from a surgical congress in Istanbul, as always in the company of friends, and was buried in the British War Cemetery, Piraeus, outside Athens. Remembered with great affection by all who came in contact with him.

CHANCE, Sir Arthur, CBE PRCSI 1904–1906

Dublin Surgeon

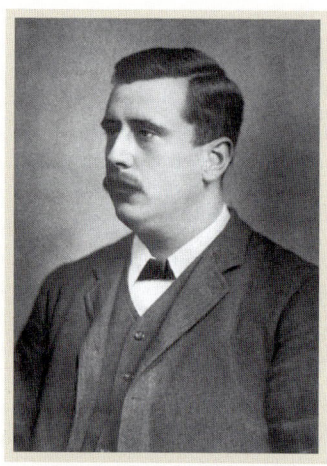

b. 1859, Dublin, son of Albert Chance (a Londoner)
Educ. Catholic University School of Medicine (Cecilia Street), Dublin
m. 1st in 1886: Martha Rooney of Belfast (d. 1891); 2nd in 1900: Eileen Murphy, daughter of William Martin Murphy (Dublin industrialist and newspaper proprietor); 8 s (3 doctors including Arthur [q.v.] who became Professor of Surgery, RCSI), 5 d (Alice (Carleton) taught anatomy at Oxford and was President of the British Association of Dermatologists)
d. 1928

LRCPI and LM, 1881; FRCSI 1991; FRCS Ed (Hon.), 1905; FRCPI (Hon.), 1914, a rare distinction for a surgeon

Surgeon-in-ordinary to Lord Lieutenant of Ireland, 1892–95 and 1906–15.
Surgeon, Jervis Street Hospital, Dublin.
Senior surgeon, Mater Misericordiae Hospital.
Consultant surgeon, Dr Steevens' Hospital; Orthopaedic Hospital Ireland; St Michael's Hospital, Kingstown; Dental Hospital Ireland.
Member, Council, RCSI; General Medical Council.
Visitor in Lunacy, High Court, Chancery Ireland.
Temporary Colonel, Royal Army Medical Corps AMS. Inspector, Special Military Surgical Hospitals, Irish Command.
Vice-President, Leinster branch (President, Dublin Division, 1903–4), BMA.
Senator in NUI.
Examiner in clinical surgery, TCD.
President, RAMI, 1921–24.

Author of 'Operative Treatment of Enlarged Prostate', Transactions of the *Royal Academy Medical Ireland*, 1893; 'Cancer of Male Breast,' Ibid.; 'Surgical Treatment of Empyema', Ibid., 1906; 'Choledochotomy', *Dublin Medical Journal* 1902.

Chance was a forceful and logical speaker who would have made a fine lawyer. He had a cheerful breezy manner, which gave great confidence to patients and relatives. While establishing himself in practice he became an accomplished anaesthetist. A multi-talented thoroughgoing Catholic gentleman.

COPPINGER, Charles Phillip

Dublin Surgeon

b. 1846, Dublin, son of Joseph William Coppinger
Educ. Clongowes Wood; Trinity College, Dublin; Catholic University School of Medicine (Cecilia Street), Dublin
m. Agnes Cooke
d. 1908

MD, RUI; MCh (*hon. causa*), 1885; FRCSI, 1881; MRCPI, 1881

Surgeon, Mater Hospital, 1869–1904; St Michael's, Dún Laoghaire; National Lying-in-Hospital
Professor of Physiology, Institute of Medicine, Catholic University, Dublin.

Coppinger was an enthusiastic disciple of Lord Lister (1827–1912) and his antiseptic method, and his operations were most successful. For many years, he went to London and assisted Lister at operations. He died of Bright's Disease (glomerulonephritis).

CORCORAN, John (Johnny)

Dublin Surgeon

b. 1910, youngest of 11 children
Educ. O'Connell Schools; University College Dublin
m. 1945: Dr Freddie Mitchell; 3s, 3d (3 doctors: Darach, a gynaecologist; Eleanor, a psychiatrist; David, a neonatologist)
d. 1986

MB, UCD, 1933; LM, MCh, 1936; FRCSI (Hon.), 1972

Postgraduate appointments as orthopaedic house surgeon, Ancoats Hospital, Manchester (with Harry Platt).
In 1938, spent six months visiting North American Clinics in Boston (Drs Lahey and Cattell); New York (McCarthy and Sheehan); Baltimore (Babcock); Rochester, Minnesota (Chuck Mayo and Thompson); St Louis (Graham).
Assistant surgeon, Children's Hospital, Temple Street.
Assistant surgeon, Mater Hospital, Dublin, 1938; surgeon, 1955–81.
President, surgical section, RAMI, 1964–65.

Johnny Corcoran's family had been in the Castleknock area of Dublin for almost 200 years. His parents died when he was young but he went through UCD on County Council scholarships and won many prizes. He was trained on the spot in the Mater Hospital, Dublin, by Harry Barniville [q.v.] and Charlie MacAuley [q.v.]. He worked at the Mater for seventeen years before going on the full staff.

He was one of the last of the truly general surgeons who took on everything. He operated on patients with mitral stenosis, did portocaval shunts and in 1955, on the death of Andy Butler [q.v.], he went on the senior staff of the Mater and inherited Butler's urological practice. He was involved with the Knights of Malta and became Chief Medical Officer to the Order.

Johnny collected oriental snuffboxes and Dublin pottery and was interested in all aspects of Dublin's history. Never, ever, even in the operating theatre, without a cigarette ('sterile ash'), he became ill in 1976 and his memory began to fail.

Above medium height, broad shouldered, sharp featured but kindly, balding from early days, always immaculately turned out, he had a great sense of humour and had a fund of self-deprecating anecdotes which partly concealed a fine intelligence. He was highly popular in the profession.

CORRIGAN, Thomas Peter (Tom)

Dublin Surgeon

Educ. University College Dublin

MB, UCD, 1964; FRCSI, 1968; MCh, NUI, 1973

Postgraduate appointments as surgical tutor, UCD; Mater Hospital Pfizer Research Fellow; senior surgical registrar, King's College Hospital, London (with Prof. V. V. Kakkar).
Senior Research Fellow in vascular surgery, Cleveland Clinic, Ohio.
Lecturer in surgery, UCD.
Consultant surgeon, Mater Hospital, 1975–2004.

HEDERMAN, William Patrick (Billy) PRCSI 1990–1992

Dublin Surgeon

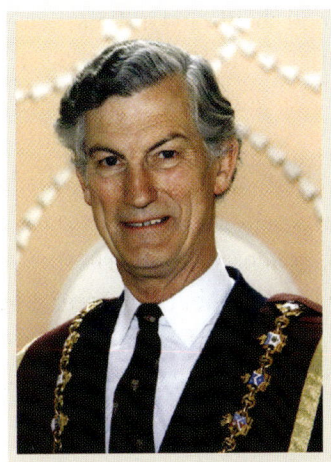

b. 1928, Croom, Co. Limerick, only son of Dr William Hederman and Ethel Hederman (*née* Hannigan); 3 sisters; his grandfather was Dr William Hederman
Educ. CBS Charleville; Crescent College, Limerick; Glenstal Priory School, Murroe, Co. Limerick; University College Dublin
m. 1964: Carmencita Cruess Callaghan, MA, DL, NUI (*hon. causa*); DL, DU (*hon. causa*). (Alderman, Dublin City Council for 25 years; Lord Mayor of Dublin 1987–88); 2 s, 3 d (Wendy elected to Dublin Corporation)

MB, UCD, 1951; FRCSI, 1957; MCh, 1958; FRCS Ed (*ad hom.*), 1991; FRCP&S Glas (Hon.); FCS South Africa (Hon.)

Postgraduate appointments as house surgeon, Mater Hospital (with Andrew Butler [q.v.]), 1951; senior house officer, Prince of Wales Hospital, Tottenham, London (with A. Dickson Wright and Ted O'Malley, 1952); casualty officer, Mater Hospital, 1953–54; surgical registrar, Mater Hospital (with Prof. Henry Barniville [q.v.] and Mr Charles McAuley [q.v.]) 1955–57. Senior surgical resident, Colorado University Hospital, Denver, Colorado (with Prof. Henry Swan and Prof. Ben Eisman, two of the most productive surgeons in the US at that time). Surgeon, Mater Hospital; St Ann's Hospital, 1957–92.
President, Vascular Surgery Society of Great Britain and Ireland, 1991–92.
Honorary Fellow, College of Medicine, Malaysia; American Academy of Medicine, Bahrain.
Member, James IV Association; Medical Council; Dental Council; Bord Altranais (Nursing Board).
PRCSI 1990–92.

Much influenced by Andrew Butler, Dickson Wright, Charlie McAuley, Henry Swan and Eoin O'Malley [q.v.]. General, vascular, head and neck surgery interests.

Billy Hederman is a hugely popular professional, much loved by his junior staff. A gifted, deft but apparently unhurried, superbly trained operating surgeon, he never ever took on more than was appropriate. Denver added something to the talent already there. He promoted good working relationships in his hospitals with his easy manner and unfailing courtesy, and he enjoyed teaching and training. His motto was 'Get it right first time and avoid complications.' With Eoin O'Malley, he developed the vascular unit, and the open-heart unit in the Mater Hospital

Tall and angular, he has something of the grandee about his physiognomy, and would not be out of place as a master of foxhounds or the scion of very old Anglo-Irish landed gentry. He rode horses from childhood and later his bicycle. Energetic, diligent, meticulous, generous and public-spirited, he enjoys a hectic social round and family life. He also skis, dives, fishes, hill-walks in his beloved Connemara, loves driving at or near the speed limits and took easily to bridge. A model citizen and surgeon.

HEFFERNAN, Seán Joseph ('The Heff')

Dublin Surgeon

b. 1923, Dublin, eldest son of John and Margaret Heffernan
Educ. CBS, Dún Laoghaire, Co. Dublin; University College Dublin
m. 1967: Mary Heffernan (*née* Reid); 1s, 3 d (Anne is a consultant anaesthetist, Dublin)
d. 1996

MB, UCD, 1948; FRCSI, 1952; MCh, 1954; FACS, 1981

Postgraduate appointments at Mater Hospital, Dublin; St Michael's, Dún Laoghaire, Jervis Street Hospital; St Mary's Chest Hospital, Dublin.
Senior house officer, GU and thoracic surgery, St James's Hospital Balham, London (with the legendary Norman Tanner: 'Get it right now so that you won't be worrying about it in bed tonight'). Registrar, GU & general surgery, Princess Beatrice Hospital; St John's & Elizabeth Hospital, London.
Tutor and lecturer, Mater Hospital, Dublin.
Consultant surgeon, Mater Hospital, Dublin, 1959–90; James Connolly Memorial Hospital, Blanchardstown, 1973–90. Consultant surgeon, three private Dublin hospitals.
Member, Council, RCSI, 1983–93.
President, Irish Society of Gastroenterology; surgical section, RAMI. Uniquely twice President of UCD Medical Society, a tribute to his interest in teaching the undergraduate students.
Chief medical officer to Dublin Diocesan Pilgrimage to Lourdes for over 20 years.
Member, Comité Internationale de Lourdes (which adjudicated on claims of miracles).
Appointed Papal Knight of St Gregory, 1988.

His main interests were in gastric surgery and he published several papers on highly selective vagotomy for peptic ulcer and on thyroid and parathyroid surgery. He wrote an invited leader for the *Lancet* on peptic ulcer.

Seán Heffernan had a large, carefully tended, private surgical practice all over Dublin, often visiting patients twice or three times a day, even when on 'holidays' in Donabate, Co Dublin. He was interested in music, art, literature and the theatre.

Seán was an exemplary Catholic, and the Church, together with his family, was at the centre of his life. Tall, bespectacled, broad shouldered, he had an episcopal look and demeanour, as if constantly worried about his flock of patients. He needn't have been. They were in safe hands.

LAVELLE, Edward Francis (Eddie)

Dublin Surgeon

MSc, NUI, MB (first class hons), UCD, 1929; MCh, NUI, 1934.

Postgraduate appointments as resident surgical officer, North Middlesex Hospital; clinical assistant, Royal Chest Hospital, London.
Assistant surgeon, Mater Hospital, Dublin.
Surgeon, St Michael's Hospital, Dún Laoghaire.

A brilliant natural operator, Eddie Lavelle developed stomach cancer in his late forties and went to London to Norman Tanner, the leading abdominal surgeon of his time. Going down for surgery he requested to be allowed to keep his watch on, 'for luck', as he said. Awakening from the anaesthesia, he looked at the watch and, from the short elapsed time, knew that he was inoperable.

LENTAIGNE, Sir John PRCSI 1908–1910

Dublin Surgeon

b. 1855, son of John Francis O'Neill Lentaigne (doctor, Privy Councillor, Knight, CB and Knight of the Order of Pio IX) and Mary Lentaigne (*née* Magan)
Educ. Clongowes Wood College; Catholic University, Dublin; Trinity College, Dublin
m. 1882: Phillis Coffey (d. 1893); 6s, 2d
d. 1915

BA, TCD, 1880; LRCP&SI, 1881; FRCSI, 1886

Surgeon, Jervis Street (1883–87); Mater Hospital; Children's Hospital, Temple Street; National Maternity Hospital, Holles Street.

The Lentaigne family, originally from Normandy, came to Dublin in 1792, after which there was a doctor in each generation. A painstaking rather than graceful surgeon, Sir John lacked diplomacy but was without bitterness and was highly popular. He died of angina pectoris, aggravated by severe influenza.

MacAULEY, Charles John (Charlie)

Dublin Surgeon

b. 1887, son of Charlie and Ann MacAuley; brother Harry MacAuley [q.v.] was Mater Hospital orthopaedic surgeon
Educ. St Malachy's College, Belfast; Royal University, subsequently renamed University College Dublin
m. Clare Spain (d. 1925); eldest son Niall died aged 14 years from tuberculous meningitis; son Patrick MacAuley [q.v.] became Mater Hospital orthopaedic surgeon
d. 1956

MB, UCD, 1912; FRCS Eng, 1921

Postgraduate training in surgery in Glasgow.
Surgeon, the Children's Hospital, Temple Street.
Lecturer in applied anatomy, UCD.
Surgeon, Mater Hospital, Dublin; St Mary's Hospital, Cappagh.

Charlie MacAuley read Classics for two years but was then advised by Professor John McNeill, a cousin, to change to Medicine. He went to UCD because the then Bishop of Down and Conor prohibited Catholics from attending Queen's University Belfast.

On Wednesday, 19 April 1916, just before the Easter Rising, Charlie operated on Joseph Plunkett (1887–1916), poet and patriot, for tuberculous glands of the neck (he had advanced pulmonary tuberculosis as well). He later got an urgent message from Mrs Desmond FitzGerald (Mabel), Garret FitzGerald's mother, to go to check on Plunkett in the General Post Office. Plunkett spent his week in the beleaguered Post Office, confined to his cot, attended by his aide, Michael Collins. Charlie stayed to treat other wounded until Seán T. O'Kelly (subsequently President of Ireland) told him to leave or he would 'never get a practice in Fitzwilliam Square'. Plunkett was executed by firing squad on 4 May 1916.

Charlie was a member of the All-Ireland Polo Club at the Phoenix Park for twenty years. To his great distress, the Polo Ground was the first piece of the Park dug up to grow vegetables during the 'Emergency' of 1939–45. Every Tuesday, he hunted with the Fingal Harriers, and on Saturday with the Ward Union.

In the words of his son Paddy, Charlie 'was a typical, outspoken, Northern, Catholic, Republican.'

O'SULLIVAN, John Frederick (Jack or Jacko)

Dublin Surgeon

b. 1916

Educ. O'Connell's Schools; University College Dublin

m. Marie Stanford (whose two doctor brothers had a big general practice in Scunthorpe, Yorkshire, where O'Sullivan went to train); 10 children (no doctors)

d. 1961

MB, UCD, 1939; MCh, NUI, 1943; FRCSI

Postgraduate appointments as house officer, War Memorial Hospital, Scunthorpe; resident surgical officer, Crumpsall Hospital, Manchester; surgical assistant, Mater Hospital, Dublin. Assistant Surgeon, Mater Hospital; St Mary's Orthopaedic Hospital, Dublin.

Jack O'Sullivan built up a huge practice quickly on the basis of the three As: Affability, Availability and Ability. He was a fast, confident operator, and was one of three founder members of the Irish Surgical Travelling Club.

Short, chubby, friendly, good humoured, he was great company and an accomplished storyteller, complete with pregnant pauses. His juniors remember his generosity. Constantly on the move, he was at the centre of an incident in which he was urgently called to see a patient who was experiencing postoperative complications in a big private hospital. The unavailable operating surgeon was a Mater surgical registrar who should certainly not have been doing private practice there or anywhere else. Exile followed.

Jack developed fatal malignant hypertension and kidney failure in his forties. Eoin O'Malley [q.v.] said, 'He was one of the brighter lights in Irish surgery and his early death prevented his realising his full potential…He was active in the Association of Surgeons of Great Britain and Ireland, the International Society of Surgeons, the Royal Society of Medicine and the Ulster Surgical to which he had been introduced by his senior, Charlie McAuley [q.v.], with whom he was really close.'

O'CONNELL, Francis Xavier (Frank or FX)

Dublin Surgeon

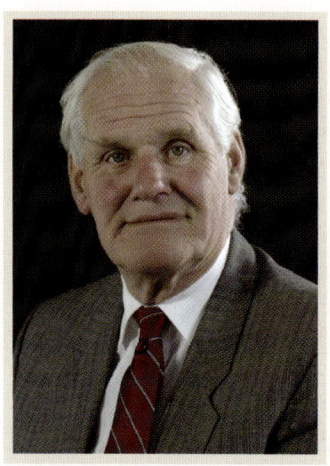

b. 1926, second son of Michael O'Connell [q.v.] (County Surgeon, Laois) and Agnes O'Connell
Educ. Clongowes Wood, College; University College Dublin
m. 1953: Enid B. Carton, MSc; 2 s, 3 d (2 doctors)
d. 1996

BSc (hons; anatomy), UCD, 1948; MB (hons), UCD, 1951; MCh, UCD, 1956; FRCSI, 1956

Postgraduate training posts in the Manchester area (with Anthony [Tony] Anscombe).
Assistant surgeon, Mater Hospital, Dublin, 1957.
Consultant surgeon, Mater Hospital, 1958–91.
Surgeon, St Luke's Hospital; Bon Secours Hospital, Glasnevin; St Joseph's Hospital, Raheny; Mount Carmel Hospital, Rathgar.
President, surgical section, RAMI; Surgical Travellers Club.
Dean of Students, Mater Hospital; examiner, UCD and RCSI finals and Primary and Fellowship of the RCSI at home and in the Middle East.

At school, Frank O'Connell excelled as an athlete but once he went on the staff of his various hospitals, he found little time for any sport. He gave the highest possible level of care, visiting all patients daily, and was always available and encouraged all staff to contact him if there was any concern. He was a superb operating surgeon who worked his way through crushing operating lists. There were occasional eruptions in theatre, which could be measured only on the Richter scale, but it is doubtful if anyone in these islands did more operative surgery during his thirty-four years at the 'table'. He loved the challenges.

Frank took a great interest in teaching his house surgeons and registrars, and he was a considerate, knowledgeable examiner with a profound knowledge of the realities of surgery and a deep-rooted sense of fairness.

He was a man of deep faith and a devoted husband and father. Tragically, in his so well-earned retirement, he was beset by a series of serious vascular problems ('cheroots'), including a successfully replaced thoracic aneurysm, and he did not live long to enjoy the fruits of what had been a heroic operating career.

He was tall (6'1"), dark, broad-shouldered, indefatigable and good-looking, and nothing except his religion surpassed his sense of duty.

SMYTH, Patrick Joseph ('Pakey')

Dublin Surgeon

b. 1891

Educ. University College Dublin

m. Married a member of the Dillon family (a sister of James Dillon, TD); a son, Nicholas, qualified MB in first place at UCD and became chief of surgery in Washington Center Hospital, in Washington DC.

d. 1962

MA, MB (hons), NUI, 1914; BSc (hons), NUI

Postgraduate appointments as senior house officer, Halifax Royal Infirmary; Mater Hospital, Dublin.

Served in Indian Medical Service before going to the Balkans as a Major, Royal Army Medical Corps, and Officer-in-Command, Surgical Division, 25th General Hospital Salonika, Greece. Surgeon, Mater Hospital, Dublin; St Michael's Hospital, Dún Laoghaire; the Cedars Hospital. President, Irish Society of Thoracic Surgeons.

Smyth early recognised the necessity for specialisation and took on the arduous duties of surgeon to the sanatoria. Lobectomies for tuberculosis were difficult, bloody procedures with dense adhesions everywhere, but even more traumatic were the thoracoplasties with the sequential fracturing and collapsing of the rib cages, with the object of collapsing the affected lung. Little was known about blood and fluid replacement in the 1930s and 1940s, and there were many deaths from inadequate blood and fluid replacement. A pint of blood might be given, but rarely two, when the requirement might have been four. Such was the mortality — and this tale probably did not involve Pakey — that there was a persistent story of a patient who, on being told that he was for surgery in a few days' time, opened the window of the ward and escaped into the grounds and was gone.

A large, smart, aldermanic, somewhat military figure, Pakey Smyth was always well dressed. He had a reputation for frugality in the matter of assistants' fees and general entertainment, a reputation that lost little in the telling. He had seen terrible carnage in the First World War and was quite stoic about his own mishaps, the number of which might have brought him just above average for the time. His considerable courage was put to the final test when he was being wheeled down to the operating theatre for possible repair of a ruptured aortic aneurysm. He knew that, at that time, no patient in these islands had survived this condition. He looked up at the blood 'drip' going as fast as possible and his last words to the surgeon were, 'Good luck; you may need it.'

Meath Hospital

MONTGOMERY, Douglas Wellington ('Monty') PRCSI 1968–1970

Dublin Surgeon

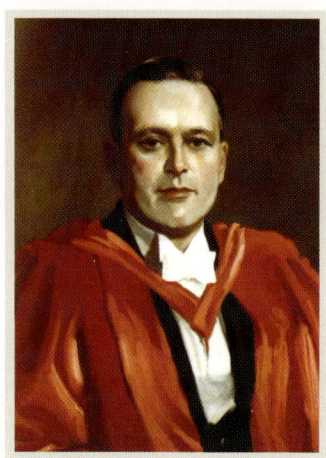

b. 1913, Fort Wayne, Indiana, USA, son of Mr and Mrs T. W. Montgomery

Educ. USA; CBS Omagh; Trinity College, Dublin

m. 1st: Brenda Boydell; 1 s, 2 d (Dr Gillian (O'Kane) became an anaesthetist); 2nd: Sheilah Hession

d. 1974

MB, TCD, 1940 (Haughton medal, Bennett medal and surgical prize); FRCSI

Postgraduate appointments as house surgeon and acting assistant surgeon, Sir Patrick Dun's.
Royal Army Medical Corps, 1942–44.
Surgeon, Meath Hospital 1945–74.

Montgomery was the first Allied surgeon ashore at Normandy on D-Day, 6 June 1944. His first operation there was on a German soldier. He and his team of four others set up an operating theatre about a mile and a quarter inland and gave their first blood transfusion (Group 4 0) an hour and twenty minutes after landing. He damaged his back wading ashore carrying his 80lb of equipment and was subsequently invalided out of the army.

Perhaps the most memorable event of his presidency of the RCSI was a lecture given on 11 November 1968 by Dr Christiaan Barnard on 'Cardiac Transplantation', less than a year after he had done the first such operation in the world. The charismatic, handsome surgeon spoke to an overflow audience. Monty went to South Africa as part of a successful team who raised funds for the College, mostly though 'Surgeons' graduates.

In surgery, he had been presciently impressed with the potential of the peritoneoscope, which was to become so much part of surgical practice thirty years later. He was retained by a number of British-based insurance companies as a really expert medical witness. He was always beautifully groomed and spoke in a low voice with carefully chosen words. Having qualified as a teacher of shorthand before studying medicine, he used his somewhat unnerving shorthand skills to record witnesses' statements for possible refutation. There was a view that you were far better off being in front of Monty as a patient than as a plaintiff. As might be expected, he was cool when 'under fire' from those disputing his findings.

ORMSBY, Sir Lambert Hepenstal PRCSI 1902–1904

Dublin Surgeon

b. 1849, Auckland, New Zealand, only son of George Ormsby (civil engineer and deputy surveyor-general of the 'colony') and Selina Ormsby (*née* Hepenstal); there were clergymen on both sides of the family

Educ. Local schools, New Zealand; Royal School, Dungannon, Co. Tyrone; apprenticed to Mr George Porter at the Meath Hospital at 15 years of age, and by 19 he was a qualified physician and surgeon at the Meath and the RCSI

m. 1st in 1874: Anastasia Dickenson; 2 s, 2 d. 2nd in 1921: Geraldine Matthews

d. 1923

BA, MB, TCD; FRCSI, 1875; MD, 1879

Surgeon, Meath Hospital.
Senior surgeon, National Orthopaedic and Children's Hospital.
Honorary consulting surgeon to the New Zealand Expeditionary Force, First World War.

Author of a number of semi-promotional articles on common subjects and a *Medical History of the Meath Hospital* (1888).

Ormsby invented a pocket ether inhaler which was widely adopted (1877). He proceeded MD 1879 with a thesis on anaesthesia. He established the National Orthopaedic and Children's Hospital, the forerunner of the National Children's Hospital, Harcourt Street, where he was senior surgeon. He had a flair for teaching and may have been one of the last to have anatomy pupils residing with him. Later, he resigned all teaching appointments and concentrated on expanding his large practice, which he serviced from a smart carriage drawn by a pair of grey cobs.

He was particularly interested in advancing the nursing profession and was involved in various charitable and other public-spirited activities.

Sir Lambert was of an expansive nature and his arrogance spread close to advertising, for which he was censured by the College, but the censure was later withdrawn. His presidency of the RCSI was noteworthy for a number of events rather than initiatives: Dr Tom Crean VC was given an honorary FRCSI (six votes to five), the College was told it was liable for income tax (it did not become a charity with tax exemption until 1965), and the Irish language was allowed as an optional entry examination subject. He was notably outspoken on a number of issues and was completely oblivious of any offence caused. One doesn't have to be popular to become President of the RCSI.

ROBINSON, Derek Lyster

Dublin Surgeon

b. 14 February 1923, Dublin, eldest child of Dr Cecil and Kathleen Robinson
Educ. Sandford Park School; Trinity College, Dublin
m. 1965: Pamela Matthews; 1 s, 1 d

MB, TCD, 1946; FRCSI, 1951; MA, 1952

Postgraduate appointments as casualty officer, Meath Hospital; resident surgical officer, General Hospital, Cheltenham; clinical assistant, subsequently assistant surgeon to Douglas Montgomery [q.v.].
Medical Officer, Merchant Navy; P&O Line.
Consultant accident and orthopaedic surgeon, Meath Hospital, 1956–89.
Consultant surgeon, Leopardstown Park Hospital.

Influenced by Henry Stokes [q.v.], Robinson Henry and Bourdillon in Cheltenham and subsequently Douglas Montgomery and Brandon Stephens [q.v.] in the Meath Hospital.

Cecil Robinson, Derek's father, was secretary of the medical board of the Meath Hospital for over sixty years, and Derek played an active part in the administration of his beloved hospital. He was a keen teacher of medical students and nurses, and was also in great demand as an expert court witness.

Strongly built and very athletic, he skied for over fifty years, hunted with the Meath Hunt, played snooker, squash and tennis. He is uniquely a Life Member of Portmarnock Golf Club and sailed in Dublin Bay and beyond. He has a beautiful speaking and singing voice and was President of the Hibernian Catch Club for three years. He is an energetic Commissioner of the St John Ambulance Brigade of Ireland.

STEPHENS, Brandon Edward

Surgeon, Meath Hospital Dublin

b. 1919, Dublin, second son of Edward Stephens (lawyer) and Lily Stephens (*née* Day); his father was a nephew of playwright John Millington Synge; his mother was involved in the clean milk bill in the 1920s
Educ. Newtown School, Waterford; Sandford School, Ranelagh; St Andrew's College, St Stephen's Green, Dublin; Trinity College, Dublin
m. 1946: Diana Moore (social worker, d. 2000), daughter of George and Irene Moore; 3 s (eldest, Richard, surgeon, St James's Hospital, Dublin), 1 d (occupational therapist)

MB (first class hons in surgery), TCD, 1942 (Wheeler gold medal, Royal City of Dublin Hospital); FRCSI, 1946

House posts at Royal City of Dublin Hospital (RCDH); assistant surgeon (resident surgical officer), Adelaide Hospital, 1944–46; assistant surgeon, RCDH (Baggot Street), 1946–55.
Consultant surgeon, Meath Hospital, 1955–83.
Surgeon, Guinness medical department, 1973–83.
Visiting surgeon, Mount Carmel Private Hospital, 1953–83.
Consultant surgeon, Arthur Guinness & Sons.

Brandon Stephens trained on the job with experienced 'chiefs'. His appointment to the Meath Hospital was made at the time of the attempted takeover of the governing body of the Meath by the Knights of St Columbanus, a stormy chapter in the hospital's history. (With the exception of T. D. J. Lane [q.v.], appointed as a pathologist, there had never been a Catholic appointed to the staff in almost 200 years). Stephens did everything from pinning the neck of the fractured femur to removal of the toxic colon. On busy nights, there were stretchers between beds. The Meath's urology unit made it the national centre for stone disease, some of which were caused by parathyroid disease, and Brandon Stephens became the country's expert in parathyroid surgery.

Described by a colleague: 'Tall, well dressed, punctual, expected team on its toes. At times short fuse causing some crack!' Very much a man of his time. Always completely professional, with an old-world courtesy, he put patients 'first, last and always'.

STOKES, Henry PRCSI 1940–1941

Dublin Surgeon

b. 1879, India, son of Henry John Stokes and Mary Anne Stokes (*née* MacDougall); his grandfather was William Stokes (1804–78) of Cheyne-Stokes breathing and Stokes Adams syndrome; Barbara Stokes, FRCPI, paediatrician, was his niece
Educ. Strangeways School, St Stephen's Green; Trinity College, Dublin
m. Kathleen Elizabeth Franks, daughter of Sir John Franks; 4 children (Elizabeth, FRCSI)
d. 1967

MB, TCD, 1903; MD, TCD, 1905; FRCSI, 1907

Post graduation travelled to Leiden, the Netherlands; Berne, Switzerland; and the Mayo Clinic, Rochester, Minnesota, where he must have been one of the earliest Irish Fellows. Like almost all their alumni, he kept in touch with 'the Clinic' throughout his life.
Surgeon, Meath Hospital (fourth generation of his family to be on the staff); National Children's Hospital, Harcourt Street, St Ultan's Infant Hospital.
Lieutenant-Colonel, Royal Army Medical Corps, First World War.

Henry Stokes was the first Irish surgeon to advocate and use blood transfusion. He was the first in Dublin to remove a parathyroid tumour and, as the Meath's Department of Urology grew, with parathyroid-related kidney stones being sent there, he became the nation's expert. He was a fair, judicious examiner.

Bob Collis (1900–75), Ireland's most distinguished paediatrician, said that Stokes was too kind to charge the poor and too grand to charge his friends and, in consequence, was exceedingly poor. But while others were boastful, Stokes was candid and gave talks on his mistakes.

He was a country man at heart, loving 'outings', elaborate picnics, rough shooting, fishing the Boyne for salmon, and archaeology. He had an abiding interest in the extinct Giant Irish Elk. He played billiards and was a member of a 'Periatetics' card school, which moved from house to house in turn. He had ascetic habits and was a regular walker. He was a keen Rotarian.

With the passing of Henry at the age of 89, there ended the century-long honourable and fruitful association of the Stokes family with the Meath Hospital.

MERCER'S HOSPITAL

BOUCHIER-HAYES, Thomas Adrian (Tommy, Tom, 'The Bouch')

Senior Surgeon, Mercer's Hospital, Dublin

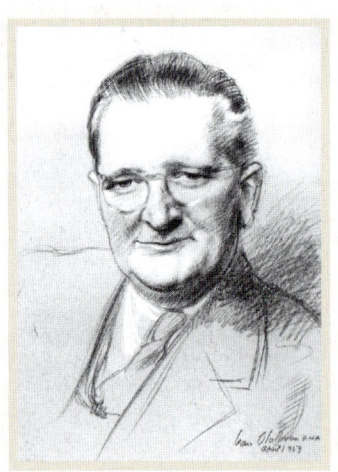

b. 1907, Rathkeale, Co. Limerick, grandson of Thomas Hayes MD (1832–1913) Edinburgh (MRCP, JP, medical officer of health and consultant sanitary officer for the Rathkeale No. 1 Dispensary District); one of 7 children, 4 of whom became doctors (Henry was a GP in Charleville, Co. Cork; John was a GP in Rathkeale) **Educ.** Rathkeale Secondary School; Trinity College, Dublin

m. 1935: Mona Graham, daughter of Dr Matthew Graham, Limerick GP (first cousin of 'Surgeon Extraordinary' John Benjamin Murphy of Chicago, the pre-eminent surgeon of his day); 7 s (David [q.v.] became Professor of Surgery, RCSI, and was consultant surgeon at Beaumont Hospital), 5 d
d. 1960

BA (Mod), TCD, 1929; MB, TCD, 1930; FRCSI, 1934
Postgraduate appointments as house surgeon and surgical registrar, Richmond Hospital. He was encouraged to go to the Richmond by Sir Thomas Myles [q.v.].
Senior surgeon, Mercer's Hospital.

Assistant surgeon, Richmond Hospital.
Consultant surgeon, Vergemount Fever Hospital, Clonskeagh.
Consultant surgeon to the National Health Insurance Society.
Honorary surgeon to Leopardstown Racecourse.
Close association with the Irish Red Cross. Chief medical adviser to Aer Lingus.
Medical adviser to the Irish Municipal Employees Trade Union, 1935–60.
Member, Council, RCSI.

His father had been a teacher, so that dominant gene was to continue to express itself. He had studied in London and was an MRCS. He married Elizabeth Bouchier and her maiden name was incorporated into the family surname. Tommy Bouchier Hayes's grandfather, Thomas Hayes, had been a respected surgeon whose skills were much in demand all over Munster and was active, operating, right into his eightieth year. He had seen James Young Simpson (1811–70) administer chloroform and used it extensively in his practice. He was a facile writer and a frequent contributor to the medical literature of the time. A Gaelic scholar, he translated *The Odes of Horace* into Irish. He was a talented linguist, mastering, amongst others, both Welsh and Hebrew. He had been President of the Munster branch of the British Medical Association. He was described by a contemporary obituarist as 'High-minded, honourable and upright.'

Following a brilliant undergraduate career in the competitive atmosphere of Trinity, where he won many prizes and medals, Bouchier-Hayes started in practice in Dublin and rapidly built up a huge reputation. He was a prodigious worker and did many smaller operations as day cases, which was most unusual at the time. On one occasion, his patients occupied seventy beds in the Richmond Hospital, when his allocation was two. Hugely popular within and without the profession, he often wore morning clothes on rounds and at clinics. His first paid appointment had been as medical adviser to the Irish Municipal and Electrical Trade Union (IMETU), and, out of loyalty, he did house calls to beneficiaries until the end.

He attended the victims of the North Strand bombings of 31 May 1941, when an off-course German aircraft over Dublin came under fire and dropped a landmine, killing thirty-four and injuring over sixty. His reputation extended beyond the country and he had been made a Freeman of Louvain for his services to aviation surgery.

He was a brilliant clinical teacher (his hero was Abraham Colles, 1773–1843, who regularly got standing ovations at the end of a lecture), and gave a daily free five o'clock grind in surgery at the Dixon Theatre, Trinity College. He was much in demand as a perceptive examiner.

As a young man, he had been interested in athletics, an interest he transferred to horse racing, and he owned some horses given to him by grateful patients. Racing proved an expensive hobby. He was a music lover and was President of the Bohemians Musical Society. This brought him into contact with the rising stars of the day, including Dermot Troy and Veronica (Ronnie) Dunne, whose Covent Garden début he attended as a guest of the Dunne family. Card playing — bridge, poker and whist predominating — was a major domestic and social activity until overtaken by television about 1955, with the 'card school' rotating through the participants' homes and the men's clubs, and Bouchier-Hayes was a sharp poker player.

He was kind and charitable, both in failing to bill for his services and in giving 'loans' to impoverished students. The drawing by Seán O'Sullivan was done in gratitude for rescuing himself and Myles na gCopaleen (Brian O'Nolan) from Pearse Street Garda Station following a 'misunderstanding' with the guardians of the law. Perhaps 5'10", he was burly with legendary energy. His wife, Mona, was a nurse at the Richmond Hospital, and, because she looked delicate, Sir Thomas Myles [q.v.] advised that she not do night duty. She lived to be 91. Four of her brothers played on the same Munster rugby team, which is still a record.

Tommy was doctor to the Jewish Old Folk's Home and it was said that there were more promises of olive trees for Israel than Mass cards at his funeral. As a measure of the man, the President, Eamon de Valera, two senior cabinet ministers and the Lord Mayor of Dublin attended.

COOLICAN, John Edward Francis (Jack)

Dublin Surgeon

b. 25 March 1924, Dublin, second son of John and Helen Coolican
Educ. Xavier's; Belvedere College, Dublin; Clongowes Wood; Trinity College, Dublin
m. Dr Joan McGill (his first intern); 3 children

MB, TCD, 1948; MCh, TCD, 1951; FRCSI, 1951; FRCS Eng, 1954

Postgraduate appointments at Mercer's Hospital, Dublin; St John and Elizabeth's, London; Leicester General Hospital; Harefield Hospital. Courses in postgraduate surgery in Middlesex and Westminster Hospitals.
Surgeon, Mercer's Hospital, 1953–83; Sir Patrick Dun's, 1983–86; Meath/Adelaide, 1986–89; Hume Street 1965–83; Newcastle Sanatorium, Co. Wicklow, 1956–62; St Bricin's Military Hospital, 1963–83; Peamount Sanatorium, 1965–80.
Associate professor, RCSI.

Main interests were in general and thoracic surgery. Influenced by J. H. Coolican (father) [q.v.], Thomas Bouchier-Hayes [q.v.], Sir M. J. Smyth and Sir Thomas Holmes Sellors.

Appointed to Mercer's Hospital at 29, Jack Coolican had been trained in lung surgery, especially the surgery of tuberculosis. New sanatoria had been built to cope with the scourge but new antibiotics such as streptomycin meant that the disease went into rapid decline and, with that, the need for the mutilating operation of thoracoplasty.

Tall, athletic ('slicing golfer') and ruggedly handsome, with a shock of white hair, he is a quiet, retiring gentleman.

COOLICAN, John Henry (Jack)

Dublin Surgeon

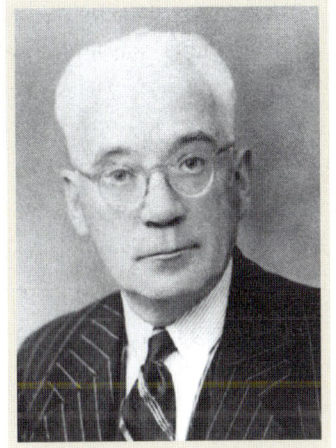

b. 1896, second son of Edward Coolican, Ballina, Co. Mayo
Educ. Our Lady's Bower, Athlone; Clongowes Wood College; Trinity College, Dublin (medical scholar)
m. Helen; (second son, John, a Dublin surgeon [q.v.])
d. 1964

MB, TCD, 1919; FRCS Ed, 1929; FRCSI, 1932

Postgraduate studies at New York City Medical School; Edinburgh Medical School; clinical assistant, West London Hospital, with Prof. Finsterer (Vienna), Prof Kock (Bratislava).
Consultant surgeon, Mercer's Hospital; Peamount Hospital (TB); St Luke's Hospital; City of Dublin Skin and Cancer Hospital, Hume Street.

Influenced by Prof. Finsterer and Sir William Wheeler RCSI [q.v.]

Coolican was a general surgeon who latterly took on the surgery of pulmonary tuberculosis, an exhausting and dangerous specialty in which the fluid and blood losses were gravely underestimated at the time, resulting in severe shock and some deaths following thoracoplasty, even in the best hands. He devised a pubofemoral bone graft for TB hip. He was in great demand as a second opinion on a variety of problems.

Spruce, of middle height, humorous and convivial (captained Portmarnock Golf Club), he was totally sincere and genuine. Carelessness and imprecision annoyed him, particularly when he was overworked. At such times, he could be irritable and impatient. But his moods mellowed. A pillar of the profession, an excellent teacher and a wise operator.

MATTHEWS, Joseph Gerard (Joe)

Dublin Surgeon

LRCP & SI, 1936; FRCSI, 1940

Surgeon, Mercer's Hospital; St Michael's Hospital, Dún Laoghaire.
Examiner, Primary and Final Fellowship, RCSI. Member, Council, RCSI.

Handsome, hardworking, shrewd and successful, Joe Matthews was at his best with a major problem in abdominal surgery. He was also in great demand as a medico-legal opinion.

MAUNSELL, Charles PRCSI 1924–1926

Dublin Surgeon

b. 1872, son of Robert Maunsell of Ballinasloe, Co. Galway
Educ. High School; Trinity College, Dublin
m. 1911: Eleanor (Nell) Hanna; 1 d
d. 1930

MB TCD 1894. FRCSI 1900

House surgeon, Sir Patrick Dun's Hospital.
Honorary visiting surgeon, Mercer's Hospital, 1898–1930.
Consulting surgeon, Royal Hospital for Incurables, Donnybrook, Dublin; Cottage Hospital, Drogheda.
Major, Royal Army Medical Corps at Dublin Castle; Red Cross Hospital; General Hospital, Boulogne.

The main event of his presidency of RCSI was the decision of the newly established Irish Free State government to set up a separate Irish Medical Register. Maunsell was against this on the grounds that it might damage medical education in Ireland, and there were fears that Irish graduates might not be able to practise in Britain. However, there was little fear of this as Irish graduates were required as general practitioners particularly in the heavily industrialised north of England, but also in the armed forces. The best interests of the Irish medical schools were preserved and, in 1926, he became a member of the Irish Medical Registration Council.

Maunsell worked hard to restore Mercer's reputation. He was calm, self-confident and unruffled. Reserved in manner, he had no small talk and could remain disconcertingly silent. A colleague called him 'a great surgeon and a great gentleman'.

PRINGLE, Seton Sidney, OBE PRCSI 1934–1936

Dublin Surgeon

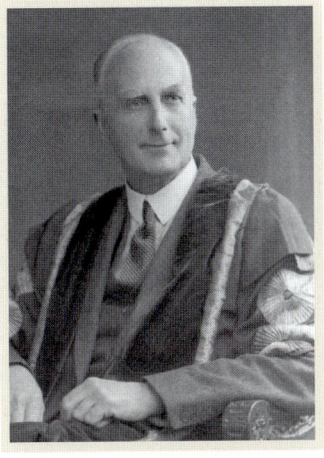

b. 1879, Clones, Co. Monaghan, son of John Pringle (businessman)

Educ. Coleraine Academical Institute; Trinity College, Dublin

m. 1st: Ethel, daughter of Dr Andrew McMunn of Ballymote, Co. Sligo; 5 children. 2nd: Eileen Florence Blandford (lady district superintendent, St John Ambulance Brigade)

d. 1955

BA, Dublin (1st Respondent), 1902; MB (stipendiary conditions), 1903; FRCSI, 1905 (TCD); MCh (Hon.), TCD; Fitzpatrick medical scholarship, Stewart medical scholarship.

Surgeon, Dublin Castle Red Cross, Mercer's Hospital, Dublin.
Demonstrator in anatomy, TCD.
Lieutenant Colonel, Royal Army Medical Corps; Officer-in-Command, Urgency Cases Hospital, with the French Army.
Surgeon, Royal City of Dublin Hospital (succeeded Mr Henry Moore [q.v.] who had died at the Front); Drumcondra Hospital; Cork Street Hospital, 1918–45 (succeeded by his cousin J. Seton Pringle [q.v.], later Regius Professor of Surgery, TCD).
Consultant surgeon, Princess Patricia Hospital.
President, RAMI, 1939–43; Council of the St John Ambulance Brigade.

Author of 'Appendico-Enterostomy', *Medical Press*, c.1906; 'Sacrococcygeal Teratoid Tumour', *Lancet*, 1907; 'Case of Pancreatic Abscess', *Lancet*, 1909; 'Transperitoneal Cystotomy for Tumour of Bladder', *Lancet*, 1910; 'Radical Operation for Malignant Disease of Testes', *Lancet*, 1913; 'Acute Unilateral Pyelonephritis', Practice, 1911; 'Chronic Intestinal Stasis', *British Medical Journal*, 1914; 'Radical Operation for Chronic Osteomyelitis', *British Journal of Surgery*, 1914.

Seton Pringle was a strikingly handsome man with bushy eyebrows, piercing eyes, florid complexion, pleasant manner, northern accent and an immense capacity for work. He was a daring, dauntless operator, regarding no patient as hopeless, and did radical surgery on advanced cancers. He did a lot of urology but it was as an abdominal surgeon that he excelled. His *tour de force* was abdominoperineal resection for rectal cancer. He had a massive private practice from all over Ireland. His speed meant that surgery was not always entirely bloodless but he was one of the most skilful of his day. He was always chuckling behind his operating mask.

WHEELER, Sir William Ireland de Courcy (Billy) PRCSI 1922–1924

Dublin Surgeon

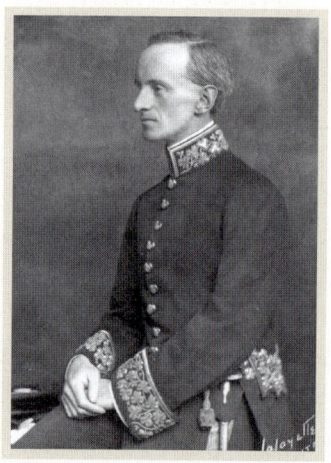

b. 1879, son of William Ireland de Courcy Wheeler (1844–99) MD, PRCSI (1883) and Victoria Wheeler (*née* Shaw — a relative of Bernard Shaw); one of 9 children
Educ. Mr Strangeway's School; High School; Trinity College, Dublin
m. 1909: Elsie Shaw, eldest daughter of Lord Shaw of Dumferline; 1s, 1d
d. 1943

MB, TCD, 1902; FRCSI, 1905; FACS (Hon.); MCh, Cairo (Hon.), 1928

Surgeon, Mercer's Hospital, Dublin, 1904–32.
Surgeon, Southend-on-Sea, Essex, from where he also worked at smaller London hospitals.
Surgeon Rear Admiral and consulting surgeon to the Admiralty, 1939–43.

Billy Wheeler visited Doyen's clinic in Paris and spent three months with Theodor Kocher (Nobel Prize in Medicine, 1909, and a founder of modern scientific surgery) in Berne. He was appointed to Mercer's Hospital in 1904, aged 25. At the time, many of the appointees to Mercer's were youthful, and it became known as 'the children's hospital', but Wheeler was a fine operator and teacher. He was particularly adept at thyroidectomy, using the technique that he had learnt from Kocher. When he resigned in 1932, Sir John Lumsden spoke of him as 'the man who made Mercer's'.

Wheeler was a man of great personal charm even if he did not always exercise it. As a student, he had lost the sight of one eye, and he could be demanding, irascible and overbearing. However, he had a fund of stories and was a master of after-dinner speaking. He was dismissive of any real competition in his practice and, although a Protestant, said that he wore a crucifix under his clothes so that in case of an accident he would not be taken to the Protestant Adelaide Hospital and come under the care of his arch enemy, Professor William Pearson [q.v.]. His enmity with Sir Arthur Chance [q.v.], who outranked him in the army, far outstripped the usual

He retired at 65 to Co. Meath, where he kept a 'Georgian Gem' of a house and where he entertained graciously. He worked hard and endlessly on his property, as well as fishing on the Boyne and shooting. He was buried in his native Monaghan. A master surgeon.

Protestant and Catholic antagonisms of the time. Wheeler nurtured imagined slights and was petty in his crusades.

During the First World War, he gave his private nursing home at 33 Upper Fitzwilliam Street as a hospital for wounded officers. He was mentioned in dispatches for his courage and skill during the Easter Rising. Later that year, he went briefly to the front in France.

He wrote on a great variety of subjects and his papers were often cited, and he was an invited speaker at BMA meetings in England. The American College of Surgeons had given him their Honorary Fellowship and gave him another of their highest distinctions, the John B. Murphy Oration in Surgery, in 1932. He was the sixth son of a President of the RCSI to be elected to the office.

In 1932, he left Dublin, which understandably had not felt the same for him since the newly independent state had come into being in 1922, for a new hospital in Southend-on-Sea in Essex from where he worked at smaller London hospitals also. At the outbreak of the Second World War he became consulting surgeon to the Admiralty with the rank of Surgeon Rear Admiral. His sudden death in Aberdeen occurred when he was dressing for dinner.

Billy Wheeler was a great character, as well as a skilful, well-rounded surgeon who nurtured and displayed the qualities required for success in the wider world. His entire career was a microcosm of the times.

Richmond Hospital (St Laurence's)

BROWNE, Harold Joseph

Dublin Surgeon

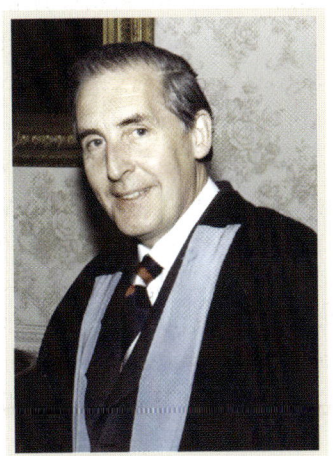

b. 1922, Dublin, eldest child of Frederick and Helen Browne
Educ. St Michael's National School, Longford, 1927–36; St Mel's College, Longford, 1936–40; University College Dublin
m. 1st in 1955: Dr Aileen McClancy (d. 1982); 3 s, 2 d (Ingrid is a consultant anaesthetist). 2nd in 1999: Vivienne Nash, SRN

MB (hons and second place), UCD, 1946; DA (RCSI), 1948; MS, surgery, Mayo Clinic, 1952; MCh, UCD, 1953; FACS, 1961; FRCSI (Hon.), 1977.

House surgeon, resident anaesthetist and surgical registrar, Richmond Hospital, Dublin, 1946–49.

Fellow in surgery, Mayo Clinic, Rochester, Minnesota, 1950–54; honorary visiting professor, 1983.
Consultant surgeon, Richmond Hospital, 1955–87; St Michael's, Dún Laoghaire, 1964–77.
President, Medical Council (Ireland), 1989–94 (member, 1984–94); surgical section, RAMI, 1976–77.
Founder and governor, American College of Surgery chapter in Ireland, 1982–88. Appointed Bar Council for 5 years. Examiner at Fellowship level in UK, Bahrain and Sudan.
Carmichael lecturer, RCSI, 1983; Widess memorial lecture, RCSI, 1988; William Doolin memorial lecture, IMO, 1995.

Career influenced by Drs John Waugh, Mark Coventry, Oliver Beahrs and S. Harrington, all of the Mayo Clinic (all of whom remembered him with great affection), and AB Clery [q.v.] of the Richmond Hospital. Special interest in upper abdominal surgery, as well as parotid dissection.

Harold Browne is one of the most popular, loved and trusted figures in Irish surgery and has been for forty years. He was at the Mayo Clinic in Rochester during its apogee. He rotated on to eleven 'firms' at the Mayo, a training system that contrasts with many in Ireland at that time, where a really good 'resident' was sometimes kept on one firm to 'give a hand'. His superb training was a lifelong influence and was reinforced by frequent subsequent visits. He returned to Ireland and the Richmond Hospital 'gift-wrapped'.

In the late 1960s, a colleague from the Mayo Clinic was staying with the editor's family in Dublin. A few local Mayo Clinic alumni were invited to meet the visitor, who commented, 'That guy Harold Browne asked to be remembered to every last nice guy in the Clinic while that other Fellow [name withheld for legal reasons] was asking to be remembered to every pain in the butt we have there'. Unsurprising and revealing.

Harold was an immaculate operative surgeon who loved technical refinement and taught his juniors to appreciate tissue. He rarely presents papers at meetings but he is an assiduous attendee, and all wait on his courteous and carefully considered, succinct summing up. He has written generous appreciations of many deceased colleagues and is a great source of lore on surgical subjects, much of it delivered in a wry, yet kindly manner. He is the ultimate Irish surgical sage.

Of medium height, he looks vaguely like a member of the Spanish nobility, with black hair intact. Slightly stooped from surgery and golf (he twice won the Dublin Hospitals Cup), he has a clear voice with great diction, and continues, in his middle eighties, to teach anatomy to appreciative students. In his eighty-fourth year, while he was still lecturing, the RCSI designated the anatomy theatre in the College 'The Harold Browne Theatre'. A fitting celebration of a most admirable professional.

BROWNE, Hyacinth Ignatius ('Hy')

Dublin Surgeon

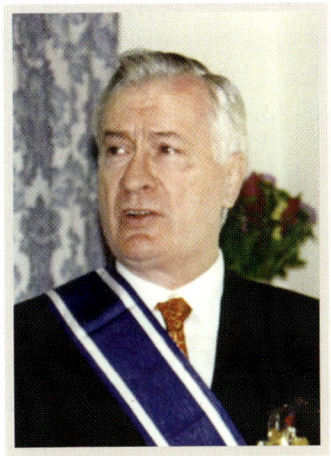

b. March 1932, youngest of 8 children of John and Loretta Browne, Rathronan Castle, Co. Wexford
Educ. Teirmohan National School, Co. Kildare; Catholic University School, Dublin; Royal College of Surgeons in Ireland.
m. Olive Jennings; 2 s, 1 d (Amanda, a trainee ophthalmologist)

LRCP & SI, 1956; FRCSI, 1969; FCCP, DSc, Khartoum University, Republic of Sudan

Postgraduate training posts at Mercer's Hospital Dublin; Jervis Street Hospital, Dublin. Consultant surgeon, James Connolly Memorial Hospital and Richmond Hospital, 1973–99.
Medical administrator, James Connolly Memorial Hospital, 1974.
Postgraduate Dean, RCSI 1989–93; Dean, Faculty of Medicine, RCSI, 1993–98.
Medical director and consultant surgeon, Armed Forces, Kuwait, 1999–2000.
Order of the Two Niles, Republic of Sudan, 1996; Albert Schweitzer gold medal, Albert Schweitzer Academy of Medicine.

As a skilled general surgeon, Hy Browne was equally at home with vascular, thoracic and trauma surgery. He travelled as lecturer, assessor and demonstrator of operative technique to many countries in the Middle East, the Sudan, Libya and Malaysia. He was a popular teacher and lecturer to generations of RCSI graduates and undergraduates.

Above medium height, dark, with black hair going gracefully grey, he is always impeccably dressed as for an important meeting. He has a relaxed manner and a good sense of humour and is greatly devoted to the College. He was a loyal servant. His leisure activities include shooting and private flying.

BURKE, Michael Plunkett (Mick) PRCSI 1952–1954

Dublin Surgeon

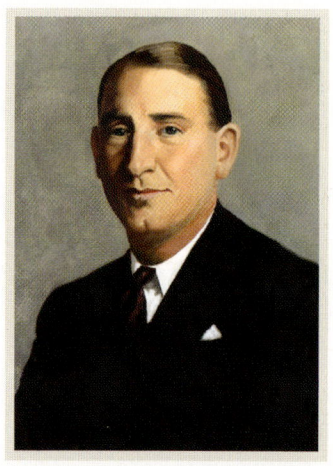

b. 1893, Longford, son of Peter Burke and Mary Anne Burke (*née* Plunkett); his nephew, Harold Browne [q.v.] was an iconic Richmond Hospital surgeon
Educ. St Mel's College, Longford; University College Dublin
m. Maude Naughton of Tuam
d. 1964

LRCPSI, 1915; FRCSI, 1929

Postgraduate house posts, Richmond Hospital.
Was out on the streets with a Red Cross armlet during 1916 Easter Rebellion, and went to France in 1917 as médecin-major [medical officer] with the Croix Rouge Française.
Assistant surgeon, Richmond staff (with Sir Thomas Myles [q.v.]).
Irish Army Medical Service, on leave of absence from the Richmond.
Surgeon, Richmond Hospital; St Michael's Hospital, Dún Laoghaire; Peamount Sanatorium, 1928–64.
Member, Council, RCSI, 1934–64; President, 1952–54.
President, surgical section, RAMI, 1957–60 (he wrote a history of the section).

Mick Burke had a close, almost paternal, relationship with Sir Thomas Myles, with whom he worked at the Richmond. He had a huge practice, perhaps based more on his immense charm than on his operative delicacy. His unpunctuality was legendary but he expected his resident staff to be standing in line, awaiting his arrival, no matter when 'the Late Mr Burke', as he was called, swept in from his Bentley. (This standing in line was still the rule, affecting house surgeons only, at the Hospital for Sick Children, Great Ormond Street, London, in 1952.) He put a great deal of time, effort and influence into the upgrading and extension of St Michael's Hospital, Dún Laoghaire, and was a most loyal colleague.

He lived in great style at 67 Lower Baggot Street, and loved entertaining in the grand manner. His home was one of the last outposts of the black-tie dinner for friends. His real interests, outside surgery, were golf and gossip. He was captain of both Portmarnock Golf Club in Dublin and Lahinch Golf Club in Clare. When he visited Lahinch, 'he was greeted like a royal personage being the uncrowned king of golfing revels'. He collapsed in Portmarnock clubhouse a few weeks before he died.

A burly figure with a fine head, he rarely stopped talking and was hugely popular in the profession.

CLERY, Anthony Burton (AB or Tony) PRCSI 1956–1957

Dublin Surgeon

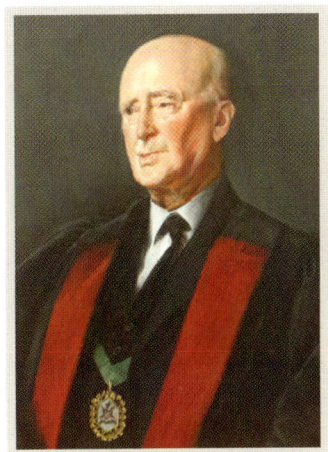

b. 1899, Bantry, Co. Cork, fourth child and youngest son of Francis Patrick Clery (Provincial Bank, Kilmallock, Co. Limerick) and Gertrude Clery (*née* Dolan) of Cootehill, Co. Cavan
Educ. Clongowes Wood College; Royal College of Surgeons in Ireland
m. 1928: Mary Gabriel (Gay) Hogan [q.v.]; 3 s (Anthony Patrick Tully (Tony) [q.v.], retired colorectal surgeon; Gerald (Geróid), Irish Ambassador; John, orthopaedic surgeon, New South Wales, Australia), 1 d (Mary, medical laboratory technologist, Connecticut, USA)
d. 1979

LRCP & SI, RCSI, 1920 (first in class; gold medal in operative surgery); FRCSI, 1923

Postgraduate appointments as house surgeon, Richmond Hospital, 1920; resident anaesthetist, Richmond Hospital, 1921; assistant surgeon (to A. A. McConnell [q.v.]), 1923. Senior visiting surgeon, Richmond Hospital, 1937.
Consultant surgeon, St Anne's Hospital; St Luke's Hospital; St Bricken's Military Hospital.
Director of surgery, Our Lady's Hospital for Sick Children, Crumlin, Dublin, from its opening in 1956 to his retirement in 1974.
Member, Council, RCSI, 1947–79; President, 1957–58.
General Medical Council, 1967 onwards.
President, Medical Register Ireland.
External examiner for NUI.

As he was under 25 years when he became FRCSI, AB's diploma was handed to him outside the Boardroom and he had to return the following year for conferring.

He continued as an expert medical witness until the very day he died. Beginning as a completely general surgeon, he took an increasing interest in plastic and reconstructive work, influenced by T. P. Kilner (Oxford), Archie McIndoe (East Grinstead) and Harold Gillies (Basingstoke). With them he was a founder member of the British Association of Plastic Surgeons. He was a first-rate natural technical surgeon who enjoyed cleft-lip and palate surgery and was a superb freehand cutter of skin grafts for burns. He was easy to assist and a very good assistant. He was a well-organised teacher, had a large surgical practice and gave careful postoperative care. He was one of the last surgeons to consult, and live over the 'shop', in an elegant house in 59 Fitzwilliam Square. Thirty years as a compassionate, unobtrusive Secretary of the Royal Medical Benevolent Fund typified AB's attitude to service within the profession.

He could be patronising and, as he did not retire from surgery until aged 74, he slipped a bit behind the times towards the end. However, he was a great favourite with the nursing staff. His reactions were always calm, fair and measured. Careful to the point of hospital pantomime parody ('Is it raining, Mr. Clery?' (to a dripping figure), 'Well it was when I came in.'), he was a fine chairman and accomplished at defusing confrontations. (When the editor complained in colourful detail to AB about the multiple shortcomings of a trainee AB had appointed, AB's reply was 'What you are telling me is that he's no Barry O'Donnell…and sure isn't that a great thing?')

A keen history student, he published articles on the O'Clery family in the Journal of the *Royal Society of Antiquaries of Ireland*. His family sept was rooted in east Limerick, and, despite his place of birth, he regarded himself as a Limerick man, with a deep inbred aversion to all things and people of Cork origin. (He was a traceable relative of the editor but he denied this!) He also wrote a history of the Richmond Hospital.

Tall (6'1"), balding, neatly dressed, conservative and somewhat Victorian in appearance, he was austere on first meeting. His wit was somewhat wan. He was physically strong, could swim long distances, and had a prodigious capacity for work of all kinds. He was deeply religious. He played golf to an eight handicap at his best. Holidays were spent in a family bungalow at Rosslare, Co Wexford.

Though he held no academic post, AB had much influence in Dublin surgical affairs for over thirty years because of his sustained, detached integrity. There is a splendid portrait of him by Leo Whelan in the RCSI boardroom, which completely captures the man. A superb surgeon and an adornment to the profession.

CLERY, Anthony Patrick Tully (Tony)

Dublin Colorectal Surgeon and Hospital Administrator

b. 1929, Dublin, son of Anthony Burton Clery [q.v.] and Mary Gabriel (Gay) Hogan [q.v.]
Educ. Clongowes Wood College; University College Dublin
m. 1955: Pauline Dolores McElroy, SRN (Gold medallist, St Vincent's Hospital, Dublin School of Nursing and widely regarded as a secular saint); 1 s, 1 d

MB, UCD, 1953; MS, Minnesota, 1960; FRCSI, 1961; FACS, 1967

Postgraduate appointments as senior house officer, Richmond Hospital, 1953–54; Fellow, Mayo Clinic, Rochester, Minnesota, 1956–60, rotating through six surgical units as well as general medicine and pathology; senior registrar, Richmond Hospital, Dublin, 1960–62.

Consultant surgeon, Richmond Hospital and subsequently Beaumont Hospital, 1963–89; chairman, surgical division and medical administrator, 1987–89.

Consultant surgeon, Ibn-Al-Bitar Hospital, Baghdad, 1989–91.

Consultant surgeon and medical director, Military Hospital, Tabuk, Kingdom of Saudi Arabia, 1991–92.

Professor of Surgery, RCSI, 1991.

Many offices in general medical and specialist colorectal societies, including presidencies, Surgical Specialist Society of London and Irish Society of Colorectal Surgeons.

Tony was the first to return to the Republic as a fully trained colorectal surgeon. The systematic and almost monastic training at the Mayo Clinic in those days was unsurpassed anywhere, and it remained his spiritual home. He was a meticulous operator whose low anterior resection anastomoses did not leak. He was attentive to the finest detail and was honest about his results. He was also interested in minor anorectal surgery and developed some personal techniques. The Mayo Clinic convinced him of the importance of clinical research and he kept careful notes for national and international presentation and publication. He was a keen and clear teacher, and passed his expertise on to his registrars, most of whom remained friends over the years.

Of slim build, balding, 5'9", wiry constitution and a dapper dresser, he has a direct and forthright manner, which has left some scars, most of which healed with time.

A devoted family man, he spends some of his retirement in Majorca. He was a competitive dinghy sailor (really a competitive everything), fishes and is a fine shot. He will not and should not be forgotten.

HOGAN, Mary Gabriel (Gay)

Private Practice Assistant to AB Clery, PRCSI

b. 1900, daughter of Thomas Hogan and Mary Hogan (*née* Murnane)

Educ. Convent of the Sacred Heart, Roscrea; Royal College of Surgeons in Ireland

m. 1928: AB Clery [q.v.]; 3 s (Anthony Patrick Tully (Tony) [q.v.], retired colorectal surgeon; Gerald (Gearóid), Irish Ambassador; John, orthopaedic surgeon, New South Wales, Australia), 1 d (Mary, medical laboratory technologist, Connecticut, USA)

d. 1970

Dip Public Health, 1923; FRCSI, 1927 (first woman to obtain first place in her final examination at the RCSI)

Postgraduate appointments as house surgeon, Royal Victoria Eye and Ear Hospital, 1922–23; house surgeon, Children's Hospital, Temple Street, 1924; resident surgical officer, General Hospital, Bridgetown, Barbados, 1924–26.

Sir Thomas Myles [q.v.] encouraged Gay Hogan to train in surgery. Louis Werner [q.v.] and Lawrence Curtin [q.v.], both of the Royal Victoria Eye and Ear Hospital, also encouraged her. On marriage, she gave up all thoughts of another career but subsequently returned to the College Anatomy Department as a graduate demonstrator, and read all the medical and non-medical literature she could lay her hands on.

She created a precedent by coming, as the first women ever, to the white-tie Charter Day Dinner, in her own name of Gabriel Hogan FRCSI, when her husband, AB Clery, was President in 1959. A talented, warm, petite, vivacious woman with striking blue eyes, she brought up her children to consider the sexes with equal respect.

FITZSIMONS, John Joseph

Dublin Surgeon

b. 1892, Baldoyle, Co. Dublin, only son of John Fitzsimons and Jane Fitzsimons (*née* Doyle)
Educ. Belvedere College; College of Veterinary Surgeons; Royal College of Surgeons in Ireland
m. 1st in 1917: Margaret Smyth (d. 1946); 2 s (elder, John, was a doctor in USA), 4 d. 2nd in 1949: Aline McGuinness, widow of Surgeon Ned McGuinness
d. 1956

LRCPI & LM, LRCSI & LM (gold medal in operating surgery), 1921; FRCSI, 1936; MRCVS, 1915

Postgraduate appointments as house surgeon, Richmond, Whitworth and Hardwicke Hospitals; hospital surgeon, Metropolitan Race Course at Phoenix Park and at Baldoyle Race Course; senor demonstrator in anatomy and examiner in surgery, RCSI; Examiner, Nurses' Council; examiner in anatomy, Apothecaries Hall.
Surgeon, Richmond, Whitworth, and Hardwicke Hospitals, Dublin, 1931–59.
Surgeon, St Patrick's Hospital.

John Fitzsimons was of the no-nonsense school of operative surgery. He had been a veterinary surgeon before qualifying as a surgeon and this gave birth to a number of pretty obvious cross-references. To the undergraduate class, out of the patient's hearing: 'The last time I saw anything like this, the whole herd had to be put down.' (It has been difficult to provenance this story.) He enjoyed teaching and was popular with the students. He had great loyalty to his hospital, which was not the most fashionable, but which he maintained was 'the best'. He was really collegiate, openly admiring contemporary colleagues (that's a defining quality) such as AB Clery [q.v.]. He assisted neurosurgeons Adams A. McConnell [q.v.] and John Lanigan [q.v.], as required.

His passion was horses and he had a splendid 'country' residence, 'Stapolin', a large farm of 250–300 acres near Baldoyle, Co. Dublin, on which he was born. His father had pressed him to become a vet, but when his father died during his veterinary studies, he turned to medicine, and then surgery, which was what he had always wanted to do. He never practised as a vet except on his own farm.

John's life is a microcosm of a surgeon's life in Dublin between 1930 and 1960. During the Second World War, the family moved into a house in Fitzwilliam Square in the city centre. He and his wife attended all the home rugby internationals, golf championships at Portmarnock and Davis Cup matches at Fitzwilliam Lawn Tennis Club. Going to the theatre or cinema in Dublin, he would let the attendant or usherette know where he was sitting, so that he could be called out to the hospital should he be required. He would spend two weeks in London every October, visiting hospitals by day and going to the theatre at night. They took motoring holidays on the Continent with friends. He was deeply but quietly religious, and his home was a respite for the local clergy where they could play low-stakes card games. He seldom drank and probably had not been in a pub in his life. There is a JJ Fitzsimons Model for Operative Surgery based on the results of the final surgical examination at the RCSI. An appropriate tribute.

Of medium height, 5'10", and clean-shaven, he was very handsome in his youth. Perhaps a Victorian father to his children, he could be witty and jovial with his contemporaries. Panache was a characteristic and, when told that he had a fatal carcinoma of the prostate, he reacted by buying a Rolls Royce. Colleague surgeon Tommy Bouchier-Hayes [q.v.] asked him, 'How is the Squire of Baldoyle?' 'Fine. And how is the Sire of Leeson Street?'. A reference to Bouchier-Hayes' family of twelve children.

LYNCH, Gearóid

Dublin Surgeon

b. 1932, Dublin, youngest of 7 children of Fionan Lynch (former cabinet minister) and Bridget Lynch (*née* Slattery)
Educ. St Mary's College, Rathmines; Royal College of Surgeons in Ireland
m. 1966: Fredericka Dempsey; 3 s, 2 d

LRCP & SI, RCSI, 1955 (gold medal in surgery); FRCSI, 1959; FRCS Eng, 1960; FACS, 1972 (Governor, Irish Chapter, 1992–98)

Interned in Buffalo, New York State, 1955 (a measure of the bleakness of the medical scene and the entire national psyche in Ireland at that time).
Worked at St Anne's Cancer Hospital and Our Lady's Hospital for Sick Children in Dublin.

London, 1959–64: casualty officer, Royal Free Hospital; orthopaedic senior house officer and surgical registrar, Hammersmith Hospital (with Prof. Ian Aird and R. H. Franklin); surgical registrar, Whittington Hospital, North London (with Paul Savage); plastic surgery registrar, the London Hospital (with Charles Heanley and John Watson).

First senior registrar in plastic surgery under J. B. Prendiville [q.v.], 1964.

Consultant surgeon, Richmond Hospital, Dublin, 1968–97; went immediately to Houston, Texas, to spend nine months in vascular surgery with Michael DeBakey and Denton Cooley. WHO Fellowship to US, to study micro-vascular surgery, 1971.

Surgical tutor, RCSI; Dean of postgraduate studies, 1975–85.

Established Primary Fellowship courses in Kuwait, Dhammam and Jeddah, Kingdom of Saudi Arabia. Examiner in London, Glasgow, Cairo, Khartoum and Abu Dhabi.

President, Association of Graduates, RCSI, 1972–73; surgical section, RAMI, 1992–94. Council, RCSI, 1996–2000.

Honorary member, surgical section, Royal Society of Medicine, London 1992.

His main interest was in plastic surgery and he was the ultimate national resource for managing Dupuytren's contracture.

Gearóid Lynch was a fine operator and a superb teacher. He organised primary and Fellowship courses for the RCSI for twenty years, and many good judges who benefited from these courses speak highly of the quality of the teaching, but particularly of the tuition by G. Lynch himself. He was a loyal servant of the College and defended the institution against all-comers in a firm, articulate fashion. He enjoyed the cut and thrust of 'parliamentary' debate. He remains a generous host, particularly to all his hospital personnel.

A fit, energetic 'live wire', 6'3", he played rugby for St Mary's RFC, good club championship tennis and golf to single figures for fifteen years.

Gearóid was one of the last surgical apprentices to plan his own training. His illustrious career was solidly built on almost thirteen years of postgraduate work in many good places and some great units. Would that the future generations of patients might be so well served.

MacCARTHY, Hugh

Dublin Surgeon

b. 1915, Dublin
Educ. Royal College of Surgeons in Ireland (brilliant student career with his name on many merit boards in the RCSI)
m. Patsy (MB, UCC); 1 d (Patricia, graduated RCSI, 1974)
d. 1985

LRCP & SI, 1938; FRCS Ed; FACS; FRCPI

Postgraduate appointments in Manchester (with Peter McEvedy); resident surgical officer, Royal Infirmary, Newcastle upon Tyne during the Second World War.

Assistant surgeon, Richmond Hospital, Dublin, 1945–53.

Director of Surgery, St James's (formerly St Kevin's) Hospital; St Columcille's Hospital, Loughlinstown, 1953–85.

An interim year was spent at King Edward VIII Hospital, Durban, South Africa.

Brainy and talented, Hugh MacCarthy passed the MRCPI after the Fellowship. On his return to Ireland in 1945, he was appointed assistant surgeon to the Richmond, aged 29. He was the first general surgeon on the staff to have been trained abroad and, with his youthful appearance, he was known as 'The Boy Surgeon'. A master technician with meticulous operating skills, he was a real 'bloodless surgeon'. His *tour de force* was the 50-minute partial gastrectomy for peptic ulcer. This was the 'signature' abdominal operation for forty years (1945–85).

Hugh was easy to work with and easy to assist, another mark of the master technician. He would come in, do the operation and leave, and perhaps not see the patient again, because he felt he didn't need to, until the follow-up clinic. Although, (or maybe because), his father had a prosperous general practice in Monkstown, Co. Dublin, he disliked private work and took a fully salaried post to escape it. He became director of surgery at St Kevin's Hospital (now St James's) at €3,750 per annum. When he transferred there, he decided that he would not refer any surgical problems out of the hospital. A bold decision. He held this post until his sudden death.

Hugh was a gentle, courteous person, a dapper dresser and handsome to boot. His hobby was motorcars and he had a pit at home for car maintenance. He painted to exhibition standard. Admired by all who knew him well, he published regularly.

McKEE, Frederick Francis (Freddie)

Surgeon, Dublin and Belfast

b. ?1916

m. Simone (native of France); 3 children

d. ?1962

LRCPI & LM, LRCSI & LM, 1939 (many prizes including gold medal in operative surgery), RCSI; FRCSI, 1942; MRCPI, 1943

Postgraduate appointment as resident surgical officer, Royal Victoria Hospital, Belfast.
Surgeon, St Laurence's Hospital and Drumcondra Hospital.

A big, larger than life, wholesome, chattering, popular, colourful, quick surgeon who knew his own mind, Freddie McKee was a superb technician, a rapid and safe operator with good clinical judgment, and an excellent and popular teacher. In the 1950s, the hospitals were still purely voluntary and assistant surgeons, of whom he was one, survived by doing county surgeon locums, giving grinds and lecturing. But Freddie built up a significant private practice in the then newly built private hospital, the Bon Secours, Glasnevin, and at the Drumcondra Hospital on Whitworth Road. He had a special interest in thromboembolic problems and did many lumbar sympathectomies by the injection technique.

At the end of the Second World War, he went with the Irish Red Cross to St Lo in France, with a group of Irish doctors (and Samuel Beckett). It was there he met a French dental student, Simone, who became his wife. The glamorous Simone was high maintenance and Freddie drove a Volkswagen, which contrasted with the two Rolls Royces (Adams McConnell [q.v.] and Colman Byrnes [q.v.]) and Michael Burke's [q.v.] polished Daimler in the Richmond car park.

He was a most amusing man with a huge fund of stories told in his inimitable Northern accent. He died suddenly in mid-forties (probably a tobacco-related coronary thrombosis) and his widow brought the three children back to France.

MYLES, Sir Thomas, CB (Tom) PRCSI 1900–1902

Dublin Surgeon

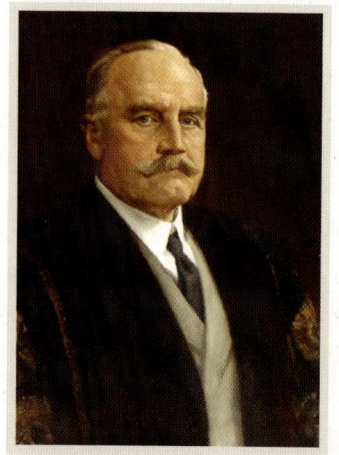

b. 1857, Limerick (probably in a premises now occupied by Flannery's Public House), son of John Myles (corn merchant) and Prudence Bradshaw, Myles's second wife; third of 10 children, six of whom survived to school-going age
Educ. Trinity College, Dublin
m. 1888: Frances Elizabeth, daughter of Rev. George Ayres, a canon of St Patrick's Dublin; no children
d. 1937

BA, TCD, 1880; MB, TCD, 1881; MD, TCD, 1889; FRCSI, 1885; Fellow American Surgical Association, 1907; FACS (Hon.), 1918

Postgraduate appointments as resident surgeon, Dr Steevens' Hospital, 1881–85; in 1882, he received into the hospital the victims of the Phoenix Park murders, the Chief Secretary for Ireland and the Undersecretary. Visited Vienna.
Honorary surgeon, Jervis Street Hospital, 1885–1900.
Surgeon, Richmond Hospital, 1900–retirement.

Professor of Pathology, RCSI, 1889–97 (first chair of pathology established in Ireland).
RCSI Representative to GMC, 1905–10.
Honorary surgeon to King George V in Ireland.
Temporary Lieutenant-Colonel, Royal Army Medical Corps, Irish Command.

There are many who would say that Thomas Myles was Ireland's greatest surgeon of the twentieth century. There is much evidence on their side. He was one of the first to introduce Listerian antiseptic methods to Ireland. His instruments were boiled in the hospital kitchen, 'to soften them, I suppose,' said the cook. He was one of the first in Dublin to wear surgical gloves, initially cotton and later rubber. (The tradition of ophthalmologists not wearing gloves lasted into the 1940s.) He published widely and had a perfect memory. He was widely read in French literature and history, and quoted freely from Shakespeare. As a surgical grinder, he was incomparable. 'The lucidity, brevity, accuracy and virility of his descriptions of disease were unique,' said a pupil.

A skilled, fast surgeon sometimes operating with a stopwatch, he had a ready wit and dramatic eloquence. 'With his massive shoulders and determined features, he worked with the care and dexterity of a needlewoman,' observed one contemporary. He was charming and even-tempered. He was also an outspoken anti-vivisectionist.

During the Boer War, which was a defining cause for the then small number of nationalist Irish, he is alleged to have produced an Irish Bull quoted as 'Why should Irishmen stand with their arms folded and their hands in their pockets when England calls for aid?' He was a lifelong nationalist, a member of the Protestant Home Rule Party (there were many such, all with slightly different aims and leadership), and ran guns for the rebels into Kilcoole, Co. Wicklow, from his own motor yacht, Chota (a Tamil word for fish). However, he opposed the Easter Rising in 1916 because Home Rule had been agreed. He treated patients from both sides of the great divide in that historic week.

In his late teens, when he was thought to have been developing 'consumption' (tuberculosis), he had spent some time 'before the mast' on a large sailing ship, and he subsequently became one of Ireland's most experienced sailors in a series of large motor yachts. He had an immense physique and there is a persistent story that he was physically strong enough to have boxed a few rounds with John L. Sullivan (1858–1918), sometime heavyweight champion of the world, around the time when the champion was at his prime, possibly when he visited Ireland in December 1887, and offered the equivalent of $50 to any man who could spend four rounds in the ring with him. (It has been difficult to provenance this colourful tale.) At Trinity, he was an oarsman and on the rugby team.

A knighthood was normally conferred on Presidents of the RCSI at that time and his was on the Coronation Honours list of 1902. The Companion of the Order of the Bath was for services during the First World War. He was also made a Freeman of the City of Limerick. One glowing obituary was by Dr Donald Balfour, Director of the Mayo Clinic.

The family had been in Limerick for many generations and there is a street named Myles. The family summered in Kilkee, Co. Clare, and there are two establishments named 'Myles's Creek', one a diving pool and the other a 'night club'. There is a wonderful portrait of him, by Leo Whelan, in the RCSI.

Sir Patrick Dun's Hospital

GILL, Frederick (Freddie) PRCSI 1946–1948

Dublin Surgeon

b. 1895, Saintfield, Co. Down
Educ. Trinity College, Dublin
d. 1960

MA, TCD, 1917; MB, TCD, 1918; MD, 1921; FRCSI, 1921

Resident medical officer, British Hospital, Port Said, for a time.
Assistant to the Professor of Surgery, TCD.
Surgeon, Sir Patrick Dun's Hospital, 1924–60.
President, RCSI, 1946–48.

His special interest was in thyroid surgery, and he was meticulous in this trying discipline.

Choleric and tempestuous in the operating theatre, Freddie Gill was attentive to his patients. He enjoyed teaching and the students liked him. He was an exponent of the Northern direct mode of address with unmistakable regional accent.

He was always well dressed, and Angela Butler, long-time assistant registrar at the RCSI, said that 'he was a good ambassador for the College'. During his presidency, Sir Alfred ('Beery Alf') Webb-Johnson, PRCS England, was made an honorary FRCSI. (It was Webb-Johnson, with Lord Moran, who led the UK consultants into the National Health Service. For this 'service' he was raised to the peerage. Gill and he had a close friendship.)

Slightly below average height, Freddie Gill was burly and energetic. He really loved turning his Rolls Royce into his reserved parking spot at Dun's, and also held a pilot's licence from the British Air Ministry. He had a great interest in all sports, especially rugby, boxing and athletics. (Boxing was still a university sport into the 1960s but was stopped when evidence of brain damage accumulated.) He was 'surgeon' to the Trinity rugby team.

Freddie was gregarious and enjoyed his membership and presidencies of the Hibernian Catch Club, the Dublin convivial choral and dining club whose foundation dates back to 1680. He was an enthusiastic Freemason and was raised to the thirty-third degree.

HEATLEY, Seymour Frederick, OBE (Mil.)

Vice President (effectively President-Elect) RCSI at the time of his death

b. 1903, son of Frederick Charles Heatley (farmer) and Elizabeth Heatley (*née* Fahy); eldest of 6 children; his niece Hazel is married to Gordon Watson, surgeon, Waterford
Educ. Mountjoy School, Dublin; Trinity College, Dublin
m. 1933: Kathleen Foley (1915–84), daughter of Patrick and Elsie Foley (*née* Shipton); 2 d (Wendy married James Clinch, Master, Coombe Hospital)
d. 1967

BA, MB (hons, first place), Dub, 1926; FRCSI, 1930

Postgraduate training: Commissioned Flying Officer in RAF Medical Branch, 1926; assistant to director of pathology; surgical assistant to the Central Hospital.
Visited surgical centres at Lausanne, Bonn, Heidelberg and Brussels, 1929.
Registrar, Baggot Street Hospital; assistant surgeon, Baggot St Hospital, 1930.
Honorary visiting surgeon, Mercer's Hospital, 1932.
Consultant surgeon, Sir Patrick Dun's Hospital; Ministry of Pensions, 1938–67.
Lieutenant-Colonel, Royal Army Medical Corps, 1942–46.
Awarded OBE (Military), 1946

Seymour's forte was abdominal surgery, where he was known for his skill and gentleness in dissecting tissues with his fingers, rather than clamping and cutting. He could operate extremely quickly. One of his students assisted him during a chyloecystectomy on an elderly, admittedly thin, lady which took seven minutes from 'skin to skin'.

He was 5'8", of medium build, with dark hair and grey-green eyes. Boxing was his main sport but he also played rugby and rowed on the junior eight. After qualification, he was commissioned as a Flying Officer in the RAF medical branch. He was welter-weight champion of the RAF in the days when officers did not fight against 'other ranks'. His other recreations included golf and fishing.

Though anxious to join the 'colours' at the outbreak of war (1939), his wife persuaded him to defer enlistment until 1941. He served with the army in Tunisia.

Seymour did not talk about the hardships of war — most of the stories were amusing, such as the time when the tent was stolen, leaving his exhausted colleagues sleeping and unaware until the sun rose. He also served in Europe, following the troops fighting through France and on to Belgium where he was appointed Chief of the 1,500-bed military hospital in Brussels, the clearing station for casualties when the Allies crossed the Rhine.

His relationship with his senior colleague, Freddy Gill [q.v.], was legendary in its acrimony. The pair did not speak to one another, or to each other's staff. The basis of it was that when Seymour, having done the 'right thing' at the time, came back from the War, he found that 'his beds' at Dun's Hospital had been subsumed into Gill's, and he could not get them back.

He always wore a suit when doing rounds, never a white coat. When lecturing, he chain-smoked but on occasions gave up smoking for several months at a time. He would question students as often as giving didactic lectures, perhaps an early form of 'interactive' education. Seymour was immensely proud of Dun's and the Trinity connection.

Although his wife drove a Jaguar, his own car was an ancient Ford Anglia — he liked to think he was known for surgical skills rather than for flamboyance. He was well known for growing roses and won many prizes both at home and in England. He spent his retirement years in Oughterard, Co. Galway. He and his wife created a beautiful garden from what had been poor soil and hazel scrub on a four-acre site on the shores of Lough Corrib. But no roses!

Agnostic in belief until he retired, he then became interested in religion and, at the end of his life, he derived great comfort from it.

LANE, David Amyrald Armstrong

Surgeon, Sir Patrick Dun's Hospital, Dublin, 1966–1993

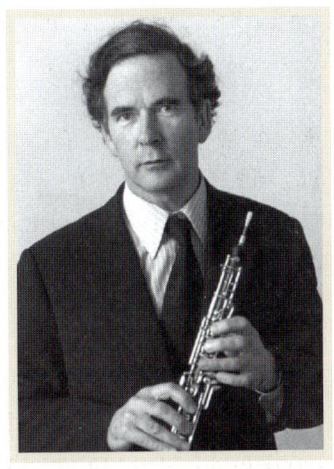

b. 1927, youngest son of Dr S. A. Lane (Royal Army Medical Corps, First World War; GP and surgeon, Bognor, Sussex, England)

Educ. Aravon School, Bray, Co. Wicklow; Oakham School, Rutland, England (Head boy); Trinity College, Dublin

m. 1956: Marjorie Hammond of Leicester Royal Infirmary; 2 children

MB, TCD, 1950; FRCS Eng, FRCSI, 1954

Postgraduate posts at Sir Patrick Dun's, Leicester Royal Infirmary, Royal United Hospitals, Bath, and back to Leicester as registrar to E. R. Frizelle ('Friz') and George Sawyer. ('Friz', a QUB graduate, had an immaculate operating style with a 'leading man' appearance, was the star of a distinguished staff and was a lifelong influence).

Assistant surgeon, Meath Hospital; National Children's Hospital, Harcourt Street, 1956–66.
Consultant surgeon, Federated Voluntary Hospitals, Dublin, at Sir Patrick Dun's, 1966–88; Monkstown Hospital, 1957–87.
President, surgical section, RAMI, 1988–89.

Interested in general surgery and gastroenterology.

Retiring and undemonstrative, David Lane was a superb technical surgeon (gold standard). Passionate about surgery and his oboe, he was, for over thirty years, oboist with the Dublin Baroque Players. He played with the RTÉ Symphony Orchestra and broadcast as soloist. Having captained his school rugby and shooting teams, he went on to be a Trinity Athletics Pink 100 yards champion. His interests in later life include fly-fishing, dinghy sailing and photography.

Of middle height, spare build and calm, with dark hair flecked with grey in his late seventies, he was greatly loved and admired by patients, staff, trainees and colleagues, and still is. A peerless professional.

MILLIKEN, James (Jimmy)

Dublin Vascular Surgeon

b. 1930, Belfast, eldest son of Augustus Milliken and Maud Milliken (*née* Copeland)
Educ. St Andrew's College Dublin, Trinity College, Dublin
m. 1956: Brenda McMechan, daughter of Captain J. McMechan, MC, and May McMechan; 2 s, 1 d

BA, TCD, 1951; MB, TCD, 1953; MA, MD, TCD, 1962; MCh, TCD, 1965; FRCS Ed, 1959; FRCSI, 1965; FACS, 1968.

Postgraduate posts at Sir Patrick Dun's Hospital, Dublin; Moyle Hospital, Larne; Great Yarmouth General Hospital, East Anglia; Stockport Infirmary, Cheshire; and Musgrave Park Hospital, Belfast.
Surgical registrar, Belfast City Hospital; RVH Belfast; Sir Patrick Dun's Hospital.
Research Fellow in cardiovascular surgery, Harvard Medical School, 1963–64.
Senior surgical registrar and tutor, TCD; Sir Patrick Dun's Hospital.
Consultant vascular surgeon, Federated Dublin Voluntary Hospitals to include Sir Patrick Dun's, Royal City of Dublin (Baggot Street), Adelaide and St James's Hospitals, 1967–87.
WHO Travelling Fellow, North America (eight centres), 1969.
Following retirement from the Health Service, continued to act as surgeon in the private and charity sectors, including service in Mostar, Bosnia and Chechnya until retirement in 1991.
President, Irish Surgical Travellers Club, 1983.

Published more articles after appointment than before it.

Jimmy Milliken was a highly competent, much liked, agreeable colleague. Looking at his numerous junior appointments in different places, he must have had involuntary changes of address at least eight times. In the 1950s, there were no training ladders and trainee surgeons had to find a new post every six months, usually though the advertising pages of the BMJ. Patients survived the endless changes of junior medical staff because of wise, experienced, senior nurses drawing the young doctors aside and advising them what not to do. (The editor, having worked at eight hospitals by age 28, was asked on arrival at the Lahey Clinic, Boston, USA, 'Doctor O'Donnell, couldn't you hold down a job *anywhere*?')

Jimmy retired to the Mullet peninsula, Co. Mayo, to garden, read and play bridge.

O'NEILL, Tom (Tom)

Surgeon, Sir Patrick Dun's Hospital

b. 1912, near Newmarket, Co. Cork
Educ. Presentation College Cork, University College Cork
m. 1945: Dr Dorothy Moriarty; 5 s
d. 2000

MB, UCC, 1935; MD, MCh, NUI, 1943; FRCS Eng, 1941; FRCSI (*ad eundem*), 1967

Postgraduate posts at Halifax Royal Infirmary; surgeon, Emergency Medical Service, London, during London Blitz, 1940–41; surgical chief assistant, Royal Infirmary, Manchester.
Surgeon, Sir Patrick Dun's 1949–77.
Lecturer in surgery, Trinity College.
President, surgical section, RAMI, 1988–90.

Publications mainly on partial gastrectomy for peptic ulcer, for which he invented a useful modification.

Tom burst upon the Dublin scene as a Catholic appointment to a Protestant hospital, an appointment that was unheard of in Dublin in 1948. He had come through London and Manchester, where he had been superbly trained. Life was difficult for such an interloper but his high intelligence was applied to all difficulties, in and out of the operating theatre. He was a skilled, no-nonsense operator who gave great attention to his patients and to his referring general practitioners. He was not easy to assist at surgery and it was not unknown for trainees to request a transfer to another unit.

He was retained by leading insurers as a medical expert and, when asked what his area of expertise was, he said, 'I am an expert at giving medical evidence', a statement which was absolutely correct in all respects. Malingerers, or those thought to be malingerers, or who had been associated with malingerers, got short shrift.

A combative corner forward in the all-conquering UCC Fitzgibbon Cup hurling team of 1930, he transferred his volcanic energies to golf and won many prizes, playing down to a handicap of 8 at his beloved Portmarnock.

Of medium height, round faced and balding, he had athletic shoulders and sustained drive and energy. Plain speaking, with an expertise on a huge range of topics he was the subject of a massive range of anecdotes, some apocryphal, but the majority bore a seal of authenticity because of his unique, self-deprecating, use of language. Those who never met him really missed something special.

St James's Hospital (formerly St Kevin's)

BOLAND, Charles Richard (Charlie)
Dublin Surgeon

Educ. Trinity College, Dublin

BA (gold medal), TCD, 1924; MSc, 1926; MB, TCD, 1926; MD, 1928; FRCSI, 1929

Postgraduate post at Royal National Orthopaedic Hospital, London.
Chief assistant, surgical unit, British Postgraduate Medical School, Hammersmith.
Research student, TCD.
Surgeon, County Hospital, Cashel, Co. Tipperary.
Surgeon (orthopaedics), St Kevin's Hospital, Dublin.

When he returned to Ireland, Charlie Boland had been trained with the best people in England, but he could not get a teaching hospital post and was briefly a county surgeon. He was a talented member of a talented family; his brother, Freddie Boland, was a diplomat who became Chairman of the United Nations General Assembly and Chancellor of Trinity College, Dublin.

St Michael's, Dún Laoghaire

ASHE, Matthew Peter (Peter)
Dún Laoghaire Surgeon

b. 1921, Dublin, only son of Dr Paddy Ashe of Dingle and May Murphy, daughter of Martin J. Murphy (Nationalist MP for East Waterford, 1913–18, and owner of Tramore race course. He had been a Captain in the Royal Army Medical Corps in the First World War)
Educ. St Mary's College, Rathmines; University College Dublin
m. Eva Walsh; 1 s, 1 d
d. 1983

MB, UCD, 1945; FRCSI, 1949; MCh, NUI, 1953

Postgraduate posts at Mater Hospital, Dublin; Croydon Hospital Group, Surrey.
Senior surgical registrar, Beckenham Hospital, Kent.
Resident surgical officer, St Michael's Hospital, Dún Laoghaire.
Surgeon, St Michael's Hospital, Dún Laoghaire, 1955–83.

Recognised by all as having superb clinical judgment and refined operating skills, Peter Ashe was one of the last of the truly general surgeons who 'pinned hips' as well as doing urology, but he was most at home operating in the abdomen. A perfect gentleman in all his actions, he was dark, handsome and impeccably dressed, with a private, complex, gifted personality. Though self-assured, he lacked assertiveness in a thrusting specialty.

He picked winners at race courses, was an enthusiastic rally driver, and a more-than-useful sail-boat crew on Dublin Bay. At home, he was keen on sketching, woodcarving and landscape gardening. He became a first-class shot but his passion was salmon fishing on the Slaney, where he displayed the same patience and skill as he did at the operating table.

Following two bitterly cold nights of operating into the small hours, he got his first coronary thrombosis, and he died two months later.

St Vincent's Hospital

DOOLIN, William (Bill) PRCSI 1950–1952

Dublin Surgeon

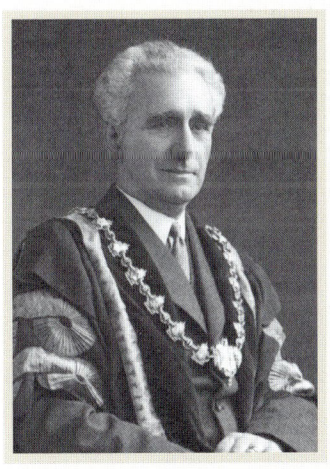

b. 1888, Ely Place, Dublin, son of Walter Doolin (architect)
Educ. Catholic University School, Dublin; St Mary's College, Dundalk; Clongowes Wood College, Kildare
m. 1st. Clare Kennedy, 2nd. Maureen Clinton
d. 1962

MB, NUI, 1910 (the first medical honours graduate in the NUI, founded 1908); FRCSI, 1912, FRCS Eng (Hon.); DLitt (*hon. causa*), TCD and UCD.

Postgraduate visits to Edinburgh, London, Paris, Berlin.
Assistant surgeon, St Vincent's Hospital, 1914–28 (with Johnny McArdle as Senior).

Surgeon, St Vincent's Hospital, 1928–62; Children's Hospital, Temple Street.
Honorary Professor of Medical History, UCD.
Editor, *Irish Journal of Medical Science*, 1925–62; *Journal of the Irish Medical Association*, 1954–62.

A good, rather than a great, operating surgeon, it was said that the breadth of Bill Doolin's knowledge contributed to his indecision in the theatre. A warm, widely read man, fluent in many languages, he had an ornate style of speaking at all times, with quotations, usually in the original form, endlessly interpolated. The ultimate surgeon scholar and renaissance polymath, he was a man of many parts. As a surgeon, he was remarkably self-deprecating, always extremely critical of his own results. As he was particularly interested in cleft lip and palate surgery, where perfection was not then and could not now be achieved in every patient, these criticisms were largely unwarranted.

He was an indulgent editor, frequently rewriting an entire article himself before publication. He was also a most generous book reviewer. Sir Gordon Gordon-Taylor (1882–1960), the ultimate arbiter in these matters, said, 'Doolin is the best writer of English in surgical literature today.' The English College made him an honorary Fellow and, uniquely for an Irishman, a Vicary Lecturer.

There was a good deal of the actor in Bill's make-up and he played the part that was expected of him, both as a lecturer, where he excelled, and in his attire. His deeply lined face, mane of silvery hair and beautiful speaking voice made him an unforgettable figure, such as one would hope to meet in a literary or artistic salon. He loved quoting William Osler, and was the nearest Ireland has come to producing a similar figure. Admired and held in great affection by all who knew him.

FAGAN, Patrick Joseph

Dublin Surgeon

b. 1864
Educ. Castleknock College, Dublin
d. 1910

LRCPI & LM, LRCSI & LM, 1891; LM, Rotunda Hospital Dublin, 1891 (Catholic University, Dublin); FRCSI, 1896

Surgeon, St Vincent's Hospital, Dublin.
Chief demonstrator in anatomy and lecturer in elementary physics, Catholic University Medical School; examiner in anatomy, Apothecaries Hall, Ireland and RCSI.
Fellow, Royal Academy of Medicine, Ireland.

Contributor to 'An Irregular Distribution of Nerves on the Dorsum of the Foot', Transactions of the Royal Academy Medicine Ireland vol. X; 'Arrangement of Branches of Right Bronchus and Their Relations to the Pulmonary Artery', Ibid.

He died suddenly at his fireside at the age of 46.

MEHIGAN, John Augustine (Gussie)

Dublin Surgeon

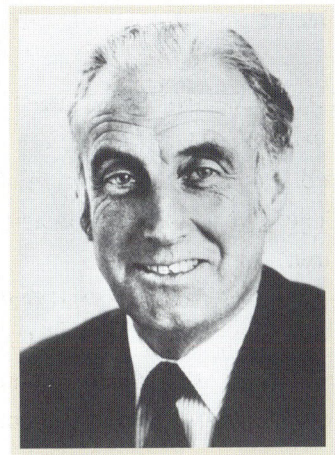

b. 1926, Dublin, son of Paddy Mehigan ('Carbery'), a famous *Irish Times* sports journalist
Educ. Catholic University School; University College Dublin
m. Unmarried
d. 1981

MB (hons), UCD, 1950; FRCSI, 1954.

Postgraduate post at Royal Postgraduate Medical School, Hammersmith Hospital, London (with the great Prof. Ian Aird).
Assistant surgeon, St Vincent's Hospital, Dublin, 1957.
President, Irish Medical Association, 1978.
Council, RCSI, 1972–81; would undoubtedly have become President of the College.

Gussie was a favourite son of St Vincent's Hospital and, when sent to work at the Hammersmith in London, he was immensely popular, and Professor Aird clearly thought highly of him. When he returned to St Vincent's in 1957, he immediately threw himself into helping Bob O'Connell [q.v.] organise the first cardiac surgery unit in the country. The specialty was going through an exciting time, with patients for open-heart surgery being operated on under moderate, and later profound, hypothermia, while the concept of extra-corporeal oxygenation was being developed.

Gussie's gifts lay particularly in organisation, and he it was who masterminded the actual move of St Vincent's from St Stephen's Green to Ballsbridge in 1970, though its planning had begun in 1934. He became a spokesman for the hospital at home and for the Irish medical profession abroad. He was a good example of a man who did a great deal for surgery without having written many papers, but worked tirelessly for his chosen institutions, St Vincent's Hospital and the Irish Medical Association.

Dynamic (5'6"), dark, warm, smiling, conciliatory, charming, articulate, vastly amusing and without an enemy in the world, he remained a bachelor despite some near 'misses'. He had lost count of his appearances as best man and godfather. He was a fitness fanatic and died of a 'heart attack' while running in his green tracksuit, in which he was a familiar sight all over south Dublin. Gussie was one of the great Dublin surgical personalities of the second half of the twentieth century.

KEAVENY, Thomas Vincent (Vincent or 'TVK')

Dublin Surgeon

b. 1937, Moville, Donegal, youngest of twelve children and seventh son of James Keaveny (active in the War of Independence)
Educ. St Columb's College, Derry, where there has been a strong family link for over fifty years; University College Dublin
m. Phyl Dowling as an undergraduate; 3 s (Andrew is a Mayo Clinic hepatologist in Jacksonville, Florida; 2 lawyers)

BSc, UCD, 1957; MB (hons), UCD, 1961 (gold medal in surgery); FRCSI, 1964; FRCS Ed, 1964; MCh, 1966; FACS; KLJ

Postgraduate training at St Vincent's Hospital (with Prof. Patrick Fitzgerald [q.v.]; England (under Mr Sol Cohen, a London area vascular surgeon); Edinburgh Royal Infirmary (under Sir John Bruce and Sir James Fraser); San Francisco (under Dr J. E. Dunphy, one of the greats of the time). Returned to St Vincent's to continue under Prof. P. Fitzgerald.
Consultant surgeon, St Vincent's Hospital, 1971–2002; National Maternity Hospital; Blackrock Clinic.
President, European Society of Surgical Research, 1976.
Governor, Irish chapter, ACS.
Chairman, Association of Vascular Surgeons of Ireland.

Vincent Keaveny built up the vascular surgery unit at St Vincent's and was an internationally recognised authority on carotid surgery for stroke prevention, a subject on which he published widely. He was an early enthusiast of video presentations and intensive care units for vascular patients. He was a vivid teacher.

Probably his most controversial decision was to turn down, at the eleventh hour, the offered Chair of Surgery at Trinity College. Trinity had 'gone the extra mile' and offered the Chair to a Catholic for the first time in three centuries, and there was some hand wringing on both sides of the ever shallower divide.

A keen swimmer, he enjoys outdoor activities and keeps up with the Classics. He fundraises for hospitals, international charities, the World Mercy Fund and the Order of St Lazarus of Jerusalem.

Of medium height, dark and handsome, charming to all, with an ever-present smile, he was superbly trained and acknowledged to be one of the outstanding surgical technicians of his time. A most admirable man.

KENNEDY, Denis ('The Doc')

Dublin Surgeon

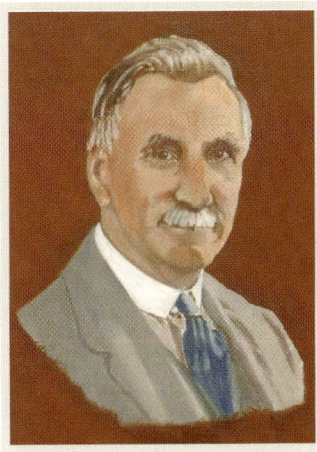

b. 1866
Educ. CBS Nenagh, Royal University of Ireland
m. 1st: Mary Francis (d.), daughter of Richard Langan of Tara, Co. Meath; 2nd in 1944; 5 s (Theo and Dermot, surgeons), 6 d (Eileen, ophthalmic surgeon; Kathleen, GP; Maeve, anaesthetist, m. John 'Mac' McAuliffe Curtin [q.v.])
d. 1954

Surgeon, Jervis Street Hospital, 1896–1906; St Vincent's Hospital, 1906–54.

Special interests were abdominal and neck surgery.

A big, tall man with a strong, almost overpowering personality and a bristling moustache, Denis Kennedy was a skilled and courageous surgeon. He presented the first case of parathyroid adenoma removal to the RAMI in the 1930s. He had remarkable diagnostic flair. Those he trained held him in great affection. He had a no-nonsense style of operating, which once led one of the Mayo brothers, who were watching, to say to the other, 'God, what a gash', and demanded nothing but the best of care for his children and grandchildren, which meant that he operated on them himself, frequently with his daughter, Dr Maeve, giving the anaesthetic; they bear the significant scars of his successful operations.

Stories abound of his 'luck'. Once, when visiting a nursing home for an operation, he was informed that the patient had died and was actually being laid out for burial. The Doc said, 'I am here to operate on her,' and demanded that she be put on the operating table and that his faithful accompanying anaesthetist, Dr Mick O'Hea, give her an anaesthetic. O'Hea held an anaesthetic mask, without any ether or chloroform, over the patient's face and the Doc did one of his trademark 'all layers at once' abdominal incisions, whereupon the patient sat up and the surgeon admonished the anaesthetist: 'Deeper, O'Hea, deeper.'

For recreation, he enjoyed golf. In the days of heroic surgeons, he was a role model.

MAHER, James Gerard (Jamsie)

Dublin Surgeon

b. 1912, Cahir, Co. Tipperary
Educ. Local national school; Blackrock College; Rockwell College; University College Dublin
m. Unmarried
d. 1975

FRCSI, 1954

Assistant surgeon, St Vincent's Hospital, 1948 (with the MAO as his single postgraduate qualification).
Assistant master, Coombe Hospital.
Surgeon, St Anne's, Northbrook Road; Coombe Hospital.
Surgeon to the Irish Rugby Football Union.
Council, RCSI, 1968–75 (always elected on an early count).

A real character, Jamsie Maher was of the no-nonsense school of operating. He had been personal assistant to Professor 'Harry' Meade and Bob O'Connell [q.v.], and was a surgeon who gave wonderful care to his patients, whom he might visit in the middle of the night, coming from a 'social' event. Strong as an ox, he had been on the fringe of the Irish rugby team during his training. He wrote almost no papers but was much sought after as a sound clinical opinion, and he was a prodigious worker, wading briskly through long operating lists, which might last into the night. His surgery was anything but delicate. When he finished an operation, still in theatre garb, he went straight to the telephone to tell the referring doctor the outcome; then, and only then, would he speak to the relatives.

Above average height, with a huge mane of hair, white from an early age, he was a bachelor of the old school, and delighted in late nights with students, hospital staff and rugby players. The basement of his rooms and home at 32 Fitzwilliam Place was a nidus for many a party from which there was no escape, as Jamsie locked the doors from the inside and would allow no one to leave until the party was over, usually at or about dawn. Ironically he died of carcinoma of the colon, which had been his area of greatest expertise. He was hugely popular at all levels. It has been said that every hospital needs a Jamsie Maher. The nuns, the nurses and everybody else loved him.

McMULLIN, Joseph Patrick O'Byrne ('Shos' or 'Joe Mac')

Dublin Surgeon

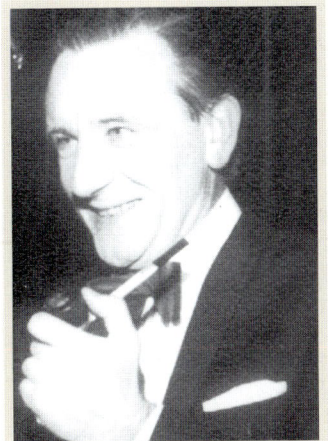

b. 1921, eldest son (fourth of 12 children) of Joseph Columba McMullin [q.v.] (surgeon at Sheil Hospital, Ballyshannon, and later County Surgeon, Cavan) and Mary Frances O'Byrne

Educ. Clongowes Wood College, Kildare; University College Dublin

m. 1949: Raphael Aglaia Devlin, youngest daughter of Liam and Margaret Devlin, Monkstown, Co. Dublin; 3 s (eldest, Liam, is surgeon, County Hospital, Roscommon), 2 d (both nurses)

d. 2003

MB, UCD, 1947; FRCSI, 1952; FRCS, 1954; MCh, 1954

Postgraduate posts as house officer, St Vincent's Hospital, Dublin; casualty officer, Westminster Hospital, London; surgical registrar, St John and Elizabeth's Hospital, London.
Travelling Scholarship, Lahey Clinic, Boston, 1957 (worked with Dr Ken Warren, master pancreatic surgeon).
Surgeon, St Vincent's Hospital, St Stephen's Green/Elm Park, 1956–85; St Luke's and St Anne's Hospital, Dublin.
Medical director and general/transplant surgeon, Ibn Al Bitar Hospital, Baghdad, 1985–90.
President, Irish Society of Gastroenterology, 1983–84.

Joe Mac was a superb natural technician, whose main surgical interests were biliary, pancreatic, thyroid and parathyroid surgery. Other surgeons came to watch him and, on one memorable occasion, he operated on a professor of surgery in a London surgical 'cathedral'. In Baghdad, he carried out over 300 live-donor renal transplants, with excellent results. His stories about the families' choice of who would be the live donor were memorable — the first choice was often the youngest *daughter-in-law* who, whatever her personal qualities, was the 'relative' least likely to have a compatible tissue type. Not interested in medical affairs, he was an energetic and tireless worker always available to patients and colleagues.

He had been a rugby scrum-half for Clongowes and later for Lansdowne RFC. He then switched to tennis, squash and skiing. Five foot nine, broad shouldered, muscular, with a receding hairline, he had piercing grey eyes, which could transfix a dreamy assistant. Perhaps he was more admired than loved by his trainees. He loved his family and worked on his home, building a pool and tennis court himself. He loved parties and had a fine tenor voice but will be best remembered as a great gentleman and a master surgical craftsman.

MORRIN, Francis Joseph (Frank or 'Pops')

Dublin Surgeon

b. 1893
Educ. University College Dublin
m. married
d. 1967

MB, UCD, 1916; MCh, NUI, 1926

Surgeon, Jervis Street Hospital, Dublin; Medical Service, Free State Army and surgical consultant.
Consultant surgeon, St Anne's Skin and Cancer Hospital; Coombe Maternity Hospital.
Surgeon, St Vincent's Hospital, Dublin.
External examiner in surgery, UCD.

Pops Morrin had been with the British Army in France and Belgium during the First World War and proudly wore the French Legion of Honour ribbon in his buttonhole. He had the reputation of being tough on 'shirkers, scrimshankers and malingerers'. He kept a watchful eye on a subordinate 'who was twice the only survivor on a raft'.

As a surgeon, he was somewhat radical and revelled in displaying his skills with the Dejardins suturing needle. Tall, wiry, with a certain military precision, he was proud of his small incisions and, when operating for appendicitis, he would deliver the appendix by putting a long forefinger into a tiny wound and free it up by blind dissection and then, 'out it pops'. When an operation ended rather before it had been expected to, he laconically said, 'The patient quit.'

An honourable, old-fashioned character, he was extremely kind to his much younger, invalid wife.

O'CONNELL, Thomas Columba James ('Bob')

Dublin Surgeon and Professional Leader

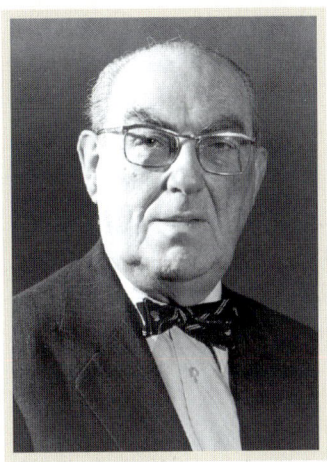

b. 1906, Co. Westmeath, son of Thomas James O'Connell (secretary, Irish National Teachers' Organisation)
Educ. Belvedere College, Dublin; University College Dublin
m. 1933: Nance; 5 s (2 doctors; Diarmuid a GP in Dublin)
d. 1985

MB, UCD, 1930; MD, MCh, NUI; FRCSI (Hon.), 1962; FACS; BSc

Postgraduate studies in Britain, Germany and Austria, 1930–34.

Appointed consultant staff, St Vincent's Hospital, 1934; St Kevin's Hospital, 1941; consultant thoracic surgeon to many hospitals. President, Irish Medical Association, 1955; Irish Nursing Board, 1954–61 (a career enthusiasm), and many other national bodies.

Over fifty publications including first operation in Ireland for patent ductus arteriosus, coarctation of the aorta and, uniquely, a world first when he did a mitral valvotomy on a patient in labour.

Bob O'Connell was the most colourful character in Irish surgery from 1940 to his death. A rampaging rugby forward in his early days, he later became doctor to the Irish rugby team. He was, in every sense, larger than life. In the bloody battles with various Ministers of Health in the early 1950s, Bob was the undoubted leader and true tribune of the profession. He was a magnificent orator, whose Churchillian appearance and demeanour were well and worthily cultivated, down to the throat clearings and the polka-dot bow tie. He was an expert on the pregnant pause. Nobody, absolutely nobody, before or since, was in more demand as an after-dinner speaker, and he had hundreds of stories and anecdotes, many about characters in his beloved Co. Galway, which were just as funny each time he told them as at the first time of hearing.

Much teased that his surgical 'firsts', and there were many, usually appeared in the newspapers before the medical journals, he was the epitome of the 'courageous' surgeon who would take on really bad-risk patients. His operative surgery was of the no-nonsense variety, but his technique in delicate thyroid work was outstanding. He had a determination that cardiac surgery would blossom in Dublin, and was a true pioneer with inevitable headlines and heartbreaks marking his progress.

The fact that he was the total antithesis of his near contemporary, Paddy Fitzgerald [q.v.], who had effectively beaten him for the chair of surgery, made this symbiotic and complementary pairing the most powerful duo in Irish surgery in the 1950s and 1960s, and St Vincent's prospered. Bob had been the heir apparent to succeed Professor Harry Meade, but lacked the vital academic credentials, and the outcome worked well for Irish surgery and the wider profession. Like Paddy Fitzgerald, Bob had not taken the FRCSI, 'banned' by UCD, thus denying the Royal College a certain electoral poll topper and a charismatic President. But Bob continued to teach as only he could, and his undergraduate audiences loved him. He was a terrifying but compassionate examiner. His was a warm, generous spirit, who gave and generated enormous loyalties within the profession.

The system of payment, or indeed the absence of anything approaching a fair salary for public work and little in the way of a pension forthcoming, meant that Bob, when he was really over the hill in the private sector, had to go on working and doing some careful surgery long after he had earned a decent retirement.

An icon and role model. An Irish giant.

TOBIN, Richard Francis (Dick or 'Daddy')

Dublin Surgeon

b. 1843, Waterford, son of Patrick Tobin, Waterford
Educ. Catholic University, Dublin; Royal College of Surgeons in Ireland
m. 1887: Fanny, daughter of James Costello, Raheny, Co. Dublin

LRCP, 1882; FRCSI 1882

Surgeon, St Vincent's Hospital.
President, Irish Medical Association.
Surgeon in Ordinary to the Lord Lieutenant.
Assistant Professor of Surgery, Army Medical School.

12
CORK, GALWAY AND LIMERICK SURGEONS

CORK, GALWAY AND LIMERICK SURGEONS

CORK SURGEONS

ATKINS, Thomas Gelston

Cork Surgeon and Obstetrician

Educ. Queen's College, Cork

BA, RUI, 1874; MD, MChir, LM, 1878 (senior scholar in surgery and midwifery and first exhibition in the practice of medicine, surgery and midwifery)

Consultant surgeon, Cork Maternity Hospital.
Surgeon, Cork Street Infirmary and County Hospital.
Medical referee, Scottish Union and other assurance companies.
President, Cork Medical and Surgical Society.
Senior physician and joint lecturer in midwifery and gynaecology, QCC.

Author of 'Successful Hysterosalpingo Oopherectomy for Pelvic Suppuration and for Double Ovarian Papilloma and Carcinoma of Cervix Uteri', *British Gynaecology Journal*, 1904; 'Surgical Treatment of Chronic Gastric Ulcer and Dilation of Stomach by Gastrojejunostomy and Jejuno-jejunostomy', BMJ 1905; 'Surgical Treatment of Malignant Disease of Rectum', *BMJ*.

BARRETT, John Gerard (Jack)

Cork Surgeon

b. 1911, Cork, second twin son of John V. Barrett and Mary Barrett (*née* Magner)
Educ. Christian Brothers College. Cork; Castleknock College, Dublin; University College Cork
m. 1941: Moira O'Hanlon, daughter of Dr O'Hanlon, Mallow, Co. Cork; 1 s (Jack, consultant anaesthetist and pain specialist, Cork University Hospital), 1 d (Jill, BA, UCC, 1966)
d. 1996

MB, UCC, 1934; MCh, FRCS

Postgraduate work included house surgeon, St James's Balham, London; surgical registrar, St Andrew's Hospital, London; St Mary's Hospital, London.

Surgeon, Bon Secours Hospital, Cork; Cork Military Hospital.

Jack Barrett had been a Major in the Irish Army during the 'Emergency'. He worked as a general practitioner and obstetrician/gynaecologist while applying for surgical posts. He was surgeon at the Bon Secours Hospital, Cork, which, for many years, was the largest private hospital in these islands. He built up a large private surgical practice by assiduous patient (and doctor) care and modest fees. He was naturally adept in many surgical fields and prospered without a public appointment, a difficult feat before the days of Voluntary Health Insurance (introduced 1956). He was highly rated as an operating surgeon, and was completely ambidextrous, which is an advantage in some operations such as thyroidectomy.

An expert shot, he was the founding member of a number of gun clubs, as well as being a keen fisherman and gardener. Jack Barrett was a dark, handsome charmer with what a number of ladies described as 'Hollywood good looks' and 'great presence'.

BURKE, Thomas (Tom)

Cork Surgeon

b. 1919, youngest child of Edward and Mary Burke
Educ. St Brogan's School, Bandon, Co. Cork; Presentation College, Cork; University College Cork
m. 1975: Kathleen (Kay) Lynes, MCS Physiotherapy

BA, UCC, 1937; MB, UCC, 1942; MCh, NUI, 1948; FRCS Eng, 1951; FRCSI (*ad eundem*), 1975

Postgraduate training involved more than eight years in English hospitals. Junior training posts at Royal Hospital, Sheffield (with John B. Ferguson Wilson); surgical registrar, Royal Victoria Infirmary, Newcastle on Tyne (with Norman Hodgson and John Gilmour); senior surgical registrar, Royal West Sussex Hospital, Chichester (with John Brookes). Consultant surgeon, Bon Secours Hospital, Cork, 1952–89; St Finbarr's Hospital, Cork, 1953–55 (where the late, great John Kelly [q.v.] was a beacon of what one could do in Cork); Mount Alvernia Hospital, Mallow, 1954; South Infirmary, Cork, 1952.
Surgeon, Military Hospital, Cork, 1970–90.

Tom returned to Cork as a consultant and, like many of that time, he had never had a junior post in Ireland. When he qualified, there were only two house surgeon posts in Cork each year. He was a most patient man who became an excellent technical surgeon with a great respect for tissues. He was at his happiest doing an almost bloodless thyroidectomy. He also excelled in skin grafting for injuries and burns.

Retiring by nature, he enjoyed his daily piano practice (great hands) and attending symphony concerts. Widely read, he was an enthusiastic walker. Kay and he knew every path in West Cork. Spare, studious, bespectacled, perhaps 5'10" in height, in retirement he was in demand as a medico-legal expert, giving a clear irrefutable opinion. A most admirable professional.

CAHILL, Joseph (Joe)

Cork Surgeon

b. 1940, Dublin, son of Tim and Mary Cahill
Educ. Terenure College, Dublin; University College Dublin
m. 1970: Pamela Pixie Anne, MB, Liverpool; 3 s, 2 d
d. 1988

MB, UCD, 1963; FRCSI, 1969; FRCS, 1970

Postgraduate junior appointments as intern, St Vincent's Hospital, Dublin; house officer, St Michael's Hospital, Dún Laoghaire. senior house officer, Regional Hospital, Galway, 1964–66; registrar, Our Lady's Hospital, Cashel, 1967; surgical registrar, Walton and Warrington Hospitals, 1968–70; senior registrar, Dr Steevens' Hospital, Dublin, 1970–73.
Tutor, Mater Hospital, Dublin, 1974; lecturer in surgery, TCD, 1975–77.
Consultant surgeon, North Infirmary, Cork, 1977–81; South Infirmary, Cork, 1981–88.
President, Medical Union, 1982; formerly executive council member, IMA.

Joe chaired what may have been the biggest medico-political meeting ever held in Ireland when the Irish Medical Union and the Irish Medical Association amalgamated to become the Irish Medical Organisation. This was decided in 1982 in Killarney. He gave the performance of his life in the chair and there were many who felt that the vital merger would have failed were it not for Joe Cahill. He was a first-class operating surgeon and, at the time of his death, he had built up one of the biggest practices in Cork (not ever easy, but coming from Dublin didn't make it easier). He was hugely popular at all levels of the greater medical profession.

Charismatic, energetic and enthusiastic, he had captained the Terenure Junior rugby team to win the Leinster Junior Cup in 1956. His premature death was a huge loss to the profession at many levels.

CREEDON, Francis (Frank)

Cork Surgeon

b. 1934, Tralee, eldest son of Francis Creedon (MB, UCC, 1926) and Grace J. Creedon (*née* Riordan), Brockton, Massachusetts, USA
Educ. Christian Brothers College, Cork; University College Cork
m. 1963: Margaret Murphy, only child of Tadg Murphy, Cork; 3 s, 4 d
d. 2000

MB, UCC, 1957; FRCSI, 1964; MCh, UCC, 1965

Postgraduate training: South Infirmary and St Finbarr's, Cork; Jervis Street Hospital, Dublin; Manchester Royal Infirmary; registrar in thoracic surgery, Hammersmith Hospital, London.
Tutor in surgery, RCSI.
Consultant general surgeon, Bon Secours Hospital, Cork.

Frank Creedon was described by himself as: 'Stocky, extrovert, sociable, opinionated, mathematically minded. Great social skills. Strong religious convictions.' He had a marked attachment to his ancestors' rural origins in mid-Cork. His wide interests included beagling, mountain-climbing, trout fishing and stamp collecting.

DONOVAN, Edmond (Ned, nickname 'Dongo')

Cork Surgeon

b. ?1899

MB, UCC, 1922; LM, Coombe Hospital, Dublin, 1924; MD, NUI, 1927; MCh, NUI, 1930; MAO, 1932

Radiologist, South Infirmary, Cork.
Part-time assistant in anatomy, UCC.
Honorary surgeon, Bon Secours Hospital; South Infirmary, Cork.
Visiting surgeon, St Finbarr's Hospital, Cork.
Lecturer in surgery, UCC.

'Dongo' was the only doctor of his time to hold major degrees in the three disciplines of medicine, surgery and obstetrics, but surgery was his main interest. He enjoyed teaching undergraduates the very basics of physical signs. He was not a great one for detailed history taking and his surgery was of the 'no-frills' variety. 'Every patient has his own disease,' was his somewhat enigmatic watchword.

Very well read in a wide variety of topics, he was a scrupulously fair examiner and was much loved (and imitated) by the students.

Short, tubby, ruddy faced, with a full moustache, he spoke slowly and carefully, measuring his words, which sometimes contained literary and classical allusions.

DUNDON, John Conor

Cork Surgeon

b. 1914 eldest son of Prof. John and Mary Dundon; younger brother, Charles (Charlie), worked with Terence Millin [q.v.], became an urologist, and emigrated to Ontario, Canada
Educ. Clongowes Wood College; University College Cork
m. 1940: Dr Anna ('Johnnie') Gallagher, UCC, Royal Army Medical Corps; 3 d (incl. Carol Dundon, FFARCSI, consultant anaesthetist, Midland Health Board)
d. 1985

MB, NUI, 1938 (first class hons, Pearson medal); MSc (anatomy), Manchester, 1941; FRCS Ed, 1943; FRCSI (*ad eundem*), 1976

Postgraduate appointments as assistant lecturer in anatomy, University of Manchester, where he worked with Professor Frederick Wood-Jones, arguably the leading anatomist of the twentieth century, and a lifelong influence; resident casualty officer, Ancoats Hospital, Manchester; house surgeon, Manchester Royal Infirmary; resident surgical officer, Royal Victoria Infirmary, Preston.
Consultant Surgeon General, Military Hospital, Collins Barracks, Cork; North Infirmary; Bon Secours Hospital; Mercy Hospital; St Patrick's Franciscan Hospital, Mallow.

John Dundon had a real interest in teaching undergraduates and had considerable expertise in thyroid surgery (always an anatomist's focus). He did faciomaxillary work at the Cork Dental Hospital. He retired in 1968.

Tall, elegant, handsome and very dark, he was well read and somewhat reserved, but a very kind man with an excellent sense of humour. He was a keen gardener, specialising in roses, which he grew in profusion in an old city garden behind the family home at 16 St Patrick's Place.

HEGARTY, Daniel Francis (Dan)

Cork Surgeon

b. 1877, eldest son of William and Mary Hegarty
Educ. Miss Kelly's School, South Mall, Cork; Queen's College, Cork
m. Ita Magner; 1 s (Billy, RIP, consultant anaesthetist, Harefield Hospital, London who worked with Sir Magdi Yacoub, the premier heart surgeon of the day. Billy undoubtedly saved the editor's life by acting as enforcer in the front row of the schoolboy scrum, aged fifteen), 2 d (Patricia, GP, London; Una, Dublin)
d. 1950
MB, Queen's College, Cork, 1900 (Charles medal in surgery); FRCS Ed

House surgeon and outpatient surgeon, North Infirmary, Cork (under Professor Charles Yelverton Pearson [q.v.]).
Surgeon, North Cork Charitable Infirmary, 1908–48.

His principal interest was abdominal surgery.

Of medium height, with a moustache, Dan Hegarty was gentle, popular and the soul of kindness. Good humoured and keen on basic surgery teaching, he had an aristocratic limp, always thought to be of military or equine origin, but which was, in fact, poliomyelitis. He summered in Ballycotton, Co. Cork where he had a close medical association with the gallant, decorated (at Buckingham Palace) Sliney family who had three generations of bemedalled Lifeboat men.

HEGARTY, George F.

Cork Surgeon

b. 1881; younger son of William and Mary Hegarty; nephew of Sir Daniel Hegarty, first Lord Mayor of Cork
Educ. Christian Brothers College, Cork; Blackrock College, Dublin; University College Cork
m. 2 d (Eleanor and Mary, both doctors)
d. 1967

House surgeon, South Infirmary, Cork (1912) and then successively radiologist, junior surgeon, senior surgeon and honorary secretary of the medical staff to the hospital which he served for over fifty years.
Royal Army Medical Corps, First World War.
Chairman, Irish Red Cross Society; founder member, Cork Blood Bank.

A tall (6'1"), kindly, distinguished figure, with a military moustache, and always formally turned out, George Hegarty was rarely without a Gold Flake cigarette in hand. He had been a fine athlete with UCC Rugby Club (played for Blackrock College against a Rockwell College team which contained Éamon de Valera), and UCC Rowing Club. Indeed, the rumour was that he stayed on a year or two extra at UCC so that he could continue to qualify for the rowing eight.

KEARNEY, John Joseph (JJ)

Prof of Obstetrics and Gynaecology, UCC (1926–1948) and Cork Surgeon

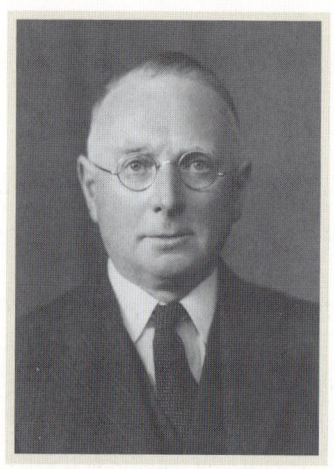

b. 1885
Educ. Royal University of Ireland
m. 3 s (William (Billy) succeeded him as an extrovert, progressive Professor of Obstetrics; 'JB' was a polished gynaecologist; Kevin was a hugely popular Cork surgeon)
d. 1962

MB, RUI, 1907; MD, NUI, 1910 (first class hons & gold medal); DPH (first class hons), 1910; FRCS Ed, 1921; FRCOG, 1946

Dispensary doctor, styled medical officer of health (MOH), Roscarbery, West Cork, before moving to Cork as an obstetrician and surgeon. Clinical assistant, Chelsea Women's Hospital.

Consultant surgeon, Mercy Hospital; Bon Secours; Erinville Maternity Hospital, to his first retirement in 1948 and after.

JJ did much general surgery as well as the 'carriage trade' obstetrics. This utterly charming man, who had the priceless reputation of being unfailingly lucky, enthralled the patients, and the nuns, in all hospitals. He had an optimistic attitude towards patients' problems and was a gifted operator. He was kind, genial and approachable. His appearance was straight from Hollywood Central Casting. He was above average height, with sleek, white hair and gold-rimmed spectacles. His working clothes consisted of striped 'pepper and salt' trousers, black jacket, white shirt and dark tie, and he always wore them, even lying on Youghal beach with his shoes and socks off.

Referring 'country' doctors invariably made the 'right diagnosis'. This was partly on the basis that he too had once been an exposed solo practitioner, and realised that the mantle of infallibility was crucial to survival in a small remote community, but also on the basis that there were plenty of patients in the country, but referring doctors were an endangered species to be cultivated and kept happy. At his peak, before anaesthesia became safe, he was a rapid operator and many lives were saved, and JJ's reputation kept intact, by his escaping to safety from a complex abdominal problem through the lumen of a large drainage tube.

He had developed a few simple phrases, which covered almost all adverse situations: 'He had a bug in the blood.' Obviously nothing could be done (before 1940) for such a tragedy and no further questions were asked.

'It was a dirty, rotten, nasty thing and she's better off without it.' This covered much between appendicitis, 'early' (perhaps twenty years early) or late, a twisted ovarian cyst or a perforated diverticulitis.

'He had it all the time.' This was ominous and was associated with the never mentioned 'Big C' word. But grieving relatives would realise that once more Dr Kearney was right. The deceased had been acting 'strangely' or 'crankily' for some weeks (or months or years — take your pick) and his demise was softened by the knowledge that he could not have been in better hands anywhere in this world. They were probably right.

As for hands, he was missing a ring finger on his right hand, presumably 'blood poisoning' (there I go again…ed) following a farming accident followed by amputation. This gave him an advantage as a gynaecologist but also enabled him to slip away easily from a handshaking patient who wished to know when she was going home. She knew she was going home because Dr Kearney was looking after her. She just didn't know when. Neither did Dr Kearney. She would be discharged when her bed could be filled and not before, thus fulfilling the nuns' Fourth Law of Thermodynamics that a bed must be kept warm. His trademark was the handshake (just like the Mayo Clinic in its early days) and one small, retiring nun claimed to have had her hand shaken and wished 'Happy Christmas' eleven times on that same day.

His approach to his professorial duties was disarmingly simple. The lectures were read out from typescripts that were never, ever circulated and were guarded like irreplaceable religious relics or original signed Mozart scores. A prying student (the editor, who should be ashamed of himself) discovered that they had been copied word for word from a small book, *Aids to Obstetrics and Gynaecology* (seven shillings and sixpence), written by a hard-headed London obstetrician. But this book title did not appear on the short list of recommended texts, all of which cost three times as much, or more. Never mind. The chosen work was full of simple classifications and common sense and contained enough to get honours in the BAO. JJ augmented 'his' notes with a series of colourful anecdotes, illustrating the perils of life at the coalface. The practical teaching at the maternity hospital was memorable and one realised that one was seeing a master at work.

He had a vast practice at 24 St Patrick's Hill, and queues outside the door were not uncommon. The consultation fee of one guinea (a pound avoided the change problem) was always accompanied by the considerate phrase: 'I'll see you again for that.' He never left town...or so it appeared. The secretary (who may have been his sister) stayed at her post and would give a telephone appointment for one, two or three weeks' time until the first of the three daily *Cork Examiner* notices that 'Dr Kearney has returned to No. 24 St Patrick's Hill' appeared, to the relief of all. But then he had never really been away...

Vernon O'Hea Cussen [q.v.], his contemporary, an ophthalmologist, and a man not given to exaggerating the exceptional qualities of colleagues, said, 'John Kearney is a remarkable man.' He understated the reality by an order of magnitude.

(The editor must enter a caveat...JJ delivered me, took out my tonsils, set my upper and lower limb fractures, gave me boiled sweets for my measles (he took them out of his doctor's Gladstone bag in our home and what works better in childhood measles? ... as always with JJ, the patient was impressed), drained my mother's empyema (1932), successfully closed a huge spina bifida cystica in a three-week-old close relative who became a front row rugby forward (early 1930s), advised my mother on the garden ('Those roses need pruning') and gave my father advice on the stock exchange ('You should buy some Great Universal Stores, Mr O'Donnell). You just couldn't make him up. The ultimate refutation that warm kindly manners and gold medals do not co-exist. An easy winner of the best doctor I ever met.)

KEARNEY, Kevin Victor Joseph

Cork Surgeon

b. 1919, Cork, third son of Prof. John ('JJ') Kearney [q.v.] and Mary Kearney
Educ. Christian Brothers College, Cork; St Gerard's, Bray; University College Cork
m. 1950: Ann Kinmonth, daughter of Dr George and Mrs Delia Kinmonth; 6 s (Michael, b. 1953, palliative care physician, Santa Barbara, California; Peter, b. 1963, cardiologist, Cork University Hospital), 1 d
d. 1996

MB, UCC, 1942; MCh, NUI, 1950; FRCS Eng, 1951; FRCSI (*ad eundem*), 1972

Postgraduate appointments as house surgeon, Bolingbroke Hospital, London; surgical registrar, St Giles Hospital, London, and General Hospital, Nottingham.
Ship's surgeon, Royal Navy in the latter years of the Second World War; his ship struck a mine off Walcheren Island and was sunk in the Battle of the Scheldt (near Antwerp), November 1944. He suffered a left ankle injury from which he made a slow but good recovery, following which he returned to Ireland.
Surgeon, Bon Secours Hospital; Mercy Hospital, Cork, 1951–84.

Kevin was a very keen clinical teacher, much loved by his students. He is remembered by his students and junior colleagues as addressing them as 'Doc'. His teaching was characterised by memorable anecdotes, and his approach consisted of whirlwind tours through the tortuous stairwells and corridors of the Mercy Hospital, punctuated by multiple instructive vignettes and encounters with patients, illustrating a variety of conditions. He stressed the importance of courtesy and had learned from his father the importance of the handshake. He told the story of an occasion soon after returning to work in Cork when he worked largely on a charitable basis in a number of the city's hospitals, including St Patrick's on Military Hill. Having spent many hours rounding, he was joined by his father, JJ, who visited the hospital for his regular but much shorter visit. When JJ had left, a patient asked Kevin might he not take the time his father did in meeting with his patients! On reflection, Kevin realised that unlike his father he did not always start each consultation with a handshake, something which thereafter became as much a part of his character as his father's.

In his early years, he enjoyed playing rugby and golf, and in mid and later years, was a keen rugby supporter, and passionate and persistent, if not very successful, fly fisherman. An avid reader and collector of books, he had a large library, dominated by war history, biography, aviation, and sport. He loved his dogs. Paradoxically a most affable and sociable man, on the one hand, but retiring and shy on the other, particularly in the setting of public engagements, Kevin was hugely popular within and without the medical community. He retired to Union Hall, West Cork. A man of great compassion, who did not undertake surgery lightly.

KELLY, John

Cork Surgeon

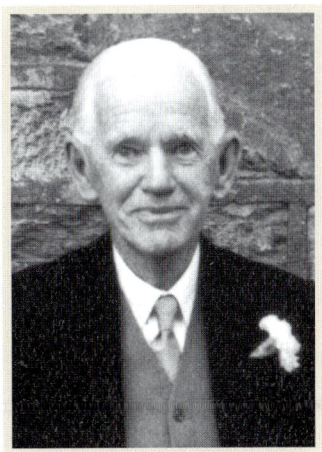

b. 1901, Kilrush, Co. Clare; father had been in the British Army and spent some time in India but returned to be garrisoned in Youghal, Co Cork.
Educ. Christian Brothers School, Youghal; University College Cork
m. 1937: Alice Glanville (medical student); son John is a Cork surgeon
d. 1973

MB, UCC, 1925 (clinical prize in surgery; Blayney scholarship); FRCS Eng, 1931

Postgraduate appointments as casualty officer and house surgeon, St John's Hospital, Lewisham;

assistant medical officer, London County Council; senior casualty officer, house surgeon and senior resident medical officer, General Hospital, Nottingham; junior surgeon (temp.), North Middlesex Hospital, Edmonton, North London; assistant in Neurosurgical Department, London Hospital.
Surgeon, St Finbarr's Hospital; Bon Secours Hospital; Mercy Hospital, Cork.
Honorary senior consultant surgeon, Mount Alvernia, Mallow.

John Kelly was hugely admired by generations of students of UCC. He had been away ('England' for seven years) and it showed in all sorts of ways, but most of all it showed that 'going away' made a massive difference. Since all knew that they were going to go away, usually for good in those days, his every slow, careful word was digested and dissected. It was said of this painstaking surgeon that the time spent in neurosurgery had left its mark. He was calm, cool, sage and undemonstrative and, above all, immensely practical. The diagnosis of a fractured forearm was based not on history or appearances but 'across the yard and down the slope' (to Nottingham General Hospital's X-ray Department). Like Joyce and Dublin, many felt that they could find their way around that hospital from what he told them of it. He sent many favoured sons there and gave practical encouragement to a greater number.

Not altogether welcomed by the Establishment on his return to Cork and St Finbarr's Hospital, which was very much a Poor Law premises, complete with rodent population, he gave the students hope for the future. Extremely modest and shunning the limelight, he would not accept a retirement gift subscribed to by a large number of medical admirers, and eventually the 'radiogram' (1965) was just delivered to his home. It is still in the family in 2006.

Perhaps 5'8", with trademark white hair and centre crease, he often wore an overcoat on teaching rounds because of the unheated wards. A powerful, sustaining role model.

KIELY, John ('K John')

Cork Surgeon and Lecturer in Surgery

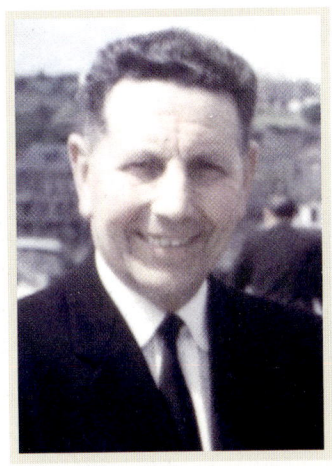

b. 1899, Stradbally, Co. Waterford, son of John Kiely and Mary Kiely (*née* Moloney), seventh of 10 children; younger brother of Patrick Kiely ('PK') [q.v.]
Educ. St Augustine's, Dungarvan; St Colman's College, Fermoy; University College Cork (scholarship)
m. 1931: Helen Goggin (dentist); 4 s (David [q.v.], urologist, capped as wing forward for Ireland five times; Patrick Edward [q.v.], vascular surgeon; Edward, paediatric surgeon, Hospital for Sick Children, Great Ormond Street, London; Roger, FRCS, RIP), 2 d (Helen a pathologist)
d. 1996

MB, UCC, 1922; MD, MCh, UCC, 1930; FRCS Ed, 1938

GP, Ballyduff, Co. Waterford, 1922–27.
Consultant surgeon, North Infirmary; Mercy Hospital; Bon Secours Hospital, Cork.

'K John' began in Cork as anaesthetist to his elder brother 'PK'. His first consultant appointment was to St Finbarr's Hospital, which was then still a workhouse/infirmary.

He was hugely popular and much loved by the students as he was most helpful, rather than 'putting them down', and one can well believe that in retirement what he missed most was 'the bedside teaching of students', at which he was a master. His signature phrase 'd'ye see' still raises a smile amongst his far-flung graduates. He gave the Doolin Lecture 1973 at the RCSI on 'The Golden Era of Surgery'.

His idea of a holiday was to visit the Mayo Clinic and the Lahey Clinic in Boston, where he was a well-known and welcomed figure. He was an excellent natural operating surgeon who could slow down to demonstrate a feature or speed up if needs be.

Of medium height, broad shouldered, handsome, tireless, dark (in his nineties) and faultlessly groomed, he always wore a bowler hat. His interests outside surgery were golf (to a low handicap), Gaelic games (he had played football for Waterford) and breeding Holstein Friesian cattle. He adopted the nom de plume 'K John', an inversion of his name, so that the public would not see his real name on the golf prize list too often and draw the wrong conclusions. This he did in a city where everyone knows what everyone else is doing and buys the (Cork) *Examiner* newspaper only to see if they got caught doing it. His most famous patient, whom he repaired after many 'close encounters' of every kind, was the greatest hurler of all time, Christy Ring (1920–79). They were well met.

Three of K John's four sons became distinguished consultant surgeons, all excellent operators. A fourth son, Roger, died during his training. All four had the FRCS Eng, which is probably a sibling record. A unique but unsurprising legacy of a most admirable man.

KIELY, Patrick Bartholomew ('PB')

Cork Surgeon

b. 1931, Cork, youngest son of Prof. Patrick Kiely ('PK') [q.v.] and Mary Kiely
Educ. Christian Brothers College, Cork; University College Cork

MB, UCC, 1953; FRCSI, 1960

Postgraduate appointments as house surgeon, Postgraduate Medical School, Hammersmith; surgical registrar, Redhill and Netherne Hospital Group; surgical registrar, SS John & Elizabeth, London.
Surgeon, Bon Secours Hospital; Mercy Hospital, Cork.

PB coped very well with the difficult task of following on his charismatic father and an elder brother, John, also a brilliant surgeon, with striking good looks, who died prematurely. He had a loyal following of referring doctors and never stepped outside the boundaries of his capabilities. Popular with the students because he simplified so much, he is a man of profound religious faith, with his father's gift of the pithy phrase — 'A surgeon needs the nerves of a burglar and the fingers of a pickpocket.'

KIELY, Patrick Edward ('PE', Paddy)

Cork Vascular and General Surgeon

b. 1937, Cork, son of Surgeon John Kiely ('K John') [q.v.] and Helen Kiely BDS
Educ. Christian Brothers College; University College Cork
m. 1966: Leonie, daughter of Prof. Gus Albregts and Leonie Albregts-Evers of the Netherlands; 2 s (Patrick J., FRCS Orth), 4 d

MB, UCC, 1960; BSc Physiology (hons), UCC, 1962; FRCSE, 1967; MCh, NUI, 1968; FRCS Eng, 1968

Postgraduate appointments as surgical registrar, St Anthony's Hospital, Cheam, England; lecturer in surgery, St Bartholomew's, London (four years with Prof. Gerry Taylor); Fellow in Vascular Surgery, University of California (with Prof. John Connolly).
Consultant general and vascular surgeon, Bon Secours Hospital; Mercy University Hospital, Cork.

Tall, dark and handsome, Paddy was a superbly trained, gifted technical surgeon and the one of four surgical sons who is most like his admired father, John Kiely.

He is still, in retirement, a natural athlete, and he was one of three undergraduate brothers (David and Edward were the other two) to captain UCC RFC (1962–63). He ran the Dublin and Cork marathons in 1984 and 1985, at 47 and 48 years of age! He enjoys tennis, golf, cycling and swimming, as well as his vegetable patch in his home near Oysterhaven, Co. Cork.

LINEHAN, Gerard Martin ('Gus')

Cork Surgeon

b. 1924, son of Daniel ('Chalky') Linehan MSc and Mary Hamill (both schoolteachers)
Educ. Christian Brothers College, Cork; University College Cork (entrance scholarship: first place, 1942)
m. Dr Eleanor Murphy; 1 s, 2 d
d. 1996

MB, UCC, 1948; FRCS Eng, 1952; MCh, NUI, 1953

Surgical registrar, St Finbarr's Hospital Cork, 1953–55; Ainsworth Travelling Scholarship from UCC to London, 1955–56; clinical assistant, Royal Postgraduate Medical School, Hammersmith (Mr R. H. Franklin) and St Mark's Hospital for Disease of the Rectum. Surgeon, Mercy Hospital, Cork, 1955–84; South Infirmary, Cork, 1957–86.

His main interest was large bowel and breast cancer.

An enthusiastic teacher of all who came in contact with him, Gus was careful, meticulous and caring. A founder member of Munster Surgical Group, he was actively involved with developing surgical services in the Cork Voluntary Hospitals.

He enjoyed golf and squash and was formerly a completely reliable rugby out half with great hands. He spent summers at a holiday home in Beara, Co. Cork.

Of average height, stocky but slim, he was always immaculate (tie every day). Alert, calm and calming, he had a cerebral approach to clinical problems and a wry sense of humour. A difficult twilight was softened by wonderful family support.

MACKILLOP, Neil Campbell

Cork Surgeon

b. 1920, Karachi to Scottish parents
Educ. Glasgow High School; University of Glasgow
m. Barbara; 1 s (doctor), 3 d
d. 1980

MB, ChB, Glas, 1943; FRCS Eng, 1950

Postgraduate appointments: Royal Navy, 1944–47; resident surgical officer, Harrow Hospital, London; senior registrar, Salisbury Infirmary.
Surgeon, Iraq Petroleum Company.
GP, Leicester.
Surgeon, Victoria Hospital, Cork, 1969–80.
Surgeon, Mallow County Hospital.

'Mac the Knife' was a colourful, robust, confident, competent addition to the scene. He had captained the University of Glasgow rugby team. An able teacher, he was a fine general surgeon and was deeply committed to his work.

O'DONNELL, Joseph Anthony (Joe)

Cork Vascular Surgeon

b. 1943, eldest son of Wilfred O'Donnell and Lelia O'Donnell (*née* Kirby)
Educ. Rockwell College, Co. Tipperary; University College Cork
m. 1969: Avril O'Neill, daughter of Raymond (pathologist) and Marie O'Neill; 2 s, 2 d

MB, UCC, 1967; FRCSI, 1971; MCh, NUI, UCC, 1976; American Board of Surgery, 1976; FACS, 1978

Postgraduate work in St Finbarr's Hospital, Cork; St Vincent's Hospital, Dublin; Our Lady's Hospital for Sick Children, Crumlin, Dublin.
Resident and chief resident, St Vincent's Hospital, Worcester, Massachusetts, USA, 1971–75 (Ainsworth scholarship from UCC for the first year).
Fellow in vascular surgery, Beth Israel Medical Center, Newark, part of New Jersey College of Medicine and Dentistry, 1975–76.
General and vascular surgeon, Cork Regional Hospital, 1979–2002.
Clinical lecturer in surgery, UCC, 1979–2002.
Examiner in Primary and Final FRCSI. Member, Council, RCSI, 1988–93.

Career influences included M. P. Brady [q.v.] and Tom Hennessy [q.v.] in Cork and H. Bronwell Wheeler, UMASS Medical School, Worcester.

Joe O'Donnell was the first fully trained vascular surgeon to be appointed in Cork. He has a sharp intelligence, a very impressive natural technical skill, with excellent outcomes, and a polished manner, all of which combined to make his services in great demand. His premature retirement from the health service, at under 60, highlights one of the dilemmas of medical practice in a small country with a low population density. He was very fit and 'full of work' at the time of his departure and he left a huge gap in the surgical resources of Cork and Munster. At the time he left, he was the only vascular surgeon in the university hospital and was, in theory and in practice, always on call for the entire year. This included being called while on leave in his holiday home in Schull over 70 miles west. His colleagues understandably did not wish to undertake work for which they had not been trained, and vascular surgery was advancing rapidly but the advance planning could be criticised. It is ironic that now, five years later, there are five vascular surgeons in Cork.

Cork neurosurgeon Michael O'Sullivan did some of his training with Joe and was impressed by his professionalism and manual skill: 'He was very supportive of his staff and if a mistake occurred all he would ask is "What did you learn?" In nearly 30 years, I have never heard a bad word about him from anybody. The porters and his peers held him in the highest esteem. His patients adored him. This is some record.' Gerald McGreal (now a Cork vascular surgeon) praises his persistence, care and attention and the way he explained every step of management of the current problem using apt analogies from his vast experience. Past trainees frequently quote his aphorisms.

Tall, dark and handsome, Joe looks a decade younger than his years ('beautifully maintained by one careful owner', Avril). In retirement, he plays golf, paints and keeps a close eye on the UCC rugby team. He liked going home. He is admired outside Cork as well as in it.

WHELTON, William Francis (Frank)

Cork Surgeon

b. 1909, Cork, youngest child of Michael Whelton and Johanna Whelton (*née* Kelleher)
Educ. Presentation College, Cork; Clongowes Wood College, Kildare; University College Cork
m. 1944: Anne Lynch (d. 1994), daughter of Patrick and Ellen Lynch; 1 s (Frank Jnr a dental surgeon), 3 d (Anne a dental surgeon)
d. 1991

MB, UCC, 1932 (Charles gold medal for anatomy); MCh, NUI, 1939; FRCS Ed, 1942

Postgraduate training in English hospitals, 1934–44.
House surgeon, Northampton General Hospital; Leicester Royal Infirmary.
Consultant surgeon, Limerick County Hospital, Croom.
Surgeon, Bon Secours and North Infirmary Hospitals, Cork, 1944–75.

Frank's great interest, outside of surgery, was the scouting movement in which he worked both as a surgeon and as an author of scouting textbooks. He was a keen teacher of undergraduates.

Galway Surgeons

Galway (pop. 66,163)
Galway County Hospital established 1786 (60 beds)
In 1920, there were five medical officers but still no mention of a surgeon.

COLOHAN, Nicholas Whistler, JP

Surgeon, Galway County Hospital

Educ. Queen's College Galway and Dublin

MD, MCh, RUI, 1872 (Queen's College Galway and Dublin)

Professor, Materia Medica and Therapeutics and lecturer in clinical surgery, QCG. Surgeon, Galway County Hospital.
Certified factory surgeon.
Attending surgeon, Royal Irish Constabulary; Post Office.
Surgeon, Naval Sick Quarters Galway.

PYE, Joseph Patrick, JP

Honorary Surgeon, Galway County Hospital

DSc, RUI (hon. causa), 1882; MD (Peel scholarship and gold medal), MCh, 1871; LRCS Ed, 1870 (QCG, London and Paris)

Honorary surgeon, Galway Hospital.
Professor of Anatomy and Physiology, UCG; examiner in anatomy, RUI.

BRERETON, William Westropp

Galway Surgeon and Professor of Surgery

LRCPI & LM, 1865; LRCSI & LM, 1865 (RCSI); MRCPI, 1890

Professor of Surgery, UCG; examiner in surgery, UCG.

KINKEAD, Richard J JP

Galway Obstetrician

Educ. Royal College of Surgeons in Ireland; Trinity College, Dublin

AB, Dub, 1867; MD, 1873; LRCSI & LM, 1865 (RCS, TCD)

Publications include *Proofs of Virginity* and *Vaginal Hysterectomy: 4 Cases of Laparotomy*.

Galway Regional Hospital

MAHON, Ralph Bodkin

Professor of Practical Medicine, UCG

MD, RUI (first place, first class hons); MCh, 1885; FRCS Eng, 1896; LM Coombe (Galway, London, Dublin, Berlin)

Temporary Captain, Royal Army Medical Corps.
Surgical specialist, Southern Military Hospital, Dartford, Kent.
Professor of Practical Medicine, UCG.

McHUGH, Thomas Francis (Tommy)

Galway Surgeon

b. 1920
Educ. University College Dublin

MB, UCD, 1943; MCh, NUI, 1946

Postgraduate training: resident medical officer, Nuffield House (private wing), Guy's Hospital, London; resident surgical officer, Royal United Hospitals, Liverpool; house surgeon, Royal National Orthopaedic Hospital, Stanmore, London.
Visiting Surgeon, Central Hospital, Galway.

McDERMOTT, Edward Neale (Neil) PRCSI 1966–1968

Galway Surgeon

b. 1902, England, son of John McDermott (an officer of the Inland Revenue)
Educ. Ursuline Convent, Cheltenham; Kendal Grammar School; St Ignatius College, Galway. University College Galway (scholarship)
m. 1947: Anna 'Bea' Geraghty of Ahascragh, Co. Galway; 2 s (John is a medical graduate)
d. 1972

BS (first class hons; anatomy and physiology), 1922; Primary FRCSI, 1923 (Primary FRCSI examination could be taken as an undergraduate up to about 1950); MB (first place, first class hons), UCG, 1924; FRCSI, 1929; MD, 1931; MCh, 1940

Postgraduate work: research in medicine in Edinburgh.
Staff surgeon, Galway Central Hospital, 1930; St Enda's Military Hospital, Galway with the rank of Major (Reserve) Army Medical Service; Portiuncula Hospital, Ballinasloe.
Thoracic surgeon, Woodlands Sanatorium; Galway and City Hospital; Limerick.
Professor of Pharmacology, UCG. Member, governing body UCG and NUI Senate
President, IMA, 1958.
Knight of Malta, Knight of St Gregory.

A man of great energy, dextrous and decisive, Neil McDermott was a model of integrity, probity and dignity. He was unsuccessful in his spirited bid for the Chair of Surgery at UCG in 1957. He took a legal action against the NUI for its decision not to appoint him, but lost. He is remembered by some of the nurses as an appalling male chauvinist. He was most active in medical affairs and was completely against any state intervention in medicine, even for the shrinking numbers with tuberculosis. He was vigorous in his defence of the Irish medical schools, some of which were threatened with closure in that terrible decade of the 1950s. He justified the huge medical emigration that was taking place at that time by saying that the departing doctors' role was akin to that of the missionary priests.

His fine intellect allowed him to master Irish, English, French and German, with a competency in Spanish, Portuguese, Latin, Italian, Dutch and Danish. He read Greek and Russian. With these qualifications he was an inveterate traveller and joiner of international surgical organisations. A stern man, he could never have been accused of levity about anything, ever.

Perhaps 5'7", but broad shouldered, stocky and impressive, he gradually became more aldermanic as the years passed. He lived in great style, and he and his warm, laughing wife were generous hosts and entertained on a lavish scale.

GALVIN, Colm

Consultant Surgeon, Galway

b. 1921
Educ. Belvedere College, SJ, Dublin; University College Dublin
m. Mary; 4 d
d. 1997

BSc, 1944; MB, UCD, 1947; MCh, NUI, 1953; FRCS Eng, 1954; FACS, 1970; FRCSI (*ad eundem*), 1972

Postgraduate training at St Vincent's; St John and Elizabeth's Hospital, London; Harrow Hospital, Middlesex; Queen Mary's Hospital, Roehampton; St Mark's Hospital, London.
Senior surgical registrar, United Norwich Hospital Group, Norwich, for two years.
Consultant surgeon, St Catherine's Hospital, Tralee 1957–69.
Consultant surgeon, University College Hospital, Galway and lecturer in surgery, University College Galway, 1970–86.
Member, Medical Council, Council of IMA and the ground-breaking Consultative Council on General Hospital Services (Fitzgerald Report), 1968.
Council of Europe Fellowship, Sweden, 1962; World Health Organisation Fellowship, USA, 1967.

Colm had a shining intelligence, was a superb technical surgeon and returned to Ireland having had a full training in surgery, particularly in colorectal work, at his beloved St Mark's, London, where he subsequently served as President of the St Mark's Association. He had a certain reserve and an occasional spikiness of manner, which may have cost him an appointment at his alma mater, but nobody questioned his integrity. He became involved in medical affairs in both the IMA and the Irish Medical Union, and was always heard with great respect. He was an early negotiator on the Consultants' panel and it was he who coined the vital term 'Common Contract', which was to dominate discussions with government for twenty years. There was an understandable sense of incomplete fulfilment about his career, but his patients benefited from superb care.

MURPHY, Bernard (Bernie)

Galway Surgeon

b. 1926

Educ. St Vincent's, North Monastery, Cork; University College Cork

MB, UCC, 1948; FRCS Eng, 1954; FRCSI (*ad eundem*), 1963; FACS, 1972

Postgraduate posts of increasing responsibility in various hospitals in the Liverpool area for seven years, finishing with four years as registrar and senior registrar, Broadgreen Hospital, Liverpool (James Moroney and S. V. Unsworth were his best-known chiefs). Registrar, Ennis County Hospital.
Surgeon, Donegal Town and Lifford Hospitals.
Temporary consultant surgeon, Galway Regional Hospital, 1958–69.
Consultant surgeon, University College Hospital, Galway, 1969–88.
Lecturer in surgery, UCG.
President, surgical section, RAMI, 1988–89; Council RCSI, 1986–94.
Revived Western Surgical Club.
Chairman, Galvia Private Hospital, Galway. Inaugural Chairman, Galway Lions Club.

Bernie Murphy had prodigious energy in tackling long operating lists, was greatly admired by the trainees, and carried out his work in a no-nonsense style. Although a well-trained surgeon, he was kept as 'temporary' for eleven years; this disgraceful situation was common at the time.

A big man (6'2"), in every respect, amusing and intelligent company, he played Sigerson Cup football and Fitzgibbon Cup hurling at UCC and was on the Senior Cork football team. Affectionately known to the entire hospital staff as 'The Duke', after John Wayne — this really says it all.

Ballinasloe
See Chapter 10: Surgeons by County in the Republic of Ireland

Limerick Surgeons

Limerick (pop. 86,998)

Barrington's Hospital and City of Limerick Infirmary founded 1829 (60 beds)

1900	Honorary visiting surgeons	Dr Graham Holmes
		Dr Fogarty

County Infirmary, Limerick established 1765 (40 beds)

1900	Surgeon	R. R. Gelston
	Assistant surgeons	Dr Fogarty
		F. Kennedy
		Dr Humphries

St John's Hospital established as Fever Hospital 1778, General Hospital 1888 (65 beds)
1905–1964

DEVANE, John Francis

Limerick Surgeon

b. 1883, son of Cornelius Devane and Joanna Devane (*née* McCormack)
Educ. University College Dublin
m. 1916: Vera Keogh, daughter of Andrew Keogh and Julia Keogh (*née* Brennan); 2 d (Joan m. Frank Duff PRCSI; Virette m. William Finlay, Governor, Bank of Ireland), 4 s (Dermod John [q.v.], surgeon; Barry, GP; Leonard, GP; Andrew, distinguished architect)
d. January 1964

MB, RUI, 1905; MD; FRCSI (first place); MD (gold medal)

Postgraduate posts in medicine, surgery, gynaecology and obstetrics and as senior house physician, Mater Hospital, Dublin.
Postgraduate studies in British Postgraduate Hospital, London; Allgemeines Krankenhaus, Vienna.
Worked at St John's Hospital Limerick 1905–64.
Consultant to local institutions, schools and to Shannon and Foynes air bases.
Surgeon, Limerick County Infirmary; Barrington's Hospital.

John F. Devane was an immensely knowledgeable and capable doctor who devoted much of his life to the improvement and upgrading of medical facilities in Limerick, and particularly in St John's Hospital. The sisters relied on him as much more than general surgeon, and he worked tirelessly on their behalf to bring their charitable institution into the first rank, chosen above others for its efficiency and standards. It was he who introduced surgery to St John's, which had formerly been a fever hospital. He carried out a wide range of work both as GP and surgeon, and had an immense interest in the history of the hospital and of the wider Limerick area. He wrote the *History of St John's Hospital*, which was privately published in 1970.

His practice covered a large area, and he was one of the first doctors to attend to his rounds by car, attended by a young helper. Emergency operations were sometimes carried out on kitchen tables. A sister would join him, or a nurse from the County Infirmary, in cases where moving the patient would have resulted in their death. Even in hospital, there were no blood transfusions, antibiotics or modern anaesthesia.

He was on the Council of the RCSI for some years, which was huge recognition for a surgeon from outside Dublin at that time.

A great traveller, he was also a fine cameraman, and made quality movies of the various canoeing and walking trips made in Europe with his family. Tall, distinguished appearance with a courtly manner allied to great, admirable professionalism, he was a wonderful role model at many levels.

1920

GRAHAM, Patrick F.

Limerick Surgeon

Educ. Queen's College, Cork and Dublin

MD, MCh, MAO, RUI, 1881 (QCC, QCD)

Physician, Limerick Lying-in Hospital.
Surgeon, Barrington's Hospital, Limerick.
Physician, St John's Hospital, Limerick.

FOGERTY, William A.

Limerick Surgeon

Educ. Queen's College, Cork

MA, RUI, 1880; MD, MCh, MAO, 1885 (QCC)

Honorary surgeon, Barrington's Hospital.
Visiting surgeon, County Infirmary, Limerick.
Surgeon *accoucheur*, Lying-in Hospital, Limerick.

ROBERTS, James

Limerick Surgeon

Educ. Catholic University School of Medicine (Cecilia Street), Dublin

LRCPI & LM, LRCSI & LM, 1905 (Catholic University, Dublin)

Visiting surgeon, Barrington's Hospital.
Honorary visiting physician, Lying-in Hospital; St John's Hospital, Limerick.

1944–1983

DEVANE, Dermod John ('Derry')

Limerick Surgeon

b. 1921, son of John F. Devane [q.v.] (Limerick surgeon) and Vera Devane (*née* Keogh)
Educ. Clongowes Wood College, Kildare; University College Dublin
m. 1st in 1944: Kathleen Ryan (d. 1985; a stunning, raven-haired beauty who became a leading film actress. Her most famous role was in *Odd Man Out*), daughter of Senator Séamus Ryan and Agnes V. Ryan; 2 d, 1 s. 2nd in 1973: Catherine Maguire
d. 1985

MB, UCD, 1944; FRCSI; FICS.

Postgraduate appointments at Mater Hospital, Dublin, 1944; resident surgical officer, Jervis Street Hospital, 1944–46; Postgraduate Medical School of London, 1948–49; 1951–52.
Study tour, North American Clinic of Plastic Surgery at Mayo Clinic.
Assistant surgeon, Barrington's Hospital, Limerick 1951–56.
Acupuncture courses in various countries including China.
Surgeon, Limerick County Infirmary, 1946–56; Barrington's Hospital, Limerick, 1956–73; St John's Hospital, Limerick, 1944–83.
Lecturer in surgery, Little Company of Mary School of Nursing, Limerick, 1951–56.
Surgeon to Irish Red Cross Hungarian Refugee Camp, Limerick, 1958.

A strikingly handsome, athletic, warm, charming man, beloved of his patients, Dermod Devane travelled widely in pursuit of his twin greatest loves — medicine and wildlife. A born naturalist, his knowledge of wildlife both in Ireland and throughout the world was as extensive as his medical know-how. He chose to remain in the relatively quiet waters of Limerick in order to assist his father's practice, but brought the most up-to-date surgical methods to St John's Hospital, where he was greatly admired. A brilliant diagnostician and meticulous surgeon, he performed a wide range of operations from complex plastic surgery to appendectomy. He became interested in acupuncture when it was disregarded by most of his profession, and found it a useful adjunct to his work. After an early self-diagnosis of motor neurone disease, he successfully concentrated on acupuncture in 1983 when surgery became too physically demanding.

County Infirmary established 1765 (42 beds)

1920	Medical and surgical staff	W. A. Fogerty
		F. W. Kennedy
		T. K. Mulcahy
		J. F. Devane
		J. Roberts

St John's Hospital, Limerick

	Consultant surgeon:	W. A. Fogerty

Limerick County Hospital, Croom

See Chapter 10: Surgeons by County in the Republic of Ireland

Regional Hospital, Limerick

KENNEDY, Dermot Patrick ('DP')

Limerick Surgeon

b. 1907, fifth of 11 children of Surgeon Denis Kennedy [q.v.] ('The Doc', St Vincent's Hospital) and Mary Kennedy (*née* Langan)
Educ. Belvedere College, Dublin; University College Dublin
m. 1946: Andree Hetzel; 7 children (2 doctors: Phillip, neurologist, Atlanta; Colette, radiologist, Auckland)
d. 1986

MB, UCD, 1932; FRCS, 1936

Postgraduate training in Berlin, 1936.
General surgeon, Southlands Hospital, Sussex, 1937–40; 1946–51
Royal Army Medical Corps, 1940–46; 1st Army, Algeria, November 1942; North African and Italian campaigns.
County Surgeon, Cashel, Tipperary, 1951–56.
Surgeon, Regional Hospital, Limerick, 1956–75.
Demonstrator, Anatomy Department, RCSI, 1978–82.

Influenced by his father, surgeon Denis Kennedy, and Howard Hanley, London, who stimulated his interest in urology.

Tall and lean, modest and unassuming, DP Kennedy was a keen, dedicated surgeon and teacher, appreciated by all who came in touch with him, from patients to students. He met his future wife in Djebel, Hallouf, Tunisia, where his Royal Army Medical Corps surgical unit was stationed just behind the front line. In retirement in Greystones, he gardened (grapes and strawberries), walked, shot, golfed and fished. A full, well-spent life.

MURPHY, Michael

Limerick Surgeon

b. 1917, Cork, son of Mary and Joe Murphy; a brother, Barry, is a retired gastroenterologist
Educ. University College Cork
m. 1946: Nuala (physiotherapist); 1 s (Stephen, a paediatric gastroenterologist), 3 d (Gillian, a dermatologist; Michelle, a dentist; Deirdre, a social worker)

MB, UCC, 1937; FRCS Ed, 1944

Trained at Mansfield District General Hospital 1938–44 (with E. Nichol and Mr Millward. Mansfield was the heart of coalmining country and Nicholl fundamentally changed the management of compression fractures of the vertebrae, calling on his vast experience of mining injuries).
Major, Royal Army Medical Corps, 1944–48.
Consultant general surgeon, Mansfield District General Hospital, 1948–56.
Consultant surgeon, Limerick Regional Hospital, 1956–82.

Matriculating at 15, Michael Murphy went straight to UCC and qualified while still not 21. As was the norm at the time, he went straight to England and Mansfield, where he was quickly appreciated. While in the Royal Army Medical Corps, he was posted firstly to Moira in Northern Ireland and then to Berlin, where his duties included checking the health of prominent prisoners of war in Spandau Prison. These included Admiral Erich Raeder, Walter Funk (former Minister of Finance) and Admiral Karl Donitz (briefly German head of state, 1945).

In Limerick, he quickly built up the hospital's Surgical Gastroenterology Department ('Mick the Knife'). He was a highly skilled operator, completely ambidextrous, including tying knots with either hand, and enjoyed teaching undergraduates and trainees. A talented administrator (the RAMC experience was not wasted), he was a member of Comhairle na nOspidéal for years and became a full-time 'surgeon in charge' for four years, 1978–82.

Of distinguished appearance, he is a talented gardener, interested in music, photography and travel.

EGAN, Thomas Joseph Mary (Joe)

Limerick Surgeon

b. 1929, The Commons, Co. Tipperary, fourth child and second son of Thomas Egan and Kathleen Egan (*née* Wall)
Educ. Rockwell College, Co. Tipperary; University College Galway
m. 1964: Patricia Ann Finn of Mallow, Co. Cork; 3 d (Margaret Ann is specialist registrar in cardiology), 1 s
d. 1999

MB, NUI, UCG, 1954; FRCSI, 1961; MRCPI, 1965; FRCS Canada, 1969; FRCPI, 1973; President & Fellow, International College of Angiology, USA

Postgraduate appointment as registrar, St Kevin's (now St James's) Hospital (with Hugh McCarthy).
Surgeon, Walwyn Hospital, Newfoundland, 1969–70; St John's General Hospital, Newfoundland, 1970–74.
Surgeon, Limerick Regional Hospital, 1974–96; chief, Surgery Department, 1984–96.
Lecturer in surgery, UCC.
Comhairle na nOspidéal.

Special interests were vascular and thoracic surgery.

Joe Egan was a keen teacher and followed the careers of his junior staff. He introduced day surgery to Limerick and specialised, where he did at all, in thoracic, vascular and thyroid work. He was a dedicated operating surgeon well able for long hours at the table.

A Rowing Blue at UCG, Joe later enjoyed skiing, cycling and jogging. He had an abiding intellectual curiosity, with a fascination for philosophy and history. He enjoyed music, art, and travel. It was in Nigeria that he met his future wife. He brought his family to work in Canada twice. Despising golf, he was a gold-standard armchair gardener, achieving unheard-of levels of inertia while practising this avocation. He loved company and was an inventive storyteller, particularly of the 'shaggy dog' genre. He had also a dangerous wit.

Tall (5'11"), broad-chested (rowing), blue eyed, with dark short hair and receding hairline, bespectacled, fit and trim, he was calm under pressure and good at keeping up hospital morale.

DELANEY, Peter Vincent

Limerick Surgeon

b. 1936, youngest son of Peter Delaney and Lillian Delaney (*née* O'Reilly)
Educ. O'Connell's School, Dublin; University College Dublin
m. 1965: Mary O'Loughlin, daughter of Patrick and Ethel O'Loughlin; 1 s (Conor, colorectal surgeon, Cleveland, Ohio), 4 d (Miriam is MRCPI)
d. 2002

MB (hons), UCD, 1964; BSc (hons), UCD, 1966; FRCSI, 1968; MCh, UCD, 1969.

Postgraduate positions as house physician and house surgeon, Mater Hospital, Dublin; senior house officer to surgical registrar, Mater Hospital (Eoin O'Malley [q.v.], FX O'Connell [q.v.], Seán Heffernan [q.v.]), 1966–69; surgical registrar, General Hospital, Leicester (J. B. Self, R. K. Greenwood), 1969–71; clinical assistant and resident surgical officer, St Mark's Hospital, London (Sir Hugh Lockhart-Mummery, Sir Alan Parks), 1972–73; senior registrar and tutor in surgery, Mater Hospital, Dublin, 1973–75.
Consultant surgeon, General Hospital, Castlebar, Co. Mayo, 1975–76.
Senior lecturer, Department of Surgery, TCD and St James's Hospital, 1976–79.
Consultant general and colorectal surgeon, Regional Hospital, Limerick, 1979–2002.
Member, Council, RCSI, 1985–97.
Examiner for Royal Colleges of Surgeons, Ireland, Edinburgh, Glasgow and England. Founder of Sylvester O'Halloran Surgical Meeting, Limerick, 1993.
Inaugural President's Medal, University of Limerick.

Peter Delaney brought academic surgery to Limerick. His successor (the graceful Pierce Grace) was given a Chair, and the University of Limerick has established a medical school, beginning with a graduate intake. This happened, at least in part, because Peter established a research laboratory to study the molecular biology of colon cancer. He founded the Mid-Western Development Trust to encourage local generosity and investment. It, in turn, procured major hospital equipment for the region. He built up a postgraduate centre and raised the funds to house it. From this start, the University sponsored a National Institute of Health Science and the appointment of medical academics. He was awarded the University's first President's Medal in 2002.

He loved music and had taken all eight grades, with honours, at Trinity College of Music, London. He played tennis at inter-provincial level, was many times club champion at Glasnevin Tennis Club, Dublin, and captained the UCD tennis team. He won an all-Ireland hurling medal with Dublin and was a natural golfer.

Surgery was his life but he was a dedicated family man. He is remembered as 'a generous, gentle, warm, kind, good, religious man of vision and a faithful friend and colleague'. Of medium height, spare build, wiry and tireless, he had a great desire to give something back to surgery. He made a difference. This is high praise in Ireland.

13
CARDIAC SURGERY IN THE REPUBLIC OF IRELAND

Mr Maurice Neligan

CARDIAC SURGERY IN THE REPUBLIC OF IRELAND

Writing history is, for a non-historian, a challenging and onerous task. The allocation of 'firsts' and/or primacy, in this field or that, has always seemed to me to be detached from the progression of the core issue.

I am well aware that somebody may produce 'well-authenticated' cases of open-heart surgery amongst the Fianna or the Tuatha De Danann, but I feel if such were found to exist, that they were hardly planned as therapeutic. I shall accordingly restrict myself to describing the speciality in the Republic, how it started and how it developed. In this I am fortunate, as the development of cardiac surgery has been contemporaneous with my lifetime, and I have been privileged in knowing personally very many of the pioneers, both here and abroad.

Cardiac surgery is one of the later surgical disciplines and really commenced its growth period only in the 1950s, with the understanding that the correction of cardiac abnormalities, both internally and externally, was best achieved in a bloodless field and with a motionless heart.

The surgeons had first dealt with some congenital conditions such as patent ductus arteriosus (1938) and coarctation of the aorta (1944). The first attempts were then made to apply surgical solutions to acquired heart disease, both valvular and ischaemic. All of this was made possible by the great advances in anaesthesia, including the advent of positive pressure ventilation and endotracheal intubation. The name of the German surgeon Sauerbruch, and also those of Magill, Rowbotham (two anaesthetists) and Janeway were to the fore in these advances.

In Ireland, as in many smaller, poor, countries outside the mainstream, surgeons watched new developments with great interest. Here as elsewhere, the specialty developed on a rather ad hoc basis, with many institutions and surgeons involved and doing limited amounts of closed cardiac surgery. The majority of these surgeons were generalists and coupled the new discipline with already onerous operating schedules. Trained thoracic surgeons were few; Maurice Hickey [q.v.] in Cork, Keith Shaw [q.v.] in Dublin, and Des Kneafsey [q.v.] in Galway were amongst the first. Maurice Hickey performed the first mitral valvotomy in Ireland in St Kevin's Hospital, Dublin, in 1949. Hickey it was who performed the first series of closures of hole in the heart (closure of atrial septal defect) in the country, in ten consecutive patients, in the unsophisticated ambience of St Finbarr's Hospital, Cork. The majority were general surgeons with varying interest in the new discipline: Eoin O'Malley [q.v.], TCJ (Bob) O'Connell [q.v.], W. A. L. McGowan [q.v.], Jack Coolican [q.v.], amongst others. Bob O'Connell had a world first in doing a successful mitral valvotomy on a woman in labour.

In the US, the surgical landscape had changed in 1952, when, in Minneapolis, Dr C. Walton Lillehei and Dr John Lewis performed the first successful correction of an intracardiac defect at the University of Minnesota, using the technique of moderate hypothermia, in which the patient was cooled in a bath and cooling blanket to a surface temperature of 28°C. This gave a period of 7–8 minutes in which the heart could safely be stopped. Given the inexactitude of diagnostic methods at the time, many surgeons grew prematurely old within this time limit, and results left much to be desired. However, in 1953, in Philadelphia, Dr John Gibbon had reported successful surgery using his prototype pump oxygenator. He himself abandoned the technique, disappointed by subsequent results. In the Mayo Clinic, the man now regarded by most as the Father of Cardiac Surgery, Dr John Kirklin, seized the torch and carried it forward. Using a modification of Dr Gibbon's machine, he had a stream of successful procedures and thus the specialty was truly born.

The world, especially its medical component, took notice. Ireland was no different. Some rationalisation of the units that had dabbled before was obviously necessary. These had included the Mater, St Vincent's, Baggot Street, Mercer's, Sir Patrick Dun's and St Kevin's in Dublin, as well as the children's hospitals, Our Lady's, Crumlin, and Temple Street. St Stephen's Hospital in Cork, Merlin Park in Galway, Ardkeen in Waterford and Ripley-like, 'Believe or Not', Castlerea Sanatorium in Roscommon were also sites. In the middle and late 1960s, there was a small, successful series of closures of atrial septal defects in children under moderate hypothermia at Our Lady's Hospital for Sick Children, with Barry O'Donnell [q.v.] as surgeon and W. S. (Bill) Wren [q.v.] as anaesthetist. Pulmonary valvotomies were carried out there with cardiac arrest at normotherma, which gave the surgeon just three minutes to split the congenitally narrowed valve under direct vision.

The new specialty of open-heart surgery, with its dedicated teams of surgeons, anaesthetists, perfusionists and nurses, on the one hand, and full-time cardiologists on the other, mandated change. When did change ever come easily in Irish medicine? This was no exception, and reason and inescapable logic were sometimes conspicuously absent. Eventually the field narrowed to those institutions that could maintain such teams on a more permanent basis and that, more importantly, selected the appropriate technique for the task ahead. The Baggot Street team, led by Keith Shaw, initially favoured the so-called Drew technique, in which the patient's own lungs acted as the oxygenator. It was difficult and time-consuming and was soon abandoned. The team in the Mater, led by Professor Eoin O'Malley, preferred the Kirklin and Melrose modifications of the original machine. This was the key decision and developments soon vindicated Eoin O'Malley's choice. Ultimately, many moons later, it led to the Mater becoming the National Cardiac Surgical Centre. It quickly and painfully grew in experience.

I well remember the intensity of those times which formed my resolution to metamorphose from medical student to cardiac surgeon. I recall the professional rivalry. I remember the successes and the failures and the ever-changing field, as weekly there came new equipment and new techniques. At that stage, we had reduced to the Mater and Baggot Street, with paediatric work in Crumlin. Sporadic cases were undertaken in Cork and Galway. In the late 1960s, preliminary discussions took place between the Mater and Baggot Street, principally involving Eoin O'Malley and Keith Shaw, concerning cooperation in the specialty and the sharing of resources, techniques and personnel.

The author became one of the earliest embodiments of this venture as, on my return from my senior registrar position in England, I worked in both hospitals with the respective teams. The then Department of Health was supportive of such reorganisation and provided resources to construct a new cardiac surgical theatre block in the Mater. This opened in 1971 and the Baggot Street team, led by Mr Keith Shaw and with Dr David Hogan as anaesthetist, moved their cardiac surgical commitment to this site. They brought with them two people who were fundamental to the growth and development of the specialty in Ireland. The late Mr Cliff Dawson and the late Mary O'Hara (*née* Slevin) took over the duties of perfusionists in the Mater and developed the service enthusiastically and rapidly. Their commitment was total and infectious. They were also instrumental in the development of the Society of Perfusionists of Great Britain and Ireland, whose second annual meeting was held in the Mater Hospital. Paul Keartland and Annette McCarthy in the Mater, Martin Hargrove in Cork, and Fritz Reiter in Blackrock were amongst the trainees who expanded the role. They now not only provide the technical expertise in heart surgery, but provide staff if required for liver transplantation in St Vincent's Hospital, extra corporeal membrane oxygenation (ECMO) in Crumlin and for isolated limb perfusion in cancer treatments. Two wonderful people, they left their legacy and standards with us.

With the development of the cardiac theatres and subsequently dedicated cardiac wards and a new intensive care unit, the discipline continued to grow. I joined the consultant staff in 1971 but almost immediately went on sabbatical to the United States. At this time, very large and incrementally growing numbers of patients with valvular heart disease, many consequential on earlier rheumatic fever, and indeed adults and older children with congenital heart disease, provided the bulk of the unit's work. Many of these patients were chronically ill with organ failure and damage resulting from long-term cardiac failure, and in common with other units worldwide; this initial exposure provided its share of disappointments and difficulties. More almost than any other surgical discipline, cardiac surgery involves major teamwork. The nursing strength of the Mater in all disciplines, theatre, ward and dedicated intensive care, stood the fledgling unit in good stead, both initially and right up to present days.

Anaesthesiology, so integral a part of modern surgery, was in this discipline and for many years represented by Dr David Hogan, Dr John R. McCarthy, Dr John Magner and Professor Denis Moriarty; without their selfless input and that of the many colleagues who worked with them and succeeded them, the development of the specialty to the level of excellence it maintains today would not have been possible.

Hindsight is a gentle mirror, reflecting the best of times. Reality faces the gruelling hard work, interminable hours and frequent disappointments of the early years.

The year 1974 saw the now National Cardiac Surgical Unit at the Mater take over the provision of a paediatric service at Our Lady's Hospital for Sick Children at Crumlin. The Mater provided the surgeon (the author), the anaesthetist (Professor Denis Moriarty), and the perfusion team. Apart from emergency work, cardiac operating lists were held twice weekly. Dr Bill Wren, Mrs Pauline Ward, wife of Professor O. C. Ward, the unit cardiologist and Sr Augustine established the Intensive Care Unit at Our Lady's, the latter two having travelled to London to take the intensive care course at Great Ormond Street Children's Hospital. For me, it was a ten-year stretch as sole provider before I was joined by Mr Freddie Wood. Now there are three surgeons, Mr Wood having been joined by Professor Mark Redmond and Mr Lars Nolke. All the most complex procedures in neonates and children are undertaken with internationally comparable results. At the time of writing deficiencies of access and staffing still remain, although with the redevelopment of the hospital these should be remedied.

The development of coronary angiography and subsequently coronary bypass surgery in the Cleveland Clinic ushered in a period of unprecedented and largely unforeseen demand for cardiac surgical services. The first such operations in the Mater Hospital took place in 1974, and the initial successes, coupled with the enhanced protection afforded to the heart during surgery by the then-new techniques of hypothermia, moved cardiac services into another era. The rapid expansion to over 1,000 cases per annum in the unit unfortunately coincided with national economic downturn and a failure to invest, leading to lengthy waiting lists with their harvests of misery and suffering. This fact, coupled with similar problems throughout the medical field, led directly to the development of, first, the Blackrock Clinic, in 1984, and shortly thereafter the Mater Private Hospital. These were the first private hospitals to provide high-technology services and both continue to expand and achieve excellent outcomes. Between them they account for in excess of 1,000 open-heart procedures annually.

The year 1986 saw the first heart transplant in the Mater, by the author and Freddy Wood, and this programme has grown over the years, albeit with the usual problem of transplant units — shortage of donors. In 2005, the first lung transplant was performed, and this programme also is expanding slowly and successfully. A separate transplant theatre, promised in 1999, has, however, not materialised and, as in so many aspects of health care, *mañana* seems to be the order of the day, and even this word conveys too much urgency compared with the reality.

The year 1986 saw the resumption of cardiac surgical services in Cork, with the establishment of a unit led by Mr Tom Ahern, previously a senior registrar in the Mater. Martin Hargrove, also from the Mater, moved to head the perfusion team. This unit now has three surgeons.

In 1999 a unit was provided in St James's Hospital in Dublin, with Ms Eilis McGovern as lead surgeon. This unit now has three surgeons; Mr David Luke, one of the original Baggot Street group, chose to stay with the National Unit in the Mater and contribute his great experience to the main unit. His skills and common sense over the years provided a rock of strength. A unit for Galway, a long time in gestation, finally opened in 2007, with two surgeons.

Ironically, despite all this late development, two factors emerged which lessened the demand for coronary artery surgery and other elements of the surgical treatment of ischaemic heart disease. Firstly there has been a decline in the morbidity and mortality from coronary arterial disease throughout the developed world over the past thirty or forty years. The aetiology of this decline remains unclear but it seems to have some parallels with the decline in the use of tobacco. Secondly the availability of angioplasty and stenting for the treatment of coronary artery obstruction has reduced the requirement for surgical intervention.

It is a fact that the surgery of heart disease, both for palliation and cure, has been one of the most significant advances in medical treatment in our time. The great steps were taken in the 1960s and 1970s. The present is a time of refinement. Valve reconstruction and repair saves many patients artificial valve replacement. Minimally invasive surgery lessens the patient impact in some procedures, and robotically delivered surgery has established itself in the surgical armamentarium.

Currently in the Republic we have surgeons covering all aspects of cardiac surgery, from the womb to extreme old age. In addition, we have trained or assisted in the training of many surgeons from all over the world. India, Pakistan, Bahrain, Bangladesh, Malaysia, Singapore, Iran, Egypt, Libya, Sudan, Nigeria, Kenya, Canada, USA, Jamaica and Spain all have surgeons who worked and learned here. We are proud of them.

In 2008, the specialty is in good hands, and dare I say it, in good heart. Eoin O'Malley's pioneering work is remembered eponymously in the National Unit in the Mater. The late Keith Shaw is similarly honoured in the unit in St James's. I think that both would agree with my observation that if those who followed where we led are not better than we were, we would be deemed to have failed. Looking today at the spectrum of Irish cardiac surgery, we did not fail.

CARDIOTHORACIC SURGEONS OF THE REPUBLIC OF IRELAND

HICKEY, Maurice Desmond

Pioneer Chest Surgeon, Cork and Dublin

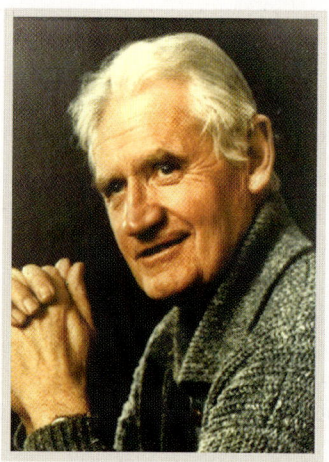

b. 1915, the fifth of 9 children of Maurice and Joan Hickey, Cork
Educ. Presentation College, Cork; Rochestown College, Co. Cork; University College Cork
m. 1945: Dr Mary Burke; 2 s, 2 d (3 doctors)
d. 2005

MB, UCC, 1941 (first class hons, Peel Memorial prize, Pearson medal for surgery, Blayney scholarship and bursary in surgery (open to all NUI graduates), Henry Hutchinson Stewart award in surgery); MCh, NUI, 1943; FRCS Ed, 1943

Postgraduate work: Nottingham City Hospital; Nottingham General Hospital; London Chest Hospital where he rose to become surgical first assistant (junior consultant). (As chief assistant, he worked with Vernon Thompson and (Sir) Thomas Holmes Sellors, the acknowledged master technician in chest surgery of his day, and who always asked other Irish surgeons, 'How is Maurice Hickey?')
First Local Authority cardiothoracic surgeon appointed in Ireland, 1948.

When he came to Dublin, trained to London standards, and in answer to an advertisement (which was a great rarity in those days), Maurice Hickey's talents were recognised by the then Minister of Health, Dr Noël Browne. The pair hit it off immediately and Browne gave instructions to the Department officials to 'give Mr Hickey whatever he wants'. Hickey operated on tuberculous, cancer and other patients throughout the country, spending two days each week in Dublin (St Mary's, Phoenix Park and Rialto Chest Hospital), two days in Cork and one day in the Castlerea Chest Hospital, Co. Roscommon. The Department of Health offered, but he did not accept, a chauffeur-driven car. This may well be a unique distinction. He worked anywhere there was an operating table, and his results set new standards.

He was the first in the country to operate successfully on a patient with mitral valve stenosis. This was carried out in what was then St Kevin's (now St James's) Hospital, in 1949.

His particular interest was congenital heart disease. When he transferred to Cork, he and his colleagues reported the first Irish series of successful closures of 'hole in the heart' in ten children. These operations were carried out in St Finbarr's Hospital, which at that time still had relatively modest facilities. He had a superb, symbiotic, relationship with the ever-genial, ever-competent Dr Desmond Gaffney, the chief anaesthetist. He subsequently worked in Sarsfield's Court Hospital in Glanmire, outside Cork, and eventually in Cork University Hospital. He was a master surgeon with flawless technique, and was West Cork Man of the Year in 1972.

Maurice Hickey was a genuine legend in his working lifetime. He was a larger than life figure with a most imposing appearance. Well over six foot tall, he was broad shouldered and always carefully groomed, with a trademark centre parting of his huge head of hair. He never baulked at any situation and thrived on the worst-case scenario. Nothing but the best was good enough for his patients; he gave them the closest possible attention. He was dogmatic, ruthless, not particularly popular with colleagues, and often rubbed people up the wrong way. However, he was a fervent Catholic and was very charitable about others. He did not make, nor did he seek to make, a lot of money in private practice.

He was an indulgent father who was greatly loved by his family. He loved the sea and, in retirement, he went to Baltimore, Co. Cork, where he sailed, fished and played golf.

Maurice was a man who profoundly changed much in his area of expertise for the better, and the people of Cork, with great insight and generosity, made him a Freeman of the City (the only surgeon ever), in 1992. This was undoubtedly the honour he treasured most, and it was so well deserved.

KNEAFSEY, Desmond Vincent (Des) PRCSI 1988–1990

Thoracic Surgeon, Galway and Ardkeen Hospital, Waterford

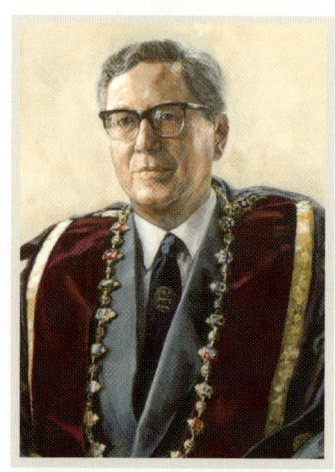

b. 1920

Educ. Royal College of Surgeons in Ireland, where he took many undergraduate prizes

m. Bernie; 1 s (Paul, pathologist, deceased), 1 d

d. 2002

FRCSI, 1948

Postgraduate training posts in St Laurence's, Dublin; Northampton General; Frenchay Hospital, Bristol. Appointments at St Mary's, Phoenix Park; Rialto Hospital, Dublin.
Consultant thoracic surgeon, Merlin Park Hospital, Galway; Ardkeen Hospital, Waterford, 1954.
Statutory lecturer, UCG.

A well-trained, skilful surgeon with apparently boundless energy, Des Kneafsey was one of the last of those with a huge experience of surgery for tuberculosis of the lung. Always emphasising standards, he was an excellent teacher. He had great empathy with patients. He would drive from Galway to Waterford (140 miles), do a huge operating list, and then drive home, all in the one day.

Personally he could be charming, irascible, highly argumentative and disarmingly discursive, and all within a few minutes. An extremely competitive sportsman, he was self-critical of much of his performances. He was an accomplished musician, and it speaks much for his popularity that his beloved guitar, 'Harvey', was made an Honorary Member of the Western Surgical Club.

The wavy hair remained dark to the end; he was 5'10", bespectacled, stooped from long hours at the operating table, broad shouldered, amusing and indefatigable.

LOGAN, Patrick John ('Paddy')

Dublin chest surgeon

b. 1923, eldest son of Patrick and Mary Logan of Mohill, Co. Leitrim
Educ. St Mel's College, Longford; University College Dublin
m. 1952: Maura McGuiness of Mohill, Co. Leitrim; 1 s (Mark, radiologist), 3 d (Máirín, radiographer; Patricia, ophthalmic surgeon; Brenda, public health nurse)
d. 1975

MB, UCD, 1950; LM 1951; FRCSI 1961.

Postgraduate posts in Derby, Blackburn, Wrightington Hospital (Wigan), County Hospital, Mullingar and Royal City of Dublin Hospital, Baggot Street, Dublin. Influenced by Prof. Dobson, Wrightington, Keith Shaw and Seton Pringle of Baggot Street.
Consultant surgeon, Baggot Street Hospital, Drumcondra Hospital. Clinical tutor, Trinity College, Dublin.

Paddy was a handsome, well-dressed west of Ireland man. He enjoyed the outdoors and outdoor pursuits. He fished, shot game and played golf at Newlands golf club. He loved animals and trained his gun dogs.

He was quiet and contemplative, taking his work very seriously and always with his patients' interests at heart. He is remembered for having had the 'common touch' and past patients and students still appear thirty-three years later with fond memories of him; former assistants recall him as a really fine operating surgeon who was easy to assist, a discerning accolade. He was very active in the St Vincent de Paul Society. He certainly would have been proud that all his children are working in medicine and in Ireland.

LYNCH, Vincent Patrick

Dublin Chest Surgeon

b. 1934, Belfast, only son of James Lynch and Elizabeth Lynch (*née* Nugent)
Educ. St Malachy's College, Belfast; Queen's University Belfast
m. 1974: Geraldine O'Halloran, daughter of William and Margaret O'Halloran; 2s, 1 d

MB, QUB, 1960; FRCS Ed, 1964; FRCSI (*ad eundem*)

Postgraduate appointments as intern and senior house officer, Belfast City Hospital; demonstrator in anatomy, QUB; registrar in cardiothoracic surgery, RVH, 1964–65; registrar general in surgery, RVH, 1966–68; registrar in surgery, Our Lady's Hospital for Sick Children, Crumlin, Dublin, 1966–68; senior resident in cardiothoracic research, Mayo Clinic, Rochester, Minnesota, 1968–70; lecturer in cardiac surgery, Royal London Medical School; first assistant, Royal London Hospital, 1970.
Registrar and tutor, St Laurence's (Richmond) Hospital (with Prof. W. A. L. MacGowan [q.v.]); registrar, Jervis Street Hospital, (human kidney transplants with Mr Peter McLean[q.v.]). Consultant cardiovascular and thoracic surgeon, St Vincent's Hospital, and Dublin Federated Group of Hospitals, 1975–99; left cardiac surgery in 1977 and continued as a pure thoracic surgeon.
President, Irish Surgical Travellers Club, 1984.

Co-authored many papers relating to lungs, mediastinum, cardiovascular system, and oesophagus and tumour cell culture.

Vincent Lynch has been continuously involved in research, from 1966 to the present. He was involved in experimental transplantation of heart and liver and was the first ever to transplant the oesophagus successfully. At the Mayo Clinic, with the legendary Dr 'Bunky' Ellis, he reproduced Barrett's oesophagus in dogs. He also had a huge series of mediastinoscopies. He worked with Prof. Martin Clynes at the National Cell and Tissue Culture Centre at Dublin City University, now a large unit with over fifty full-time scientists. He stayed on as clinical adviser when he retired from surgery.

A natural speedy, but careful, operating surgeon, he has been entrusted with the care of many of his colleagues. He was one of the few in these islands to remain a purely chest surgeon and he had a large referral practice.

He has also been active in trying to bring peace to Northern Ireland and was a 1984 founding member and later chairman of Conciliation Ireland. He played hurling at QUB, and now goes hill-walking and jogging, does some gardening and has trained as a basketball coach.

Tall, loose limbed, open, affable, charming and concerned, he can go from smiling to serious and back again quite quickly; a really acute intelligence is just under the soft surface.

NELIGAN, Maurice Christopher ('Maurice')

Cardiac Surgeon

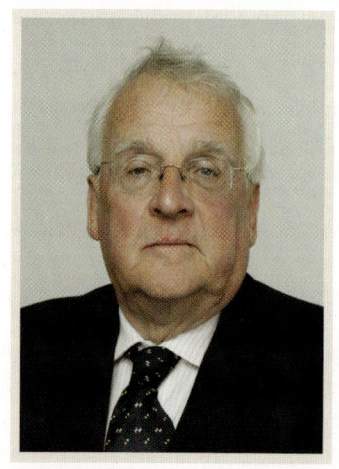

b. 1937, Dublin
Educ. Willow Park School; Blackrock College, Dublin; University College Dublin
m. Patricia O'Brien, MB; 7 children (Maurice Fitzmaurice is a consultant orthopaedic surgeon at Tallaght Hospital, Dublin; Sara, SRN, d. 2007)

MB, UCD, 1962; BSc, UCD; FRCSI, 1966

Postgraduate training as surgical registrar, Mater Hospital, Dublin; senior registrar (cardiothoracic), Queen Elizabeth Hospital, Birmingham (with Leon Abrams).
Consultant cardiac surgeon, Mater Hospital; Our Lady's Hospital for Sick Children, Crumlin, Dublin; Blackrock Clinic, to 2002.

One of the first fully fledged 'new era' cardiac surgeons to begin work in Dublin, Maurice had been selected by Professor Eoin O'Malley [q.v.] for further training in cardiac surgery in Birmingham and was well prepared for the snowballing of the discipline that occurred when obstructed coronary arteries began to be treated by putting in vein grafts. A man of great energy and drive, with huge populist appeal, he recruited a strong team to deal with the expansion. During a heroic surgical career of more than thirty years, he did 18,000 cardiac operations, mostly coronary artery bypass procedures, using the heart lung machine, 'the pump'. Probably nobody in these islands has done this number and, because much of what was surgical is now treated in a less invasive way, it seems that nobody ever will. He launched a free-to-all heart transplant programme in the Blackrock Clinic, a private hospital where he was a substantial foundation shareholder and where he worked until he retired. He seldom published scientific articles outside the country and as a result he has rarely been asked to speak from platforms abroad. They missed something special.

To the Irish public, because of his frequent appearances on TV shows, and the huge number of patients nationwide on whom he has carried out life-saving surgery, he is easily the most recognisable surgeon in the country. He was and is an outspoken tribune of the people in campaigning for more resources to be made available for patients. He has never run for office within the wider profession but he writes a regular, polemic column, sometimes almost a 'data-free zone', in the Health Supplement of Tuesday's *Irish Times*, in which he draws attention, in a colourful manner, to the foibles and failings of various government agencies. The health service, the state of the roads, traffic lights, the helicopter services and the management of the broader economy continue as targets. The country he describes is not always recognisable to all of his readers but he continues to generate a loyal readership. When, in the summer of 2007, his daughter Sara, an intensive care nurse, was brutally murdered, he received over 12,000 messages of condolence, including letters from the President, the Taoiseach and his peppered target, the Minister for Health. This is some measure of his standing in the eyes of the people.

Perhaps 5'11", with massive shoulders, he has great reserves of stamina. He played rugby in his youth and is now a big hitter of the golf ball in Portmarnock and at his holiday home in Dooks, Co. Kerry. A really amusing, well-read, knowledgeable companion with a marked sense of irony and humour. A surgical icon of our times.

O'NEILL, Brendan

Dublin Thoracic Surgeon

b. ?1913
Educ. University College Cork

MB, UCC, 1936; MCh, NUI, 1940; FRCSI, 1942

Worked at St Mary's in the Park (Phoenix Park); St Kevin's Hospital, Rialto
Member (Chairman), Irish Surgical Travellers Club.

Brendan O'Neill is remembered as a safe, rapid surgeon who had a big experience of lobectomy for tuberculosis and bronchiectasis.

SHAW, Keith Meares PRCSI 1978–1980

Dublin Chest and Cardiac Surgeon

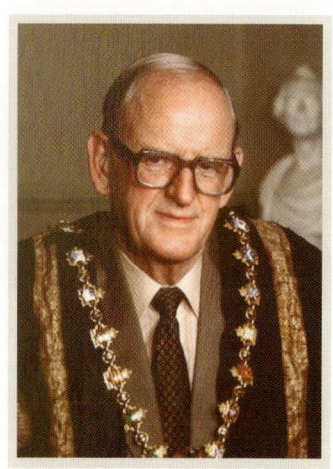

b. 1919, Dublin, son of William and Anne Shaw
m. Dorothy ('Dot') May, daughter of Mr and Mrs A. Poignand of Jersey, Channel Islands; 1 s
d. 2001

MB, TCD, 1942; MD, TCD, 1953; FRCSI, 1945; MCh (*hon. causa*)

Postgraduate junior posts at the Adelaide Hospital, Dublin; West Kent General Hospital; Grantham Hospital; resident surgical officer at Preston Royal Infirmary; surgical first assistant, London Chest Hospital (to Sir Thomas Holmes Sellors, the finest chest technician of his time and who always asked after Keith, Vernon Thompson and Russell C. Brock, subsequently Lord Brock); St George's and Colindale Hospitals.
Surgical specialist, Royal Army Medical Corps, 1847–1949.
Surgeon, Royal City of Dublin Hospital, Baggot Street Hospital.
Thoracic surgeon, National Children's Hospital; Dublin Corporation; Adelaide Hospital; Meath Hospital; Mater Hospital; Sir Patrick Dun's Hospital.
Lecturer in thoracic surgery, TCD.
World Health Organisation Fellowships, 1966 and 1973

Keith Shaw developed a department of experimental surgery in TCD and worked on the development of cardiac bypass ('the pump oxygenator') before carrying out the first successful open-heart operation, under heart lung bypass, in Ireland, in 1960. He developed his unit at Baggot Street Hospital under the most severe of constraints. His subsequent fusion with Professor Eoin O'Malley [q.v.] and appointment to the Mater Hospital heart unit was a turning point in the development of cardiac surgery in Dublin. The dedication of the unit at St James's Hospital as the Keith Shaw Cardio-vascular Unit is a worthy tribute to his achievements by those who knew him best, his trainees. He was a first-rate colleague and a really competent chairman.

Tall (6'2"), slim, quietly spoken (except in the cauldron of the operating theatre), this charming man was the first fully trained cardiac surgeon to come back to Dublin, and his skills, when translated into fine results, made a huge difference to the professional and public perception of the specialty.

He enjoyed golf, gardening, fishing, bridge and sailing.

14
NEUROSURGEONS IN THE REPUBLIC OF IRELAND

NEUROSURGEONS IN THE REPUBLIC OF IRELAND

BUCKLEY, Timothy Francis ('Ted')

Cork Neurosurgeon

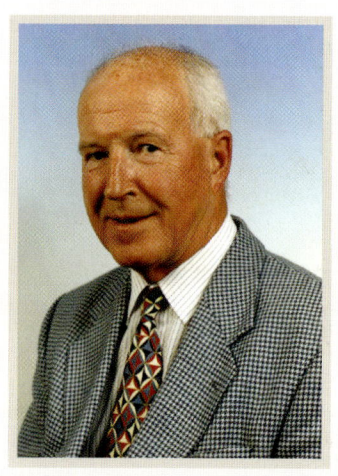

b. 1935, Millstreet, Co. Cork, second son of Timothy Buckley and Anna Sullivan (*née* O'Sullivan)
Educ. Sullivan's Quay, CBS, Cork; University College Cork
m. 1962: Maeve Ryle, daughter of Thomas and Maud Ryle; 5 d (Deirdre a dermatologist)

MB (first class honours), UCC, 1959; MD, NUI, 1970; FRCS, 1963; FRCSI (*ad eundem*) 1980.

Training posts: St Finbarr's Hospital, Cork; North Middlesex Hospital London; registrar in general surgery, Churchill Hospital, Oxford, 1962–64; researcher in neuroanatomy, University of Oregon, Portland, Oregon, USA, 1964–65.

House surgeon, registrar and senior registrar, neurological surgery, Radcliffe Infirmary, Oxford, 1965–68; senior registrar, neurosurgery, Royal Infirmary, Manchester, 1968–70.
Consultant neurosurgeon, Liverpool Region, 1970–71.
Consultant neurosurgeon, St Finbarr's Hospital; Cork Regional Hospital, 1971–2000. Lecturer in neurosurgery, UCC.
Honorary Professor, University of Santo Domingo, Dominican Republic, 1984.
Member, Medical Council, 1999–2004 (Chairman, Fitness to Practice Commission).

Influenced by John Kelly [q.v.], Cork; Joe Pennybacker and John Potter, Oxford; and Richard Johnson, Manchester.

Ted Buckley brought modern neurosurgery to Cork where, with patience and tenacity, he built up a unit of international quality. Perhaps his biggest contribution was that he influenced six Cork graduates to become neurosurgeons and, at time of writing, there are more Cork graduates than Dublin graduates in neurosurgery, a remarkable tribute to his role-model status. Despite his best efforts, in the early years, there was not much collaboration with the established Dublin unit, where there was little tradition or interest in teaching local juniors, and the Cork graduates had to get much of their training in the UK. Dozens of others from the Third World received a major part of their training in Cork.

An oarsman and squash player in his youth, he is now a golfer, a sailor and a traveller, with a modest, retiring personality. Short, stocky, 'brainy', determined, Ted Buckley is hugely admired within the profession and is recognised as a man who made a big difference to his chosen specialty.

CAREY, Patrick Cyril Joseph (Paddy)

Dublin Neurosurgeon

b. 1920, Dublin, son of a GP who moved to London shortly after Paddy's birth
Educ. St Joseph's Academy, Blackheath, London; Douai Benedictine Abbey, near Reading; University College Dublin
m. Breda
d. 1993

MB, 1944, UCD; MCh, NUI, 1950; Hon. FRCSI, 1976

Postgraduate appointments as intern, Mater Hospital, Dublin and Royal Infirmary, Leicester; surgical registrar, Mater Hospital, Dublin; registrar, neurosurgery, Salford Royal Hospital, and Royal Manchester Children's Hospital, for five years; senior surgical registrar, National Hospital for Nervous Diseases, Queen Square, London.
Neurosurgeon, St Laurence's (Richmond) Hospital, Dublin, 1959–85; Mater Hospital, Paraplegic Unit; National Rehabilitation Centre, Dún Laoghaire.
Lecturer in neurosurgery, RCSI.
President of the Irish Neurological Association.

In 1945, Paddy joined the Irish Red Cross surgical staffing at St Lo, Normandy, in the company of Dr Alan Thompson, Surgeon Freddie McKee [q.v.] and the storekeeper/ambulance driver Samuel Beckett. It was there that he met his future wife Breda. He introduced to Dublin stereotactic surgery for Parkinson's disease and microsurgical repair of cerebral aneurysms. He was one of the first to perform epilepsy surgery and the surgical decompression and bone grafting for paraplegia complicating Potts (tuberculous) Caries of the spine.

For a short time, he was the only consultant neurosurgeon in the unit as there were unfortunate delays in making replacement appointments. There had been a series of, mostly overseas, assistants but no real training programme. He carried out a crushing operating schedule, often at the operating table five days a week. A heavy smoker (one on either side of the mouth before a posterior fossa tumour exploration), he epitomised nervous energy.

He enjoyed gardening, horse racing and fishing. Sadly a couple of years before retirement, he developed visual problems, which eventually resulted in total blindness.

DONOVAN, Patrick Feargus (Feargus)

Dublin Neurosurgeon

b. 1919, Darjeeling, India, second of 4 children of John Thomas Donovan (Indian Civil Service, CIE Barrister-at-Law) and Sara Donovan (*née* Devane; sister of John Devane, grandee father of Limerick surgery); sister Deirdre an anaesthetist and brother, the late Desmond, beloved paediatrician, Galway

Educ. Governess in India; Hodder Preparatory School; Stonyhurst College, Lancashire; University College Dublin (entrance scholarship in Classics, 1937; medical scholarship every year)

m. 1st in 1951: Claire Ouellette (d. 1963), daughter of Hermas Ouellette and Alda (*née* Perrier); 2 d (Denise, academic public health physician, Sherbrooke, Ontario; Estrie m. in Sherbrooke)

d. 2002

MB, UCD, 1942 (first class hons, McArdle prize and O'Ferrall gold medal); FRCSI, 1946; MCh, NUI, 1947.

House surgeon, St Vincent's Hospital, Dublin; Guy's Hospital London.
Surgeon-Lieutenant, Royal Naval Volunteer Reserve, 1944–45 ('cruising the Mediterranean at His Majesty's expense', but later hit a mine).
Surgical registrar, Jervis Street Hospital, 1945–46; assistant surgeon to John Devane [q.v.], St John's and Barrington's Hospitals, Limerick; senior registrar (to Prof Ian Aird), British Postgraduate Medical School, Hammersmith, London, 1946–47.
Assistant Professor of Surgery, University of Ottawa, Canada, 1947–51.
Fellow in Neurosurgery, Mayo Clinic Foundation, Rochester, Minnesota, USA, 1952–55.
Neurosurgeon, St Vincent's Hospital; Children's Hospital, Temple Street, Dublin, 1955–84.
EEG consultant, St Vincent's Hospital, 1984–96.
Lecturer in neurosurgery, UCD.

Feargus Donovan started the Neurosurgical Department at St Vincent's Hospital, then still in converted Georgian houses in St Stephen's Green. He built up a splendid unit with a national reputation for excellence. His ward was named after the founder of the Order, the Mother Mary *Aikenhead* ward, a nominal conjunction which did not escape the new arrival. He was the invincible combination of a hugely talented intelligence with a superlative training, and it showed.

He was dedicated, precise and known for causing the minimum of tissue damage and blood loss. He was the major national resource for the treatment of spinal dysraphism. Perhaps the nurses enjoyed him more than the surgical trainees who did not see him as a role model. Always up to date with the literature and practice, he was one of the first in Dublin to employ the operating microscope, which revolutionised neurosurgery. Sadly he had made no plans for succession. He felt it to be none of his business, though there were those who felt otherwise. The upshot was that there were no young, trained Irish neurosurgeons available for appointment in the early and mid-1980s. Despite his best efforts and those of his talented colleague, Chris Pidgeon, who joined him in 1978, the unit closed after he retired. He maintained his subscriptions to his medical journals in retirement — a typical touchstone of a surgeon's obsession.

Feargus loved sailing and boats. He was a superb photographer, always appropriately illustrating his lectures. He cycled well into his seventies. A family member described him as 'tall, slim, handsome, dapper with an acerbic wit'. His interest in punctuation pursued him to the end. He passed away with a 'semi-colon'.

LANIGAN, John Paul (Johnny) PRCSI 1970–1972

Dublin Neurosurgeon

b. 1915, Dublin, son of John Lanigan (Kilkenny solicitor) and Katherine Lanigan (*née* Lean) of Dungannon

Educ. Our Lady's Bower, Athlone; St Gerard's School, Bray; Royal College of Surgeons in Ireland

m. 1st: Nancy Egan (died in childbirth, 1950); 1 s (Dr Patrick, qualified RCSI community physician, Kilkenny, 1973), 2nd: Dr Mary Dunworth (anaesthetist), 1 d (Jane, solicitor)

LRCP & SI, 1938; FRCSI, 1941; FRCSI (Hon.), 1994 (a rare honour for a surgeon)

Postgraduate junior posts: Richmond Hospital; demonstrator in anatomy, RCSI.
Consultant neurosurgeon, Richmond Hospital; Mercer's Hospital; Rotunda Hospital; National Children's Hospital; St Ultan's Hospital; British Ministry of Pensions, 1945–83.
PRCSI, 1970–72.

Johnny Lanigan gave a massive commitment to his patients and he developed tuberculosis in 1950, which took a year to resolve. For many years, he was the only neurosurgeon in the country. He served the patients devotedly but it was a situation which should not have been allowed to occur.

Of middle height and balding, he was a careful operator with a mild disarming manner, and a great colleague.

McCONNELL, Adams Andrew (Adams A) PRCSI 1936–1938

Dublin Neurosurgeon

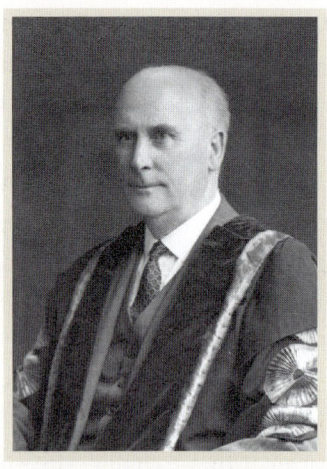

b. 1884, Lisburn, Co. Antrim, son of Dr Andrew McConnell and Margaret McConnell (*née* Adams)
Educ. Royal Belfast Academical Institute, Trinity College, Dublin
m. 1st in 1914: Nora Boyd (d. 1968); 2nd: Gladys Danesfield; no children
d. 1972

MB (first place), TCD, 1909; FRCSI, 1911, Hon. Fellow, TCD, 1956

Junior training posts at Sir Patrick Dun's Hospital. Assistant surgeon, Richmond Hospital, 1911; surgeon, 1914.
Council member, RCSI, 1923–26; again 1930; President, RCSI, 1936–38.
Professor of Surgery, RCSI, 1926–29.
Regius Professor of Surgery, TCD, 1946–61.
Founder member (later President), Society of British Neurological Surgeons.
President, RAMI, 1946–47.
Chairman, Board of Governors, St Laurence's (Richmond) Hospital, 1943–58.

Published many papers, particularly on operative techniques and management of head injury.

Although acting as a general surgeon, McConnell was already interested in neurological surgery and when Dandy introduced ventriculography, in 1918, McConnell was the first surgeon outside the USA to use this diagnostic technique. He presented a paper on the subject to the Association of Surgeons of Great Britain and Ireland, in 1920.

On a working visit to the United States in 1923, he spent time with both Harvey Cushing in Boston and Walter Dandy at Johns Hopkins. He brought back from the US a Hudson Brace for use as a trephine. Many surgeons had invented trephines, all claiming that his was the fastest to get into the cranial cavity. Up to perhaps 1950, many unconscious head-injury patients had trephining as the only available intervention. If there was an extra dural haemorrhage, it could be life saving. Sometimes it relieved intracranial pressure and the patient improved. If the patient improved, the trephining, and the surgeon, got the credit. If not, well, it was a bad brain injury. Much of the time it conferred no real benefit.

One of his most important contributions was the number and quality of his assistants. They included A. K. Henry, A. B. Clery [q.v.], Shalto Douglas (who became a brilliant radiologist) and Colman Byrnes [q.v.]. All admired his surgical skills. Indeed, all who worked with him said that he was a superb operating surgeon and an outstanding teacher. He was a strict disciplinarian and an unyielding antagonist. Promising trainees were not retained. He was the unquestioned 'Father of Irish Neurosurgery' and one of the few Irish surgeons with a genuinely international reputation. The unit achieved international status largely as a result of his drive, foresight and skills. It is a wonderful heritage of a great man.

In the early days of the Richmond Hospital-based neurosurgical unit, there was inevitably a high mortality and a significant number of death notices in the press included the ominous words 'at the Richmond Hospital'. The other surgeons at the hospital felt that it was becoming a reflection on their work and the relatives of the deceased neurosurgery patients were asked to put in the words 'at a Dublin hospital' instead of naming the Richmond. Thenceforth, whenever 'at a Dublin hospital' appeared in a death notice, the doctors of Dublin chorused, 'That's the Richmond.'

He continued to visit the Neurosurgical Department at the Richmond Hospital into his eighties and the neurosurgical operating list continued to include his name, although he had long since given up surgery. To the very end, the Department of Neurosurgery notepaper listed the three consultant surgeons, but the top billing, and this really included billing, was 'A. A. McConnell to whom all correspondence should be addressed'. He died in the Richmond Hospital in 1972, aged 88.

PATE, Alexander Roberts ('Sandy')

MB, Glas, 1952; FRCS, Glas, 1962
Assistant in neurosurgery, Richmond Hospital, 1964.

SAYED, Kamaludeen ('Kamal')

Dublin Neurosurgeon and Surgeon Prosector RCSI

b. 1934, India, eldest son of Aminoodin and Kamilla Sayed
Educ. Johannesburg High School for Boys (first in class and scholarship to RCSI); RCSI
m. 1961: Monica Bonnie, Dublin (musician); 1 s; 3 d (Camilla, ENT surgeon; Jacintha, occupational health physician; Safia, GP)
d. 2006

LRCP&SI, 1960; FRCSI, 1972

Postgraduate senior house officer, Wexford; registrar, paediatric surgery, Our Lady's Hospital for Sick Children, Crumlin, Dublin; registrar in orthopaedics Navan (Willie de Witt) 1963–1967, registrar in general surgery, Navan (Ruari Lavelle) 1967–71.
Assistant neurosurgeon, St Laurence's Hospital, Dublin 1971–86; medical director and chief of neurosurgery, King Fahad Hospital, Kingdom of Saudi Arabia 1986–92; surgeon prosector, RCSI, 1997–2006.

He was an excellent technical surgeon with a real interest in its craft and its art. Kamal deputised for his teacher John Lanigan while he was President of the RCSI for two years, and he was sometimes the only neurosurgeon on duty in the country. At all times he gave a mature, considered opinion. He had a great intellect, integrity, trustworthiness and common sense. His approach to anatomy was practical and hugely appreciated by all the students, particularly those from abroad to whom he spoke in their own language.

Six foot three, he had a surgeon's stoop and a splendid handsome appearance. As a student he excelled in rowing and cricket. He loved military music. His own roses were proudly displayed in his buttonhole. Philosophical to the end, he battled his worsening emphysema with humour and bonhomie.

He is remembered with great affection in the RCSI who have created an anatomy prize in the joint names of him and Sean Hanson — the Sayed Hanson Memorial Medal. No one deserves it more.

15
OBSTETRICIANS AND GYNAECOLOGISTS

Dr John F. Murphy and Barry O'Donnell

OBSTETRICIANS AND GYNAECOLOGISTS

INTRODUCTION

BACKGROUND

At the beginning of the twentieth century, Ireland, especially Dublin, was noted for a high standard of obstetric practice. In Dublin at that time, as at present, there were three large maternity hospitals: the Rotunda, founded in 1746; the Coombe, founded in 1826; the National Maternity Hospital, just six years old in 1900. It is worth examining the foundation of these hospitals as so much concerning the practice of obstetrics and gynaecology developed from them and their associated general hospitals and universities.

Bartholomew Mosse (1712–59) founded the Rotunda Hospital in 1746 as a charitable institute for the relief of poor women in childbirth. Mosse was a man of unique energy, compassion, foresight and skill. Following his establishment of the Rotunda and its initial success in small premises, he engaged the famous architect, Richard Cassells (1690–1751), to design a large hospital building, which, while considerably expanded, to this day houses the activity of that famous hospital. Mosse instituted the concept of the Mastership system, which has served the practice of obstetrics and gynaecology so well and which was copied as the administrative structure of the two other hospitals. He decreed that the Mastership should be for seven years.

The second Dublin maternity hospital, the Coombe Lying-In Hospital, the name to be changed towards the end of the twentieth century to the Coombe Women's Hospital, was founded by a benefactress to look after the poor women on the southside of the Liffey. Hilary Boyle came upon a woman lying dead in the snow; the woman had been in labour and trying to make her way to the

Rotunda Hospital. Hilary Boyle was so moved by this that she founded a hospital for the relief of labouring women. The Coombe Hospital, which has always enjoyed the support of the Earls of Meath and the Guinness family, had two locations until it settled into its present site in Dolphin's Barn, in 1967. At the turn of the century, the Coombe Hospital was delivering about 500 women each year. In the 1900 report, it is stated that special congratulations were due because of the low (maternal) mortality, with only two such deaths recorded.

The National Maternity Hospital, colloquially known as Holles Street, was founded in 1894 to serve the women in the south-eastern aspect of the city. The joint founders were Dr Patrick Barry and Dr, later Sir, Andrew Horne. Over the course of the twentieth century, it grew to be one of the busiest hospitals in Europe.

There were also maternity hospitals of significant size in Belfast, Cork, Galway and Limerick, and many other maternity homes attached to county hospitals throughout the country, or indeed as stand-alone institutions.

Gynaecology

Obstetrics and gynaecology have traditionally been part of the same collective subject. Gynaecology was also well developed, certainly in Dublin, by the turn of the century. St Vincent's Hospital, founded in 1834, had its first gynaecologist, John A. Byrne, appointed in 1876. Alfred Smith was gynaecologist at the hospital and Professor of Obstetrics and Gynaecology at University College, Dublin, between 1891 and 1922, and there has been an unbroken line of visiting gynaecologists on the staff to the present day.

At the Mater Hospital, while not involved in obstetric practice, Thomas Moore Madden was appointed obstetric physician in 1878. Robert Farnan was gynaecologist to the Mater between 1902 and 1942. (He was part of the Irish delegation which accompanied de Valera to London in July 1921 in an effort to negotiate a treaty giving independence to Ireland.) There were Chairs of obstetrics and gynaecology in all Dublin medical schools in the early part of the century.

Gynaecology in the Rotunda was very active at the turn of the century, with many of those associated with the Rotunda acting as visiting gynaecologists to the hospitals subsequently amalgamated as the Federated Dublin Hospitals, now situated in St James's Hospital and Tallaght Hospital. These other hospitals included Mercer's Hospital, Dr Steevens' Hospital, Sir Patrick Dun's Hospital, the Adelaide Hospital, the Meath Hospital, and the Royal City of Dublin Hospital (Baggot Street).

In 1900, the report of the Coombe Hospital details lists of gynaecological problems treated during that year. There were ten cases of fibroids, twelve cases of uterine retroversion, three cases of uterine prolapse and five ectopic pregnancies. Six cases of malignancy are reported: three of the cervix and three of the uterine corpus.

The National Maternity Hospital was just six years old at the turn of the century. Sir Andrew Horne [q.v.], who was joint Master with Patrick Barry until 1926, was noted for his gynaecological surgery.

Gynaecological Surgery at the Turn of the Century

In company with other branches of surgery, gynaecological surgery showed spectacular advances in the second part of the nineteenth century, as a result of the establishment of anaesthesia and an understanding and acceptance of the principles of antisepsis and later asepsis. Blood transfusion and antibiotics were another century away.

The principles of many current gynaecological operations had been well established by 1900. Removal of large ovarian cysts, then ovariotomy (first described in 1812), was a well-established procedure with Lawson Tait (1845–99) of Birmingham (who had some training in the Coombe Hospital) and Spencer Wells (1818–93) of London being the main proponents. There was considerable professional and personal rivalry between these two surgeons, each trying to outdo the other as regards numbers of operations and death rates. It is impossible to verify the data they published, but the numbers were considerable. By 1872, Spencer Wells had a series of 500 such operations. The operation had first been described in detail by McDowell (1771–1830) in 1812, in the United States. Lawson Tait was also the first to carry out salpingectomy for ruptured ectopic pregnancy (1883), an operation that has since saved the lives of countless young women. It was, however, anaesthesia and the sterilisation of ligatures, as recommended by Lister, that allowed the surgery to become safer.

Hysterectomy, by the year 1900, was also an established procedure. The first hysterectomy, carried out vaginally, was probably done in error as the surgeon was trying to amputate the cervix.

Gross uterovaginal prolapse is a most disabling condition. Because it was so common in women who worked in industry around the midlands and north of England, it was surgeons in Manchester who devised successful operations to deal with it. One of the best known was by William Fothergill (1865–1926) who, in 1888, described what is now known as the Manchester repair.

Malignant Disease

By the turn of the century, surgery for certain types of malignant disease in the female genital tract had been well established. Ernest Wertheim (1864–1920) of Vienna had developed his radical hysterectomy for cancer of the cervix by 1899. He believed that it was important to dissect out as far as possible towards the pelvic sidewall and to take a large cuff of vaginal epithelium. This necessitated dissecting out the ureters, and he described how to do this and at the same time preserve the vascular bundles. He also described the dissection of the pelvic lymph nodes. His early cases had a high mortality. He persevered and, in the early decades of the twentieth century, his operation as practised by Wertheim himself and by other experts like Victor Bonney of London (1872–1953) and Joe Meigs of Boston (1892–1963) had a low mortality.

Wertheim's hysterectomy, with or without additional chemo radiation, still represents the treatment of choice for early invasive cervical cancer. It is also interesting to note that the therapeutic uses of radiation for cervical cancer were described in the same year, 1899.

Practice in Ireland

With obstetrical and gynaecological surgery being well established in 1900, and recognising that there were significant numbers of obstetricians and gynaecological surgeons practising at that time, the focus of the rest of this chapter will be to select who in Ireland were the 'Weather Makers' who most influenced practice during the century and what significant advances were made or were developed. There were many practising gynaecologists during the century. Centres of academic gynaecology had been established in the medical schools. What will be examined is who stood out, who wrote the textbooks and who developed opinion.

In the first twenty-five years of the century, those who stood out include Horne and Ernest Tweedy [q.v.]. Between 1925 and 1960, those who stood out include Bethel Solomons [q.v.], C. H. G. Macafee and J. F. Cunningham [q.v.]. Arthur Barry, Alex Spain, J. K. Feeney and Éamon de Valera were also prominent at this time. Between 1960 and 1980, the weather makers in obstetrics and gynaecology were Kieran O'Driscoll at the National Maternity Hospital and Alan Browne at the Rotunda and the Royal College of Surgeons in Ireland. From 1980 onwards was the era of development of subspecialisation. Gynaecological oncology was practised between the National Maternity Hospital and St Vincent's Hospital, between the Coombe and St James's, and between the Rotunda and the Mater. Assisted fertility was developed at the Rotunda and Galway. The prevention of cancer of the cervix by screening cytology backed up by colposcopy and conservative treatment was developed in the Coombe, the National Maternity Hospital and also in Galway, Cork and Belfast.

HORNE, Sir Andrew

Dublin Obstetrician and Gynaecologist

b. 1856
Educ. Clongowes Wood College; Carmichael School of Medicine, Dublin
m. 1884: Margaret Norman, daughter of Francis Norman (solicitor); 2 s, 2 d
d. 1926

LRCP & SI, 1877; MRCPI, 1889

Postgraduate training at Mater Hospital and St Vincent's Hospital.
Assistant to Arthur P. Macken, Rotunda Hospital.
Private practice in obstetrics and gynaecology, from 1884.
Joint Master, National Maternity Hospital, Holles Street, 1894.

Andrew Horne was without doubt one of the leaders in obstetrical and gynaecological thought in the early decades of the twentieth century. He joined the Carmichael School of Medicine in Dublin in 1873 and during his studentship in the Rotunda was greatly influenced by the then Master, Arthur P. Macken. He became a dresser in St Vincent's Hospital and later in the Mater Hospital and in 1889 was awarded membership of the Royal College of Physicians of Ireland. He was attracted to obstetrics and gynaecology and following his assistantship at the Rotunda he decided to travel and studied gynaecology at the Krankenhaus in Vienna where he became interested in aseptic techniques and in the prevention and treatment of pelvic infection. There he also gained experience in the operation of salpingectomy for ectopic pregnancy and the removal of pyosalpinx for acute pelvic inflammatory disease. He published his observations in the *Dublin Journal of Medical Science*. He married in 1884 and commenced practice in obstetrics and gynaecology in 28 Harcourt Street. He was constantly drawn to the Rotunda Hospital and, in 1888, applied for Mastership of that hospital but was beaten by Smiley who went on to be a noted Master. Horne and Smiley remained friends and frequently consulted each other about difficult cases. This was an early example of the collegiality for which the Dublin maternity hospitals are justly proud. Horne became a Member of the Dublin Obstetric Society, which had been founded in 1938 by Dr Evory Kennedy (another Master of the Rotunda) and this developed into the obstetric section of the Royal Academy of Medicine in Ireland. Horne became Secretary of the obstetric section.

In 1884, Dr Rowe founded a small hospital in Holles Street, again to look after the poor women in the southeast of the city. This hospital, however, failed and closed. In 1894, Dr Patrick Barry, who had failed to be elected Master of the Coombe, joined with Dr Horne and they became the first Masters of the new National Maternity Hospital. The hospital had a number of objectives, the third of which was to establish gynaecological beds for the treatment of disorders peculiar to women. The hospital prospered and was granted a Royal Charter in 1903. The noted St Vincent's surgeon, John S. McArdle, was present at the opening and became visiting surgeon. As regards practice, the hospital went from strength to strength, with 112 gynaecological cases treated in 1906, and this went up to 225 by 1910. Horne carried out the first caesarean section in the hospital in 1901.

Horne was way ahead of his time and stressed the importance of asepsis in vaginal surgery, and his publications discussed ectopic pregnancy and the removal of abdominal tumours. He also described cases of cervical cancer occurring during pregnancy, pyosalpinx and mastitis. His interests in obstetrics were most general and at the Transactions of the Royal Academy of Medicine in Ireland he discussed the induction of labour and the management of breech presentation. He became President of the Obstetric Section of the Academy in 1911. He was genuinely interested in women's health and became a member of the Women's National Health Association and the Dublin Babies Club. He was also interested in the Royal College of Physicians, becoming a Fellow in 1885 and thereafter a Censor, Vice-President and was elected President in 1907, the eighth obstetrician to be President of that College. He was knighted for his services to obstetrics in 1913 when King George V visited Dublin. It was Horne who, with Solomons, fostered the relationship between obstetrics and the Royal College of Physicians, a relationship that prospers to this day.

Horne was a golfer, a gifted pianist and a member of a dining group called the Phagocytes Club. He was really interested in children and was a founder member of the Society for the Prevention of Cruelty to Children.

The activities of the National Maternity Hospital were the subject of the section in *Ulysses*, the Oxon and the Sun, with the hospital famously being called 'the House of Horne'.

TWEEDY, Ernest Hastings

Dublin Gynaecologist and Professor of Obstetrics and Gynaecology

b. 1862, to a prominent Dublin professional family; grew up in a large house in North Frederick Street
Educ. Wesley College; Carmichael Medical School of Medicine, Dublin
d. 1945

LRCP & SI, 1885

Postgraduate posts: resident surgeon, Birmingham; Dr Steevens' Hospital, Dublin; assistant to Dr (later Sir) William Smiley, Rotunda Hospital, Dublin.
Gynaecologist, Dr Steevens' Hospital; Royal City of Dublin Hospital, Baggot Street.
Master, Rotunda Hospital, 1903.
Professor of Obstetrics and Gynaecology, RCSI, 1917–26.

There can be little doubt but that Ernest Hastings Tweedy was one of the 'weather makers' in the advance of obstetrics and gynaecology in the early part of the twentieth century. It was his appointment as assistant to Dr William Smiley (later Sir William) in the Rotunda that was to shape his career. Smiley (1850–1941) was related to Tweedy through marriage. He was pivotal in bringing many concepts of the then modern midwifery to the Rotunda, and his clarity of teaching greatly impressed the young Tweedy.

A man of boundless energy, Tweedy was recognised as a superb clinician. He introduced many innovations and modernisations of clinical practice during his Mastership of the Rotunda and during that time maternal mortality fell to record low rates. He introduced many other advances including his method (subsequently termed the Dublin method) of treating eclampsia. He recognised the need to regard eclampsia as essentially a disease of the first-time mother, and described in detail the steps in managing the epileptiform fits and also the mother's general condition. In a celebrated history of the Rotunda Hospital, a subsequent Master, O'Donnel Browne (who had married Tweedy's daughter), placed Tweedy among the great Masters of that hospital because of 'his originality of thought in all branches of the specialty, but especially in his treatment of eclampsia'. He was also author of a popular textbook *Practical Obstetrics*. Following his Mastership, he returned to Dr Steevens' Hospital and then transferred his work to the Royal City of Dublin

Hospital in 1919. He retained his position of Professor of Obstetrics and Gynaecology at the RCSI until blindness, due to glaucoma, forced him to retire.

1825–1960

In addition to the well-known advances of medicine during these years one of the seminal events was the founding in London of the Royal College of Obstetricians and Gynaecologists, in 1929. This College put a structure on clinical practice and training that endures to this day.

SOLOMONS, Bethel

Dublin Surgeon and Master of the Rotunda Hospital

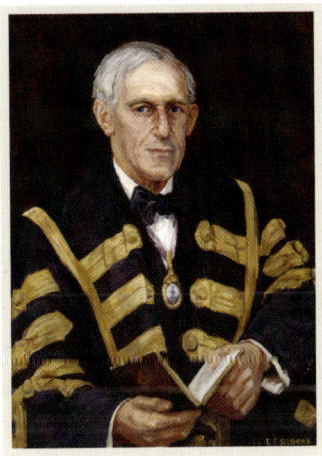

b. 1885, Dublin, the third of 4 children
Educ. Trinity College, Dublin
d. 1963

Postgraduate studies, Rotunda Hospital.
Assistant Master, Rotunda Hospital, 1911.
Surgeon, Mercer's Hospital.
Master, Rotunda Hospital, 1926–33.
Fellow, American College of Obstetricians and Gynaecologists.
Foundational Fellow, Royal College of Obstetricians and Gynaecologists; member of Council and third vice-president.
President, College of Physicians in Ireland, 1946.

Bethel Solomons was undoubtedly another of the obstetrical and gynaecological 'weather makers' of the twentieth century. Like Andrew Horne [q.v.] he was alluded to by James Joyce, this time in *Finnegans Wake* — 'In my bethel of Solomon's I accouched their rotundities'.

His mother's obstetric history, commenced at the age of 36, was complicated by several miscarriages and the successful removal of an abdominal tumour by Spencer Wells of London. His parents were both English and Orthodox Jews yet assimilated and completely identified with the Irish Victorian society in which they moved.

Bethel's eighty-year span was filled by a life of wide interests and activities. His early interests, apart from medicine, were acting and rugby football. He was capped ten times for Ireland at rugby.

On graduation from Trinity College Dublin in 1907 he had a view to taking up general practice in England. However, a postgraduate course in the Rotunda changed all that. He showed a great interest in obstetrics and gynaecology and, prior to taking up his post as Assistant Master, studied and observed practice in various European centres. On completing his Assistantship, he set up in practice and was appointed to the staff of Mercer's Hospital. One of his colleagues there was the famous surgeon Sir William de Courcy Wheeler [q.v.] (PRCSI 1922–1924). In Mercer's Solomons insisted on gynaecological practice not being part of general surgery and, in his somewhat egocentric autobiography (*One Doctor in his Time*), describes surgery on abdominal tumours and ruptured ectopic pregnancies. His practice was successful as was his prowess as a teacher. He was always teaching and was popular at grinds for postgraduate students. He was author of a book on gynaecological practice — *Handbook of Gynaecology* — first published in 1919, which went into four editions. He was also author of many clinical papers. In addition, he wrote *Practical Midwifery for Nurses* in 1930 and edited three editions between 1925 and 1937 of Tweedy's *Practical Obstetrics*.

In 1926, he was elected Master of the Rotunda and, during the ensuing seven years, focused his considerable energies on the advancement of that hospital. He recognised the need for laboratory services, X-ray services and specialist paediatricians. A true internationalist, he established the Rotunda as an international teaching centre. He was a member of the Gynaecological Visiting Society (GVS) from which the Royal College of Obstetricians and Gynaecologists developed. As a Foundation Fellow of that College in 1929, he insisted that Ireland should be part of its constituency. He travelled extensively in Europe, Britain and North America.

His *Handbook on Gynaecology* showed the breadth of his knowledge and practice. In this book, there are descriptions and illustrations of vaginal and abdominal hysterectomy, of repair procedures and uterine suspension procedures popular at that time. With regard to the Gilliam Suspension, he described his own modification of that operation. He also described in detail the repair of genital tract fistulae. There are also in his book descriptions of how best to sterilise suture material.

His thoughts were not confined to surgical techniques. He wrote about thromboprophylaxis and in this was well ahead of his time. He was one of the first advocates of early ambulation in the postoperative period.

During his presidency of the RCPI, he hosted a huge reception for the visit of the British Congress of Obstetrics and Gynaecology. His wonderful portrait, painted by his sister Estella, adorns the main corridor of the College.

Professionally, in addition to competence and innovations, he was forward-looking and brave. The Dublin in which he practised obstetrics and gynaecology was dominated by high parity with all its attendant problems for mothers and families. Yet there were then, as now, some 10 per cent of couples unsuccessful in achieving a pregnancy. He was not afraid to address the subject of fertility. He set up a service dedicated to this problem and helped to found what is now recognised as an important subspecialty of obstetrics and gynaecology.

In addition to his undoubted clinical skills and energy, Solomons was all the more remarkable because of his ability in many other fields. He was a sportsman of note and he was on friendly terms with many of the literary giants of the time. Bethel Solomons was a professional giant on the obstetrical and gynaecological stage during the first and second quarter of the twentieth century.

CUNNINGHAM, John F.

Dublin Gynaecologist and Professor of Obstetrics and Gynaecology

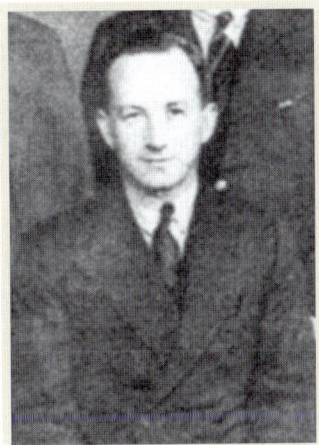

b. 1895
d. 1982

Assistant Master, National Maternity Hospital, to Sir Andrew Horne [q.v.].
Gynaecologist, St Vincent's Hospital.
Master, National Maternity Hospital, 1932–42.
Professor of Obstetrics and Gynaecology, UCD, 1942–62.

Another who must be regarded as one of the 'weather makers' is John Francis Cunningham. His term as Master of the National Maternity Hospital was extended to ten years by Act of Parliament, in order that he might oversee the building in Holles Street. In addition to being a superb clinician and teacher, Cunningham oversaw, in a most meticulous fashion, the building and equipping of the new hospital. When it opened in 1938, it was the most modern hospital in the city, the first all-electric hospital, and was partially funded by the profits of the Hospital Sweepstakes.

Cunningham succeeded Robert Farnan to the Chair of Obstetrics and Gynaecology in UCD. He in turn was succeeded, in 1963, by Éamon de Valera. Cunningham authored a very popular textbook of obstetrics. This was a highly individualised text based on the practice of obstetrics at the National Maternity Hospital during his Mastership, and updated with the help of the consultant staff of that hospital.

He was a tall elegant man who was a most fashionable obstetrician at that time and usually referred to by his patients as 'Divine John'. He died in 1982 following a prolonged illness.

The Mid-Century

The 1940s, 1950s and 1960s were dominated in obstetric practice by concentrating on anaemia in pregnancy, abruption of the placenta and its consequences and the care of the highly multiparous woman. It was the era when a change occurred from a concentration on maternal mortality to the emerging touchstone of perinatal mortality. Perinatal mortality was, in turn, in later decades of the century, to give way to perinatal morbidity.

The practitioners who dominated these decades were: John Kevin Feeney and Joseph Stuart in the Coombe; Alex Spain and Arthur Barry in Holles Street; T. D. O'Donnel Browne and E. W. L. Thompson in the Rotunda. These were years when the ordinary operations of gynaecological practice continued with little innovation. Obstetrics was the main focus of the hospitals. Women giving birth in the three Dublin hospitals were often poorly nourished, and iron deficiency anaemia was common. It was the era of uncontrolled fertility with often relatively young women being regarded as grand multiparae. At the Coombe, being pregnant for the sixth time designated the mother a grand multipara, while being pregnant for the eighth time defined the women as 'great grand multipara'. It was Feeney, Barry and O'Donnel Browne who recognised the influence of social class on obstetric performance and attempted to benefit the plight of the highly parous, possibly chronically anaemic woman. The conditions in the homes of many of these women were truly appalling. The conditions in parts of the hospitals were also poor. A sense of hopelessness was often present in both the carers and those for whom they cared. In these decades, the problem of disproportion exercised the minds of the Masters of the three maternity hospitals, and there were frequent debates on how to ensure a live baby while doing as few caesarean sections as possible. It was to try and address this balance that operations to enlarge the pelvis re-emerged.

Operations to Enlarge the Pelvis

Surgery aimed at enlarging the pelvis for cases of disproportion or suspected disproportion have recently attracted public concern. This concern has been generated by pressure groups who regard the performance of these operations in the middle decades of the century as 'barbaric' and are seeking redress for some of the women still alive and who, it is claimed, still suffer the consequences of the surgery. It is important to judge such procedures in the setting of the time in which they were carried out and the thinking behind their advocacy.

From time immemorial, one of the most challenging features of childbirth has been cephalopelvic disproportion as a result of pelvic deformity, often following childhood rickets. Delivery was achieved only by the deliberate destruction of the foetus by an operation called craniotomy. Obstetric museums are full of gruesome-looking instruments for such destructive procedures. While the problem could in many instances be solved by caesarean section, such operations were not without considerable problems prior to antibiotics and safe blood transfusions. Repeat caesarean section can pose considerable risk to the mother.

Symphysiotomy, which entails splitting the symphysis pubis, was first reported in Paris in 1777. These operations, while used in the nineteenth century, fell into disfavour in English-speaking countries in the early part of the twentieth century. However, with the development of X-ray pelvimetry, accurate pelvic measurements could be made, and the operations were re-introduced largely by Cunningham, Spain and Barry at the National Maternity Hospital, Feeney and Stuart at the Coombe and Thompson at the Rotunda.

Spain published a series of symphysiotomies in the *Journal of Obstetrics and Gynaecology of the British Empire* in 1949. In the fourth edition of the much-used textbook by Cunningham, *Textbook of Obstetrics*, published in 1964, six pages are devoted to the indications for symphysiotomy and the techniques of the operation.

The last symphysiotomy at the National Maternity Hospital was performed in 1970. The operation was designed to spare young women, often small and poorly nourished, the risks of repeated caesarean operations. The subsequent availability of improved nutrition, better understanding of the management of labour, safer caesarean section and a willingness to advise on and accept family planning has rendered the operation of no value in this part of the world. It is of interest, however, that in the *British Journal of Obstetrics and Gynaecology* (BJOG), there was a review published in 2003 on the uses of symphysiotomy, which included analysis of 5,000 cases in the twentieth century. Because of the controversy, the results and commentary on this retrospective analysis deserve attention. In an editorial in that journal in 2003, it was said that the paper on symphysiotomy was probably the most important paper that that prestigious journal had ever published because symphysiotomy was an operation with the potential to save thousands of women's lives each year. The controversy will probably continue.

The Belfast Experience

Obstetrics and gynaecology in Northern Ireland during the twentieth century is inseparably linked with the Royal Maternity Hospital in Belfast and its staff. Two towering figures stand out: C. S. Lowery and C. H. G. Macafee.

The hospital from which the Royal Maternity evolved was founded by a group of women who called themselves 'The Humane Society for the Relief of Lying-In Women' and was opened on 4 February 1794. It was a house in Donegal Street with six beds. The hospital subsequently moved on three occasions, with the present Royal Maternity Hospital being opened on 21 October 1933 by Mrs Stanley Baldwin, wife of the then British Prime Minister.

In 1907, when the hospital was in Townsend Street, Dr C. S. Lowery was appointed house surgeon. This man, more than any other, was responsible for the building of the present Royal Maternity. Following his training, he was appointed Professor of Midwifery at Queen's University in 1920, succeeding Professor Byers who was Professor of Midwifery between 1893 and 1920. At that time, the Chair was divided into two, with Professor R. J. Johnston occupying the Chair of Gynaecology.

From 1925 onwards, Professor Lowery, with much help and encouragement, conceived a campaign to secure a site for a new maternity hospital in the proximity of, and amalgamated to, the Royal Hospital. Lowery travelled to the United States and Canada to see the then state-of-the-art maternity hospitals there. He encouraged the Marquis of Dufferin and Ava to do the same. On his return, the Marquis was interviewed by members of the press who were astonished by his statement: 'Belfast should be ashamed of its City Hall.' When asked to expand, he replied, 'The city that has a maternity hospital like Townsend Street and a City Hall like it is should be ashamed.' Professor Lowery was a tireless campaigner and rightly appalled at the high maternal mortality. In 1925, 150 women in Northern Ireland died during pregnancy and childbirth. With the advent of the new hospital and a developing enthusiasm for keeping up with medical advances, the maternal and infant mortality rates dropped significantly.

While Lowery used his energies in developing the hospital and its service, it was his son-in-law and successor to the Chair, C. H. G. Macafee, who made important clinical strides of world importance. Macafee revolutionised the treatment of placenta previa. Until about 1940, any woman admitted with antepartum haemorrhage believed to be due to placenta previa was immediately delivered, irrespective of foetal maturity, because it was considered that the mother could bleed to death. Macafee believed that the first haemorrhage from placenta previa was not necessarily life-threatening and therefore not an emergency. He believed that in many mothers delivery could be delayed until the foetus was more mature. His treatment was to put the mother to bed in the hospital until 38 weeks, and to avoid pelvic examination until a decision had to be made as regards delivery. This 'expectant treatment of placenta previa', practised to this day, revolutionised the outlook for mothers and babies. In Belfast, the maternal mortality associated with placenta previa in Macafee's time fell from twenty-six to five per thousand and the foetal loss from 500 to twelve per thousand. In his publications on the subject, Macafee was characteristically unselfish in acknowledging the co-operation and involvement of paediatricians, nurses and, of course, the mothers themselves.

Macafee held the Chair of Midwifery and Gynaecology in Queen's University Belfast, from 1945 until he retired in 1960. He was regarded as an accomplished obstetrician, was a Foundation Fellow of the Royal College of Obstetricians and Gynaecologists, and at one time its Vice-President.

Since Macafee's time, obstetrics and gynaecology in Northern Ireland has grown from strength to strength. Many centres have been established throughout the province. The hub continues, however, to be the Royal Maternity Hospital. Notable during the last twenty-five years of the twentieth century was Professor J. M. G. Harley, for his work on diabetes in pregnancy and his renowned skill as a pelvic surgeon. Harith Lamki founded colposcopy services in Northern Ireland and is noted for his interest in postgraduate medical education. Professor James Doran has developed the internationally renowned centre for foetal medicine at the Royal in Belfast and has brought that subject of foetal medicine to new heights.

Mater Infirmorum Belfast, Obstetricians and Gynaecologists

DEMPSEY, Sir Alexander

Belfast Obstetrician and Gynaecologist

b. 1852, a son of Bernard Dempsey of 'Coldagh' near Ballymoney, Co. Antrim
Educ. Catholic University School of Medicine (Cecilia Street), Dublin; Queen's College, Galway
m. his son, Alexander Joseph Dempsey [q.v.], succeeded him in his medical practice at the Mater Infirmorum
d. 18 July 1920

MB, QCG

Obstetrician and gynaecologist, Mater Infirmorum Hospital, 1883.
Chairman, Mater Infirmorum Hospital Medical Staff Committee, 1883–1920.

Sir Alexander Dempsey graduated in Medicine at Queen's College, Galway, and later specialised in obstetrics and gynaecology. He was the first medical doctor appointed to the small twenty-eight-bed hospital in 1883, when he was 31 years old. He was knighted in 1911 for his services on the Universities Commission, which finally settled the University question in 1908. He died from diabetes.

DEMPSEY, Alexander Joseph

Belfast Obstetrician and Gynaecologist

b. a son of Sir Alexander Dempsey [q.v.]

Obstetrician and gynaecologist, Mater Infirmorum Hospital.
Honorary secretary, treasurer and representative, BMA Council in London.
President, Ulster Medical Society.
Fellow, Royal Society of Medicine, London; British Gynaecological Society.
Member, Governing Body of UCD; National University Senate.

Alexander Joseph Dempsey succeeded his father, Sir Alexander Dempsey, in his medical practice as obstetrician and gynaecologist in the Mater Infirmorum Hospital. Along with Dr William McKeown (ophthalmologist) and Dr John Moore, he established the Northern Ireland Branch of the British Medical Association.

KENNEDY, Frank

Belfast Obstetrician and Gynaecologist

Educ. Queen's University Belfast
m. married (his wife predeceased him); 3 s (Joseph [q.v.], late consultant genitourinary surgeon; Hugh, QC, barrister in Belfast; Fr Frank, priest in the Diocese of Down and Connor)
d. 1972

MB, QUB

Junior resident doctor, Mater Infirmorum Hospital, ?1924–26.
Consultant obstetrician and gynaecologist, Mater Infirmorum Hospital, Belfast.

Frank Kennedy's father died prematurely when Frank was very young. One brother was a bank official and the other was a consultant psychiatrist, based in England. Frank was a clerk in Caffrey's Brewery, Glen Road, Belfast, before studying medicine. He died as a patient in St John's Private Nursing Home, facing the Mater Infirmorum Hospital, Crumlin Road, Belfast.

From the 1970s

By the 1970s, perinatal mortality had replaced maternal mortality as the yardstick of excellence in obstetrics, with perinatal morbidity being the developing interest. The weather makers were undoubtedly Kieran O'Driscoll at the National Maternity Hospital and Alan Browne in the Rotunda.

While, by the 1970s, it was accepted that the mother was by and large safe from a physical standpoint, the process of labour was still dominated by thoughts of pelvic measurements, foetal malpresentations, and skill with the obstetric forceps. The experience of labour for many mothers, especially first-time mothers, was horrific. This experience was helped, though not in a fundamental fashion, by the development of techniques of regional anaesthesia and analgesia. The most significant advance in the management of labour was made at the National Maternity Hospital by the work of O'Driscoll in what he entitled the Active Management of Labour.

KIERAN O'DRISCOLL (1923–2007) AND *THE ACTIVE MANAGEMENT OF LABOUR*

In his introduction to the manual entitled *The Active Management of Labour*, and co-authored by his colleague Declan Meagher, O'Driscoll states, 'In orthodox medical circles recognition has come slowly that labour, especially first labour, is the most disturbing emotional event in the lifetime of one half of mankind.' O'Driscoll and Meagher changed all this with a programme for the management of labour in primigravidae which aimed to decrease the duration of labour initially to 24 hours and then to 12 hours.

In several important publications, and in their manual, they set out principles that would ensure a safe and rewarding experience for the mother and the safety of the baby. These principles clearly state that there must be an active participation in the management of labour from senior obstetricians and midwives. There must be a clear distinction between primigravidae and multigravidae, to the extent that from the perspective of labour they are regarded as 'separate biological species'. There should be efforts made to establish robustness in the diagnosis of labour, based on objective criteria. There should be a clear distinction between the management of women whose labour started spontaneously and that of those who had labour induced. There should be early recognition of slow progress and, when this could be attributed to inefficient uterine action, that action should be corrected by the use of Oxytocin. Simple partograms, colour coded for primigravidae and multigravidae, were used and designed so that poor progress could be easily detected.

Active Management has excited much debate and comment, and not a little hostility, since the first publication in 1970. It has frequently been misunderstood, with many misconceptions that the word 'active' meant just the liberal and possibly indiscriminate use of Oxytocin. In fact, 'Active Management of Labour' is a package and, when properly applied, has achieved results unimaginable just a few decades ago.

O'Driscoll and his co-author Meagher graduated from University College, Dublin. Meagher succeeded O'Driscoll as Master of the National Maternity Hospital in 1970. Since that time, subsequent Masters and staff at Holles Street have developed and refined aspects of the Active Management of Labour, such as the introduction of foetal monitoring and epidural anaesthesia. The principles of Active Management, however, remain enduring. They were based on clinical observation and deep original thought. O'Driscoll, following his Mastership, became Professor of Obstetrics and Gynaecology at UCD, and introduced a scheme of teaching that is regarded by the undergraduates as superb and has encouraged so many to enter the specialty. The Active Management of Labour, however, will remain as his most important memorial as it was probably the most important piece of clinical research carried out in Ireland in the second half of the twentieth century.

ALAN BROWNE (1923–   )

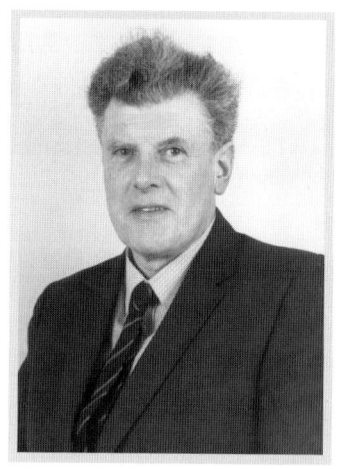

Another of the undoubted weather makers from 1970 on was Alan Browne. Browne was Master of the Rotunda Hospital between 1966 and 1972 and, following the completion of his Mastership, was elected Professor of Obstetrics and Gynaecology at the Royal College of Surgeons in Ireland. Browne, a Trinity graduate, and a gifted clinician, advanced the clinical practice in the Rotunda Hospital during his Mastership of that hospital. However, it is as Professor at the Royal College of Surgeons in Ireland, as first Chairman of the Institute of Obstetricians and Gynaecologists, as President of the Royal Irish Academy of Medicine in Ireland and as an indefatigable encourager of the undergraduate and postgraduate students that he has left an enduring legacy. Possessed of an enquiring mind and enthusiasm, he was the first to introduce colposcopy to Ireland. He recognised the great importance of cervical mucous and studied its components. He developed a surgical procedure — Target colporrhaphy — for stress incontinence long before the advent of urodynamics. He also researched the value of amnioscopy and hysteroscopy before the recent revolution in technology.

Alan Browne belonged to that small group of enthusiastic academics who changed the whole aspect of the Royal College of Surgeons in Ireland and paved the way of its development into the world-class institution it has now become. During the final two decades of the century, subspecialisation developed. Gynaecological oncology became more concentrated in a few centres, with Éamon de Valera, Anthony Keane and Michael Foley at the National Maternity Hospital and John Bonnar at St James's having a significant influence in this regard.

In obstetrics, electronic foetal monitoring had become possible and the largest randomised trial to assess its value was conducted by Dermot MacDonald at the National Maternity Hospital. Ultrasound, now an essential part of obstetric care, was developing and, at the Coombe Hospital, John Drumm and Joseph Stuart were the first to develop Doppler flow studies in the umbilical cord vessels.

John F Murphy, initially at the Coombe, and from 1980 at the National Maternity Hospital, introduced colposcopy, which plays such a huge part in gynaecological practice. The mainstay of treatment of premalignant lesions of the cervix is now the LLETZ (large loop excision of the transformation zone), a procedure first described by Walter Prenderville at the Coombe Hospital.

The last two decades of the century were unfortunately coloured and to a significant extent marred by the rapidly developing medico-legal crisis.

INTO THE TWENTY-FIRST CENTURY

The current century will see huge changes. It is probable that subspecialisation will so develop that the generalist with a special interest will become a thing of the past. The specialty may well split at a postgraduate level. Exciting times are ahead and it is likely that the specialists at the turn of the next century will look back at our practice in a similar way to the way that we regard the practice of the 'weather makers' of the 1900s.

MURPHY, John Francis (John)

Dublin Obstetrician/Gynaecologist

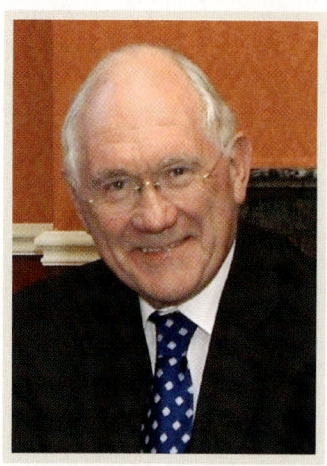

b. 1942, Dublin, son of John J. and Carmel T. Murphy (*née* O'Donnell)
Educ. Gonzaga College, Dublin (first intake); University College Dublin
m. 1972: Anne Tweedle, a midwife at Birmingham Maternity Hospital; 3 s, 2 d

MB (hons), McArdle Medal in Surgery, UCD, 1966; MRCPI, 1971; MRCOG, 1971; MD, Birmingham, 1974; FRCPI, 1979; FRCOG, 1983

Basic postgraduate training St Vincent's Hospital, Dublin; Registrar, Obstetric and Gynaecology Professorial Unit, Birmingham; research fellow, Department Obstetrics and Gynaecology, University of Birmingham for three years.

These posts were most demanding, time off and any concept of rest during the days or nights were unknown.
Assistant Master, Coombe Hospital, 1976–79.
Consultant gynaecologist, National Maternity Hospital, Holles Street and St Vincent's Hospital, Dublin, 1979.

John Murphy wanted to be a gynaecologist since his undergraduate years and most of his training years were in Birmingham with the legendary Professor Hugh McLaren. McLaren, a Scottish Presbyterian, was a vocal opponent of abortion, a view that probably cost him the Presidency of the Royal College of Obstetricians and Gynaecologists with the accompanying knighthood. John Murphy's research was mainly into the early detection of cervical cancer. This work resulted in many significant, durable publications, an MD degree and the award of the prestigious Blair-Bell Lectureship at the Royal College of Obstetricians and Gynaecologists. He pioneered colposcopy in Dublin.

He has had a long involvement with RCPI, serving as Hon. Librarian, Treasurer, Vice President and President; he has also been active in the Irish Cancer Society. He has been a visiting lecturer in the UK, USA, South Africa and Australia. His recreations include reading political biographies, some fair weather golf and an enduring interest in Irish art.

John Murphy is a greatly talented, cerebral operating surgeon and hugely respected both as a leader of his specialty and as someone who has made considerable personal sacrifices in devoting himself unstintingly to the entire profession.

16
OPHTHALMIC SURGERY

Dr John Nolan

OPHTHALMIC SURGERY

INTRODUCTION

The start of the twentieth century in Ireland found eye surgery well established in the three major cities, Belfast, Cork and Dublin, in alphabetical order.

BELFAST

Belfast had four eye departments, situated in the Royal Hospital, the Ophthalmic Hospital, the Benn Ulster Hospital and the Mater Infirmorum Hospital. The Royal Hospital had started in 1845 as the General Hospital, with an eye ward being instituted by Dr Samuel Browne in 1850. It became the Royal Hospital in 1897. The Ophthalmic Hospital was founded in 1844 by Dr Samuel Browne, and replaced by a new building in 1867. Dr William McKeown opened the Benn Ulster in 1874, sponsored by the philanthropist Edward Benn.

The eye departments of the Royal, the Ophthalmic and the Benn Ulster were amalgamated into one eye department, in the new Royal Victoria Hospital, in 1964. The Mater Infirmorum was opened in 1883 and replaced by a much larger foundation in 1900. Eye departments were subsequently opened in Londonderry and Armagh.

CORK

In 1897, the Cork Eye Infirmary, which had opened in Caroline Street in 1818, moved into the new Eye and Throat Hospital ('de Iron Trote') on Western Road. Lady Arnott, who resurrected the Enniscorthy Fair, renaming it the Cork

Festival and producing £7,000, raised the funds for this hospital. She was the step great-grandmother of Eric Arnott, FRC Ophth who would introduce phacoemulsification cataract surgery into the UK and Ireland in the later part of the twentieth century.

The Cork Eye Infirmary, together with the above eye hospitals in Belfast, reflected the conceptual enlightenment of the eighteenth century and the philanthropy of the nineteenth.

Dublin

In the south of Ireland, the ophthalmic twentieth century really began in 1897 with the opening of the Royal Victoria Hospital in Adelaide Road, Dublin. In that year, the National Eye and Ear Hospital, which had been founded in 1814 by Commander Isaac Ryall, RN, amalgamated with St Mark's Hospital, founded in 1844 by Dr William Wilde, to form the new hospital.

Ophthalmology and otorhinolaryngology had gradually developed as a combined branch of general surgery and, at the start of the twentieth century, was a somewhat esoteric minor specialty. Its practitioners would gravitate to one side or the other and, after the Second World War, Eyes and ENT finally divided completely into distinct disciplines.

As the twentieth century progressed, eye surgery was established in Galway followed by Limerick, Waterford and Sligo.

It was after the Second World War that ophthalmology developed rapidly from a Cinderella specialty into the one which transformed the whole of surgery in a white-hot technological revolution, pioneering the use of the operating microscope, transplant surgery, implant surgery, prosthetic surgery, laser, ultrasound and phacoemulsification surgery, small-incision and day-case surgery.

None of these developments could have occurred without the intelligence, dedication and enthusiasm of the surgeons themselves. Those who worked in twentieth-century Ireland are listed below in chronological order under the heading of the hospital to which the major commitment was given. The hospitals are listed by city, in alphabetical order, except for Northern Ireland.

Northern Ireland

Belfast

The year 1900 found Belfast with four eye units, situated in:
- The Belfast Royal Hospital; this became the Royal Victoria Hospital in 1903
- The Belfast Ophthalmic Institution Eye and Ear Hospital (the Ophthalmic Hospital)
- The Benn Ulster Hospital
- The Mater Infirmorum Hospital

In 1949, the Ophthalmic Hospital amalgamated with the Benn Ulster Hospital and this joint body amalgamated with the Royal Victoria Hospital in 1964, to become the new Royal Victoria Hospital Eye Department. The surgeons appointed to these three hospitals prior to 1964 are listed under the hospital to which the major commitment was given. After 1964, they are listed under the Royal Victoria Hospital.

The Belfast Royal Hospital (BRH) Eye Department (1900–1964)

NELSON, Joseph

Ophthalmic Surgeon

b. 1840, son of Rev. S. Craig Nelson of Downpatrick
Educ. Royal Belfast Academical Institution; Queen's College, Belfast
m. married twice; 5 children
d. 1910

MD, RUI; LRCSI, 1863.

Postgraduate training in Dublin and Vienna (with von Arlt and Ernst Fuchs).
Ophthalmic Surgeon, BRH and Belfast Hospital for Sick Children, 1882–1905.
President, Ulster Medical Society, 1898.

Generous and extroverted, Joseph Nelson broke his medical studies in 1860 and joined Garibaldi's volunteer army. He was commissioned lieutenant, fought in Sicily and Volturno, received a sword of honour from Garibaldi and two medals from the King of Sicily, and returned home to finish his medical studies. He worked as surgeon in an Indian tea plantation and was awarded a further medal in an expedition against the Manipuris. He came back to Ireland in 1880. An inspiring teacher and a flamboyant host.

CRAIG, James Andrew

Belfast Ophthalmologist

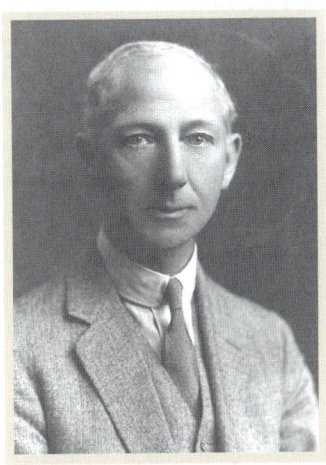

b. 1872, Ballymoney
Educ. Coleraine Academical Institution; Queen's University Belfast
m. 1917: Blanche Waldron (d. 1952); 2 s (Maurice, elder son, was an historian)
d. 1958

MB (first class hons), RUI, QUB, 1895; MRCS, 1898; FRCS, 1902; Hon. MD, QUB, 1951

Postgraduate work: three years, Royal Southern Hospital in Liverpool, and then studied eye and ear diseases in Vienna; demonstrator in anatomy, QUB, 1899; honorary assistant, Eye, Ear and Throat Department, RVH, 1901.

Lecturer in ophthalmology and otorhinolaryngology, QUB, 1913–37.
President, Irish Ophthalmological Society; Ulster Medical Society.
Editorial committee, *British Journal of Ophthalmology*.
Returned to hospital work in 1939, at age 67, to allow younger men to do war service.

Craig was a generous benefactor of QUB, and the college established the James Craig Prize. A keen golfer, he was twice Captain of the Royal County Down Golf Club (Newcastle). A man of great presence and wide knowledge, he was highly respected, not least for his ability on skis. He loved the sea and retired to Cultra on the shores of Belfast Lough.

HANNA, Henry

Belfast Eyes and ENT Surgeon

b. 1874, son of Henry Hanna (merchant), Belfast
Educ. Belfast Royal Academy; Queen's College, Belfast; St John's College, Cambridge

MA, BSc, 1896; MB, 1903

Postgraduate studies in Vienna.
Eyes and ENT surgeon, RVH, 1915–39.

A biologist before studying medicine, Henry Hanna was a kind man with a strong sense of justice. Basically shy, he loved fly-fishing and collected old Irish glass and porcelain.

JEFFERSON, Fred

Belfast Eye Surgeon

MB, BCh
Assistant, 1920–30.
Surgeon in charge of outpatients, RVH, 1930–1934.

Fred Jefferson retired in 1934, due to ill-health.

WHEELER, James R.

Belfast Eye Surgeon

MB; FRCSE; DOMS; DLO

Clinical assistant, 1923–28.
Assistant surgeon & surgeon, Belfast Ophthalmological Hospital, 1928–65.
Clinical assistant, 1930–34; assistant surgeon, 1934–37; surgeon, RVH, 1937–65.
University lecturer in ophthalmology, 1937–65.
President, ophthalmology section, Royal Society of Medicine, 1957.
Colonial Office Visitor to the Fiji Islands, 1957.

SINCLAIR, Samuel R.

Belfast Ophthalmic Surgeon

d. 1960 (suddenly)

BSc; MB; FRCSE

Major, Royal Army Medical Corps, 1939–45.
Ophthalmic surgeon, RVH and BOH, 1946–1960.

COWAN, Eric Cecil

Consultant Ophthalmic Surgeon, Belfast

MB, QUB, 1952; FRCS Ed, 1959; FACS, 1977; MCh, QUB, 1972

Senior registrar, Benn Hospital, Belfast; registrar, corneo-plastic unit, Queen Victoria Hospital, East Grinstead; senior house officer, Royal Eye Hospital, Manchester.
Consultant Ophthalmic Surgeon, 1960–97.

Belfast Ophthalmic Hospital (BOH) (1900–1964)

SHAW, Cecil

Belfast Surgeon and Lecturer in Ophthalmology and Otology

Educ. Queen's College, Belfast
d. 1913 (from pernicious anaemia)

MB, QUB, 1885

Postgraduate training: Moorfield's Eye Hospital, London; Paris; Vienna.
Assistant surgeon, 1895–1913.
Lecturer in ophthalmology and otology, QCB, 1904–13.

BROWNE, Sir John Walton

Belfast Consulting Surgeon

b. 1843, son of Dr Samuel Browne, MRCS, RN, JP (founder of the Belfast Ophthalmic Hospital, 1845; ophthalmic surgeon 1847–75; Mayor of Belfast, 1870, and first Chief Medical Officer of Health)
Educ. Queen's College, Belfast
d. 1923

BA, QUB, 1863; MD, MRCS, 1867; LLD, RUI, 1908

Postgraduate studies in London and Vienna in ENT and Eyes.
Attending surgeon, 1875–1921.
Consulting Surgeon 1921–1923, BOH.
President, N of I branch and also of ophthalmic section, BMA.
Senator, QUB; Deputy Lieutenant, City of Belfast, 1913; KB, 1921.

Sir John began as an eye surgeon but moved to general surgery in 1883. In July 1903, he welcomed King Edward and Queen Alexandra to the opening of the new hospital. A memorial plaque in the Royal Victoria Hospital remembers him as 'A great surgeon, a great philanthropist and a great citizen'.

CUNNINGHAM, Herbert Hugh Blair

Ophthalmic Surgeon

Educ. St Mary's Hospital London; Brussels; Trinity College, Dublin

LRCP, Lond, 1903; BA, MB, TCD; MD, Brussels, 1904; FRCSI, 1905

Postgraduate training: Moorfield's, London; ophthalmic surgery, Ulster Hospital for Women and Children, Belfast; clinical assistant, Ophthalmic Hospital, Belfast.
Clinical assistant, 1908–1913; assistant surgeon, 1913–14.
Examiner in ophthalmology and otology, RCSI.
Honorary demonstrator in anatomy, QUB.
Chief clinical assistant, Royal London Ophthalmic Hospital; senior clinical assistant, Royal Ear Hospital, London.
Senior ophthalmic clinical assistant; ophthalmic house surgeon; resident casualty officer; assistant demonstrator in anatomy and physiology, St Mary's Hospital, London.
Prosector in anatomy. RCS Eng; surgical clinical assistant, Hospital for Sick Children, Great Ormond Street; clinical assistant Samaritan Free Hospital, London.
Lieutenant-Colonel, Royal Army Medical Corps. Ophthalmic Specialist, British Army of Occupation, Germany.

Publications include: 'Remarks on the Use of Electro Magnet in Ophthalmic Surgery, with Rep. of 3 cases', *St Mary's Hospital Gazette*, 1906; 'Ein Fall von Empyem der Keilbeinhohle mit Augensymptom nebst Bemerkungen über die Anatomie der Keilbeinhohle', *Zeitschrift für Augenheilkunde*, 1907; 'Case of Streptococcic Conjunctivitis', *British Medical Journal*, 1907; 'Some Complications of Chronic Ottorhoea', Ibid. 1908; 'Acid Intoxication Following Ethyl Chloride Anaesthesia', *Lancet*, 1908; 'Deafness resulting from Epidemic Cerebro Spinal Meningitis', Proceedings of the Royal Society of Medicine, 1908.

McCREADY, Wyclif

Ophthalmic Surgeon

b. 1880
Educ. Royal Belfast Academical Institution; Trinity College, Dublin; Queen's College, Belfast
d. 1944

MB, FRCSI

Postgraduate training: Vienna; clinical assistant, 1908–12; assistant surgeon, 1913–14.
10th Battalion, Royal Irish Rifles, 1914–16; Captain, Royal Army Medical Corps, 1916–18.
Surgeon, BOH, 1918–33.
Ophthalmic surgeon, Belfast Hospital for Sick Children, 1908–14; 1918–33.

Wycliff McCready dressed informally and was noted for his courtesy.

LYNN, Beatrice

Ophthalmic Surgeon

MB, FRCSE

Clinical assistant, subsequently surgeon, BOH, 1923–64.
President, Irish Ophthalmological Society, 1960.

Benn Ulster Eye, Ear, Nose and Throat Hospital

McKEOWN, William Alexander

Ophthalmic Surgeon

b. 1844, elder son of Dr William McKeown of Ballyclare, Co. Antrim; a descendant of King Robert II of Scotland
Educ. Ballyclare; Queen's College, Belfast
d. 1904

MB, 1869 (first class hons and gold medal); MD; MCh

Postgraduate training in Paris.
Surgeon, 1871–1903.
First lecturer in ophthalmology and otology, QCB.
Senator, Royal University of Ireland.

In Belfast, McKeown founded a dispensary for the free treatment of eye and ear disorders, which attracted the attention of the philanthropist Edward Benn and was transmuted into the Benn Ulster Hospital.

KILLEN, William Marcus

Ophthalmic Surgeon

b. 1863, son of Very Rev. T. Y. Killen, DD
Educ. Royal Belfast Academical Institution; Queen's College, Belfast
d. 1945

MD, MCh, MAO, 1887

Postgraduate training in Dublin and Vienna.
Surgeon, 1904–35.

DAVIDSON, Isaac

Ophthalmic Surgeon

b. 1869, France
Educ. Methodist College, Belfast; Queen's College, Belfast
d. 1942

MB, 1892; MD, 1898; DPH (Cantab), 1902

Assistant surgeon, 1913–14.
Royal Army Medical Corps, 1914–18.
Surgeon, 1918–39.
President, Irish Ophthalmological Society; Ulster Medical Society.

ANDERSON, William Arthur

Ophthalmic Surgeon

b. 1885
Educ. Royal Belfast Academical Institution; Clare College, Cambridge
d. 1956

MA, MB, 1910; MRCS, MD

Postgraduate training in Moorfield's Eye Hospital, London.
Assistant surgeon, 1913–14.
Royal Army Medical Corps, 1914–18; mentioned in Dispatches and Medaille d'Honneur d'Or
Surgeon, 1918–50.
Deputy Lieutenant for Belfast, 1942.
Vice-President, Ophthalmological Society of the United Kingdom.
President, Irish Ophthalmological Society; Ulster Medical Society.
Chairman, combined Board of Management of the Belfast Ophthalmic and Benn Ulster hospitals.

CORKEY, J. Allison

Ophthalmic Surgeon, 1933–1964

See also Royal Victoria Hospital, 1964–2000, below.

MARTIN, Victor A. F.

Ophthalmic Surgeon, 1950–1964

See also Royal Victoria Hospital, 1964–2000, below.

Royal Victoria Hospital (1964–2000)

ARCHER, Desmond, OBE

Ophthalmic Surgeon and Professor of Ophthalmology

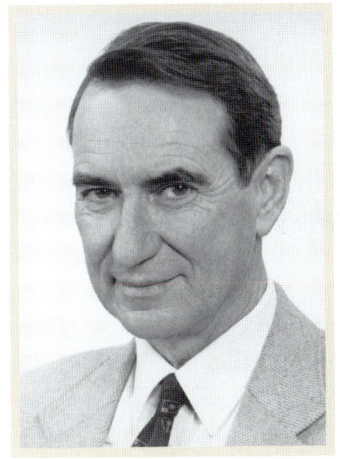

MB, QUB, 1959; FRCS, 1968; FRC Ophth, 1990; FMed Sci, 2000

Consultant Eye Surgeon, RVH, 1971–2003.
Founder and first Director of the Ophthalmic Research Centre, RVH.
Professor of Ophthalmology, QUB 1971–2003; Emeritus Professor, 2003 to date.
Vice-President, Royal College of Ophthalmologists; Chairman, Education Committee, 1990–94.
Visiting Professor, USA, Australia, Europe and China.
Doyne Lecturer, Oxford Ophthalmological Congress, 1992.
Bowman Lecturer, Royal College of Ophthalmologists, 1999.
Montgomery Lecturer, Irish Ophthalmological Society, 1986.
Chang Lecturer, Hong Kong Ophthalmological Society, 1991.
McKenzie Lecturer, University of Glasgow, 2004.
OBE for services to ophthalmology, 2000

Desmond Archer is a renowned authority on diabetic retinopathy, who developed his department into one of worldwide esteem. He is a prolific author of research papers of quality, relevance and durability.

CORKEY J. Allison

Consultant Eye Surgeon

MD, FRCSI, DOMS

Consultant Eye Surgeon, Benn Ulster Hospital, 1933–64; RVH, 1964–68.
President, Irish Ophthalmological Society, 1964–66.

MARTIN, Victor A.F.

Consultant Eye Surgeon

MB, FRCSE

Consultant Eye Surgeon, Benn Ulster Hospital, 1950–64; RVH 1964–77.
President, Irish Ophthalmological Society.

BAIRD, Robert Hamilton

Consultant Eye Surgeon

Educ. Queen's University Belfast

MB, QUB, 1939; FRCS Eng, 1955; DO Eng, 1950

Consultant Eye Surgeon, Benn Hospital and RVH, 1950–70.

COWAN, Eric Cecil

Consultant Eye Surgeon

MB, FRCS, FRC Ophth
Consultant Eye Surgeon, RVH, 1960–96.

MAGUIRE, Charles James Frederick

Consultant Eye Surgeon, Bermuda

Educ. Queen's University Belfast

MB, QUB, 1954; FRCS, FRC Ophth

Consultant Eye Surgeon, RVH, 1964–96.

LOGAN, William Caskey

Consultant Eye Surgeon

Educ. Queen's University Belfast

MB, QUB, 1953; FRCS Ed, 1962; FRCS Eng, 1963; FRC Ophth

Resident surgical officer, Birmingham and Midlands Eye Hospital.
Senior registrar, RVH, Belfast; Ophthalmic Hospital, Belfast.
Consultant Eye Surgeon, RVH, 1964–96.

JOHNSON, Stewart

Consultant Eye Surgeon

MB, FRCS
Consultant eye surgeon, RVH, 1975–94.
First President, Irish College of Ophthalmologists, 1992–94.

Belfast City Hospital

HART, Patricia

Ophthalmic Surgeon

MA, MB, FRCS, FRC Ophth

Armagh Hospital

WARE, Charles Francis Wakefield

Associate Specialist Ophthalmic Surgeon

Educ. Queen's University Belfast

MB, QUB, 1958; FRCSE, 1965; FRCSI, 1974; FRC Ophth, 1991

Coleraine Causeway Hospital

HANNA, Mary E. A.

Ophthalmic Surgeon

MB, FRCSI, FRC Ophth

Mater Infirmorum Hospital

This hospital was opened by Sir Robert J. McConnell, Lord Mayor of Belfast, on 23 April 1900. It replaced the smaller building which had been opened in 1883 by Bishop Patrick Dorrian. Dr Marcus Killen (see under Benn Ulster Hospital) was appointed to the Visiting Medical Staff as Eye and ENT specialist on 6 November 1900 but resigned in 1904 when appointed to the Benn Ulster Hospital. His place was taken by his assistant, Dr P. J. H. Mulholland.

MULHOLLAND, Patrick Joseph Haydn

Eye and ENT Specialist

b. 1856

Educ. Royal University of Ireland, Queen's College, Belfast; Royal College of Surgeons, Edinburgh

d. 1940

Mus. Bac. 1893; LRCP, LRCS, Edin; LFPS, Glas, 1898

Postgraduate studies in Vienna and Cairo.
Assistant surgeon, Mater Infirmorum Hospital, 1902–04; Surgeon, 1904–40.

An excellent musician, Patrick Mulholland was organist in St Patrick's Church, Donegall Street, Belfast.

McCAUGHAN, David Vincent

Consultant ENT Surgeon

b. 1897
Educ. St Malachy's College, Belfast; Queen's University Belfast
d. 1984

MB, 1920

Postgraduate training in Manchester, Cheltenham, Bristol and Liverpool.
Assistant surgeon in eyes and ENT, Mater Infirmorum Hospital, 1923–50.
Consultant ENT surgeon, Ballymena, Antrim, Larne and Carrickfergus, 1950–62.

GORMLEY, Peter John Anthony

Consultant Eye Surgeon

b. 1920, Ballygawley, Co. Tyrone
Educ. St Patrick's College, Armagh, 1932–37; Belfast Technical College, September 1937–March 1938; Queen's University Belfast, 1938–44.
m. son, Peter Gormley, FRCS, is consultant ENT Surgeon, Galway

MB, QUB, 1944; DOMS (E), 1948

Junior resident house officer, Mater Infirmorum, 1944–45; honorary clinical assistant (to Dr David Vincent McCaughan) in Eye, Ear, Nose and Throat Department, Mater Infirmorum, 1945–47.
In September 1947, granted a year's leave of absence to do postgraduate training in London: junior clinical assistant in ophthalmology, Moorefield's Eye Hospital, including attendance at Institute of Ophthalmology for preparation for Diploma in Ophthalmology (Conjoint Board of Examiners) half the number from the RCS (London) and the other half from the Royal Society of Medicine (London).
Junior clinical assistant in laryngology and otology, Royal National Throat, Nose and Ear Hospital, London January–June 1948, including attendance at the Institute of Laryngology and Otology (based in the hospital).
Mater Infirmorum, 1948–87: junior resident house officer; assistant surgeon, eyes and ENT (1950); surgeon (1964).
Fellowship in Ophthalmology, Royal College of Surgeons in Ireland.
Clinical lecturer and examiner in Ophthalmology, QUB.
Clinical examiner for Diploma in Ophthalmology, RCSI.
Member, Irish Ophthalmological Society; Irish Faculty of Ophthalmology.
Foundation Fellow, Royal College of Ophthalmologists in England.
Committee member, Irish Ophthalmological Society.

CAMPBELL, Brian J. Campbell

Consultant Ophthalmic Surgeon

b. 15 August 1920, Omagh, Co. Tyrone; older sister, Molly, an ophthalmologist in Omagh in community medicine and private practice (she trained in Wolverhampton, England, and had her Diploma in Ophthalmic Medicine from Oxford University); older brother, Edward, FRCS (general surgery) was a GP in England
Educ. Christian Brothers School, Omagh; University College Dublin
m. Eithne (primary school teacher; died prematurely); 2 d (one a consultant psychiatrist in Reading, England; the other a consultant radiologist in Altnagelvin Hospital, Derry), 1 s (a chemist in England)

MB, BCh, BAO, UCD, 1945; MCR (in ophthalmology), UCD (?1955); DOMS (E), 1949 (DOMS); FRCS (1) in ophthalmology, 1965

Consultant surgeon in Eye and ENT Department, Mater Infirmorum Hospital, Belfast, 1950–66.
Consultant ophthalmic surgeon, Altnagelvin Hospital, Derry, 1966

Brian retired at 65 years of age and is living in Derry.

SHAW, Cyril

Ophthalmic Surgeon

Educ. Queen's College, Belfast
d. 1915

MB, RUI

Clinical assistant, Moorfield's Eye Hospital, London; Golden Square Hospital, London, for ear, nose and throat diseases.
Postgraduate training continued at Marburg, Vienna and Paris.
Assistant surgeon (to Dr Walton Browne [q.v.]), Belfast Ophthalmic Hospital, 1895.
Assistant visiting surgeon (to Dr Hayden Mulholland [q.v.]), Mater Infirmorum Hospital, 1904.
Lecturer in ophthalmology and otology, QUB, 1904.

Produced a small book on *Diseases of the Eye*, 1895; contributed papers to the scientific literature at that time, on 'Sympathetic Ophthalmia', optic neuritis, following a perforating wound to the eyeball and toxic amblyopic.

Cyril Shaw and Hadyn Mulholland [q.v.] were the two ophthalmic and otology surgeons in 1909 in the Mater Infirmorum Hospital. Shaw succeeded Dr William McKeown [q.v.] as lecturer in ophthalmology and otology at Queen's University, Belfast. On his death from pernicious anaemia in 1915, he was succeeded by Dr James Craig [q.v.].

REPUBLIC OF IRELAND

CORK

The Cork Eye, Ear & Throat Hospital, 1900–1988
AND
Cork University Hospital, 1988–2005

The Cork Eye, Ear and Throat Hospital opened in Western Road in 1897, replacing Dr H. McNaughton Jones' 1868 Eye, Ear & Throat Hospital in Nile Street. The Cork Eye, Ear & Throat Hospital served the people of Cork for 91 years until it, in turn, was replaced by the new Cork Regional Hospital at Wilton, in 1988. The Cork Regional Hospital was subsequently renamed the Cork University Hospital.

SANDFORD, Arthur Wellesley

Cork Ophthalmologist and Laryngologist

b. 1859, Kilvernon Rectory, Co. Tipperary, son of Rev. Canon Sandford (Rector of Clonmel and Chancellor of Lismore Cathedral)
Educ. Dr Knight's School; Queen's College, Cork
m. 1902: Lady Mary Carbery (widow of the ninth Baron Carbery) of Castlefreke Castle, Co Cork; 2 s
d. 1939

MD, MCh, 1882

Founder of the Eye, Ear and Throat Hospital, Western Road, Cork, 1887.
Consulting surgeon, lecturer (1890–1910) and Professor (1910–26) in ophthalmology and otolaryngology, UCC.
President of numerous learned societies, including Irish Ophthalmological Society, 1918–19; Vice-President, Ophthalmological Society of the UK, 1902–05.

Sandford practised both specialties and was honoured by the highest offices by practitioners of both. A tireless author and a 'good citizen', he was Commissioner of the Boy Scouts and a friend of Baden Powell. His sons went to school in England and he moved there to be near them, but he always returned to Cork to see patients and fulfil his academic duties. He attended hospital board meetings up to his death.

He was an adornment to his chosen specialties.

HOBART, Nathaniel Joseph

Honorary Consulting Surgeon

b. 1834, Son of Samuel Hobart, MD
m. son, Nathaniel Henry [q.v.], a consulting surgeon
d. 1909

MD, MRCS

Honorary consulting surgeon, 1868–1909.

HOBART, Nathaniel Henry

Consulting Surgeon

b. 1866, son of Nathaniel J. Hobart [q.v.], MD, MRCS
m. 1901: Edith Lane; 2s, 1d
d. 1959

MB

Anaesthetist, 1895–1911.
Consulting surgeon, 1911–22.

TOWNSEND, Thomas H. Denny

Ophthalmic Surgeon

Educ. Trinity College, Dublin

BA, MB, TCD, 1899

Assistant surgeon, 1913–26.
Senior surgeon, 1926–52.
President, Irish Ophthalmological Society.

BROWNE, James M.

Cork Eyes and Ear, Nose and Throat Surgeon

Educ. Queen's College, Cork; Cecilia Street, Dublin

MB, RUI, 1894; Diploma in Ophthalmology, Oxon 1912

Registrar and house surgeon, Royal Eye Hospital, Southwark; house surgeon, Mater Hospital, Dublin; house surgeon, Throat & Ear Hospital, Brighton.
Temporary Captain, Royal Army Medical Corps.
Visiting oculist, Union Hospital, Kanturk.
Assistant surgeon, Eye, Ear & Throat Hospital, Cork.
Ophthalmic and aural surgeon, Mercy Hospital, Cork; Cork District Hospital.

O'HEA CUSSEN, Vernon

Cork Ophthalmologist and Professor of Ophthalmology and Otolaryngology

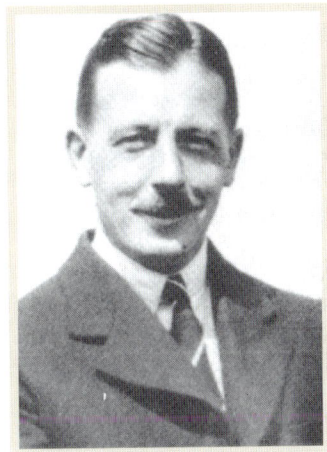

b. 1892, Cork
Educ. Christian Brothers College, Cork; University College Cork
m. 1st: Monica Bergin, Kinsale (d.); 5 children. 2nd in 1945: Mary Lehane
d. 1967

Postgraduate studies in Oxford, London and Vienna. Travelled extensively to visit European and American clinics.
Joined staff of Mercy Hospital.
Lecturer (1926) and Professor (1946) in ophthalmology and otolaryngology, UCC.

Always immaculately turned out, Vernon O'Hea Cussen cut an apparently languid figure with something of the grandee about his demeanour. Refraction was an important part of his practice and, when testing with different lenses, he was in the habit of asking the patient after each change 'Better or Worse?' This phrase got into the student folklore of the time and was part of any innocent imitation of the professor. It was perhaps inevitable that when he returned from his second honeymoon the question chalked on the blackboard was 'Better or Worse?' He gave solid, sensible advice to undergraduates, and external examiners were invariably impressed. To a student misusing the ophthalmoscope, he remarked, 'You are endeavouring to visualise your own retina.' 'Endeavouring' and 'visualise' say it all about Vernon.

He was interested in rugby and golf.

BARTER, George

Cork Ophthalmologist

b. 1896, son of Thomas Barter and Nora Barter (*née* Griffin)
Educ. Presentation College, Cork; University College Cork
m. 1921: Mary McEvoy; 2 s, 3 d
d. 1972

MB, UCC, 1921

Surgeon Sub-Lieutenant, Royal Navy, 1918 for about a year in the middle of his medical school course.
Postgraduate training at Moorfield's Eye Hospital, London; Oxford Eye Hospital; Vienna.
Surgeon, Eye, Ear and Throat Hospital, Cork, 1924–33; 1938–70.
Surgeon, South Infirmary, Bon Secours Hospital; Cork County Home (St Finbarr's).

George Barter had been everywhere there was something to learn in his specialty and it showed. The gap in his service as surgeon at the Eye, Ear and Throat Hospital was when he declined to do extern (outpatient) work, but the management, recognising his quality, enticed him back.

With an elegant appearance and completely professional, he had the 'carriage trade sewn up'. 'A man of protean interests,' he was proficient at golf, squash, tennis, sailing and angling. He was also interested in archaeology, theatre and music. Every specialty needs people who give patients complete confidence and, in his time, George Barter was such a man.

FOLEY, J. H.

Surgeon, 1928–1969

Educ. Castleknock College; University College Cork
m. Miss Murphy (the hospital matron); 3 d
d. 1969

J. H. Foley played cricket for Ireland in 1926.

HACKETT, Hawksworth

Surgeon, 1918–1922

MURPHY (ATKINS), C. M. (Nuala)

Honorary Assistant Surgeon, 1947–1962

m. 1962: Prof. H. Atkins (President of UCC)
d. 1989

CANTILLON, Charles J. (Charlie)

Consultant Surgeon

b. son of Dr Edwin Cantillon (1828–1945), MD, Lecturer in Therapeutics, UCC
Educ. Clongowes Wood College; University College Cork
d. 1985

MD, DOMS.

Postgraduate training: Oxford; Bristol; Moorfield's Eye Hospital, London.
Consultant surgeon, North Infirmary and Bon Secours Hospital, 1937–81; Eye, Ear, Nose and Throat Hospital, 1963–81.

Charlie Cantillon played cricket for Munster. He later became a highly competitive bridge player.

O'CONNOR, Ina

Consultant Surgeon, 1960–1989

MB, DOMS

Ina O'Connor was ophthalmologist to Jack Lynch TD, Taoiseach.

SULLIVAN, Jack V.

Consultant Surgeon

Educ. Presentation College, Cork; Clongowes Wood College; University College Cork

Postgraduate training: Moorfield's Eye Hospital, London and Dublin.
Royal Air Force, 1941–45.
Clinical assistant, 1956–68.
Assistant surgeon, 1968–69.

Consultant, 1969–81.

Jack was one of three Cork doctors named Jack O'Sullivan, which sometimes caused confusion. However, he was Jackie 'Eyes', while the others were Jackie 'Gas' (anaesthetist) and Jackie 'Nuts' (psychiatrist). Polished, debonair, permanently tanned, immaculate with RAF tie, whiskey voiced and wonderfully companionable, Jack was admirable and professional.

WILSON, Denis J.

Consultant Surgeon

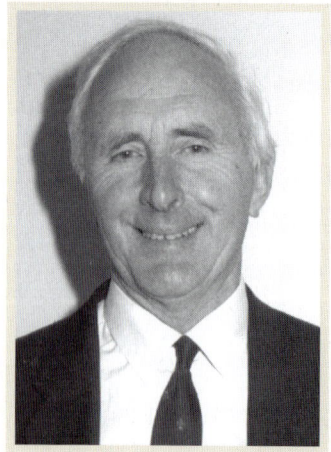

b. 1924

Educ. Presentation College, Cobh; University College Cork

m. Mary O'Flynn MSc; 3 s, 1 d (Fiona Shaw, actor)

MB, 1948; DObst, RCOG, 1952; DPH Eng, 1954; DO, 1960

Senior house officer and resident surgical officer, Royal Eye Hospital, Manchester; registrar, Department of Ophthalmology, University of Manchester. Assistant surgeon, 1968; Consultant surgeon, 1969–87, Cork Eye, Ear and Throat Hospital. President, Irish Faculty of Ophthalmology, 1980; section of ophthalmology, RAMI, 1987.

Author of *'De Iron Trote'* — *a history of the Cork Eye, Ear & Throat Hospital*

Denis Wilson played rugby (wing forward) for Munster and the Combined Universities. According to an Irish selector, he was 'too much of a gentleman to be an international wing forward'.

MADDEN, Jack G.

Consultant Surgeon

b. 1924, Cork

Educ. Christian Brothers College, Cork; University College Cork

m. Patricia Fitzgerald (d.)

MB, 1948; MCh, DO.

Assistant surgeon, 1969–76; consultant surgeon, 1976–90.
President, Irish Ophthalmological Society.
Last Chairman, Medical Board, Ear, Nose and Throat Hospital.

Dublin

Royal Victoria Eye and Ear Hospital

The Royal Victoria Eye and Ear Hospital was established in 1897 with the amalgamation of the National Eye Hospital, founded by Isaac Ryall in 1814, and St Mark's Ophthalmic Hospital for Diseases of the Eye and Ear, founded by William Wilde in 1844. The founding fathers of the new hospital were William Wilde and Henry Swanzy — 'disparate in many ways, their common ground was in owning the quality of greatness, each contributing in his own way to an amalgamated foundation whose present day sophistication neither could have imagined' (Dr Gearóid Crookes [q.v.], 1993).

SWANZY, Sir Henry Rosborough PRCSI 1906–1908

Surgeon and Professor of Ophthalmic and Aural Surgery

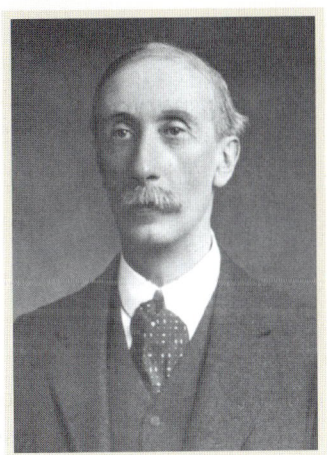

b. 1844
Educ. Trinity College, Dublin
m. Mary Knox (d. 1909), daughter of John Denham (PRCSI, 1873–74); 2 s (both died at birth); 3 d
d. 1913

BA, TCD, 1864; MB, 1865; FRCSI, 1873; DSc, Sheffield, 1908

Postgraduate training in Vienna and Berlin, including two years as personal assistant to von Graefe, a man whom he believed to be irreplaceable.
Founding father of RVEEH.
Surgeon, Prussian Army, Battle of Sadowa, 1866;
National Eye & Ear Infirmary, the Adelaide Hospital and the RVEEH, 1870–1913.

Professor of Ophthalmic and Aural Surgery, RCSI, 1877–1913, succeeding Henry Wilson, Sir William Wilde's natural son.

Bowman Lecturer of the Ophthalmological Society of the UK, 1888.
President, Ophthalmological Society of the UK, 1907.
President, RCSI, 1906–08.
Knighted 1908.

Published *A Handbook on Diseases of the Eye and their Treatment*, H. K. Lewis, London, 1884, which ran to ten editions.

When he died in 1913, Sir Henry was president-elect of the ophthalmic section of the International Congress of Medicine. Sadly, 'death robbed him of this supreme honour but already he was immortal by his lifework, an ornament to his hospital, his profession and his native land' (Dr Gearóid Crookes [q.v.], 1993)

He had a sharp tongue and was regarded as having a cool rather than warm personality, but he was probably the best-known Irish surgeon or indeed doctor outside of Ireland. A real giant.

STOREY, Sir John Benjamin PRCSI 1906–1908

Surgeon and Professor of Ophthalmic and Aural Surgery

Educ. Winchester; Trinity College, Dublin

MB 1876, MCh, FRCSI 1880.

Postgraduate training in Zurich and Vienna, under Horner, von Arlt and Jaeger.
Founder, Irish Ophthalmological Society, 1917.
Surgeon, St Mark's Hospital, 1880–97; RVEEH 1897–1922.
Professor of Ophthalmology and Aural Surgery, RCSI.
President, Ophthalmological Society of the UK, 1918–20.
President, RCSI 1906–08.
President, Irish Medical Association, 1913–14.
Honorary surgeon oculist in Ireland to HM the King.
High Sheriff of Tyrone, 1911.
Co-editor, *Ophthalmic Review*.
Knighted 1909.

Numerous publications.

Storey ranks with Wilde and Swanzy in the pantheon of Irish ophthalmologists.

BENSON, Arthur Hy

Surgeon

b. 1852, fifth son of Charles Benson (PRCSI 1854–55) and Elizabeth Benson (*née* Gray), a celebrated beauty
Educ. Trinity College, Dublin
m. 1894: Ethel Dawson of Wexford
d. 1912

MB, TCD, 1876; FRCSI, 1881

Surgeon, St Mark's Hospital 1879–97; RVEEH, 1897–1912

Arthur Benson travelled widely — India, South Africa, Canada — and published numerous papers, including the first description of asteroid hyalitis, 'Benson's Disease'. He prescribed spectacles for James Joyce.

FITZGERALD, Charles Edward

Surgeon

b. 1846
Educ. Trinity College, Dublin

MB, TCD, 1868; MD, 1878; FRCPI, 1886, subsequently PRCPI.

Surgeon, National Eye & Ear Infirmary, 1871–97; RVEEH, 1897; Richmond Hospital, 1897–1914.
Surgeon oculist in Ireland to Queen Victoria.

MAXWELL, P. W.

Surgeon

m. daughter was Dr Euphan Maxwell [q.v.]
d. 1917

MB, 1880; MD, Edin, 1888; FRCSI, 1890

Assistant surgeon, St Mark's Hospital, 1883–97.
Surgeon, RVEEH, 1897–1917.

ODEVAINE, Ferdinand

Surgeon

FRCSI, 1875

Assistant surgeon, St Mark's Hospital, 1884–97; RVEEH, 1897–1908.

WERNER, Louis J., Snr

Surgeon and Professor of Ophthalmology

Educ. Trinity College, Dublin
m. son was Louis Werner, Jnr [q.v.]

MB, TCD, 1884; FRCSI, 1898

Surgeon, National Hospital, 1886–97; Mater Misericordiae Hospital and RVEEH, 1897–1936.
Professor of Ophthalmology, UCD, 1897–1936.
Council member, Ophthalmological Society, UK.

Numerous publications.

MONTGOMERY, Robert J.

Surgeon 1897–1912

FRCSI, 1889

A respected but extremely retiring man, Robert Montgomery was a bachelor who lived with his two sisters and always wore a bowler hat. 'No matter what hat Dr Montgomery wore, when his will was read his contemporaries removed theirs with some respect when they heard he had left £5,000 to found an annual lecture in ophthalmology' (L. B. Somerville-Large [q.v.]). The lecture was named in memory of his mother, and an invitation to deliver the Mary Louisa Prentice Montgomery Memorial Lecture is now one of the great accolades in international ophthalmology.

MOONEY, Herbert Charles

Surgeon

Educ. Carmichael College; Catholic University School of Medicine (Cecilia Street)
m. son was Alan Mooney [q.v.] (ophthalmologist)

MB, RUI, 1892; FRCSI, 1893

Postgraduate training in London and Vienna.
Surgeon, Temple Street Children's Hospital & RVEEH, 1897–1942.
Oculist in Ordinary to HE, the Lord Lieutenant.

Mooney was the first of the dynasty which still serves the RVEEH with great distinction, all of whom are revered for their outstanding work and generosity.

CRAWLEY, Frank C.

Surgeon

Educ. Trinity College, Dublin

BA (Cantab), MB, TCD, 1896; MD, 1897; FRCSI, 1900

Surgeon, Royal City of Dublin Hospital & RVEEH, 1900–35.

CUMMINS, Joseph Dominick

Surgeon, Royal Victoria Eye & Ear Hospital, 1912–1926

MB, RUI, 1908

MATTHEWS, Richard H.

Surgeon

Educ. Trinity College, Dublin

BA, TCD, 1907; MB, 1910; MD, 1911

Surgeon, National Hospital for Consumption, Co. Wicklow; Dr Steevens' Hospital and RVEEH, 1913–24.

MAXWELL, Euphan Montgomerie

Ophthalmic Surgeon

b. daughter of Dr P. W. Maxwell [q.v.]

MB, Dub, 1910; FRCSI, 1914

Surgeon, Meath Hospital & RVEEH, 1913–55.

The first woman ophthalmic surgeon in Ireland, Euphan Maxwell served in the Royal Army Medical Corps, 1916–17. She gave the inaugural Montgomery Lecture (1915) and the next two as well!

MacFETRIDGE, W. C.

Surgeon, 1919–1934

GOULDING, H. B.

Surgeon, 1922–1947

MacAREVEY, J. B.

Surgeon, 1922–1950

A pioneer of successful corneal grafting, he gave the Montgomery Lecture in 1944.

CONNOLLY, Mary F.

Surgeon, 1926–1936

Originally a nursing sister in the hospital, Mary Connolly qualified in medicine and then ophthalmology, eventually being appointed to the surgical staff.

WERNER, Louis E., Jnr

Surgeon

b. son of Louis Werner, Snr [q.v.]
Educ. Trinity College, Dublin

MB, TCD; FRCSI (Hon.), 1965

Surgeon, RVEEH, 1925–65.
Lecturer in ophthalmology, TCD.
Montgomery Lecturer, 1929.
President of the Ophthalmological Society of the UK, 1974–75, one of only four Irish ophthalmologists to achieve this distinction in over 100 years.

Louis Werner was widely loved for his kindness, humour and wit and envied for his erudition and because his secretary was the most beautiful girl in Dublin.
When presented unexpectedly with his portrait in oils, painted as a reflection in the pupil of an eye, his response was 'Thank goodness I wasn't a gynaecologist'. He introduced the slit-lamp to Dublin.

MOONEY, Alan J.

Consultant Surgeon

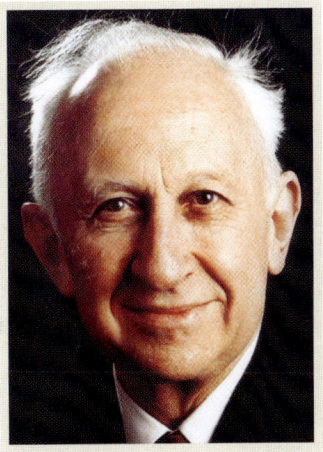

b. son of Herbert Mooney [q.v.], (ophthalmologist)
m. son was David Mooney [q.v.] (ophthalmologist)

Consultant surgeon, RVEEH, 1926–72.
Montgomery Lecturer, 1930.

Alan Mooney was one of three successive generations of noted ophthalmologists who have served the RVEEH since its foundation. He pioneered the fledgling subspeciality of neuro-ophthalmology, gaining an international reputation and bringing the greatest figures in world ophthalmology to visit Ireland. In addition, 'the single-minded determination of this most modest of men' (Dr Gearóid Crookes [q.v.], 1993) raised the money to establish the research unit at the RVEEH, together with a building to house it, designed by the architect Brian O'Connell.

The Irish College of Ophthalmologists named its annual Mooney Lecture in his honour and as a mark of appreciation for his very great help and generosity to Irish ophthalmology.

TOMKIN, Harris

Surgeon

m. son was Alex Tomkin, FRCS [q.v.]

MB, DOMS

Surgeon, RVEEH, 1928–80.

LAVERY, Frank. J.

Surgeon

m. son was Frank Linton Lavery, FRCSI, FRC Ophth [q.v.]

MD, MCh, DOMS

Surgeon, RVEEH, 1928–65.
Professor of Ophthalmology, UCD, 1946–65.
President, Irish Ophthalmological Society, 1955–57.
Montgomery Lecturer, 1930.

Frank J. Lavery was a forthright character whose dedication led to the eradication of trachoma in Ireland.

SOMERVILLE-LARGE, L. B. ('Beecher')

Surgeon

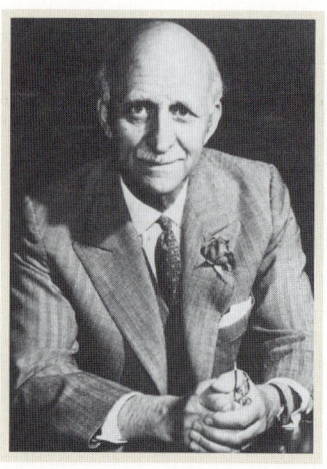

MB, DOMS, FRCSI (Hon.), 1965

Surgeon, 1934–66.
Montgomery Lecturer, 1959.
Secretary, Irish Ophthalmological Society 1935–52; President, 1952–54.
President, Ophthalmological Society of the UK, 1962–64, one of only four Irish ophthalmologists to achieve this distinction in the 102 years of its existence.

'Beecher' invited the first of many distinguished overseas ophthalmologists to deliver the Montgomery Lecture and established the international reputation of the Irish Ophthalmological Society. He commissioned a singularly beautiful presidential seal of office from the great Irish silversmith, Oisín Kelly, and presented it to the Society. It has been retained as the seal of the Irish College of Ophthalmologists.

He also endowed the Somerville-Large Award to encourage young consultants at the RVEEH to travel abroad to centres of ophthalmic excellence.

He was the proud possessor of Sir William Wilde's set of ophthalmic instruments. On joining up during the Second World War, he entrusted them to the care of the theatre sister. On returning from the war, he was informed that 'them rusty instruments' had 'been binned'.

McCREA, W. B.

Surgeon, 1937–1951

McKERNAN, R. L.

Surgeon, 1943–1965

DOUGLAS, D. H.

Surgeon, 1947–1979

d. 1979

MB, DOMS

D. H. Douglas achieved an outstanding reputation for his work on infantile glaucoma and in retinal detachment surgery.

MacDOUGALD, T. J.

Surgeon 1947–1981

MB, DOMS

T. J. MacDougald established the RVEEH glaucoma clinic.

GUINAN, Philomena M.

Surgeon 1947–1981

MB, DOMS

Ophthalmic surgeon, St Vincent's Hospital; Children's Hospital, Temple Street.

Philomena Guinan pioneered retinal photo-coagulation surgery in Dublin.

CROOKES, Gearóid P.

Consultant Surgeon

Educ. University College Dublin
m. Jean
d. 2001

MB, UCD, 1939; MCh, DOMS; BA (English and art history), 1985; MA (architectural history), 1988; PhD, UCD, 1992 (thesis on 'The Irish Builder')

Consultant surgeon, RVEEH, 1951–81.
Secretary, Irish Ophthalmological Society, 1966–81.
Montgomery Lecturer, 1981.

Gearóid P. Crookes succeeded L. B. Somerville-Large [q.v.] as an outstanding secretary of the Irish Ophthalmological Society. He furthered the reputation of the society at home and abroad and organised notable joint meetings with ophthalmological societies in the USA, Bavaria, Greece and Denmark, amongst others, a tradition that is still followed by his successors.

A delightful man, who was interested in everything and everyone, he studied the humanities after his retirement and the death of his beloved wife, Jean. His fine history of the RVEEH, *Dublin's Eye & Ear — the making of a monument*, was published in 1993. His ophthalmological swansong was a memorably witty oration at the Centenary Meeting of the RVEEH in 1997.

ROCHE, T. F.

Surgeon

d. 1969

Surgeon, RVEEH, 1952–69.

Expert in corneal grafting, T. F. Roche organised the modernisation of the RVEEH eye theatres in the 1960s.

McAULEY, Francis Desmond (Frank)

Consultant Surgeon

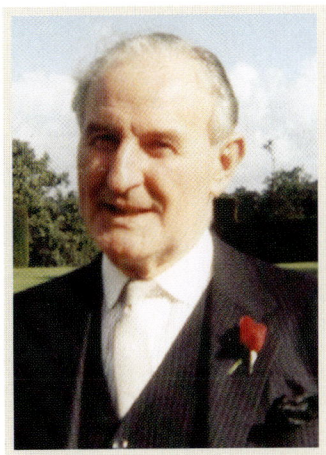

Educ. University College Dublin

MB, UCD, 1946; MCh, FRC Ophth, London

Trained and was a consultant in London before returning to Dublin.
Consultant surgeon, RVEEH, 1962–84.

A pioneer in the then newly developing area of retinal surgery, Frank McAuley founded and was the first President of the Irish Faculty of Ophthalmology, which was created to handle the increasing number of bureaucratic and other non-clinical problems faced by the speciality. It accomplished an enormous amount of largely unsung, but essential work. In 1990, the Faculty amalgamated with the Irish Ophthalmological Society to form the Irish College of Ophthalmologists.

Irish ophthalmology owes Frank a singular debt. A man of uncompromisingly high standards.

BLAKE, John

Consultant Eye Surgeon

b. 1932
Educ. Christian Brothers College, Cork; University College Cork
m. Dr Ethna Power, daughter is Alison Blake, FRCS

MB, UCC, 1955 (first place in class); MCh, FRCS, FRCSE, FRCSI, FRC Ophth

Postgraduate training in London.
Consultant eye surgeon, RVEEH, 1965–96.

John Blake was a superb operating surgeon, he is a complete gentleman and has a shining intelligence. It was as a result of his efforts in the 1980s that laminated-glass windscreens were eventually introduced on cars sold in Ireland, resulting in a 90 per cent reduction in penetrating eye injuries.

FENTON, Maurice

Consultant Eye Surgeon

MB, FRCSI, FRC Ophth

Consultant eye surgeon, RVEEH, 1967–2002.

A noted retinal surgeon, Kerry supporter and horse-racing enthusiast, Maurice Fenton also instituted the RVEEH vitreoretinal unit.

WALSH, Joseph Patrick B.

Paediatric Ophthalmologist

b. 1934
Educ. University College Dublin
m. Gloria Counihan (MB, DO)
d. 2008

MB, UCD; FRCSI, FRC Ophth

Senior registrar, Royal Eye Hospital, London
Consultant eye surgeon, RVEEH; Our Lady's Hospital for Sick Children, Crumlin, 1967–97.

His recreations included golf.

TOMKIN, Alex

Consultant Eye Surgeon

b. son of Harris Tomkin, FRCS [q.v.]
m. Julie (within two weeks of meeting her)
d. 1984

MB, FRCS

Postgraduate training at Moorfield's Eye Hospital, London.
Consultant Eye Surgeon, RVEEH, 1969–84.

Alex Tomkin was a contact lens expert and a fine cellist. His happy marriage and promising career ended with his tragically early death only three years after that of his father, Harris Tomkin, FRCS.

COLLUM, Louis

Consultant Eye Surgeon and Professor of Ophthalmology

Educ. University College Dublin

MB, UCD; FRCS; FRCSI; FRC Ophth; FEBO

Consultant surgeon, RVEEH, 1972–2005.
Professor of Ophthalmology, RCSI, 1983–2005.
President, Irish College of Ophthalmologists, 2000–2001.
Mooney Lecturer, 1997.

Louis Collum has an international reputation in corneal surgery and disease. He also has a national reputation in horse-racing!

MOONEY, David

Consultant Eye Surgeon

b. son of Alan Mooney, FRCS [q.v.]; grandson of Herbert Mooney, FRCSI [q.v.]
Educ. University College Dublin

MB, BCh, BAO, UCD, 1964; FRCS; FRC Ophth

Postgraduate training in Dublin and London.
Consultant surgeon, RVEEH, 1972–2005.
Treasurer, Irish College of Ophthalmologists, 1990–96.
Secretary, ophthalmic section, RAMI 1988–94.

David Mooney is the third successive generation of the family to have served the RVEEH since its foundation in 1897. He pioneered fluorescein angiography and established an international reputation for the RVEEH medical retina unit. As the first treasurer of the Irish College of Ophthalmologists, he is responsible for its sound finances.

CASSIDY, Hugh

Consultant Eye Surgeon

Educ. University College Dublin
m. daughter is Prof. Lorraine Cassidy, FRC Ophth

MB, UCD, 1967; FRCS; FRC Ophth

Consultant surgeon, RVEEH 1981–2003; St James's Hospital, 1990–2003.

Hugh Cassidy is a keen golfer.

Mater Misericordiae Hospital

The hospital was founded by Mother Catherine McAuley of the Sisters of Mercy, in 1861. Catherine McAuley's face graced the Irish £5 note for many years.

WERNER, Louis J. Snr

Visiting Surgeon and Professor of Ophthalmology

See also under RVEEH.

Visiting surgeon, 1897–1936.
Professor of Ophthalmology, UCD, 1897–1936.

DWYER-JOYCE, Patrick, Snr ('Robert' or 'Bob')

Visiting Surgeon and Professor of Ophthalmology

m. son was Patrick Dwyer-Joyce, Jnr [q.v.]
d. 1960

Visiting surgeon, Mater Misericordiae Hospital, Dublin.
Professor of Ophthalmology, UCD, 1936–46.

Tall, elegant, well travelled and the supreme professional, Dwyer-Joyce had a huge practice when fees were much higher than now. 'One cataract equals one housemaid for one year' (1938). He rode a bicycle into his eighties.

LAVERY, Francis J.

See under RVEEH

DWYER-JOYCE, Patrick Jnr

Consultant Ophthalmic Surgeon and Professor of Ophthalmology

b. son of Patrick Dwyer-Joyce, Snr [q.v.]

Consultant ophthalmic surgeon 1965–83.
Professor of Ophthalmology, UCD, 1965–83.

A delightful, polished gentleman, Patrick Dwyer-Joyce, Jnr, built up the Mater eye unit by bringing in a number of experienced well-trained consultants in many sub-specialties.

A classical scholar and enthusiastic race-goer.

EUSTACE, Peter

Consultant Eye Surgeon and Professor of Ophthalmology

Educ. University College Galway

MB, UCG, 1961; FRCS; FRCSI; FRC Ophth; FEBO

Consultant eye surgeon, Mater Hospital, 1973–2002.
Professor of Ophthalmology, UCD, 1983–2002.
President, Irish College of Ophthalmologists, 1993–95.
President, ophthalmology section, UEMS 1994–98.
President, International Neuro-Ophthalmological Society, 1998–99.
Founder member, European Board of Ophthalmology, 1990.

Co-author of the best-selling *Textbook of Neuro-Ophthalmolgy*.

A great enthusiast and an outstanding teacher, Peter Eustace was North of England schoolboy golf champion in 1953.

O'DONOGHUE, Hugh

Consultant Eye Surgeon

Educ. Castleknock College; University College Dublin

MCh; FRCS; FRC Ophth

Consultant eye surgeon, West Middlesex Hospital, 1965–77; Mater Misericordiae Hospital, 1977–95.

The complete gentleman, Hugh O'Donoghue was a noted teacher. He also played squash for Ireland.

BOWELL, Roger

Consultant Eye Surgeon

Educ. Trinity College, Dublin

MB, TCD, 1965; FRCS; FRCSI; FRC Ophth

Consultant eye surgeon, Sligo General Hospital, 1974–79; Mater Misericordiae Hospital, 1978–2001.
President, Irish College of Ophthalmologists, 1997–99.

A vigneron manqué, Roger is famed for winning an ophthalmological blind wine tasting in Paris in 1999, organised by Michelle Beaconsfield of Moorfield's Eye Hospital, naming five out of six wines correctly and being the only competitor who identified any! He is also a much admired professional who built up an outstanding department in the Children's Hospital, Temple Street.

KELLY (*née* BARRY) Geraldine

Dublin Ophthalmologist

b. 1943, Dublin, eldest daughter of Kevin Barry and Patricia Barry (*née* Mayne)
Educ. Convent of the Sacred Heart, Leeson Street; University College Dublin
m. 1967: Dan Kelly (urologist) [q.v.]; 3 s (Daniel deceased; Robert is a Dublin cardiologist)

MB, UCD, 1966; FRCS, 1973; FRC Ophth, 1979

Postgraduate training posts at Royal Victoria Eye and Ear Hospital, Dublin.
Consultant ophthalmic surgeon, Royal Victoria Eye and Ear Hospital; St Vincent's Hospital, 1978–2005.

Geraldine Kelly's particular expertise was in the technically demanding area of the retina where she displayed legendary calm under pressure.

Tall, elegant, always impeccably turned out as if she had just come from a salon and a spa, she continues to turn heads when she passes. In retirement, she has grown even keener on golf.

GALWAY

University College Hospital

The County Infirmary (usually called the Galway Hospital) on Prospect Hill was opened in 1802 and the Galway Workhouse in Newcastle in 1841. These were amalgamated in 1922 into a new Central Hospital, built in Newcastle on the site of the old workhouse. It was replaced in 1954 by the new Galway Regional Hospital on the same site in Newcastle, and was renamed University College Hospital in 1989.

McENRI, Seaghain Pádraig

Ophthalmologist and Professor of Ophthalmology and Otology

Educ. Trinity College, Dublin

BA, TCD, 1884; MB, 1886; MD, 1888; MA, 1908; MCh

Postgraduate training in London.
Ophthalmologist, Galway Hospital and Central Hospital, 1910–30.
First Professor of Ophthalmology and Otology, UCG, 1916–30.
President, Gaelic League; co-founder, Coláiste Connacht, Spiddal.

Numerous publications in both English and French.

Seaghain McEnri was appointed lecturer in modern Irish in UCG in 1910 and applied for a lectureship in ophthalmology in 1912, but this was initially refused on the grounds that an eye department was not needed. His perseverance paid off in 1916.

O'MALLEY, Charles Conor

Ophthalmologist and Professor of Ophthalmology and Otology

b. 1889
Educ. University College Galway

m. Dr Sarah (Sal) Joyce; sons, Patrick O'Malley MD and Conor O'Malley MD, are both eminent ophthalmologists in the USA; grandson, Simon Kelly, FRC Ophth
d. 1982
BSc, 1914; MB, UCG, 1917; MD; MCh; DOMS

Royal Navy, 1917–18.
Postgraduate training at Moorfield's Eye Hospital, London.
Radiologist, Central Hospital, 1928–32.
Ophthalmologist, Central Hospital Galway, 1922–54; Regional Hospital, 1954–63.
Professor of Ophthalmology and Otology, UCG, 1931–63.
Knight of Malta; Knight of St Lazarus; founded first unit in Ireland of the Order of Malta Ambulance Corps.

Charles O'Malley was a noted sportsman and wrote books on fishing and shooting. He was also a historian and president of the Galway Archaeological and Historical Society. He spent many vacations in India, working in cataract clinics.

HEWSON, George Everard

Ophthalmic Surgeon

MB, MCh, FRCSI, FRC Ophth

Ophthalmic surgeon, Regional Hospital Galway, 1963–92.
Statutory lecturer in ophthalmology, UCG, 1966–92.

George Hewson kept a low profile in the hospital, known only as 'the eye surgeon' and always wearing a surgical mask and hat. Well known in professional and hunting circles, a member of the Galway Blazers and a prolific letter-writer to the newspapers.

NOLAN, John

Consultant Eye Surgeon

Educ. Trinity College, Dublin
m. 1965: Ann Venables, DBO(T); 3 s (Daniel Nolan, FRC Ophth), 2 d

BA, MB, TCD, 1956; FRCS Ed; FRCSI; FRC Ophth; FEBO
Postgraduate training in Manchester.

Senior lecturer and honorary consultant, Edinburgh University & Royal Infirmary, 1965–68.
Consultant eye surgeon, St James's Hospital, Leeds, 1968–76; Regional Hospital, Galway, 1976–99.
President, Irish College of Ophthalmologists, 1996–97; ophthalmology section, RAMI, 1994–95.
Master, Oxford Ophthalmological Congress, 1995–96.
Council member, Royal College of Ophthalmologists, 1994–98.
Joint Secretary, section of ophthalmology, Union of European Medical Specialists, 1998–2006.

His subspecialty was paediatric ophthalmology and strabismus.

LIMERICK
Limerick Regional Hospital

SHORTEN, Donal

Consultant Eye Surgeon

d. 2003

MB; MCh; DOMS

Consultant eye surgeon, Limerick Regional Hospital, 1952–97.

Donal Shorten was the first consultant eye surgeon at Limerick Regional Hospital.

SLIGO
Sligo General Hospital

BOWELL, Roger

Consultant Eye Surgeon, Sligo General Hospital, 1975–83

(See under Mater Misericordiae Hospital, Dublin).

WATERFORD
Waterford Regional Hospital

CONDON, Richard A.

Consultant Eye Surgeon

> m. son is Patrick Ian Condon FRC Ophth [q.v.]
>
> MCh; DO
>
> Consultant eye surgeon, Waterford Regional Hospital, 1952–71.

Richard Condon founded the Regional Eye Department in Waterford. It started in a greyhound kennel (!) owned by the County Manager in an old derelict building, and was vehemently opposed by the Department of Health at the time. In the 1950s, he was possibly the first surgeon in Ireland to use intra-ocular lenses in cataract surgery.

RYAN, John Louis (Louis)

Waterford Ophthalmologist

> b. 1921, eldest son of Dr James Ryan and Mary Ryan (*née* O'Brien)
> **Educ.** Clongowes Wood College; University College Dublin
> m. 1958: Carmel Crotty, daughter of Raymond and Elizabeth Crotty; 2 s, 4 d (Deirdre, a doctor; Elizabeth, a nurse; Cloddah, a dentist)
> d. 1991
>
> MB, UCD, 1944; DOMS, 1947; MCh, NUI, 1958
>
> Royal Army Medical Corps, 1947–50.
> Postgraduate work at Royal Eye Hospital, London, 1951–52 (under Mr A. Cameron FRCSI); registrar, St Paul's Eye Hospital, Liverpool, 1952–54.
> Ophthalmic surgeon to Waterford County and City Infirmary, 1962–87 (closure).
> Worked at Ardkeen (Waterford Regional Hospital), 1955–91.
> Ophthalmic physician, South Eastern Health Board at Clonmel and Cashel, 1970–91.

Louis Ryan was handsome, 'romantic', full of confidence and an undaunted optimist. He loved life, which included golf, bridge, Rotary, travelling, tennis, rowing but, above all, horse-breeding. He never realised his dream of breeding the winner of the Cheltenham Gold Cup but he had a lot of fun trying.

CONDON, Patrick Ian

Consultant Waterford Eye Surgeon, 1971–2003

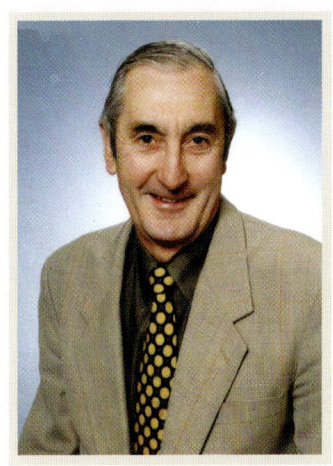

Educ. University College Dublin

MB, UCD, 1960; MCh; FRCS; FRCSI; FRCS Ed; FRC Ophth

Postgraduate training, London.
President, UK & Ireland Society of Cataract and Refractive Surgeons 1997–99.
Montgomery Lecturer, 1998. RCSI gold medal 1999.

An innovative, iconic surgeon with an international reputation, Patrick Condon introduced phacoemulsification cataract technique to Ireland, pioneered small incision cataract surgery and published original work on refractive surgery. He made his unit a place of pilgrimage and trainees beat a path to Waterford for superb training on a one-to-one basis.

A gardener, athlete, workaholic, pianist, insomniac and the life and soul of any party starting after midnight!

EYE SURGEONS IN FULL-TIME PRIVATE PRACTICE

BROWNE, Michael James ('Bomber')

Eye Surgeon

Educ. University College Galway

MB (NUI Galway), 1968; FRCS, FR C Ophth

Eye surgeon, Blackrock Clinic, Dublin.

'Bomber' Browne was a noted rugby player who captained Blackrock and played many times for Connacht. Fans felt it unjust that he never played for Ireland.

LAVERY, Frank Linton

Eye Surgeon

Educ. University College Dublin

MB (UCD),1961; FRCS; FRCSI

Eye surgeon, Wellington Ophthalmic Clinic, Dublin 4.

Frank Lavery introduced laser refractive surgery to Ireland. He is a well-known horticulturalist with a famous garden.

17
ORTHOPAEDIC SURGEONS IN THE REPUBLIC OF IRELAND

ORTHOPAEDIC SURGEONS IN THE REPUBLIC OF IRELAND

BRADY, Patrick Gerard (Gerry)

Orthopaedic Surgeon

b. 1925

Educ. Blackrock College; Royal College of Surgeons in Ireland

m. 1955: Dorothy Rowan; 3 d, 1 s (Owen, orthopaedic surgeon, Navan)

LRCP & SI, 1949; FRCSI, 1953; MCh Orth, Liverpool, 1955; FICS, 1964

Postgraduate posts included orthopaedic registrar, Royal Northern Hospital, London; orthopaedic registrar, Liverpool Orthopaedic Group.
Senior consultant orthopaedic surgeon, Jervis Street Hospital; Our Lady's Hospital for Sick Children, Crumlin, Dublin.

Gerry was a quick operator, wading through long operating lists of great variety. He was one of the first to practise hip replacement in Dublin.
Tall, fair-haired, handsome, athletic, sociable and immensely energetic, he had the remarkable distinction of representing Ireland at the Olympic Games in swimming (1948) and shooting (1960).

CHATER, Eric Harold

Galway Orthopaedic Surgeon

Educ. Calcutta; National Maternity Hospital, Dublin

MB, Calcutta, 1945; FRCSI, 1961; LM, National Maternity Hospital, Dublin, 1948

Postgraduate work: residency in surgery and orthopaedics, St Luke's Hospital, New Bedford, Massachusetts; orthopaedic registrar, Regional Hospital Galway; house surgeon, East Ham Memorial Hospital, London.

Senior orthopaedic surgeon, Western Health Board.
Lecturer in orthopaedics, UCG.

One of the early enthusiasts for the AO (internal fixation systems), Eric Chater was a pleasant colleague with a strong academic bent.

COLVILLE, James (Jimmy)

Dublin Shoulder Surgeon

b. 1940, Belfast, youngest son of James Colville and Mary Colville (*née* Orr)
Educ. Royal Belfast Academic Institute (INST); Marine Radio College, Belfast; Trinity College, Dublin
m. 1966: Ann Patterson, daughter of Samuel and Helen Patterson; 2 s, 1 d (Jane, a radiologist)

MB, TCD, 1968; FRCSI, 1972; MCh (TCD), 1979

Postgraduate training: Irish Institute of Orthopaedic Surgery senior registrar training programme; Fellowship in upper limb surgery, Heinola, Finland, 1977; Fellowship in micro-surgery/hand surgery, Canniesburn Hospital, Western Infirmary, Glasgow, 1978; Fellowship AO, St Gallen, Canton Hospital, Switzerland, 1978; visiting shoulder Fellowship, Columbia Presbyterian Hospital, New York (where modern shoulder surgery was developed by Charles Neer); Travelling Fellow, British Society of Surgery of the Hand. European visits to centres of excellence, 1978.
Consultant orthopaedic surgeon, with special interest in upper limb surgery, to the Richmond Hospital; Jervis Street Hospital (subsequently Beaumont Hospital); Cappagh National Orthopaedic Hospital, 1979–2005.
President, Irish Association of Occupational Therapists; Irish Hand Surgery Society; British Elbow Shoulder Society.
Foundation Day lecturer, Wrightington Hospital, England.
Intercollegiate Fellowship examiner in orthopaedics and trauma, 1994–2000.

Jimmy Colville, now retired to private practice, is the acknowledged leader of shoulder surgery in Ireland. His list of patients is distinguished, topped perhaps by the captain of the British Lions when his shoulder was tragically and callously dislocated on the Lions Tour of New Zealand, 2004.

Before entering medical school, Jimmy spent four years in marine radio training and at sea. He has a family history of seafaring, one uncle having been captain on a boat which regularly took linen from Belfast to North America and returned with tobacco for Gallagher's. Following internship in Dr Steevens'

Hospital, Dublin, Jimmy spent two years in Northern Canada, mostly treating patients from the Inuit Reservation.

He has a lifelong interest in horses and all matters equestrian and currently rides on a regular basis. Short, balding, wiry, highly skilled, highly organised, with great energy, he is a complete and admirable professional.

De WYTT, William Henry Hyde Joseph de Wolfe
Consultant Orthopaedic Surgeon

b. 1910, London, third child of William H. de Wolfe de Wytt (former Professor of Pharmacology, University of Aberdeen) and Mary de Wolfe de Wytt
Educ. Holloway Secondary School, London; St Bartholomew's Hospital, London, 1928–30; University College Dublin, 1930–35; Mater Hospital, Dublin, 1933–35
m. 1940: Kathleen (*née* Vickers), LRCP & SI DPH London, late Captain, Royal Army Medical Corps, 1935–46; 2 d (both doctors; Carolyn a neurologist in Brisbane)
d. 1977

MRCS, LRCP, Lond, 1935; FRCSI, 1949; FRCS Eng, 1949; MCh Orth, Liverpool, 1951

Postgraduate work: Major surgical specialist, Royal Army Medical Corps effectively 1935–1946. Pre-war and post-war resident posts in English hospitals.
Orthopaedic surgeon, North Eastern Health Board, centred on Navan, 1952.
Consultant orthopaedic surgeon and limb-fitting surgeon, National Rehabilitation Centre; Lourdes Hospital, Drogheda.
President, Irish Medical Union, 1969–70.

A well-bred Londoner, whose father died while he was at medical school, De Wytt qualified at UCD, and subsequently joined the British Army and then the Royal Army Medical Corps. He swept into the Irish orthopaedic and medico-political scene with élan and a certain swagger. His army background gave him a considerable assurance when dealing with other ranks but he was always courteous. He was a first-class orthopaedic surgeon with good judgment, even if the patients were sometimes terrified of his machine-gun-like delivery, which brooked no discussion on alternatives in management. To be fair, he was almost always right. He loved medical politics and was a forceful, fearless speaker, taking on permanent secretaries and ministers with total aplomb. His ringing voice won many a day and he was a genuine tribune of the profession.

Just above average height, dark and sometimes saturnine, always well groomed, he occasionally attended meetings with management in full riding kit. He was a bright comet in those dreary years of the 1960s. His stated ambition was 'to pay off my income tax'. He achieved a great deal and was sadly missed.

His interests included horticulture, particularly roses, orchids and landscape gardening; medical politics; amateur drama; travel; archaeology; history; art; music and antiques.

DUNLOP, John Boyd (Boyd)

Dublin Orthopaedic Surgeon

b. 1918, Dublin, son of John (Johnny) Boyd Dunlop and Constance Mary Dunlop (*née* Moore); grandson of John Boyd Dunlop (opened the world's first pneumatic tyre factory in Dublin)
Educ. Castle Park Preparatory School, Glenageary; Uppingham College, Rutland; Trinity College, Dublin
m. Evelyn Nesbitt, daughter of William Nesbitt (MD, Arnott's Department Store); 1 s (John Boyd Dunlop the Fourth); 2 d
d. 2005

MB, TCD, 1941; FRCSI, 1948

Temporary probationary surgeon lieutenant, Royal Navy, 1944; involved in scheduling the tugs that towed the Mulberry floating harbour to the beaches at Arromanches, Normandy, on D-Day.
Surgical registrar, Dr Steevens' Hospital, 1948–49.
Consultant orthopaedic surgeon, Dr Steevens' Hospital; Incorporated Orthopaedic Hospital of Ireland, 1950–83.
President, Irish Orthopaedic Association.
Member, Irish Institute of Orthopaedic Surgeons.

Influenced by William Steele ('Baldy') Haughton [q.v.], Arthur Chance [q.v.], Jack Cherry [q.v.], and subsequently by (Sir) John Charnley. His special interests were trauma, joint replacement, paediatric orthopaedics and poliomyelitis.

Boyd's work was highly organised and he was one of the first to have a patient questionnaire for common problems like backache, which meant that a recently arrived trainee became useful immediately. He was closely associated with the Central Remedial Clinic (CRC) founded by Lady Valerie Goulding (daughter of [Lord] Walter Monckton) and Kathleen O'Rourke (physiotherapist). This began to give in-patient treatment to poliomyelitis victims (poliomyelitis vanished overnight in 1960 when vaccines abolished the disease), but extended to the treatment of many disabilities and the provision of schooling. Importantly it developed its own transport system to avoid patients staying in hospital longer than was absolutely necessary.

Spare, slight, with never a hair out of place, Boyd was a retiring, widely liked, admired and respected figure and was, in his time, a careful meticulous conscientious operator, trusted by all. He was a hugely effective medico-legal expert in his retirement. Possessed of an intellectual enquiring mind, he had a great interest in history.

FitzPATRICK, David John

Dublin Orthopaedic Surgeon

b. 1937, son of David Collins FitzPatrick and Jean Thompson FitzPatrick
Educ. Miss Notley's Kindergarten and Preparatory School; the High School, 1945–55 (Sizarship in Mathematics, High School Exhibition at Entrance to TCD); Trinity College, Dublin
m. 1st in 1962: Joan Paul; 2nd in 1998: Felicity King (*née* Irvine); 1 s, 2 d (Heather Jane is RGN)

BA, TCD, 1959; MB, TCD, 1961 (professorial prize at graduation); DObst, RCOG, 1963; FRCSI, 1966; FRCS Eng, 1968; MCh, TCD, 1978; Entrance Common Foreign Medical Graduates (ECFMG) for USA registration, 1975; Dip in management, RCSI & IPA, 1993

Postgraduate travelling scholarship in surgery, TCD, 1966. Phillip D. Wilson Prize Hospital for Special Surgery, 1977. Postgraduate appointments at Adelaide Hospital; Mid-Ulster Hospital, Magherafelt; Edinburgh (Prof. J. I. P. James and Douglas Saville); Cardiff (Dylan Evans and Harold Richards); Dublin (J. Boyd Dunlop [q.v.]); Hospital for Special Surgery, New York, as Fellow in orthopaedic pathology, with Dr P. G. Bullough.
Lecturer in surgery, TCD, 1968–71.
Consultant orthopaedic surgeon, Federated Dublin Voluntary Hospitals (Adelaide, Dr Steevens', National Children's, Meath, then AMNCH Tallaght), 1971–2001.
Specialist orthopaedics surgeon, Nyangabwe Hospital, Francistown, Botswana (Overseas Development Administration, UK), 1989–92.
Lecturer in orthopaedics, TCD.

Influenced by Victor Graham (maths teacher), John Sugars [q.v.], Nigel Kinnear [q.v.] and Peter Bullough, orthopaedic pathologist, New York, who added a new dimension to orthopaedics. Wide spectrum of interests within orthopaedics, including metabolic bone disease.

Of medium height, stocky, with trademark prop forward's skewed nose, and a full mop of reddish grey hair, David FitzPatrick has an off-beat sense of humour: quick to be upset; quick to regret. He likes Lord Moynihan's (1865–1936) dictum: 'I am a physician doomed to the practice of surgery.'

He played rugby for Dublin University, Leinster and Irish Universities. He later enjoyed squash, tennis, hill and alpine walking. He reads everything, especially anything about Dublin, and collects books and modern art. He sang with New York Choral Society and Our Lady's Choral Society.

David's boundless energy and enthusiasm for work and play are his central characteristics. He is an enthusiastic and proficient medical historian.

FLYNN, Mark

Waterford Orthopaedic Surgeon

b. 1932, Fermoy, son of Michael (MRCVS) and Ellen Flynn
Educ. Christian Brothers Schools, Fermoy; University College Cork
m. 1970: Muriel Reidy (radiographer), daughter of William and Ellen Reidy, Kilmallock, Co. Limerick; 2 s (Sean, radiologist; Mark, barrister)
d. 1993

MB, UCC, 1955; FRCSI, 1969

Postgraduate appointments: Anatomy Department, UCC; registrar, Limerick County Hospital, Croom; senior registrar, Robert Jones and Agnes Hunt Orthopaedic Hospital, Oswestry, Shropshire, 1971–74; senior registrar, Birmingham Accident Hospital, 1974. Consultant orthopaedic surgeon, North Eastern Health Board, Hartlepool, Cleveland, UK; South Eastern Health Board, Waterford, 1977–93.

Honorary Research Fellowship in Engineering Department, Durham University, where he studied and improved theatre ventilation systems.

He had a particular interest in biomechanics, following his time in Prof. M. A. MacConaill's (1902–87) Anatomy Department in UCC.

He published on carbon fibre as an intra-articular implant in the experimental animal. He devised a technique for the reduction of sub capital fractures of the femoral head, which found its way into Watson Jones's book on fractures.

Mark was a good organiser and administrator and was seldom seen without his imposing briefcase. He was described by a colleague as: 'unfailingly hardworking and conscientious with particular sympathy towards the weak and the underdog.' A great conversationalist, he was also a fine technical surgeon and a most interesting personality. He had a great sense of humour, quick to retort and a ready wit. His west Cork accent remained intact over the years.

He enjoyed sailing (wore a sailor's cap when off duty ashore), shooting, horse riding, bird watching and fishing, and was interested in all of nature, including his garden.

GALLAGHER, Joseph Edward (Joe)

Dublin Orthopaedic Surgeon

b. 1925, son of Edward and Margaret Gallagher
Educ. Christian Brothers School, Westport; Mount St Joseph's, Roscrea, Co. Tipperary; University College Dublin
m. Married with 3 s (Joe, microbiologist), 1 d

MB, UCD, 1949; FRCSI, 1956; MCh, NUI, 1957

Senior registrar, Westmeath County Hospital, Mullingar (with Jimmy O'Connell [q.v.]); St Vincent's Hospital, Dublin.
Registrar, Royal National Orthopaedic Hospital and Institute of Orthopaedics, London, including sessions at the Hospital for Sick Children, Great Ormond Street and rotation to plastic unit at Mount Vernon Hospital, London.
Consultant orthopaedic surgeon, St Vincent's Hospital; Cappagh National Orthopaedic Hospital; Children's Hospital, Baldoyle, 1959–92.
Medical Adviser, Irish Rugby Football Union, 1980.
Trophy of appreciation presented by Irish Scoliosis Society.
Gallagher gold medal for clinical excellence, presented annually by Cappagh Orthopaedic Hospital.
Founder Member, Irish American Orthopaedic Society.

Influences included Jimmy O'Connell [q.v.], Prof. Patrick Fitzgerald [q.v.] and Prof. R. A. Hodson OBE, FRCS Ed, of Hong Kong, who introduced him to the pioneering anterior thoracic approach to the tubercular spine.
Main interest was spinal surgery and he established the surgical treatment of scoliosis at Cappagh Hospital, and encouraged the formation of the Irish Scoliosis Society, a lay body, to promote awareness and research into the condition.

Joe Gallagher established the orthopaedic and trauma unit at St Vincent's Hospital; he endlessly and unselfishly campaigned for the appointment of more consultant orthopaedic surgeons and everyone benefited. He set a great example.

A keen sailor with 'some trophies and some wipe-outs', he is also an enthusiastic golfer, and has started oil painting. He enjoys company, reading and music and has a wonderful sense of humour, with mesmerising stories told with great timing and skill.

Dark, with trademark slick of hair over his forehead, Joe Gallagher is about 5'8" and perhaps fourteen stone. He describes himself as being of a pleasant disposition — a huge understatement for a man who is one of the most popular orthopaedic surgeons in the country.

HAUGHTON, William Steele ('Baldy')

Dublin Orthopaedic Surgeon

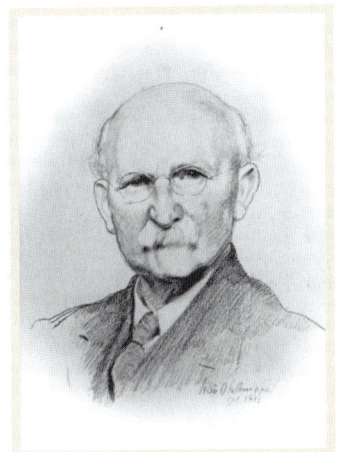

b. 1869, son of Rev. Samuel Haughton (1821–95, an innovative mathematician who developed the calculations on which the tide tables were determined, but immortalised himself by providing the grimmer calculation of the optimal height of a hanged man's fall (1875); subsequently became a doctor to reform medical education)
Educ. Portora Royal School, Enniskillen; Trinity College, Dublin
d. 1951

BA, TCD, 1891 (senior moderatorship and gold medal); MB, TCD, 1894; MD, TCD, 1901

Postgraduate appointments as assistant surgeon, Sir Patrick Dun's Hospital (with Edward Halloran Bennett of the eponymous stave fracture of the thumb); officer in charge of the X-ray Department. Consultant surgeon, Dr Steevens' Hospital, from 1899; Orthopaedic Hospital of Ireland, Clontarf, from 1907; Blackrock Military Hospital (with Sir William Wheeler [q.v.]), 1914–18. Professor of Orthopaedic Surgery, TCD.
Sole Irish foundation member, British Orthopaedic Association, 1918.

Incredibly, within six weeks of Röntgen's lecture in Würzburg in 1895, Haughton was taking radiographs in Dublin. He subsequently damaged his hands through overexposure to the X-rays. He brought back the concept of aseptic surgery to his own hospital following a number of visits to Theodor Kocher (1841–1917) at Berne (Kocher was the first surgeon to win the Nobel Prize (1909) for Medicine).

Haughton was a clear and inspiring teacher and a careful, meticulous surgeon. His writings were scientific rather than anecdotal. A man of rugged good health and infectious good humour, he was an accomplished sailor, had a fine tenor voice ('The Snowy Breasted Pearl') and the gift of easy friendship. One of his closest friends was Sir Robert Jones. He was quite happy being called 'Baldy'.

KELLY, Joseph M. (Joe)

Galway Orthopaedic Surgeon

Educ. University of Liverpool

LRCS & PI, 1963; FRCSI, 1968; MCh Orthopaedics (University of Liverpool)

Registrar, Centre for Hip Surgery, Wrightington Hospital, Wigan, Lancashire; registrar in orthopaedics, North Staffordshire Royal Infirmary, Stoke-on-Trent; Fellow in orthopaedics, Lahey Clinic, Boston.
Consultant orthopaedic surgeon, Western Health Board, based in Galway.

KENNY, Francis G ('Fred')

Regional Orthopaedic Surgeon

b. 1931, Dublin, son of Patrick and Roseanna Kenny
Educ. Christian Brothers Schools, Dún Laoghaire; Royal College of Surgeons in Ireland
m. 1959: Dr Laura Cullen (RCSI 1954; deceased); 3 s (2 in medicine, one FRCSI), 2 d (one in medicine)

LRCP & SI, 1954; FRCSI, 1961

Postgraduate appointments in Jervis Street Hospital, 1954–60; five years, 1961–66, at Sefton General Hospital, Liverpool; Nuffield Orthopaedic Centre, Oxford (eight consultant orthopaedic surgeons); Royal Infirmary, Stoke-on-Trent.
Consultant orthopaedic surgeon, Manchester region, 1966–75; North Eastern Health Board, centred on Our Lady's Hospital, Navan, 1975–96.

It is a measure of those difficult and despairing times that Fred Kenny, a man so well trained, with the polished social skills to match, and with deep Dublin roots, was not appointed a consultant in Ireland until 1975, when he was aged 44.

In his younger days, he was active in rugby. Later, he became involved in horse racing and was elected a member of the Turf Club, the governing body. Of medium height, he was dark, with trademark raised eyebrow and twinkle. Laura and he were an elegant couple at the premier race meetings.

LAVELLE, Eoghan Francis

Dublin Orthopaedic Surgeon

Educ. Trinity College, Dublin

MB, TCD, 1955; FRCSI, 1962; FRCS, 1963

Postgraduate appointments as surgical registrar, Dudley Road Hospital, the Accident Hospital, Birmingham; Robert Jones and Agnes Hunt Orthopaedic Hospital, Oswestry.
Consultant orthopaedic surgeon, St Laurence's Hospital (Richmond); James Connolly Memorial Hospital; Incorporated Orthopaedic Hospital, Clontarf.

LITTLE, Martin Gerard Aloys

Galway Orthopaedic Surgeon

Educ. University College Galway

MB, 1934, UCG; FRCSI, 1939 (UCG & Guy's Hospital, London); PhD, Lond, 1939; BSc, 1931; MCh, 1941

Postgraduate appointments as house surgeon and house physician, Galway Central Hospital; member of research staff, Sherrington School of Physiology, St Thomas's Hospital, London.
Orthopaedic surgeon, Western Region of Ireland.
Lecturer in medical jurisprudence, UCG; clinical lecturer, Galway Central Hospital.
Grantee, Medical Research Council.

Galway's first dedicated orthopaedic surgeon, Martin Little came to the post really well trained and worked hard, travelling hundreds of miles to peripheral clinics. He developed a huge medico-legal practice.

MacAULEY Henry (Harry)

Dublin Orthopaedic Surgeon

b. 1894, youngest child of Charles and Ann MacAuley; younger brother of Charles MacAuley [q.v.]
Educ. St Malachy's College, Belfast; Queen's University Belfast
m. May Brady of Belfast (a distinguished Irish scholar)
d. 1958

MCh, QUB; FRCSI

Surgeon to the Outpatient Department, Mater Hospital, Dublin.
Orthopaedic surgeon, Cappagh Orthopaedic Hospital.

The prohibition by the Bishop of Down and Conor on Catholics attending Queen's had been removed by the time Harry went there to study. When he was appointed to the Mater, the general surgeons did not want orthopaedics to become a separate specialty but the famous Sister Polycarp founded Cappagh Orthopaedic Hospital and appointed Harry as full-time orthopaedic surgeon there. He then had to give up his Mater appointment.

A Northern outspoken republican, he was deeply involved in the Irish language and culture. He holidayed in the Kerry Gaeltacht.

MacAULEY Patrick (Paddy)

Dublin Orthopaedic Surgeon

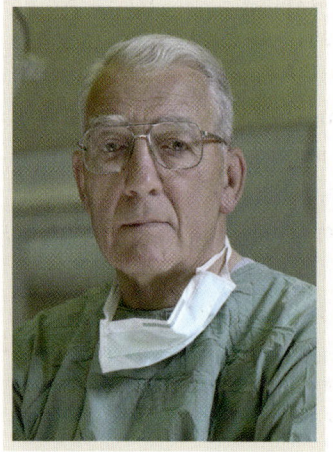

b. 1924, Dublin, youngest son of Charlie MacAuley [q.v.] (surgeon, Mater Hospital) and Clare MacAuley (*née* Spain) (d. 1925)
Educ. Catholic University School, Leeson Street, Dublin; University College Dublin
m. Lou O'Sullivan of Killarney; 1 s, 1 d
d. 2006

MB, UCD, 1948; FRCSI, 1953; MCh, NUI, 1954

Postgraduate appointments as senior house officer, Leicester Royal Infirmary, 1950–51; casualty officer, Mater Hospital (first in Dublin), 1951–52; surgical registrar (solo), Mater Hospital, 1951–54; senior registrar, Robert Jones and Agnes Hunt Orthopaedic Hospital, Oswestry, Shropshire (with Sir Reginald Watson-Jones and Sir Henry Osmond Clark who 'encouraged' him to take over musculoskeletal trauma).
Orthopaedic Surgeon, Mater Hospital, Dublin; Children's Hospital, Temple Street; Cappagh Orthopaedic Hospital, 1956–89.
Consulting orthopaedic surgeon, National Maternity Hospital; Holles Street; St Luke's Hospital, Rathgar; St Ultan's Children's Hospital; St Mary's Orthopaedic Hospital, Baldoyle.
Visiting orthopaedic surgeon, Wexford County Hospital, 1956–66.
President, Irish Medical Association, 1974.
Member (government-appointed), Comhairle na nOspidéal (Hospital Council), 1965–71 with particular involvement in the rationalisation of orthopaedic surgery nationally.
Lecturer in applied anatomy, UCD (succeeding his father); lecturer in orthopaedics, School of Physiotherapy, UCD; lecturer in orthopaedics, UCD, 1956–89.
First specialist to be co-opted to Medical Board of Mater Hospital Board of Management, Mater Hospital; St Joseph's (Children's) Hospital, Temple Street.
First Chairman of the Medical Board, Cappagh Orthopaedic Hospital.

Paddy MacAuley achieved much and his greatest monument must surely be his part in the conversion of Cappagh Hospital to Cappagh National Orthopaedic Hospital. During his time there it was changed from a sanatorium for children with tuberculosis to a 160-bed unit for elective orthopaedics, with seventeen orthopaedic surgeons on the staff. The country's only Chair of Orthopaedics, founded jointly with the RCSI, is based there. He tirelessly and unselfishly built up the staff numbers of the Orthopaedic Department at the Mater. He was the key figure in organising training in orthopaedic surgery in the Republic and was the first Irish representative on the Specialist Advisory Committee (SAC) on Orthopaedics. Throughout his career, he carried a full burden of operating on those entitled to free services, and gave excellent example in this issue. His time at the Robert Jones and Agnes Hunt Orthopaedic Hospital, Oswestry, undoubtedly influenced him about the value of a stand-alone 'cold' unit for elective orthopaedics.

As President of the IMA, Paddy was certainly not just a figurehead. He was the most tenacious, indomitable and stubborn of a triumvirate who represented the profession in stormy negotiations with the government between 1965 and 1975. His proud Northern genes enabled him to say 'No' with a wide variety of nuances, none of which meant 'maybe', but the meaning was never other than clear where the independence of medicine was involved. He was truly a tireless tribune of the profession.

A big man (6 foot), in all ways, with great presence and a deep, measured speaking voice, he had been a fearless front-row rugby forward for UCD, Lansdowne RFC and Leicester 'Tigers'. He played cricket at school and then for Merrion Cricket Club. He was a keen golfer, playing down to single figures at Portmarnock and Dooks in Co. Kerry. Deeply religious, he was a very Christian gentleman. His wife Lou was a huge support on the golf course and off. He had a tremendous capacity for work and he got the best out of all around him. A really great, admirable professional.

McDOWELL, Cecil Richard ('Cecil')

Orthopaedic Surgeon, Navan

b. 1920, Dublin, youngest son of John McDowell and Caroline McDowell (*née* McKeever)
Educ. St Columba's College, Rathfarnham, Dublin; Trinity College, Dublin
m. 1945: Doreen McKeever (d. 1998); 1 s (Carlos, consultant anaesthetist), 2 d (Melanie, physiotherapist)
d. 1969

MB, 1945, TCD; FRCSI, 1949

Postgraduate junior posts, Dr Steevens' Hospital; Kingston-upon-Thames; Hemel Hampstead Hospital, 1945–50. Senior training posts, Dr Steevens', Cavan Surgical Hospital.
Consultant orthopaedic surgeon, North East Health Board, centred on Navan, 1958–69.

Cecil's father died when he was 14 and still at boarding school. Home had been a large house in Sutton, Co. Dublin, with 20 acres, own stable and own milk. He played rugby and cricket at school but riding was his passion. As a teenager and medical student (1939–45), he hunted and rode at point to points, overcoming serious transport problems to get himself and the horse in position. Cecil rode many winners as a gentleman (amateur). One of his successful mounts on many occasions, Caughoo, won the Grand National at Aintree (1947), but there was a professional jockey in the saddle then. As a medical student, he had been part of a group who put a donkey into the third floor of the Adelaide Hospital and left him there. He sailed with his brother Jack (a jeweller), who provided the funds for a smart cruiser, while Cecil, a born helmsman, supplied the expertise.

McGRATH, Joseph Patrick (Joe)

Orthopaedic Surgeon, Navan

b. 1934
Educ. University College Cork
d. 2002

MB, UCC, 1960; MCh, NUI, 1966; MCh Orth, Liverpool, 1969; FRCS Ed, 1966

Postgraduate appointment as senior registrar in orthopaedics, Leeds Region Hospital Board.
Consultant orthopaedic surgeon, Regional Hospital, Navan.
Orthopaedic surgeon, North Eastern Health Board, Navan.

A mover and a shaker, Joe came late to medicine but was an energetic, influential figure.

MOORE, Frederick Hugh (Fred)

Cork Orthopaedic Surgeon

b. 1922, Bray, Co. Wicklow, eldest son of Frederick and Jean Moore (*née* Moir)
Educ. College of St Columba, Dublin; Trinity College, Dublin
m. 1960: Dr Elma Rankine, daughter of Dr George and Evelyn Rankine; 1 s, 2 d

MB, TCD, 1946; FRCS Ed, 1954; FRCSI (*ad eundem*), 1974

Postgraduate junior posts: Childwall Hospital, Liverpool, 1947–49; registrar, Bridge of Earn Hospital, Perthshire, 1951–55; senior registrar, Dundee Royal Infirmary, 1955–59.
Consultant orthopaedic surgeon, St Mary's Orthopaedic Hospital, Cork and Cork University Hospital.

Chairman, Irish Orthopaedic Club (before it became an association).

Prof. I. S. Smillie and the productive Prof. T. P. McMurray were main influences.
Special interest in paediatric orthopaedics, particularly congenital dislocation of the hip.

At Trinity, Fred Moore had captained the first rugby fifteen, 1945–46, and played for Leinster and North of Scotland against the Springboks and the All Blacks. He twice won the Robert Jones Cup at the British Orthopaedic Association (BOA) meeting. He was on the Council of the BOA. He valued his links with TCD and was Chairman of the Cork Association.

MULVIHILL, Cornelius Joseph ('Niall')

Dublin Orthopaedic Surgeon

b. 1934, eldest child of Tod and Kathleen Mulvihill
Educ. Killorglin, Co. Kerry; St Brendan's College, Killarney; University College Dublin
m. 1963: Emer Hargadon; 4 s (Alan, ophthalmologist, Edinburgh; Niall, cardiologist, Dublin; John, stockbroker, London; Philip, financial adviser, London)

MB, 1957; FRCSI, 1962; MCh, NUI, 1964; MCh Orth, Liverpool, 1965

Postgraduate positions as intern, Mater Hospital, 1958; senior house officer, Birmingham Accident Hospital, 1959–62; general surgical and orthopaedic registrar, Mater Hospital, 1962–64; surgical tutor, Mater Hospital.
Consultant orthopaedic surgeon, Mater Hospital and Cappagh Orthopaedic Hospital.
President, Irish Association of Orthopaedic Surgeons.

Influenced by John Corcoran [q.v.], Prof. Eoin O'Malley [q.v.] and Patrick MacAuley [q.v.].
Special surgical interests were in total hip and total knee replacements.

Within his peer group, Niall Mulvihill was a model of collegiality. Tall (6'2"), dark and handsome, he had an infinite capacity for work. His photographic memory left his undergraduate classmates envious and mesmerised. On retirement, he has played more golf and is an expert salmon fisherman. Proud of his Kerry roots, he goes there whenever he can. This quiet, undemonstrative man is greatly admired and trusted by his colleagues.

MURPHY, Michael Kevin

Cork Orthopaedic Surgeon

b. 1934
Educ. Christian Brothers College, Cork; Downside School; London Hospital Medical College
m. Dr Mary Murphy; 2 children
d. 1978

MRCS, 1959; MB, London, 1960; DA Eng,1962; FRCS, 1966

Training posts at Ascot; the Royal Free Hospital; St Thomas's; senior registrar, Luton and Dunstable and Guy's Hospital.
Consultant surgeon, Cork hospitals, 1972–78.

Michael Murphy had a special interest in scoliosis and joint replacement. He had briefly studied anaesthetics. He played rugby and tennis, and boxed for Downside. Rugby was his big interest and he subsequently played for London Irish. He also skied, golfed and played squash.

O'BRIEN, Timothy Martin (Tim)

Dublin Orthopaedic Surgeon and Professor of Orthopaedics

b. 1951, Loughrea, Co. Galway, fourth child of Frank O'Brien (well-known local politician and republican) and Kathy O'Brien (*née* Bolger)
Educ. St Brendan's, Loughrea, Co. Galway, University College Galway
m. Dr Mary Jennings (a classmate); 3 children ('No medics')

MB, UCG, 1975 (Henry Hutchinson Stewart scholarship for first place in anatomy in Ireland, 1972); FRCSI, 1979; MCh, NUI, 1983.

Postgraduate Fellowships in paediatric orthopaedics at the Hospital for Sick Children, Toronto (1983–84) and the Children's Hospital, Harvard University, Boston, 1984–85.
Consultant orthopaedic surgeon, Children's Hospital, Temple Street; Cappagh National Orthopaedic Hospital; Central Remedial Clinic, 1987; Mater Misericordiae Hospital, 1989.
Chief of orthopaedic surgery, Mater Hospital, 1990–94.
Director of training in orthopaedics for Ireland, 1991–2001; Abraham Colles Professor of Orthopaedics, RCSI, 1991–2001.

Tim had been trained by two of the top orthopaedic surgeons in the world, Robert 'Bob' Salter and John Hall, and it showed. He wrote extensively on paediatric spinal deformity and hip disease, and truly brought academic orthopaedics and research to Ireland. His work was inquisitive and original. He has a great sense of humour with a conciliatory, considered, approach to problems. He enjoyed teaching and did a superb job in organising the outstanding orthopaedic training programmes.

A keen sportsman, he played hurling at provincial schools level, was a winner of the Puc Fada ('long puck'), captained Galwegians Rugby Football Club and ran several marathons.

O'CONNELL, St John Gerard

Cork Orthopaedic Surgeon

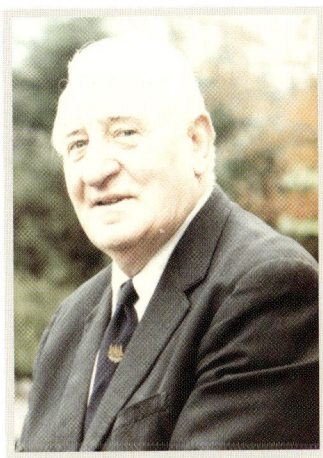

b. 1917, Mallow, Co. Cork, only son of Dominick and Nellie O'Connell (chemists)
Educ. Presentation Brothers College, Cork; Clongowes Wood College, Kildare; University College Cork
m. 1941: Madoline Horgan (MB, UCC, 1939, who worked, as a pathology trainee, under Dr (later Sir) Alexander Fleming, discoverer of penicillin), daughter of J. J. Horgan (Lord Mayor of Cork and as coroner at inquest on the victims of the Lusitania (sunk May 1915) brought in a verdict of wilful murder against the 'U boat crew and Kaiser Wilhelm II of Germany');
2 s (John, radiologist, deceased), 1 d
d. 1996

MB, UCC, 1939; FRCS Ed

Postgraduate training at Worcester Royal Infirmary; Cheltenham General Hospital; St Vincent's Orthopaedic Hospital, Pinnar, Middlesex (with J. S. Batchelor); Royal Air Force (Wing Commander); Halton Hospital, Germany; Royal National Orthopaedic Hospital, London.
First assistant, Orthopaedic Department, London Hospital (under Sir Reginald Watson-Jones and Sir Osmond Clarke, themselves two legends in their lifetimes).
Orthopaedic surgeon, Southern Health Board, 1950.
Consultant, St Finbarr's Hospital; St Mary's Orthopaedic Hospital; Cork University Hospital; based in Cork with clinics in Killarney, Cahirciveen, Tralee, Listowel, Mallow and Youghal.
Lecturer in orthopaedic surgery, UCC.
Founder member, Irish Orthopaedic Society.

St John O'Connell was a big man who made a big difference. He returned to Cork, arguably one of the first Irish orthopaedic surgeons to be fully trained, and by the very best people. He was a great organiser and the perfect man to get things moving quickly — which he did. Tall, well built, broad shouldered, good looking, tireless, shaggy haired, larger than life in all respects, he was always at the centre of things. Combative with a voice that could, and did, call hounds over broad acres (which was sometimes useful in committee rooms), he was an excellent communicator and lecturer but a formidable adversary. He built up a superb unit, always looking for extra consultant appointments.

He retired to a stud farm in his beloved Mallow, became President of the Irish Flat Horse Racing Breeding Association and travelled widely. Although he retired in 1982, he continued a huge medico-legal practice for another five years, where he was a clear and convincing expert. An Irish giant.

O'CONNELL, Richard John (Dick)

Waterford-Based Orthopaedic Surgeon

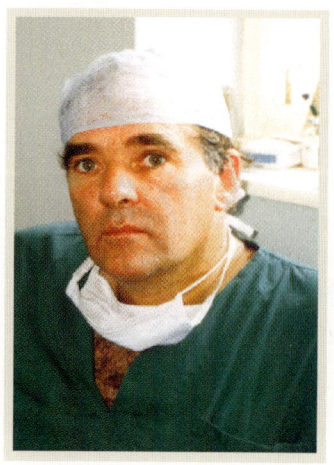

b. 1938, youngest son of Richard and Eileen O'Connell
Educ. Baltimore National School, Co. Cork; St Finbarr's College, Farranferris, Cork; Fordham University, New York; University College Galway
m. Breda Quigley (Tipperary origins); 1 s, 2 d (Fionnula is Harvard-trained pathologist at Cork University Hospital)

MB, UCG, 1966; FRCS Canada (orthopaedics), 1975

Postgraduate: entire residency programme at University of British Columbia, Vancouver (which he describes as 'a well disciplined and highly organised programme').
Consultant orthopaedic surgeon, Prince George Regional Hospital, British Columbia, 1975–78.
Chief-of-Staff and Chairman, Medical Advisory Committee, 1978.
Consultant orthopaedic surgeon, South Eastern Health Board, 1978–2003.
Chairman and clinical director, Department of Orthopaedics, 1995–2003.
Visiting Professor, University of British Columbia, 2001 (Silver Jubilee of the Department of Orthopaedics).
Chairman, Irish Institute of Orthopaedic Surgery for nine years; President, Irish American Orthopaedic Society.

Dick's biggest achievements were to bring about some centralisation of the big problems in the specialty and, even more importantly, to keep campaigning for more and more consultants for the department. In this issue, there were problems with the Department of Health, as well as some reservations from newly arrived colleagues. But there are now seven orthopaedic surgeons in the unit, to cover all specialties as well as colleagues' leave. Others followed his example but perhaps none with quite the same success. The University of British Columbia has since taken several Irish Fellows for the tertiary stage of their training.

He has a bucolic, vigorous, appearance from the great outdoors. Hurling remains his favourite game (he was surgeon to the Wexford Hurling team for some years), then football, basketball (captained College team), and athletics (winner of a New York 10-mile championship team medal).

'An increase in grey hair does not necessarily mean an increase in grey matter,' he observes. His unit is an outstanding example of what a man with a mission can achieve ('The Health of the People is the Highest Law' — Cicero).

O'DRISCOLL, Robert F. (Bobbie)

Waterford Orthopaedic Surgeon

b. 1912, Cork (fashionable Sunday's Well), youngest son of Michael and Helena O'Driscoll (leather merchants); older brother, Tim, was an Ambassador and a top civil servant
Educ. Presentation College, Cork; University College Cork
m. 1942: Dr Karen Dowling (the class beauty); 5 children
d. 1991

MB, UCC, 1935; MCh (Orth), Liverpool

Postgraduate training in the Liverpool area. (Prof. McMurray was the natural successor to the Robert Jones tradition and Liverpool was the centre of British, and possibly world orthopaedics, for many years.)
Consultant orthopaedic surgeon, South East Health Board, centred on Waterford, c. 1950–77.

Bobbie O'Driscoll was an excellent technical surgeon and particularly skilled at knee surgery before the arthroscopic revolution. He had a particular interest in sports injuries and was surgeon to the Irish and Waterford football teams for many years. He had played rugby, as an indestructible scrum half, at schools and senior inter-provincial level, as well as UCC and Sunday's Well.

He was a solo surgeon with an unbelievable workload and a certain impatience with authority. His relationship with the Health Board, who had given him a Sisyphean task, was tempestuous, and he was not allowed to act as a badly needed locum after his retirement.

Short (5'7"), stocky, sturdy, swarthy, with a mop of jet-black hair, he always looked younger than his years. He was hugely energetic, combative and feisty. He it was who founded the orthopaedic unit which serves the South East and he did a superb job for patients and colleagues.

SCANNELL, Timothy (Tim)

Orthopaedic Surgeon, Navan

b. 1940, Cork, son of Frederick J. Scannell and Esther K. Scannell (*née* Harley)
Educ. Christian Brothers College, Cork; University College Cork
m. 1968: Maureen Daly, daughter of John and Jane Daly; 4 s (John, a dentist), 2 d (Esther, an anaesthetist; Jane, a radiographer)
d. 2006

MB, UCC, 1960; BSc (pathology), UCC, 1969; FRCS Eng, 1968; MCh (orthopaedics), Liverpool, 1975

Postgraduate appointments at Birmingham Accident Hospital (PSL London); Bantry Hospital; University of Washington (with Dr Al Bleu, hand surgeon).
Fellowship in orthopaedic surgery, University Washington (Seattle), 1971–72.
Consultant orthopaedic surgeon, North Eastern Health Board, Navan, 1975–98.
Member, NE Health Board.

Tim Scannell has been described thus: '5'8½", slightly paunchy, sincere, hardworking, likes good company, good food and good wine. Most likely to say "now". Essentially a private, shy man, most at home with family and friends. A self-confessed practising bibliophile with a porous memory for names and faces. A committed Christian who "hopes that God has a sense of humour".' If he has he will get on very well with Tim.

He was Munster Under-15 tennis champion and later played golf (13).

SHEEHAN, James Michael (Jimmy)

Dublin Orthopaedic Surgeon

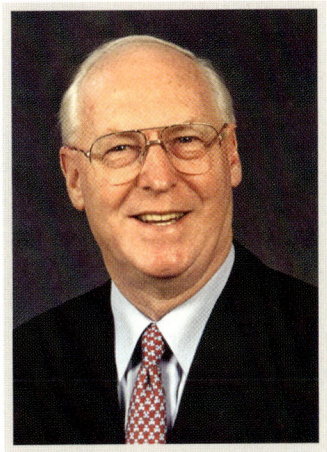

b. July 1939, eldest son of James Joseph Sheehan and Frances Sheehan (*née* Mangan)
Educ. St Mary's College, Rathmines; University College Dublin
m. 1966: Rosemary Sheehan, daughter of John and Kathleen Sheehan; 2 s, 2 d (Katherine is a doctor)

MB, UCD, 1963 (first place and gold medals in medicine, surgery and obstetrics); FRCSI, 1966; MSc (bioengineering), University of Surrey, 1970; PhD (mechanical engineering), University of Surrey, 1983 (for work on artificial knee joint replacement)

Postgraduate appointment at Wrightington Hospital, Wigan, Lancashire (with Sir John Charnley), 1968–69.
Consultant orthopaedic surgeon, St Vincent's Hospital, Dublin, 1971–87.
Honorary Fellow, Institute of Engineers in Ireland, 1985.
Trustee, AO Swiss Foundation; President, Irish American Orthopaedic Association, 1989.
Fellow Academy of Engineers in Ireland (one of few non-engineers).

Jimmy Sheehan is probably Ireland's outstanding orthopaedic surgeon of the twentieth century. His brilliant undergraduate career was followed by graduate work and academic qualifications in bioengineering, all with a view to designing better joint replacements. The 'Sheehan' knee was one of his earliest successes. A mould breaker, he established joint replacement units in Cappagh Hospital, Dublin, in 1970; Mount Carmel Hospital in 1978; and the Blackrock Clinic in 1985.

His services were in phenomenal demand as he was in on the beginning of joint replacement. His meticulous approach was reflected in superb results for his time. Over the years, the 'knee' was modified by others and, at the time of writing, the replacement part widely used is much smaller than the original but it was he who started it all. He performed about 8,000 primary and revision hip arthroplasties and 2,500 knee arthroplasties between 1968 and 2002.

Because of resource constraints, he could not operate on all the patients looking for his services in the public sector and, in frustration, he resigned his public appointments. This gave rise to persisting controversy and criticism, even amongst his many admirers, but it was disappointing that none of the institutions could provide him with a well-earned academic department.

He then entered into a second mould-breaking phase, and proved that major surgery could be carried out safely in private hospitals. With the foundation of the

Blackrock Clinic in Dublin, in 1984, he proved that a freestanding 100-bed private hospital could provide world-standard care, and people flocked to the new institution. Typically, he put much of his own capital into the new venture. 'Blackrock' became a byword for top-of-the-range medical care, and probably in itself spurred the growth of private health insurance, mostly though Voluntary Health Insurance.

Still involved in a large clinical practice until his retirement in 2002, he continued his pressures for the development of private clinics and, where possible, public-private partnerships, opening another 'Blackrock' in Galway in 2004, and yet another at Hermitage, Lucan, Co. Dublin.

Quiet, focused, determined, deeply religious, public spirited and serious (surgery is a serious matter), he has displayed admirable grit and single-mindedness at all times. He says that he has recreations ('gardening and fishing') but nobody really believes him.

He is above average height, and his lean, pale (operating theatre lamps don't give you a tan), thin-faced, stooped, bespectacled, scholarly appearance conceals one of Ireland's most driven surgeons who has broken two moulds. An admirable professional.

SUGARS, John Colvan de Renzy

Dublin Orthopaedic Surgeon

b. 1915, son of a doctor; grandson of a doctor
Educ. Trinity College, Dublin
m. Jerry; 1s, 3d
d. 1994

BA, MB, TCD, 1938; FRCSI, 1949

Surgeon-Lieutenant, Royal Naval Volunteer Reserve, 1939–45.
Postgraduate appointments at Newcastle; resident surgical officer, Gloucester Royal Infirmary; senior registrar, Winford Orthopaedic Hospital, Bristol; Bristol Royal Hospitals.
Orthopaedic surgeon, Adelaide Hospital, 1951–82; Federated Dublin Hospitals; Orthopaedic Hospital of Ireland; Rotunda Hospital.

Sugars served in many war theatres, particularly in the Mediterranean area, and escaped in the evacuation of Crete. He was taken prisoner by the Italians at Tobruk and, under an exchange scheme, was repatriated to the Isle of Man (where he met his future wife). He was deeply unhappy about how badly some of the prisoners of war were treated and never forgot the events of 1939–45.

Appointed firstly to the Adelaide, he was available day and night and saw all patients himself, which meant that clinics and outpatients were always overwhelmed, particularly as John had absolutely no idea about the time of day it was or, some said, even the day it was. The patients loved him. He was a shrewd, conservative surgeon and much sought after for committee work.

John Sugars loved sports cars and horses. Many retain a vision of him in the open MG, with his white hair and matching beard flying in the wind. He was a keen skier and regularly took the family to Norway for expeditions. When a high-ranking member of the landed gentry (a collector's item, even by John's standards) came in under his care with a broken leg, she said, 'Don't damage my beautiful Italian riding boots'. 'Italian, did you say?' he replied. 'Shears, Sister, please.'

WALSH, Martin Gabriel

Dublin Orthopaedic Surgeon

b. 1941

MB, UCD, 1965; FRCSI, 1969; MCh Orth., 1971

Postgraduate appointments as orthopaedic registrar, Our Lady's Hospital for Sick Children, Crumlin, Dublin; registrar, Robert Jones and Agnes Hunt Orthopaedic Hospital, Oswestry; senior registrar, Royal Orthopaedic Hospital, Birmingham.
Orthopaedic surgeon, Mater Hospital, Dublin; St Mary's Orthopaedic Hospital, Cappagh, 1975–2005.
Consultant surgeon, National Rehabilitation Hospital, Dún Laoghaire, Co. Dublin.

Martin was orthopaedic surgeon to the Football Association of Ireland team and accompanied the national team to the World Cup finals in 1990 (Italy), 1994 (USA) and 2002 (Saipan and Japan), when Captain Roy Keane returned home in an issue that divided the country. An unselfish, hard-working, highly respected professional.

18
EAR, NOSE AND THROAT SURGERY IN THE TWENTIETH CENTURY

Mr Andrew J. Maguire

EAR, NOSE AND THROAT SURGERY IN THE TWENTIETH CENTURY

At the turn of the century, the same specialist often treated diseases of the eye and ear. The American Academy of Ophthalmology and Otolaryngology was founded in 1904 and did not split into separate associations until 1978. The advent of the UK National Health Service in 1948 effectively separated eyes and ENT, though there were specialists in each area previously.

Surgeons in those early days were skilled enough in clinical diagnosis. However, lack of effective anaesthesia precluded major operations, and suppuration in the ears and sinuses, which often led to intracranial complications, could not be controlled. Frontal osteomyelitis and temporal lobe or cerebellar abscesses were often fatal. Some progress occurred, however, and, in 1904, Chevalier Jackson of Philadelphia introduced his bronchoscope with distal lighting. Tonsil and adenoid surgery had been introduced towards the close of the nineteenth century by Sir Morrell MacKenzie, founder of the Throat Hospital in Golden Square, London. It became more frequent in the first quarter of the twentieth century. This was also stimulated by the theory of focal sepsis. In 1930, Dr Sterling Brunnell did the first facial nerve graft and, in 1938, Julius Lempert, also in the USA, introduced the fenestration operation for otosclerosis, which regenerated otology.

Penicillin was a major advance. Though discovered by Fleming in 1929, it was not effectively available until 1941. Samuel Rosen, New York, rediscovered mobilisation of the stapes in 1952, a technique for otosclerosis that had been invented and abandoned, as being too dangerous, over half a century before. Things were different in the antibiotic era but long-term mobilisation was effective in only 25 per cent of patients. John Shea of Memphis introduced stapectomy, an operation in which the immobile stapes is removed and replaced by prosthesis. Variations of this operation have continued to be used successfully to the present day. Ear surgery had been revolutionised by the introduction of the binocular operating microscope, though strangely the Americans initially resisted it. Wulfstein's demonstration of ear surgery on a 16mm film taken through the operating microscope and shown at the World Congress of Otolaryngology in Amsterdam in 1960 led to worldwide acceptance of the microscope. The otologists had been the first to introduce various forms of microscope, and much later ophthalmologists, neurosurgeons and other specialists took up microsurgery.

Advances in anaesthesia, especially positive pressure ventilation, enabled chest surgery to develop, and operations on the lungs and heart followed. Broncho-oesophagology largely passed to the thoracic surgeons. In ENT, however, anaesthetic advances also led to the development of successful surgery for many head and neck cancers, which expanded the ENT specialty which is now renamed otolaryngology/head and neck surgery.

Advances in radiology, including CT scanning and magnetic resonance imaging (MRI) increased accurate diagnosis, for example in sinus disease and acoustic neuroma. Audiology advanced and evoked response audiometry led to earlier diagnosis of deafness in children.

While the essence of ENT is still the clinical examination and diagnosis of conditions producing myriad symptoms in the five dark recesses of the head and neck, the therapeutic potential for both common and rare afflictions in this area has multiplied. Many ENT conditions can be treated medically but some require surgery. The major divisions are otology, paediatric otolaryngology, facial plastic and reconstructive surgery, head and neck cancer surgery, rhinology and endoscopic sinus surgery.

Otology is divided into middle-ear surgery, neuro-otology and cochlear implantation. There are super specialties within other areas such as paediatric airway surgery, rhinoplasty, laser tumour surgery and skull base surgery. There is also increasing co-operation with specialists at the interface of otolaryngology, to provide the maximum beneficial patient care.

ENT/head and neck surgery has come a long way in the twentieth century and those practising today have the advantage of all that progress. However, it is probably true to say that those who preceded us with limited facilities had often a greater combination of manipulative skills and imagination to achieve so much in their eras.

Few specialities can match ENT for its all-Ireland co-operation and these brief biographies cover both jurisdictions.

GLOSSARY
IOS: Irish Otolaryngological Society
BAOL: British Association of Otolaryngologists

AGARWALA, Rasewar Prasad

Consultant ENT Surgeon

b. 1934, India, the youngest of seven children
Educ. Kalachand High School, West Bengal, India; Calcutta
m. 3 children (1 s, 1 d in medicine)

MB, BS, Calcutta, 1960; FRCS Ed, 1969; DLO Eng

Postgraduate appointments as senior house officer (ENT), Royal Hospital, Wolverhampton; registrar, Derby Royal Infirmary and Warwick Hospital; senior registrar, Tyrone County Hospital, Omagh.
Consultant ENT surgeon, Northern Area Health Board.
Member, IOS; BAOL; British Medical Association.

Main surgical interests were in general ENT, especially nasal surgery.

A very affable and supportive colleague, Rasewar retired in 1999. He describes himself as a high handicap golfer who particularly enjoys the nineteenth hole.

AITKEN, Henry

Aural Surgeon

Educ. University of Aberdeen

MB, ChB, Aberdeen, 1928; FRCSI, 1938

Training in Birmingham and Midland Ear and Throat Hospital.
Major, Royal Army Medical Corps.
Fellow, Ulster Medical Society.
Aural surgeon, Eye and Ear Clinic, Royal Victoria Hospital, Belfast.
Clinical teacher, QUB.
ENT surgeon, Ulster Hospital, Children and Women and North Down Hospitals.

Henry Aitken liked to stand when performing tonsillectomy. On the introduction of the National Health Service, he believed in the equal division of labour and that the time spent on the NHS should be equivalent to that devoted to private practice.

BENSON, Arthur

Ophthalmic and Aural Surgeon

BA, 1875; MB, 1876; FRCSI, 1881; L & LM, 1874 (RCSI, TCD, London and Vienna)

Surgeon, Royal Victoria Eye and Ear Hospital, Dublin.
Ophthalmic and aural surgeon, Royal City of Dublin Hospital.
Member, Council RCSI.

Wrote papers on 'Diphtherial Paralysis of Ocular Muscles', 'Ivory Exostosis of Auditory Meidas removed by Dental Engine' and 'The treatment of stenosis of nasal duct'.

BICKNELL, Michael Raymond

Consultant ENT Surgeon

b. 1932, only child of Rev. and Mrs L. L. Bicknell
Educ. Sherborne Preparatory School, Marlborough
m. 1966: Barbara Robinson; 3 children (one d. 1971)

MB, BS, LRCP, MRCS, 1956 (Middlesex Hospital); DLO, 1963; FRCS (Otol), 1964

Royal Army Medical Corps, 1958–1960; was RMO 2/6 QEO Ghurkha rifles.
Early postgraduate training in London hospitals, including St Thomas's and St Bart's.
ENT training continued at the Norfolk and Norwich Hospitals; senior registrar in ENT at the United Bristol Hospitals.
Consultant ENT surgeon, Altnagelvin Area Hospital, 1969–93.
Member, BMA; IOS.

A major influence on his career was Mr Angell James, a remarkable man who was a pioneer in transnasal pituitary surgery, and who lived to be 100 and farmed extensively.
His specialised interest in ENT was in microsurgery.

Michael Bicknell and his senior colleague, Ron Harvey [q.v.], ran an excellent harmonious department in Altnagelvin, as they were great friends as well. When one of his children sadly died in a cot death, Ron Harvey immediately arranged leave for him and in addition gave him fully paid tickets for two weeks in Cyprus.

Michael Bicknell was a well-built, six-foot-tall figure, with a distinguishing full beard. Retirement was not a problem for him as he had so many developed interests. A lifelong wine connoisseur, he has a cottage in the Vendée, and fishing has also been a long-time pursuit, which he gives as his motivation for coming to Northern Ireland. Entomology (the study of insects) is high on his list. His interest in forestry led to his purchase of 25 acres of rough grazing land, which he planted prior to retirement. A major interest was freemasonry in which he held several prominent offices and was elected to the thirtieth degree in 2005.

BIGGART, Hugh Gault

ENT Surgeon

b. 1919, youngest of four children
Educ. Carrickmallon PME; Royal Belfast Academical Institution; Queen's University Belfast
m. Margaret (Peggy); 2 d (Jennifer, teacher; Jane, paediatric nursing sister, Craigavon Hospital), 1 s (John, medical physicist)
d. 1976
MB, QUB, 1942; FRCS Ed, 1948

Postgraduate service in Royal Army Medical Corps, serving in France and Germany until the end of the war, by which time he had attained the rank of Major.
Trained in the Royal Victoria Hospital, following which he was appointed as ENT surgeon to the Lurgan and Portadown Hospital, from which he moved to the Craigavon Area Hospital when it opened.
Consultant ENT surgeon, County Armagh and Southdown Hospitals.
Consultant ENT surgeon to HM Forces, Northern Ireland.

Hugh Biggart practised general ENT surgery with a special interest in paediatrics. Following his army service, he continued his connection with the forces in the Territorial Army, from which he resigned in 1975, on health grounds, with the rank of colonel.

Hugh Biggart was a rugby enthusiast, both at school and later when he played for Instonians. He was also a member of Lurgan Golf Club, and later of both Portadown and Ballycastle Golf Clubs. He won many trophies and prizes during his golfing career. He enjoyed gardening, and used to grow vegetables for his family at home.

His daughter, who described him as being always smartly dressed, even at home, has no recollection of ever having seen him in his shirt sleeves without a jacket. He was 5'10" in height, of medium build, with angular bone structure and quite a stern demeanour. However, he enjoyed social gatherings and had a good sense of humour, though at times he could be a little too direct without intent.

BLACK, John Henry Artt (Ian)

Consultant ENT Surgeon

b. 1936, son of Mr and Mrs T. H. Black, Drum, Cookstown, Co. Tyrone
Educ. Rainey Endowed School, Magherafelt; Queen's University Belfast
m. Jean; 1 d, 2 s (one has completed his ENT training)

MB, QUB, 1959; DRCOG, 1961; FRCS Ed, 1967

Postgraduate career involved general surgery and obstetrics and gynaecology until 1964, when he commenced ENT training at the Royal Victoria Hospital, Belfast.
Registrar and senior registrar, Bristol General and South Meade Hospitals, Bristol. His training was influenced by Frank McLoughrin, Kennedy Hunter [q.v.] and G. D. L. Smyth [q.v.] in Belfast and by Angell James, K. Malcolmson and Mr Freeman in Bristol.
Consultant ENT surgeon, Northern Area Board United Hospitals, based at Antrim Hospital, 1967–2000.
Postgraduate tutor, Ballymena postgraduate centre; undergraduate tutor, Queen's Member, Antrim Postgraduate Centre; Ulster Medical Society; Queen's University Association; Northern Ireland Audiological Society; Northern Ireland Medical Legal Society; British Association of Otolaryngologists.
President, Ballymena Hard of Hearing Club, University Hospital, Belfast; Irish Otolaryngological Society, 2001–02 (had served earlier as a most meticulous treasurer of the society).

He practised general ENT with special interests in otology, rhinology, salivary gland and facial plastic surgery.

Ian Black has great organisational abilities and was a major contributor to the development of ENT services for the Northern Board. He developed ENT services outside Belfast, initially in Ballymena and later in Antrim. He was a keen teacher of medical students, nurses, and postgraduates for many years.

Tall, strongly built, of youthful appearance with a full head of hair, he is gregarious and good humoured with an infectious laugh. He was a great supporter of the IOS Travelling Club organised by his close friend Tony Miller [q.v.], and visited ENT centres all over the globe. Ian and his wife Jean are delightful companions, and combined ENT surgery, foreign friendships and sheer fun.

Ian retired in 2000 and one outlet for his continuing energy and skill is a twice weekly round of golf.

BLAYNEY, Alexander John Edward (Alec)

Consultant ENT Surgeon

b. 1918, only son of Neil John Blayney (County Surgeon, Maryborough, Co. Laois) and Eileen Blayney; one elder sister, Mary
Educ. Christian Brothers, Portlaoise; Castleknock College, Dublin; University College Dublin
m. Maureen Needham; son, Alexander William Blaney, is consultant ENT surgeon, Mater and Temple Street Hospitals
d. 2006

MB, UCD, 1942; DLO, London; MCh, UCD

Postgraduate house jobs in the Mater Hospital, Dublin, followed by 10 years' training in England, working in the Metropolitan ENT Hospital, London; the Royal National Throat and Nose Hospital in London; Addenbrooke's Hospital, Cambridge (chiefs included Scott Brown of textbook fame and Scott Stevenson).
In 1956, on a Council of Europe Fellowship, spent several months with Prof. Jongkees of Amsterdam and in Bordeaux with Prof. Georges Portmann.
ENT consultant, Western Health Board; Regional Hospital, Galway.
Lecturer in otolaryngology, UCG.
Founder member and past president, Irish Otolaryngological Society.
Fellow, Royal Society of Medicine; British Association of Otolaryngologists.
Irish representative of the Fondation Georges Portmann

He practised general ENT, with special interests in otology and the treatment of vertigo.

Alec Blaney was the single-handed ENT consultant to the Western Health Board. A delightful colleague, friendly, dapper and quietly spoken, he was very popular with students and with patients (about whom he worried a great deal). He regularly attended meetings of the Irish Otolaryngological Society and constantly read the ENT journals.

A keen tennis player, and a rugby enthusiast, he was also very interested in philosophy. His wife Maureen sadly died not long after he retired to Dublin. In his retirement, he remained active and interested, virtually to his death at the age of 88.

A charming individual, Alec Blaney is fondly remembered by his colleagues and friends.

BROWN, James

Ophthalmic and Aural Surgeon

BCh, BAO, RUI, 1894

Junior posts as registrar and house surgeon, Royal Eye Hospital, Southwark; Throat and Ear Hospital, Brighton.
Ophthalmic and aural surgeon, Mercy Hospital Cork; Cork District Hospital.
Fellow, RSM.

BURNS, Hugh Patrick

Consultant ENT Surgeon

b. 1944, youngest of 3 children of Patrick and Helen Burns
Educ. St Colman's School, Claremorris; University College Galway
m. Marie *née* Glynn (MB, FFA, a classmate), 4 children; (son Paul has followed his father into ENT surgery)

MB, UCG, 1968; FRCS Eng, 1974; FRCSI (*ad eundem*), 1992

Postgraduate training in Galway, the UK, Canada and Dublin.
Senior registrar in ENT, Royal Victoria Eye and Ear Hospital, Dublin; clinical Research Fellow, University of Toronto; registrar, ENT, United Liverpool Hospitals; senior house officer in ENT, Radcliffe Infirmary, Oxford.
Fellowship examiner in ORL, RCSI, 1982–94; sat on the first intercollegiate board of examiners in ORL where he served for five years as RCSI representative.
Consultant ENT surgeon, Royal Victoria Eye and Ear Hospital, 1984–2007.
Provided ENT services to Sir Patrick Dun's Hospital, 1981–84; schools for the deaf at St Mary's and St Joseph's, 1980–84; Midland Health Board area, 1980–91.
Large practice encompassed the Bon Secours Hospital and Mount Carmel Hospital, Dublin, 1980–2005.
President, Irish Otolaryngological Society, 1996–97.
First president, Irish Institute of Otolaryngology, 2004–05.

Major influences on his career were Bernard Coleman and Ugo Fisch in otology, Bob Pracy in paediatric ORL, and Philip Stell in head and neck surgery.
Special interest in stapes surgery. His other interests were functional sinus surgery and postgraduate teaching.

Hugh Burns was an outstanding otologist with a great capacity for organisation, rational thought, and forward planning. He was a prime mover in setting up and running the postgraduate training programme in ORL at the RCSI from 1977 to 1987.

Dapper, handsome with an abundance of dark hair, charm and good humour, Hugh was the best dresser since Brian O'Brien [q.v.]. A marvellous raconteur, he can deliver a word-perfect panegyric or after-dinner speech without notes. A humorous story when recounted by Hugh, with embellishments, is always infinitely better than the original. A great colleague and second opinion, he is a loyal friend with a mischievous sense of humour, and never exaggerates except in describing each week's ear for mastoid surgery as 'the worst I have ever seen'.

Hugh took early retirement in 2006. His hobbies include golf, fishing, sailing and walking.

BYRNE, John Edward Thomas

Consultant in Otolaryngology

b. 1935, son of John Byrne (d. 1979) and Violet Mary Byrne (*née* Harris) (d. 1999)
Educ. Kilkenny College; Mountjoy School, Dublin; Trinity College, Dublin
m. 1963: Margaret Elizabeth Ross; 2 d (Catherine and Joanna)

BA, MB, TCD, 1961; FRCSI, 1970

Postgraduate training at Dr Steevens' Hospital, Dublin (influenced by T. G. Wilson [q.v.] and Robert Woods [q.v.], outstanding ENT surgeons of their time); Fellow in Otology, Wayne State University, Detroit (with Ted McGee, another major influence).
Consultant in Otolaryngology, Belfast City Hospital, 1974–2000.
External examiner, NUI; examiner at the FRCSI (otolaryngology).
Member, ORS; IOS (President, 1994–95 and hon. Editor, 1974–93); Ulster Medical Society; British Cochlear Implant Group; TCD Association; Royal Society of Medicine.

His special interest was in otology and he authored various publications on blast injuries to the ears and noise-induced hearing loss.

John Byrne is an affable, relaxed colleague, with a keen insight and appreciation of the vagaries of human nature. His delineations of character and personality of generations of Irish ENT surgeons are incorporated in many of these biographical sketches. His insights and recollections, always benign, have been most helpful.

He lists his recreations as sailing, maritime history, gardening and theatre. He is a member of Strangford Lough Yacht Club. John is a keen family man, whose good-humoured, philosophical approach to life and his many interests keep him fully occupied, but he still regularly finds the time to attend the meetings of the Irish Otolaryngological Society.

CINNAMOND, Michael James

Consultant Otolaryngologist

Educ. Queen's University Belfast
m. Judy; 3 children

MB, QUB, 1967; FRCS Ed, 1974; FRCSI

Consultant otolaryngologist, Royal Victoria Hospital; City Hospital; Royal Belfast Hospital for Sick Children.
Professor of Otorhinolaryngology, QUB, 1989–95.
External examiner, FRCS Ed (otolaryngology); examiner, FRCSI.

Special interest was in paediatric airway conditions in which he had specialised in Toronto.

In the children's hospital, Michael Cinnamond built upon the work of Roy Gibson [q.v.] and John Byrne [q.v.] in intensive care situations. He performed delicate endoscopic and reconstructive operations on the paediatric larynx and trachea.

Tall, relaxed and affable, he was frequently invited as external assessor for consultant ENT posts in the Republic of Ireland. He retired in 2007.

CORBETT, Cornelius Christopher (Curly)

Waterford ENT Surgeon

b. 1921, Cork, only son of Patrick and Eileen Corbett
Educ. Christian Brothers College, Cork; University College Cork
m. 1954: Dr Sheila Boyd, daughter of Dr Thomas and Jean Boyd
d. 2002

MB, UCC, 1943; DLO, RCS Eng, 1949

Postgraduate appointments as house surgeon, North Infirmary and Mercy Hospitals, Cork; house surgeon (ENT), Nottingham General Hospital; Kent Co. Ophthalmic and Aural Hospital, Maidstone; ENT registrar, Salisbury Hospital Group; senior registrar (ENT), Warwick Hospital Group, 1950–53.
ENT surgeon, Waterford.

Warm, highly popular and enthusiastic, 'Curly' was a fearsome front-row rugby forward at UCC in his youth. Later he took up private flying with his usual élan. Shortish, broad shouldered and energetic, he was much in demand socially because he was great company.

CRAIG, David H.

Consultant ENT Surgeon

b. 1907

Educ. Queen's University Belfast

m. 2nd: Kathleen Mary Hunter (*née* McDowell; widow of colleague, Kennedy Hunter [q.v.]);
3rd: Noreen Simpson [q.v.] (another ENT colleague)

MB, QUB, 1931; FRCS Ed, 1937; FRCSI, 1968

Consultant, Benn Ulster Ear, Eye and Throat Hospital.
Consultant ENT surgeon, RVH, Belfast; Royal Belfast Hospital for Sick Children; Belfast City Hospital.
Fellow, Ulster Medical Society; Royal Society of Medicine.
Founding member and President, IOS.
Royal Army Medical Corps; attained the rank of Major.
External examiner (otolaryngology), FRCSI.

Author of report on first thousand cases which attended the ENT Department of a military hospital. Topics of various publications included cases of choanal atresia, eight cases of tuberculous mastoiditis, extra dural abscesses and explosion injuries of the ear.

David Craig was short in stature, with a moustache, spectacles and a twinkle in his eye. He bore a striking resemblance to Captain Mainwaring of television's *Dad's Army* fame, and an overseas postgraduate visitor actually congratulated him on his performance in that role. He was friendly with a great sense of humour, and a staunch supporter of the North/South Medical Association that is the Irish Otolaryngological Society.

As an after-dinner speaker, he was superb; his sense of timing was perfection and he would bring the house down at Charter Day Dinners and IOS meetings. A memorable character whose stature far exceeded his physical size.

CRAIG, James Andrew

ENT Surgeon

MB (first class hons), RUI, 1895; FRCS Eng, 1902; MRCS, NRCP, London, 1898 (QCB)

ENT surgeon, Royal Victoria Hospital, Belfast

Wrote papers on 'Surgical anatomy of the tympanum and mastoid antrum' and 'Chronic empyema of maxill antrum'.

CRONIN, Jeremiah (Jerry)

Consultant ENT Surgeon

b. 1935
Educ. University College Dublin
m. daughter is a consultant anaesthetist

MB, UCD, 1964; FRCS Eng, 1970

Postgraduate training in Oxford and Manchester.
Consultant ENT surgeon, Regional Hospital, Waterford, 1973–2000.

Jerry Cronin practised general ENT surgery, with a special interest in otology. A major influence was Albert Fagan [q.v.], whose example of great interest in his work, combined with his patient care, inspired Jerry in his choice of career. Microscopic surgery of the ear also intrigued him.

Jerry is a quiet affable individual who, as well as ENT, enjoys country life. A keen horseman and farmer, he retired in 2000.

CUNNINGHAM, Herbert Hugh Blair

ENT Surgeon

MRCS, LRCP, London, 1903; MD, Brux, 1904; FRCSI, 1905

ENT surgeon, Ulster Hospital for Women and Children, Belfast.

Wrote on use of electro magnet in ophthalmic surgery, 'Some complications of chronic otorrhea' and 'Deafness resulting from epidemic cerebral spine and meningitis', Proceedings of the Royal Society of Medicine, 1908.

CURTIN, John Michael McAuliffe ('Mac') PRCSI 1974–1976

Dublin Otolaryngologist

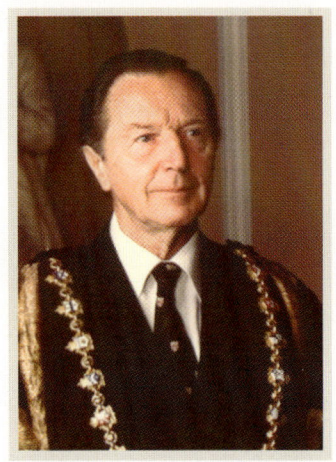

b. 1916, Dublin, son of Lawrence J. Curtin [q.v.] (ENT surgeon) and Nora Curtin (*née* McAuliffe)
Educ. Scoil Bhríde; Catholic University School; Presentation College, Bray; Royal College of Surgeons in Ireland
m. Maeve Kennedy (consultant anaesthetist), daughter of 'Doc' Kennedy [q.v.]; 6 d (Denise is consultant ophthalmologist at Royal Victoria Eye & Ear Hospital)
d. 1996

LRCP & SI (McNaughton Jones gold medal, Mercer's Hospital); FRCSI, 1945; FACS

Trained at Harrogate Infirmary; Royal Victoria Eye and Ear Hospital, Dublin.

Consultant otolaryngologist, Royal Victoria Eye and Ear Hospital; St Lawrence's Hospital (Richmond); Children's Hospital, Temple Street; Hume Street Hospital.
Honorary Fellowship, Trilological Society of America.
Member, Collegium ORLAS.
PRCSI, 1974–76; Council RCSI for 35 years (from being the youngest to being the oldest).
Founder member (and past president), IOS.

Influenced by 'Togo' Graham [q.v.] and L Ruedi, Zürich.

'Mac' took a broad view of his specialty and was well versed in the financial implications of health care in his hospitals and in the wider world. Many of the world's most distinguished otolaryngologists were invited to Dublin for lectures and honorary Fellowships of the RCSI, while 'Mac', a world traveller, gave lectures in Europe, Asia and the US. He was consulted by many actors with voice projection problems and he had been interested in amateur theatricals when young. He was endlessly caring of his patients and displayed great patience with the deaf, as well as taking an interest in the carers of his trainees.

As an RCSI graduate, 'Mac' determinedly defended the position of the institution at a time (1975) when there was a possibility of its suppression as an undergraduate medical school. The College could not have had a more articulate, knowledgeable, or formidable champion. The foundation stone of the large extension of the Medical School was laid by him in 1974, and he was one of those who made this act of faith in the future a solid reality.

Tall (6 foot) and majestic on formal occasions, he had a beautiful measured speaking voice, a head which might have been a copy of a Roman Emperor's and a mane of black hair. More importantly, he had an absolutely charming manner with a really great sense of humour. In later years, he and Maeve hunted with the Bray Harriers. As one might expect, he had a great 'seat'. He was always a prolific reader.

An outstanding professional and President.

CURTIN, Laurence John (Larry)

ENT Surgeon

b. 1884
Educ. Catholic University School of Medicine (Cecilia Street)
m. 2 s, 1 d (m. consultant obstetrician G. Gallagher)
d. 1950s

MB, BCh, BAO, RUI, 1908; MD, NUI, 1913

Authored papers on Ménière's Disease, 1914.

In the early years of the twentieth century when specialisation was less organised, it was common for would-be ENT specialists to visit the large established continental clinics such as Berlin and Vienna. Larry Curtin was clinical assistant in the Chiavi Klinik, and Poli Klinik and Urban Schitch Klinik, Vienna.

Oliver McCullen [q.v.] recalls meeting him on only one occasion, when Larry Curtin was the examiner in his final med examination. He has no bad memories of that encounter, and remembers him as being tall and resembling his son, Mac (John McAuliffe Curtin [q.v.]). There is a good photograph of him, smiling, in the library of the Royal Victoria Eye and Ear Hospital.

DELAP, John Cyril (Cyril)

Cork Otolaryngologist

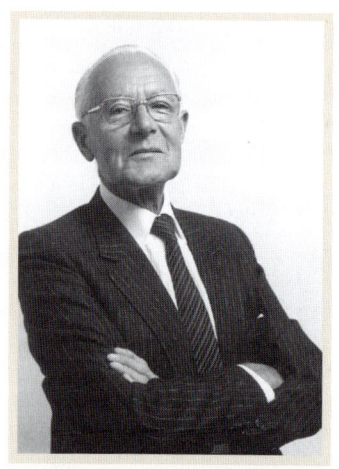

b. 1916, eldest son of Jack Delap and Elizabeth Delap (*née* Leahy)
Educ. Christian Brothers College, Cork; Blackrock College, Dublin; University College Cork
m. 1954: Helen O'Donnell, only child of David O'Donnell and May O'Donnell (*née* Lynch), Croom, Co. Limerick; 3 s (John is Dublin GP), 1 d (Libby, an optometrist)
d. 2001

MB, UCC, 1939; DLO; MCh

Postgraduate training at Gloucester Royal Infirmary and Eye Institution; Royal National Ear Nose and Throat Hospital, London (under Chapel Gill Carey).

Otolaryngologist, North Infirmary, Cork, 1946; Eye, Ear, Nose and Throat Hospital, 1950–86.

In Cork, Cyril Delap sometimes assisted JB Horgan [q.v.]. Constantly on call for 'the bone in the throat' (Christmas was a busy time) or 'the peanut in the bronchus' (Christmas again), he worked hard, and there was little in the way of a waiting list for his three successors. From his training in London, when nothing could really be done for deafness, he recalled an old chief who would remove a small quantity of wax from the ear, display it to the patient, and then, raising his voice an octave, would enquire, 'Is that better now?' He had a small ball of wax on stand-by, which could be raided if the patient had none.

Cyril told a story very well and recounted how after he had his own tonsils removed in Golden Square, London, in war time, his surgeon told him to go home in case the hospital might be bombed. He made his way down Piccadilly Tube Station, carrying two suitcases, and at the bottom started to bleed from his throat. An air-raid siren had gone off in the meantime and the crowds rushing into the subway were horrified to see Cyril coming up with blood pouring from his mouth, as they thought that the underground had been already hit.

Always immaculately turned out, with a beautiful speaking voice, Cyril is fondly remembered for his absolutely unfailing courtesy to patients of all classes, and his radiant charm, dispensed to a great circle of friends within the profession and at the racetracks. A competitive, commercial golfer, he loved Cork (and 'Paddy').

DEMPSEY, Patrick

ENT Surgeon

Educ. Catholic University School of Medicine (Cecilia Street)

FRCSI, 1901; MRCS, LRLCP Lond, 1895 (Catholic University, Dublin)

Visiting surgeon for diseases of the throat, nose and ear, Mater Hospital, Dublin.
Fellow, RAMI.

Author of 'Cancer of the larynx', 1903; 'An empyema of antrum of Highmore', 1907.

DENNIS, Augustine

Consultant ENT Surgeon

b. 1936
Educ. University College Dublin
m. Married with 8 children

MB, UCD, 1961; FRCSI, 1965; FRCS Eng, 1967

ENT training at Royal National Throat, Nose and Ear Hospital; senior registrar, Guy's Hospital.
Consultant ENT Surgeon, Our Lady's Hospital for Sick Children; St Vincent's Hospital, Dublin.

Well versed in general surgery, Gus Dennis specialised in ENT in which he trained in London. Tall and distinguished, with a commanding personality and demeanour, a mischievous sense of humour, and always sporting a bow tie, Gus built a large practice in his Blackrock Clinic rooms, with an emphasis on paediatric ENT. A precise and decisive surgeon, he was a most supportive colleague who was not involved in medical politics.

Gus has an amiable and engaging personality and, though an only child himself, has a large family of eight children. He retired in 2006.

EL-KORDI, Fatah

Consultant ENT Surgeon

Postgraduate training in Belfast.
Consultant ENT surgeon, Waveney Hospital, Ballymena.

Fatah El-Kordi practised general ENT surgery, with a special interest in otology. He was a pleasant colleague with a quiet personality. On retirement, he went to live in Egypt.

FAGAN, Albert Patrick

Consultant ENT Surgeon

b. 1899, son of surgeon Patrick Fagan (a distinguished surgeon on the staff at St Vincent's Hospital and associated with Prof. Ambrose Birmingham in the Department of Anatomy in the RUI)
Educ. Castleknock School; University College Dublin
m. Kathleen Seales (from a prominent legal family); 3 s (third son, also Albert, became a consultant cardiac surgeon in Blackpool), 1 d
d. 1966

MB, NUI, 1921 (first class hons and gold medal); MCh, NUI, 1940.

Postgraduate studies in Vienna and Berlin.
Appointment in Medical Corps, Irish Army, during civil war, 1922–23.
Consultant ENT specialist, St Vincent's Hospital.
Consultant ENT specialist, Children's Hospital, Temple Street; St Ann's Hospital, Northbrook Road.
Consultant to Peamount Sanatorium; the Lourdes Hospital, Drogheda.
Fellow, RAMI; President, section of laryngology and otology. For many years, he took an active part in its proceedings.

Albert Fagan was a warm and friendly person of high intellect, and these qualities attracted a large practice, from which he never retired. He had an innate sympathetic bond with his patients and was an exceptionally caring doctor.

Very athletic in his youth, he was a member of Castleknock Senior rugby team in the year when they reached the final (but lost). He was a keen swimmer and tennis player throughout his life and was a founder member of Old Belvedere RFC, and an honorary life member of Portmarnock Golf Club. For a time, he was also a member of Milltown, Grange and Delgany Clubs. He was also a keen race-goer.

Albert Fagan was pre-eminently a family man, and was especially reassuring to his paediatric patients. He had a quiet and unassuming personality, despite his professional eminence and distinctions.

FENELON, Robert Eric (Eric)

ENT Surgeon

b. 1921, second son of Mr and Mrs C. H. Fenelon
Educ. Earlsfort House School, Dublin; Trinity College, Dublin
m. Sylvia; 2 d (Lynda, a consultant microbiologist, St Vincent's Hospital; Sandra, an accountant).
d. 2005

BA, MB, TCD, 1944; FRCSI, 1947

Postgraduate surgical training in Manchester and Blackburn.
Assistant in general surgery, Adelaide Hospital.
Subsequently specialised in ENT and had further appointments to the Royal Victoria Eye and Ear Hospital; Dr Steevens' Hospital; Peamount Hospital; Cherry Orchard Hospital.
Founder member (and past president), IOS.

Eric Fenelon was a dextrous surgeon, and was cool and decisive in an emergency and supportive of the junior staff. He developed a particular interest in stapedectomy. He visited clinics all over the world and observed surgery. He was an able organiser and very skilful and courteous in chairing a committee. He was also prominent in the Masonic Order and represented Ireland at meetings abroad.

Socially Eric was a bon vivant and great company. He had a good sense of humour and would laugh until he almost cried. Although not too tall, he was powerfully built and had real presence. He was a delightful and enthusiastic travelling companion on many trips with the IOSTC. He and his charming wife, Sylvia, always attended the annual meetings of the IOS right up to his last illness and fostered friendships with colleagues in Northern Ireland. Sylvia and Eric were a wonderfully matched, warm and hospitable couple, in both their home in Dublin and their retreat near Parknasilla. They celebrated their fiftieth wedding anniversary only a few years before Eric passed on.

FENNELL, Francis George

Consultant ENT Surgeon

b. 1924, the tenth of 10 children of Patrick and Mary Fennell
Educ. Presentation College, Cork; Belvedere College, Dublin; Royal College of Surgeons in Ireland
m. Maura; 2 d, 1 s

LRCSI, RCSI, 1949; DLO, RCS Eng, 1955; FRCS Glasg, 1962

Following house jobs in the Richmond Hospital, Dublin, was demonstrator in anatomy for a year at the RCSI.
Commenced ENT training at the Eye and Ear Hospital.
Subsequently worked in the UK in the Metropolitan ENT Hospital, London; the Royal Sussex County Hospital, Brighton; Newcastle upon Tyne; Sheffield; Great Ormond Hospital for Sick Children, London.
Consultant, Stirling Royal Infirmary, 1962; Northern Ireland Hospital's Authority, 1963–67; Royal Victoria Eye and Ear Hospital, Dublin; Children's Hospital, Temple Street; St Bricin's Military Hospital.
Chief examiner in the FRCSI (otolaryngology) for a 10-year period.

With his wide experience and training, George Fennell had interests and practice in all areas of ENT. His quiet and unassuming demeanour concealed a mischievous sense of humour and keen observation, with non-malign appreciation of entertaining human foibles. In the FRCS examination, the candidates would search his impassive features in vain to get a clue as to whether or not their answers were on the right track. George, meanwhile, would be reading them like a book with fine print, and observing every subtle nuance. He was extremely fair minded in examinations and would always give the candidate the benefit of any doubt. He was similarly very kind to patients, and the most loyal and supportive colleague. An exhausted patient mid-morning at one of the mammoth eye and ear clinics complained to George Fennell that she had been waiting since 9.30 that morning. Always avoiding confrontation, George murmured sotto voce to no one in particular, 'I have been here since 8.30 myself'.

He has a military, athletic bearing and was a keen athlete in his youth — Irish champion fencer (foil) in 1946, and also on the swimming teams of both Belvedere College and the RCSI.

George delights in his own offspring and grandchildren. He also enjoys the companionship of old friends for an occasional beer in a Donnybrook hostelry.

FITZGERALD, Colman

Consultant ENT Surgeon

b. 14 November 1926, second child of Dr and Mrs Gerald Fitzgerald
Educ. CBS School, Tralee; Castleknock College, Dublin; University College Dublin

MB, UCD, 1950; DLO, 1954; MCh, 1956

Postgraduate training at Metropolitan ENT Hospital, London; Addenbrooke's Hospital, Cambridge (Chiefs who influenced him were Mr Frederick Boyes-Korkis and Dr A. S. Walford). Consultant ENT surgeon, Bon Secours Hospital, Tralee; Kerry General Hospital.

His area of special interest was ear surgery.

Colman Fitzgerald is an amiable and pleasant colleague with a quiet and unassuming disposition. He retired in 1980 and is a keen and expert golfer.

FURLONG, Sidney Joseph Verner, OBE

Consultant ENT Surgeon

MB, Dublin, 1920; MB TCD, 1916; LM, Rotunda, 1916; FRCSI, 1929.

Consultant ENT surgeon, Meath Hospital and Adelaide Hospital, Dublin.
Major, Royal Army Medical Corps.

As well as a general ENT practice, Sidney Furlong enjoyed aviation and driving motor cars. He built an aeroplane in his own garden and flew it successfully!

GIBSON, Roy

Consultant ENT/Head and Neck Surgeon

b. 1933, son of Robert Gibson, OBE (d. 1984) of Belfast and Mary Gibson (d. 1995)
Educ. Royal Belfast Academical Institution; Queen's University, Belfast
m. 1962: Elizabeth Deirdre (d. 1996), daughter of William Jordan Addis (d. 1981) of Belfast;
2 d (Leslie Deirdre; Jennifer Maxine)

MB, QUB, 1957; FRCS, Ed, 1962; FRCS, 1964

Postgraduate training at Royal Victoria Hospital, Belfast; clinical Fellowship in otolaryngology, Washington University in St Louis, Missouri, USA, 1965–66 (with Prof. J. Ogura, a pioneer in techniques of preservation surgery in patients with laryngeal cancer, and considered to be the most important medical figure in St Louis. This was a formative influence in his subsequent career).

Consultant ENT/head and neck surgeon, RVH, Belfast, 1972–98.

Member, central committee for hospital medical services of BMA, 1980–85; Council, BMA, 1983–85.

Chairman, Medical Advisory Committee for Eastern Health and Social Services Board, 1987–92; medical staff at the RVH, 1995–97.

Member, IOS; Association of Head and Neck Oncologists of Great Britain.

Author of various papers on general ENT and head and neck surgery.

Roy Gibson was very kind and caring to his patients, as well as giving them every benefit of his huge surgical expertise. Although he did not do private practice, he would accept telephone calls at home in the evening from anxious relatives of his NHS patients, concerning their progress and proposed surgery. His recreations include golf, gardening and reading, watching rugby and cricket.

GOGARTY, Oliver St John B.

ENT Surgeon

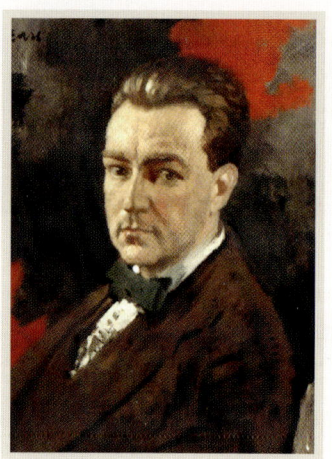

b. 1878

Educ. Mungret, Limerick; Stonyhurst; Trinity College, Dublin

d. 1957 in New York

BA, MB, TCD, 1907; FRCSI, 1910

Postgraduate training in ENT in Vienna.
Surgeon, Meath Hospital; County Dublin Infirmary.
Laryngologist and rhinologist, Richmond, Whitworth and Hardwicke Hospitals, Dublin.

Oliver St John Gogarty is widely remembered not just as a prominent ENT surgeon, but also as a poet, writer, athlete, politician and socialite. He spent a term at Oxford on the strength of having won prizes for poetry at Trinity. He was the model for the character Buck Mulligan in *Ulysses*, when he shared the Martello Tower at Sandycove with James Joyce and R. S. Chevenix-Trench.

At the time when Gogarty was in Vienna, surgery was primitive and a severe endurance test for the patients. There was a flag to be flown over the major hospital, the Allgemeine Krankenhaus, if one day should pass without a patient dying. Gogarty said that he never saw the flag flown.

He came back to Dublin and set up practice at 15 Ely Place. On his appointment to the Richmond Hospital, according to Vera Hughes, he said that it had more knights and Presbyterians on the medical staff than all the other hospitals in town. One day, a splashing sound was heard in the small stream below the operating theatre. Gogarty said that this was caused by delusional sprats from Grangegorman Hospital (the city asylum), thinking that they were salmon.

The position and priority of medicine in his multi-faceted career is uncertain, but there is no doubt that he had a successful ENT practice.

GRAHAM, Thomas Ottiwell ('Togo') PRCSI 1942–1944

ENT Surgeon

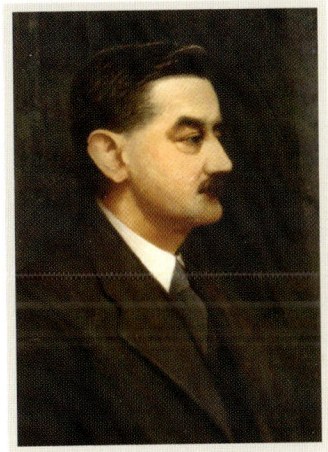

b. 1883, one of 10 children of missionary parents who left China at the Boxer rebellion
Educ. Trinity College, Dublin
d. 1966

BA, Dub, 1905 (senior moderatorship gold medal); MD, 1908; MB, BCh, BAO, TCD, 1906; DPH, 1908; FRCSI, 1912; LM, Rotunda Hospital; Bennett surgical travelling prize, 1908

ENT surgeon, Royal Victoria Eye and Ear Hospital, Dublin, 1912–60; Royal City of Dublin Hospital, Baggot Street.
Major, Royal Army Medical Corps, First World War.
Council member (and later President), RCSI; Royal Academy of Medicine.

Togo (nicknamed after a Japanese Admiral) was a man of boundless energy and enthusiasm. He was a frequent attendee at meetings and conferences, and was acquainted with the leaders in the specialty, such as Sir St Clair Thompson, Lampart and Shambaugh. He always stayed at the best hotels as he said it paid to have a good address.

Togo Graham did part of his training in Vienna, the major centre for ENT at that time. He was a likeable and charitable person, with a gracious manner. Tall, ram-rod straight, he often walked from his home in Eglinton Road to the Eye and Ear Hospital (two miles), always without an overcoat. He was on the staff of the Eye and

Ear for almost fifty years. He neither drank nor smoked and was a very charitable person. He was a member of the Synod of the Church of Ireland.

He had a place in Co. Kildare and also land at Belfield, some of which is part of the present UCD campus. Togo Graham was fearless in battle (and surgically). He personified the best of Anglo-Irish culture.

GRANT, William J. (Willie)

Consultant ENT Surgeon

b. 1930, into a prominent Buncrana, Donegal family; younger brothers, Frank and Oliver (d. 2007), both graduated in dentistry
Educ. University College Dublin
m. Maeve; 5 children (son, Will Jnr, is ENT consultant at Charing Cross Hospital, London)
d. 2003

MB, UCD, 1953; FRCS Eng, 1961

Postgraduate training was in the General Infirmary at Leeds; also worked in Blackpool (with noted otologist Ian Thorburn).
ENT consultant, Manchester.
ENT Consultant, Mater Hospital; Royal Victoria Eye and Ear Hospital, Dublin.

Willie Grant was an excellent operator whose main interest was otology. He excelled at mastoid surgery. He was a great admirer of Gordon Smyth and he had a long series of successful stapes operations over many years.

A strong personality with a mildly acidic wit, Willie was personally friendly and fair minded. He had a direct manner, which could seem slightly outspoken at times. An irate lady who was dissatisfied with her progress and Willie's concise explanation of same demanded to speak to his superior, upon which Willie, who had an imposing and magisterial presence, drew himself up and said, 'Madam, I can assure you I have no superior.' He was a wonderful second opinion for the difficult patient; after the consultation, the patient was never again to be seen around the hospital.

Tall, ram-rod straight, handsome, with a full head of hair, and always impeccably dressed, Willie was a commanding figure. He was a bon vivant who enjoyed social life enormously. He liked a good cigar and loved golf. He was a real enthusiast who played with the best and had countless lessons. His practice swing was perfect; when the ball intervened, however, the follow-through might not always be faultless. He was Captain of Portmarnock Golf Club and thoroughly enjoyed it. He was a superb after-dinner speaker, with wit and timing, and his speeches were delivered in a sonorous voice.

His wife Maeve was tall, charming and also keen on golf. Very sadly, she died just when Willie retired, and he was bereft, though he carried on. He became unwell himself a few years later and succumbed, aged 73, to prostatic cancer. Willie was courageous, outspoken and likeable, he had style and charisma and was a great otologist.

HACKETT, Edward William Ronald (Bill)

ENT Surgeon

b. 1914

Educ. Trinity College, Dublin

MB, BCh, TCD, 1938

Bill Hackett was a junior colleague of Robert Woods [q.v.] in Sir Patrick Dun's Hospital. He later moved to Athy where he continued to practise, and later retired to South Africa.

HANLON, James (Jim)

Consultant ENT Surgeon

b. 1908, younger son of John Hanlon and Claire Moyne, daughter of Thomas Moyne MP
Educ. Clongowes Wood College and Blackrock College where he was subsequently President of the Past Pupils Union; RCSI
m. 1938: Elizabeth Cullen, daughter of John Cullen and Rosanna Reilly. 2 s (John is GP in Clontarf, Dublin), 2 d (Veronica and Elizabeth), granddaughter Kelly also continues in the medical tradition.
d. 1961

LRCSI 1932, FRCSI 1937, consultant ENT surgeon, Royal Victoria Eye and Ear Hospital and St Laurence's Hospital (Richmond) and Hume Street Hospital.

Postgraduate training in ENT surgery at Eye and Ear Hospital; Richmond Hospital; Vienna.

A Dublin physician and ear, nose and throat surgeon, Jim was in Vienna in the late 1930s, but when he went back there in the late 1940s he found that all of his Jewish professors had perished in the Holocaust. A dexterous surgeon, he introduced the operating microscope for middle ear surgery to Dublin. His vision in one eye was slightly impaired after trauma. In 1950 an operation to correct this in

London was complicated by intraocular infection and subsequent sympathetic ophthalmia in the other eye, which resulted in complete blindness. To compound matters, high-dose Streptomycin resulted in deafness.

Jim Hanlon had to abandon his surgical career, but undeterred he went to London and qualified as a physiotherapist, and then returned to work in a new capacity at both the Eye and Ear Hospital and the Richmond.

Always athletic with superb co-ordination, he incredibly continued to play golf, both accurately and well. He continued as a high diver when blind. He was aided by Eddie Heron, Irish Olympian. In addition, his superb sense of touch enabled him to actually make golf clubs in his workshop, which he did for all his family. JB Carr, Ireland's greatest amateur golfer and Henry Cotton, the outstanding English player of his generation both found the clubs a delight to use. He had been Captain of the Grange Golf Club.

He had mastered Braille at high speed and the family learned sign language to keep up with him. His sense of where he was was so remarkable that people seeing him in the street or in buses (!) did not always realise he was blind. He had met Helen Keller who was deaf and blind from birth. She told him that his handicap was worse than hers because he knew what he was missing and she did not. He was also the subject of 'The most unforgettable person I have ever met', a famous section in the *Reader's Digest*.

An earlier bout of rheumatic fever had weakened a heart valve and, following a drenching when he went to the aid of a golfer who had collapsed on the course, he became ill. It was on a visit to Lourdes in 1961 that Jim Hanlon passed away at only 53. His death was first announced on French radio as he was so well known for his character and courage. Pope John XXIII was informed of his passing. He was interred in Lourdes.

Jim Hanlon was an exceptional person who faced and overcame major adversity in his life with equanimity and fortitude. Dark, handsome and with a Roman nose, he was deeply religious. He is remembered with deep affection by his family and friends.

HARVEY, Ronald Marsden

Consultant ENT Surgeon

b. 1918
Educ. King's College Hospital
m. Eustelle; 3 d
d. 2004

MBBS, King's College Hospital, 1943; DLO Eng, 1948; FRCS, 1953

Postgraduate training at King's College Hospital; research council grantee.
Major, Royal Army Medical Corps DA.
Consultant ENT surgeon, Eye and Ear Hospital, 1954.
Consultant ENT surgeon, Altnagelvin Hospital, until his retirement in 1983; chairman of the medical staff.
Chairman, Northern Ireland Central Medical Advisory Committee.
Founder member (and past president), IOS.
High Sheriff, city of Londonderry for two terms; deputy lieutenant for many years.

Ron Harvey had a charming personality, and was extremely kind and unassuming. Tall and patrician, he always dressed with panache; the breast-pocket handkerchief was never missing.

Early in his career, he was involved in the planning of the ENT Department at Altnagelvin Hospital. This was the first new general hospital to be built in the UK after the NHS came into being. He was so successful that his counsel was sought on many subsequent developments in the hospital.

He served an extended period as chairman of the medical staff, which coincided with the worst period of civil disturbance in Northern Ireland. He remained in the hospital for days on end to ensure that the frequent emergency situations were smoothly dealt with. He had not only to secure delivery of treatment to patients with severe multiple trauma, but also to ensure that the travel of staff to and from the hospital was secure enough to provide for appropriate surgical teams to be available at all times. As chairman of the Northern Ireland Central Medical Advisory Committee, he promoted the education of undergraduates and postgraduates at Altnagelvin. His service to medicine in Northern Ireland was recognised when he was appointed OBE in 1982.

In additional to his hospital work, Ron was involved with the Red Cross, for which he received the Red Cross badge of honour. He served on the committee for hearing dogs for the deaf and worked for Riding for the Disabled. He was great company on the IOS travel club visits to different countries.

Ron Harvey treated everyone with exceptional kindness and concern, from his patients and their relatives, to his staff and colleagues in the hospital. When Michael Bicknell [q.v.] and his wife suffered a cot death in their family, Ron immediately arranged compassionate leave and provided fully paid tickets for a fortnight's holiday in Cyprus.

HEFFERNAN, Daniel James (Dan)

Consultant ENT Surgeon

LRCP & SI, 1941; DLO, 1948

Postgraduate training in Sunderland, Blackburn and Birmingham.
Consultant surgeon, Birmingham Regional Hospital; Dudley Road Hospital; Sutton Coldfield Hospital; Tamworth Hospital.
Consultant ENT surgeon, Limerick Regional Hospital; St John's Hospital, Limerick.

Dan Heffernan sadly died prematurely in middle age.

HENRY, Harold Sidney Addison

Consultant ENT Surgeon

Educ. Queen's University Belfast

MB, QUB, 1930; DPH, 1932; FRCSI, 1946; DLO Eng, 1950

Postgraduate training in the UK: ENT registrar, United Birmingham Hospitals; senior ENT registrar, Middlesex Hospital and Ferens Institute of Otolaryngology at the Middlesex Hospital.
Consultant ENT surgeon at Queen Mary's Hospital for the East End of London.
Consultant ENT surgeon, South Down, South Armagh and Banbridge Hospitals.

Harold Henry was the author of papers on malignant disease in the middle ear. He drove a Rolls Royce motor car.

HINGORANI, Ram Kumar

Consultant ENT Surgeon

Educ. Rajasthan, India

MB, BS, Rajasthan, 1960; FRCS Ed, 1968

Postgraduate training in the UK.
Consultant ENT surgeon, Newry and Banbridge, Co. Down.

Ram Kumar Hingorani practised general ENT surgery. He took early retirement.

HORGAN, John Bowering ('JB')

Consultant Otolaryngologist

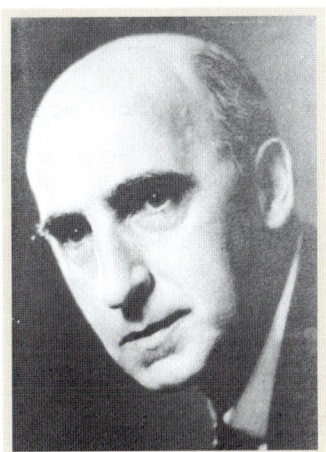

b. 1883, son of an eminent solicitor (C. S. Parnell was best man at his wedding)
Educ. 1916: Rita Wallace (a touring Scottish grand opera soprano), whom he met in Cork; 2 d
m. Clongowes Wood; University College Cork
d. 1955

Postgraduate studies in London; clinical assistant with Chiari and Widener in Vienna, and Halle's clinic in Berlin.
Consultant otolaryngologist, Eye, Ear, Nose and Throat Hospital, Cork, 1933–55.

JB Horgan's training was exceptionally long for those times. He developed new techniques in aural and nasal surgery. His operation of external frontoethmoidectomy won him international recognition; it is now reserved for extensive disease. He drowned while fishing in his beloved Blackwater.

HUNTER, Kennedy

ENT Surgeon

b. 1907, second child of William and Mary Hunter
Educ. Royal Belfast Academical Institution; Queen's University Belfast
m. Kathleen Mary McDowell; 2 d, 1 s
d. 1976

MB (hons), QUB, 1930; FRCS Ed, 1934; DLO, 1935

Postgraduate ENT training, RVH, Belfast; Throat, Nose and Ear Hospital, Golden Square, London.
Honorary assistant ENT surgeon, Belfast Ophthalmic Hospital; Benn Hospital, Belfast; Ulster Hospital for Women and Children, 1935.
ENT surgeon, Royal Victoria Hospital, 1939.
Regularly visited fever hospital in Purdysburn and Whiteabbey Sanatorium.
Foundation member (and past president), IOS.
Member, Collegium; Royal Society of Medicine; Ulster Medical Society.
Lecturer in Otolaryngology, QUB.

In his early years, particularly interested in surgery for chronically infected ears and later the surgery of otosclerosis.

Kennedy Hunter was a surgeon of wide interests and carried out many operations for malignant disease of the larynx, pharynx and paranasal sinuses. A major figure in the development of ENT surgery in Northern Ireland, he was slim, quiet, unassuming and studious. He was very conscientious in his work and was kind and generous by nature.

In recognition of his efforts in encouraging and training them, former registrars established, for medical students, a hospital prize for proficiency in otolaryngology.

He enjoyed golf, travel, photography, bridge and gardening.

JOHNSTON, Stafford

Consultant ENT Surgeon

b. Cavan
Educ. University College Dublin

BA, MB, NUI UCD, 1914

Consultant surgeon, Throat, Nose and Ear Department, Richmond Hospital (St Laurence's), Dublin; St Michael's Hospital, Dún Laoghaire; Our Lady's Hospital for Sick Children, Crumlin.
Medical adviser to John Charles McQuaid, Archbishop of Dublin.
Grand Knight of Columbanus.

Stafford Johnston was doing guillotine tonsillectomies when he was in his seventies. John McAuliffe Curtin [q.v.] was his assistant in the Richmond Hospital. Stafford Johnston lived into his nineties.

KEANE, Thomas (Tom)

Consultant ENT Surgeon

b. 1933
Educ. University College Dublin
m. Ann; 6 children

MB, UCD, 1957; FRCSI, 1963

Postgraduate training involved singular experience in neurosurgery as well as ENT.
Consultant ENT surgeon, Richmond (St Laurence's) Hospital, 1970.
Consultant in Beaumont Hospital after the transfer of services.

His area of special interest was in the interface between the two specialties, neuro-otology, which expanded greatly during his career.

Tom Keane was a meticulous and careful surgeon. He retired in 1998. Tall, athletic, good humoured and quietly spoken, he has an engaging and unassuming personality. A very keen sailor, he is also an excellent golfer and plays bowls in latter years.

KELLY, Vivian

Consultant ENT Surgeon

b. 1933, second child of Dr T. Kelly of Belmullet
Educ. Rockwell College, Co. Tipperary, 1945–52; University College Dublin
m. one son is a consultant in emergency medicine

MB, UCD, 1958; MCh 1968; ABO, 1972

Postgraduate training in the United States: residency, Wayne State Medical School, Detroit, Michigan Fellowships on head and neck surgery, Presbyterian Hospital, Newark, New Jersey; University of Chicago; University of Michigan.
ENT specialist, Saginaw General Hospital, Michigan, 1965–69.
ENT Consultant, Jervis Street, 1969–82; Beaumont Hospital, 1982–88.
Fellow, American Academy of Otolaryngology; American College of Surgeons; House Ear Clinic.

Influenced by Prof. Jan Beekhuis and Prof. James Croushose, both otologists in Detroit. Special interests were in otology and audiology and also the application of medical statistics.

Vivian Kelly was an excellent ear surgeon and colleague, with a great sense of humour and a keen intellect. He had a scientific approach and the capacity to think through a problem carefully after sound analysis. A hard worker, he was great company when relaxed, and a most entertaining raconteur.

DOYLE-KELLY, Walter

Consultant ENT Surgeon

b. 1924, younger son of Walter A. Doyle-Kelly (mining engineer in the Indian army) and Margaret Doyle-Kelly (*née* Sheehy)
Educ. Christian Brothers School, Synge Street, Dublin; University College Dublin
m. Betty; 3 children
MB, UCD, 1947; DLO, RCS Eng, 1949; MCh (otolaryngology), NUI, 1950

Postgraduate training in the UK at Kent and Sussex Hospital, Tunbridge Wells; Queen Elizabeth Hospital, Birmingham.

Consultant ENT surgeon, Sir Patrick Dun's Hospital, 1950–86, when the hospital closed; Adelaide Hospital, 1986–91.

Consultant ENT surgeon, St Luke's Hospital, 1956–91; National Children's Hospital in Harcourt Street, 1971–91.

Senior lecturer in otolaryngology, TCD.

Founding member (president, 1989–90), IOS.

Council of Europe Fellowship, 1964.

President, ORL section, Royal Academy of Medicine, 1960s (member since 1950).

The people who influenced his career were Norman Crabtree in Birmingham, and his senior colleague, Robert Woods [q.v.], Sir Patrick Dun's Hospital, Dublin.

Special surgical interest was in temporal bone surgery.

Of medium height, Walter Doyle-Kelly has a youthful appearance with a full head of hair. He is courteous, patient and unassuming, with a very droll sense of humour. Once when there had been a delay in minting the Presidential medals for the IOS, Walter was advised that his medal was now ready. He remarked, 'That's great news; I was afraid it might be awarded posthumously,' Walter is very good company with acute recall of past medical colleagues. He and Betty have what he describes as three middle-aged children and eight grandchildren. His recreations included rowing in UCD, dinghy sailing, fly fishing and clay-pigeon shooting. He was also a water colourist.

KENEFICK, Cyril

Consultant ENT Surgeon

b. 1942, Cork

Educ. Glasheen National School; Presentation Brothers College, Cork; University College Cork

MB, NUI, Cork, 1965 (several honours in his undergraduate medical career); FRCS Ed, 1969; DLO, London, 1969; FRCS Eng, 1971

Demonstrator in anatomy, UCC.
Commenced his ENT career at the RVH, Belfast.
Registrar, Middlesex Hospital; St Bartholomew's Hospital London; Royal Berkshire Hospital, Reading.
Senior registrar, North of Ireland Hospital Authority, Altnagelvin.
Ainsworth Scholarship, UCC; Marsden Fellowship.
Seconded for a year to the head and neck unit, Royal Marsden Hospital, London.
Consultant ENT private practice in Cork, 1975.
Operation lists and clinics, South Cork Charitable Infirmary; Mercy Hospital, Cork.

Locum cover, Eye, Ear and Throat Hospital; Cork Regional Hospital.

Member (and elected member of council), IOS.

Member, Royal Society of Medicine in London, section of otology and laryngology; ORL Research Society; the BEOHNS.

President, section of otolaryngology/head and neck surgery, RAMI, 2002–07.

Major influences were David Craig [q.v.], Belfast; Sir Douglas Ranger and Lancelot Dowie, London; and John McAuliffe Curtin [q.v.], Dublin

Has published and lectured on many aspects of ENT.

Cyril Kenefick's wide training and experience enabled him to cover all aspects of his specialty. He is a skilled and decisive surgeon, with wide experience. These attributes, combined with a friendly personality, ensured a large practice.

Cyril has the youthful, smartly dressed figure of the sportsman. He represented the Presentation Brothers College at cricket, tennis and rugby, and later UCC at tennis and rugby. Still an outdoors man, he concentrates on golf and sailing now. He has a keen sense of humour, and was a most popular president of the Academy of Medicine ENT section, with both his colleagues and the postgraduates. He is very good company and always a pleasure to meet. He continues in active practice.

KENNEDY, Desmond Aidan

Consultant ENT Surgeon

b. 1919

MB, NUI, 1944; MCh

Consultant ENT surgeon, Mater Hospital; St Michael's Hospital, Dún Laoghaire.

Desmond Kennedy trained initially as a physician before turning to ENT. He had a quiet, sincere personality, with old-world courtesy, and was a very loyal colleague. He was more interested in the medical aspects of otolaryngology. He retired in 1984.

KEOGH, Peadar

Consultant ENT Surgeon

b. 1941
Educ. University College Dublin
m. Sheila; 4 children (2 daughters in physiotherapy and speech therapy)

MB, UCD, 1965, FRCSI 1970, FRCS Ed. 1970.

Postgraduate training in Manchester; senior registrar, Leeds; studied otology in Nijmegen, Holland.
ENT consultant, Leeds, 1973–76; Regional Hospital, Limerick, from 1976.
Member, North of England ENT Society; IOS; ORL Travel Club (the oldest ENT group in existence).

Major influences on his career were two Leeds consultants, Oliver Lord and Tom McMaster-Boyle.

An excellent surgeon, widely experienced in all aspects of ENT, Peadar Keogh had a special interest in otology. He is tall, amiable, good-humoured, and unassuming about his exceptional abilities. A great family man, he retired in 2006. On retirement, he was about to concentrate on golf, at which he excels, when the new medical school in the University of Limerick wisely requested his services as tutor.

KEOGH, P. J.

ENT Surgeon

d. 1944

Chief surgeon, ENT Department, St Vincent's Hospital, 1930s.
Also attended Children's Hospital, Temple Street; St Ann's Hospital, Northbrook Road.

P. J. Keogh was a short, stout and bustling figure of whom it was said that his bite was almost as bad as his bark. He had a very strong personality and a large practice. Technically a good surgeon, he was a hard taskmaster to his assistants and house surgeons.

He was a keen angler and an excellent shot. Clay-pigeon shooting was his chief hobby. He did not get on with Oliver St John Gogarty [q.v.], who said that 'a hole in the hard palate is either a gumma or an adenoidectomy by P. J. Keogh.'

P. J. Keogh was wealthy, and lavished hospitality on his guests. He died suddenly, probably from a heart attack, while on a shoot on the Earl of Wicklow's Estate on St Stephen's Day, 1944, in the company of Francis 'Pops' Morrin [q.v.], senior surgeon at St Vincent's Hospital.

KERR, Alan Grainger

Otologist and Professor of Otolaryngology

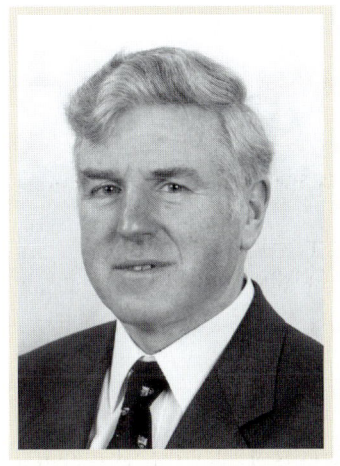

b. 1935, son of Joseph William Kerr (d. 1974) and Eileen Kerr (*née* Allen; d. 1989)
Educ. Methodist College, Belfast; Queen's University Belfast
m. 1962: Patricia Margaret McNeill (d. 1999); 2 s, 1 d

MB, DRCOG, QUB, 1959; FRCS, 1964; FRCS Ed, 1987; OBE, 2000

Trained in otolaryngology in the Belfast hospitals and Harvard Medical School.
Consultant otolaryngologist, RVH and Belfast City Hospital, 1968.
Harrison Prize at the RSM; Jobson Horne Prize of the BMA; Howell's Prize, University of London, 1988 and 1998.

President, section of otology, Royal Society of Medicine.
Member, ORL Society; National Otopathology Society; British Association of Otolaryngology; International Society of Otolaryngologic Surgery.
Member (and past president), IOS of the Irish Otolaryngological Society.
First Professor of Otolaryngology, at QUB, 1979–81.

Author of many papers on otology, often in collaboration with Gordon Smyth

Alan Kerr has had a distinguished career and is well known throughout the world as a scientific surgical otologist. An important figure in academic otolaryngology, he is an influential figure in ENT circles. He has a long association with the Royal College of Surgeons in Edinburgh. Tall, courteous and slightly reserved, with a youthful appearance and a full head of hair, he is methodical, meticulous and a clear thinker. He undertook the massive task of editing Scott Brown's *Otolaryngology*, now a work of five volumes, not once but twice, in 1987 and 1996 (the fifth and sixth editions).

Alan is athletic and his recreations include tennis, skiing and bowling. He also played football well past the age of Stanley Matthews' retirement.

In recognition of his outstanding career, Alan was elected Master of the British Academic Conference in Otolaryngology, in 2006.

KILLEN, William Marcus

Consultant Surgeon

BA (first class hons), RUI (Dub), 1884; MD, MCh, RUI

Consultant surgeon, Eye, Ear and Throat Department, Mater Infirmary Hospital, Belfast; Ulster Eye, Ear and Throat Hospital, Belfast.

KILLEN, James Wallace

Surgeon

MB, RUI, 1902; FRCSI, 1911 (QCB)

Honorary surgeon, Londonderry and NW Eye and Ear Hospital.

Author, 'Case of Optic Atrophy Treated by Opening Sphenoidal Sinuses', *BMJ*, 1911.

LAW, Kathleen

Consultant ENT Surgeon

b. 1944
Educ. Queen's University Belfast
m. John Adams (veterinary surgeon); 2 children

MB, QUB, 1968; FRCSI, 1974

Postgraduate training: senior registrar in ENT, Altnagelvin Hospital; registrar, RVH and Belfast City Hospital; senior house officer, Liverpool ENT Infirmary.
Consultant ENT surgeon, Tyrone County Hospital, Omagh; Erne Hospital, Enniskillen, Co. Fermanagh.
Member, IOS, BAOL and BMA.

Influenced by outstanding mentors: Gordon Smyth [q.v.], Ron Ballantyne, Robert Pracy, Phillip Stell, Ronald Harvey [q.v.] and Tom Wilmot [q.v.].
Special interest in otology and paediatric audiology.

Kathleen Law was the first female ENT consultant appointed in Northern Ireland, a position she held with distinction and enthusiasm. She was warmly regarded by her patients for her care and charm.

Since retiring from medicine in 2004, Kathleen has taken a new direction; she is studying Sustainable Development, with her usual full commitment.

LAW, Samuel Horace

ENT Surgeon

>**Educ.** Trinity College, Dublin
>
>BA, MD, MB, TCD, 1896; FRCSI, 1900
>
>Throat, nose and ear surgeon, Adelaide Hospital, Dublin; Stewart Institute, Chapelizod.
>Fellow, RAMI; Royal Society of Medicine.
>
>Author of 'Notes on training the voice', *Dublin Journal of Medicine*, 1906.

MACLAUGHLIN, Francis Alexander (Frank)

ENT Surgeon

>**Educ.** Queen's University Belfast
>
>MB, QUB, 1921; FRCS Eng, 1923
>
>ENT surgeon, Royal Victoria Hospital, Belfast.
>Lecturer in otolaryngology.
>Fellow, Royal Society of Medicine.

Frank MacLaughlin practised ophthalmology and ENT. He ran his private practice from home, and Oliver McCullen [q.v.] said that he got this idea from him and did likewise.

He had a large toy soldier collection, read the bible every day and drove a Rolls Royce car.

MAGUIRE, Andrew Joseph

Consultant ENT Surgeon

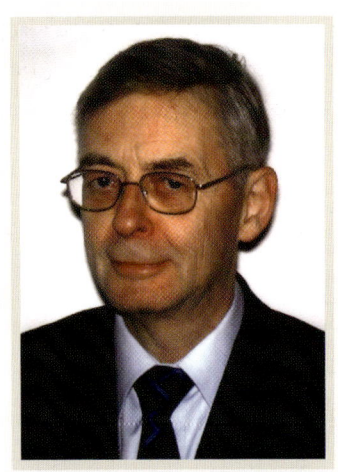

b. 1939, a younger son; grew up in the Fermanagh countryside

Educ. Clongowes Wood College, Co. Kildare; University College Dublin

m. Michelle Linnane (MA LLB (TCD), LLM (Cantab), a practising solicitor); 2 d (Ciara, TCD, medicine; Sarah, UCD, architecture)

MB, NUI UCD, 1964; FRCSI, 1970; FRCSC, 1972; Cert. Specialist Otolaryngology, Canada, 1972

Postgraduate training: senior resident, Toronto General Hospital; clinical Fellow in laryngology, Banting Institution, Toronto; registrar, Royal Infirmary and Children's Hospital, Sheffield; senior house officer, Royal National Throat, Nose and Ear Hospital, London, and Eye and Ear Hospital, Dublin; surgical registrar, Richmond Hospital (St Laurence's), Dublin.

Consultant ENT surgeon, Royal Victoria Eye and Ear Hospital, Dublin, 1973–2005; Our Lady's Hospital for Sick Children, Crumlin, 1978–2004.

President, IOS, 1992–93.

UEMS representative, Ireland, 1976–86.

Examiner FRCSI (ENT), 1976–86.

Honorary lecturer, Royal National Throat, Nose and Ear Hospital (Institute of Laryngology and Otology), London; operated (CCTV) on annual rhinoplasty and facial plastic surgery courses, 1980–2001.

Major influences in career choice were Albert Fagan [q.v.], who combined exemplary sympathetic care of patients with undiminished interest in his work; Harold Browne[q.v.], 'a physician who gently operated' and whose care was sought especially by medical families; Tony Bull, London, a master of rhinoplasty; in Toronto, Douglas Bryce and Wilfred Goodman (two giants of otolaryngology) and their younger colleague, David Briant, a great all-rounder; later in Dublin, Barry O'Donnell [q.v.], friend and mentor, who has a unique insight into matters medical, and human nature.

Andrew Maguire developed and taught head and neck surgery, and is particularly interested in plastic and reconstructive techniques in ENT, in both the adult and the paediatric patient. He has operated and lectured in several European countries, Bahrain and Pakistan. He was keen on teaching and encouraging medical students and registrars.

As Vice-President (Irel.), he invited the European Academy of Facial Plastic Surgery to Dublin for a most successful meeting at the RCSI in 2006.

Andrew Maguire retired in 2005 but continues in private consultant practice and concentrates surgically on rhinoplasty, which he finds continually fascinating. He is keenly interested in travel, and observing the best surgeons in action worldwide.

Tallish, bespectacled, with a quirky sense of humour, he enjoys walking, painting, reading biography, and Fermanagh; special concerns are facial recognition and gravity. His erudition makes him a 'dream' travelling companion.

MANNING, Kevin Patrick

Consultant ENT Surgeon

b. 1943, second eldest of 6 children of Pat and Marie Manning
Educ. Belgrove National School, Clontarf; St Paul's College, Raheny
m. Anne; 2 d (twins), 1 s

LRCSI, 1967; FRCSI, 1973; FRCS Eng, 1974

Postgraduate training in Manchester; Eye and Ear Hospital, Dublin; Richmond Hospital, Dublin. Registrar and senior registrar, Liverpool 1972–77.
Consultant ENT surgeon, Walton/Fazakerly Hospitals, Liverpool, 1977–84; Barrington/St John's Hospital, Limerick, 1984–86; Mid-Western Regional Hospital, Limerick, 1986–2008.
Desmond Lyons medal, Richmond Hospital.
Clinical lecturer, UCC; runs an excellent course in techniques of facial plastic surgery, University of Limerick.

Kevin Manning was a dexterous and decisive operator in thyroid and head and neck surgery. Dapper and youthful, he is hardworking, efficient and always good humoured. He has the capacity to see directly to the heart of the matter and is modest about his capability and achievements. He retired in 2008.

He describes himself as an avid but average golfer. Only the first adjective is true. His economy of strokes on the golf course is similar to that of his movements when operating (the mark of a good surgeon).

McCAUGHAN, Daniel Vincent

Consultant ENT Surgeon

MB, 1920

Ophthalmic and aural surgeon, Mater Infirmary Hospital, Belfast.
ENT consultant surgeon, Mid-Antrim and East Antrim Hospitals.

Daniel McCaughan was an expert in guillotine tonsillectomy.

McCREA, Robert Samuel (Bob)

Consultant ENT Surgeon

b. 1920
Educ. Queen's University Belfast
m. Married with children
d. 1983
MB, QUB, 1943; DLO Eng, 1946; FRCS Ed, 1950; BA, Open Univ, 1976

Consultant, RVH, Belfast, 1954–76.
Consultant audiological physician, RVH, Belfast.
Founding member, Northern Ireland Speech and Language Forum; Northern Ireland Society for Speech Impaired Children.
Founder member (and past president), IOS.
Fellow, Ulster Medical Society; Royal Society of Medicine; Association of Head and Neck Oncologists of Great Britain; British Association of Audiological Physicians.
Member, International Society of Audiology; several advisory medical and ENT committees in Northern Ireland.
Council member, British Association of Otolaryngologists.

Bob McCrea was unique in having two quite different careers within ENT in Belfast. During his time at the Royal Victoria Hospital, he was mainly involved in the surgery of head and neck cancer. However, ill-health forced him to retire from this post and apply for a new one as consultant audiological physician. He was interviewed for the second post by John Byrne [q.v.], amongst others whom he had previously interviewed when they were appointed.

He published many papers on both of these differing aspects of the specialty. He was a keen teacher of undergraduates and postgraduates, as well as dental students and speech therapists. He worked hard to establish a screening programme at the Belfast Hospital for Sick Children, to diagnose the difficult-to-assess children referred from all over Northern Ireland. He established Electric Response Audiometry at that time.

Bob McCrea was of average height, and was quiet but determined. He surprised everyone when he was president of the IOS by reciting a long and very funny poem of his own composition when making his presidential address; it was a great success.

Bob was dogged by ill health and sadly passed away in 1983. At his own request, he did not have a religious service.

McCULLEN, Patrick John Oliver (Oliver)

Consultant ENT Surgeon

b. 1923, son of Dr P. D. McCullen, Drogheda

Educ. CBS, Drogheda; Clongowes Wood College; University College Dublin

MB, UCD, 1947 (gold medal in medicine); DLO Eng, 1949; MCh, NUI, 1950

Postgraduate training at Metropolitan ENT Hospital, London; General Infirmary, Leeds.
Consultant ENT Surgeon, St Vincent's Hospital, Dublin, 1951; St Ann's Hospital.
Visiting consultant, Our Lady of Lourdes Hospital, Drogheda.
Member, IOS; ORL Travelling Club (which included Myles Foxen and Sir Douglas Ranger).
Vice-President, section of Otology, Royal Society of Medicine, London.

Hardworking and affable, Oliver McCullen had a huge practice which included many medical families. Bespectacled, dapper and alert, he never wasted a moment. He often did minor procedures with the patient on the trolley, to save transferral time. Highly intelligent, widely read and self-contained, he has a remarkable capacity to see to the kernel of the matter and to articulate it with brevity and unselfconscious wit: 'The only thing an ENT surgeon can do for a patient in bed is take their pulse.' He was fond of quoting, 'the only eardrops that really worked were the ones that killed Hamlet's father'. He observed that should an untoward complication befall a patient, 'the map would develop an area of alopecia regarding further referrals from that area'. An early participant in the Irish Otolaryngological Society, he also maintained his UK connection.

Oliver is a shrewd observer of human nature and character, and many of his descriptions of colleagues are integrated into these biographies. He continued in surgical practice up to age 70, and since then has been thoroughly enjoying his retirement with his many intellectual interests. He is always good company, and it is a pleasure to meet him and hear his continuing observations on life.

MATHEWS, Richard Hy

EENT Surgeon

BA, Dub, 1907; MD, MB, 1911; LM, Rotunda Hospital (TCD and Leipzig)

EENT surgeon, National Hospital for Consumption, Co. Wicklow; Royal Victoria Eye and Ear Hospital; Dr Steevens' Hospital; Drumcondra Hospital, Dublin.

MATHEWS, William

Consultant ENT Surgeon

b. 1917, second child in his family
Educ. Ballymena Academy; Queen's University Belfast
m. married; a daughter is a consultant anaesthetist in the Mater Hospital, Belfast; 3 of his grandchildren are doing medicine
d. 2007

MB, QUB; FRCS Ed, 1949

Postgraduate training in Simpson Hall's unit, Edinburgh Royal Infirmary.
Consultant ENT surgeon, Coleraine and Ballymoney, 1951; Coleraine Borough Council, 1975–80.

Bill Mathews volunteered for war service in 1940 and served two campaigns in Burma. He finished in command of a Field Ambulance with the rank of Lieutenant-Colonel. A model consultant of the old school, he was upright, courteous, modest and capable. A strong sense of civic duty and responsibility led him to volunteer in the Second World War, and also to join the Alliance Party after retirement, in which he played a major role. In recent years, his health had not been good, but he soldiered on.

For recreation, Bill enjoyed playing bridge. Always well turned out, he was a remarkable combination of charm and purpose.

MAXWELL, Patrick William

Ophthalmic and Oral Surgeon

MB, Cm., 1880; MRCS Eng,1883; LRCPI, 1884; MD, Edin., 1888; FRCSI, 1890

Ophthalmic and aural surgeon, Jervis Street Hospital, Dublin; Royal Victoria Eye and Ear Hospital, Dublin.
Surgeon aurist to HE, the Lord Lieutenant.
Ophthalmic and aural surgeon, Dr Steevens' Hospital, Dublin.

Published papers on 'Precision in squint operations' and 'The effects of nasal obstruction on accommodation'.

MILLER, Anthony Charles Michael Lindsay (Tony)

Consultant ENT Surgeon

b. 1927, Harrow, near London, son of Stanley and Isobel Miller; moved to Northern Ireland when he was 7
Educ. Portadown College; Queen's University Belfast
m. Beryl; 3 s (two qualified in medicine — Ian is training in ENT surgery; and one in dentistry)
d. 2007

MB, QUB, 1952; FRCS Ed, 1963; FRCSI (Hon.), 1984

Postgraduate training in ENT surgery in Belfast.
Consultant ENT surgeon, Belfast City Hospital and Dundonald.
Member (and past president), IOS; long-time standing Travel Club secretary.

Tony Miller practised general ENT surgery, with a special interest in nasal allergy. He had huge experience in desensitisation techniques and treated over 15,000 allergic patients. He was awarded an MBE for his medical services.

Strongly built, always well dressed with a warm good humoured personality, he was outstandingly generous. He was very hardworking and also put tremendous efforts into organising the Travel Club with great success; it most frequently went to various countries in Europe and always included observing actual surgery. Tony also organised some memorable longer trips to Australia, China and South Africa, as well as the USA. He was a wonderful companion on these trips, full of fun and with a great line of stories. One of his favourite sayings was 'Ring the bell, Nellie; I'm on.' This referred to a Belfast lady with a shopping bag in each hand, who had just managed to get on the trolley car.

Tony and his wife Beryl always gave great support and encouragement to their sons. Outside medicine, and apart from his family, his main interests were in gardening, rugby and travelling. He was an exceptional person, unassuming, warm-hearted and generous, with a sunny disposition and a great sense of fun. A rare combination.

MONTGOMERY, Robert John

Surgeon

BA, 1882; LM, 1884 (TCD); MB, 1885; LAH, 1887; FRCSI, 1889; MA, Dub, 1892

Surgeon, Royal Victoria Eye and Ear Hospital; Drumcondra Hospital.
Honorary oculist, Stewart Institution.
Fellow, RAM, Ireland.
Member, BMA.

MURPHY, William Lombard

ENT Surgeon

MA Camb, 1903; MB, 1907; FRCSI, 1906; LRCP & LM, LRCSI & LM, 1904 (University of Cambridge, Catholic University Dublin and Vienna University)

House officer, Mater Hospital, Dublin; demonstrator in laryngology and rhinology, clinic, Allgemeine Krankenhaus, Vienna.
Surgeon, Throat and Nose Department, St Vincent's Hospital, Dublin.
Fellow, Royal Academy of Medicine, Ireland.

Translator of Prof. B. Heine's *Operationen am Ohr*.

NADARAJA, Thiaga

Consultant ENT Surgeon

m. Maeve; 4 children (son is an anaesthetist)

LM, RCP & S, 1964; FRCSI, 1970

Consultant ENT surgeon, Sligo General Hospital, 1972–2006.

Thiaga Nadaraja is tall and youthful, with a full head of hair. He has an engaging personality and a great sense of humour. When he was appointed, he insisted that his department should be fully equipped before he commenced work, with the result that Sligo General ENT Department was the most up to date in the country. He also conducted clinics in Letterkenny General Hospital. He worked a huge area single-handedly for many years until he was joined by Niall Considine. Though retired from the health service (since 2006), he continues in private practice.

Thiaga was astute in medical politics and was an effective member of Comhairle na nOspidéal (the Hospital Council) for nine years. He now serves on the postgraduate Medical and Dental Board.

O'BRIEN, Brian

Consultant ENT Surgeon

b. 1909
Educ. University College Dublin
m. Mary Quinn (a stunning beauty in her day); 2 s, 2 d
d. 1978

MB, UCD, 1935; MCh, NUI, 1939

Postgraduate training, Royal National Throat, Nose and Ear Hospital, London.
Consultant ENT surgeon, St Vincent's Hospital, Dublin; Children's Hospital, Temple Street.
Our Lady's Hospital for Sick Children, Crumlin.
Lecturer in otolaryngology, UCD.
Council member, otology section, Royal Society of Medicine, London.
Fellow, RAMI.

Interested primarily in otology and paediatric ENT.

Brian O'Brien was an important figure in Irish ENT because of his strong personality and perfectionism. He was an excellent communicator and articulated ideas succinctly, rarely fudging, and sometimes uncompromisingly. He succeeded P. J. Keogh [q.v.] at St Vincent's Hospital, and when the nuns threatened to dismiss him, he dared to take them on. He informed them that he had contacts in the *Daily Express* and that the hospital's name would be in every newspaper in the land. He had a huge practice amongst the religious communities.

Brian pursued his interests in otologic surgery by making 'raids' — turning up without much notice in numerous centres abroad. He was one of the first to visit Julius Lampert in New York, to learn the fenestration operation. He had a very sociable personality and he facilitated international relations. For some years, while practising in Dublin, he continued his postgraduate association with the Royal National Throat, Nose and Ear Hospital, London. He would get the Friday-night mail boat to Holyhead, the train to London and be spruce at the outpatients clinic, which was crowded and which no one else wanted to do, at nine o'clock on Saturday morning.

Tall, handsome and always impeccably dressed, Brian did everything with style. He had charm and eloquence. The story goes that, aged 32 and a supremely eligible bachelor, he was standing on the steps of the Gresham Hotel ballroom when Mary Quinn, aged 19, danced by. One look was enough. 'I'm going to marry that girl,' said Brian. And, being Brian, he did.

Great stories abound about Brian O'Brien. He could at times be obstinate and difficult, but the overall picture is of character and charm. He did not lack courage. Once at the RSM in London, when some members from Dublin arrived a little late, the chairman made a weak and foolish joke about 'the Irish bombers' having arrived. Brian was on his feet immediately to demand a complete retraction and apology on the spot. He had a reputation of always securing payment for his work. He once asked a newly appointed consultant in anaesthetics how soon he proffered his account after an operation. The younger doctor said that he usually gave the patient a couple of weeks' leeway before he sent his bill. 'I see,' said Brian. 'Tell me, Doctor, how would you feel about paying for a meal that you had eaten a fortnight ago?'

When the death of a child in England following a tonsillectomy was reported in the newspaper, Brian cut out the article and put it in his waiting room. He wanted to inform patients that this was a serious procedure that had to be done with proper care and attention and the best possible facilities.

Brian O'Brien never retired. In his late sixties he saw the potential of the specialty developing plastic and functional surgery of the nose, rhinoplasty and septorhinoplasty and joined forces with Tony Bull in London to promote good training in this aspect of facial plastic surgery. Sadly he died prematurely from severe hypertension at age 69.

When going to the mass for Brian at St Vincent's Hospital, Willie Grant said to a colleague, 'Poor Brian is a great loss, he kept up the standards in our specialty', then as an afterthought with a twinkle in his eye, 'and most importantly, he kept up the fees.'

O'BRIEN, Michael

Consultant Otologist

b. 1916
Educ. University College Cork
m. 1944: Margaret O'Brien MB; son, Michael, a budding surgeon, died aged 30.

MB, UCC, 1942; MCh, 1947; FRCSI

Postgraduate training: General Hospital, Birmingham; Bristol Royal Infirmary; Philadelphia, USA.
Consultant to the South Infirmary and Bon Secours Hospital, Cork.
Founder member (and past president), IOS.

Major influences were J. Angell-James of Bristol and T. Scarfe.
Otology was his main interest.

Michael O'Brien was a superb surgeon and anatomist and a person of remarkable determination and resolve. When his son Michael was taking the Fellowship exam in general surgery, Michael Snr also studied for and sat the FRCSI in otolaryngology. Needless to say, both were successful. Michael was later examiner in this specialty Fellowship.

Tall, well built, quietly spoken and good humoured, Michael O'Brien was a keen low-handicap golfer and was equally fond of lake fishing for trout and salmon. He retired in 1987 and spent a good deal of his retirement near Lough Currane in Co. Kerry and has returned to live in Cork.

O'CONNELL, Cornelius Dermot (Con)

Consultant ENT Surgeon

b. 1912, eldest of 7 children of Patrick and Bridget O'Connell, Grosvenor Square, Dublin
Educ. Synge Street School; University College Dublin
m. 1940: Marie-Therese (Dolly) Murphy; 6 d (eldest, Mai, a consultant anaesthetist), 1 s
d. 1968

MB, UCD, 1936 (first class hons in all subjects); MCh, 1951

Postgraduate training in the Eye and Ear Hospital, Dublin; Yarmouth; Nova Scotia; Canada; Royal National Throat, Nose and Ear Hospital, Gray's Inn Road, London.
Consultant to the Army Medical Corps (St Bricin's Hospital and The Curragh); Dublin Health Authority children's clinics, Lord Edward Street; TB Services, Charles Street; Blanchardstown Hospital; Crooksling Ballyowen; St Clare's Hospital; Aer Lingus.
Consultant ENT Surgeon, Royal Victoria Eye and Ear Hospital; Mercer's Hospital, Dublin.
Founder member, IOS.

Con O'Connell was interested in the plastic and reconstructive procedures in ENT and was an expert in the correction of nasal injury. His interest in deaf children led to a Council of Europe scholarship. He studied these problems in the Scandinavian countries. Later he was an adviser to the government for tending to these problems. His association with public bodies gave him a clear insight in dealing with officialdom, and he was a strong advocate of preserving fairly the rights and responsibilities of the medical profession.

Personally he had a calm and friendly disposition and was a most congenial and loyal colleague, held in high regard by his peers. He was widely read, and was particularly interested in naval and military history and in boats and ships. He collected and repaired antique clocks and made and restored items of furniture.

He was 5'11", with black hair, and he chain-smoked cheroots. He was very gregarious and family orientated and encouraged his children at all times. His early demise was a great loss to his family and friends, but he had lived a full life of remarkable achievement.

O'CONNOR, Maurice Finbar Augustine ('Maurice')

Consultant ENT Surgeon

b. 1921, Cork, fourth youngest child of Peter and Connie O'Connor
Educ. Presentation School, Cork; University College Cork
m. Beatrice (Betty) McKenzie (MD, DCH), 5 s
d. 2001

MB, 1944; DPH, 1945; DLO, MCh, 1950

Postgraduate training included senior registrar, Hammersmith Postgraduate Hospital, London, and previously Central Middlesex Hospital and Golden Square Hospital, London; Addenbrooke's Hospital, Cambridge; Bristol Royal Infirmary.
ENT Consultant, Jervis Street Hospital, 1952; St James's Hospital.
Consultant to Loughlinstown Hospital; Blanchardstown Hospital.
Conducted ENT clinics in Kildare, Sligo and Donegal on a monthly basis.
Senior lecturer in ENT, Royal College of Surgeons.
Member, Royal Academy of Medicine.

Special interest was in otology.

Maurice O'Connor was a skilled surgeon and of sound opinion. He had had a Rolls Royce training and it showed. Tall, strongly built, highly individualistic and always well turned out, he had presence. A colleague, seeing him leave his consulting rooms in Fitzwilliam Square, dressed in a Norfolk jacket and plus fours, enquired if he was on holidays. Maurice advised him that he was just on his way to do a country clinic. With his strong personality, expressive face and sonorous voice he was a most entertaining raconteur, always with a definite opinion.

A skilled sailor from an early age (he went out with fishing smacks from Youghal in the summers from age 9), he raced extensively in Dublin Bay 21s, winning the Arthur Newsen Cup in 1965. He cruised in many waters, including the Caribbean, often two-handed with the supremely competent Betty as 'crew'. His extensive travels in Europe and the Middle East often related to military and archaeological history. He was keen on ornithology and the countryside.

Maurice was a family man with wide interests. He lived life to the full and enjoyed it thoroughly. He passed away unexpectedly after a brief illness, aged 80.

ODEVAINE, Ferdinand

EENT Surgeon

FRCSI, 1875

EENT Surgeon, St Vincent's Hospital, Dublin.
Examiner in ophthalmic and aural surgery, RCSI and Apothecaries Hall, Ireland.

O'DOHERTY, Edward

Consultant Otologist and Professor of Otorhinolaryngology

Educ. Cecilia Street Medical School

MB, Cecilia Street, NUI, 1925; LM, Rotunda; MCh, NUI, 1946

Consultant ENT surgeon, Mater Hospital, Dublin.
Visiting laryngologist, Our Lady of Lourdes Hospital, Dún Laoghaire and Drogheda; St Mary's Hospital, Cappagh.
Consultant laryngologist, Royal National Hospital for Consumption, Newcastle, Co. Dublin.
Consultant otologist, St Mary's Audiological Clinic, Cabra.
Director, National Organisation for Rehabilitation in Dublin.
Professor of Otorhinolaryngology, UCD.
Member, RAMI.
Fellow, Royal Society of Medicine in London.

Eddie O'Doherty, a quiet Donegal man with a cautious approach, practised general ENT surgery. He sometimes had a cigarette in the corner of his mouth when he was examining a patient. When he gave his lectures to medical students in UCD, he would walk continuously from side to side across the room, behind the desk, speaking away, never appearing to look up at the audience, even for a second.

When Eddie O'Doherty passed away, the chair of otorhinolaryngology in UCD was discontinued; it was restored only in the twenty-first century in St Vincent's Hospital.

O'LOUGHRAN, Francis (Frank)

Consultant ENT Surgeon

b. 1930, second child of Dr Frank (GP in Manchester) and May O'Loughran
Educ. Stonyhurst; Trinity College, Dublin
m. Jan (d. 2004); 3 children

MB, TCD, 1962; DObst. RCOG, 1964; FRCS Ed, 1969.

Postgraduate training, including internship, mainly in the UK, including Liverpool and Wolverhampton; returned to the Eye and Ear Hospital, Dublin.
Consultant ENT surgeon, Sir Patrick Dun's Hospital, 1972; Meath Hospital, 1974. When these hospitals closed, he transferred to St James's and Tallaght Hospitals.

His career interests in ear surgery were stimulated by Bob Farrier in Florida and Malcolm Graham in Ann Arbour, Michigan; and in head and neck by Philip Stell, Liverpool.

In his early career, Frank O'Loughran concentrated on head and neck surgery and later developed a special interest in the surgery of cholesteatoma. He is very courteous, with a great sense of humour and is great company. When he retired in 2002, he hired a large room in the Stephen's Green Club (of which he was not a member) and threw a great party for the people he had worked with over the years, and some close friends. It was his way of saying thank you to everyone. It was a memorable evening.

Frank loves golf, reading and travel, and so is at no loss to occupy his time. He is tall, strongly built and bespectacled, with a studious air. He is a low handicap golfer.

O'MAHONY, John J.

Consultant ENT Surgeon

b. 1941

m. Dr Helen Kiely (a pathologist)

MB, NUI, 1965; FRCSI

Postgraduate training in Dublin and Birmingham.
ENT surgeon, Our Lady's Hospital for Sick Children, Crumlin.
Consultant ENT surgeon, Bon Secours Hospital, Cork.

John O'Mahony practised general otolaryngology but had special interests and experience in paediatric otolaryngology having worked for several years in Crumlin. Strongly built and always good humoured and unhurried, he had excellent rapport with his patients. He retired early in 2002.

O'MALLEY, Conor

Professor of Ophthalmology and Otorhinolaryngology

b. 1889
d. 1982

Professor of Ophthalmology and Otorhinolaryngology, UCG.
Founder, Order of Malta Ambulance Corps, 1937.

O'MEARA, Patrick Anthony

Consultant ENT Surgeon

b. 1920; son of David O'Meara (LLD, solicitor, Mallow, Co. Cork) and May O'Meara (*née* Egan); eleventh or twelfth in the family (identical half twin!)
Educ. Presentation Brothers School, Mallow; Clongowes Wood College, Co. Kildare; University College Cork
m. Eileen Dowling; 4 s, 1 d

MB, UCC, 1944; DLO, RCS Eng, 1954; MCh, NUI, 1957

Postgraduate training in the UK at Northampton and London, including the Institute of Laryngology and Otology, Great Ormond Street Children's Hospital and St James's Hospital, London.
ENT consultant, Mallow General Hospital, 1962–97; Mount Alvernia Hospital, Mallow, 1957–75; University College Hospital, Cork, 1975–90.
President, section of otology and laryngology, Royal Academy of Medicine.

Influenced by Sir Terence Cawthorne of ear surgery fame, and Gilbert Honell, an expert in lachrymal drainage procedure.

Paddy O'Meara practised general ENT work, especially sinus and laryngeal surgery. A quiet and resourceful colleague, a gentleman of the old school in every sense of the word, he was widely experienced in all aspects of ENT and unfailingly courteous and friendly. His presidential address at the Royal Academy of Medicine was a brilliant dissertation on the Onodi of sinus anatomy collection.

Paddy had a large practice for forty years, an unusual feat nowadays. A countryman at heart, with keen sporting interests, he not only ran his own farm but excelled as a huntsman and fisherman (as well as rugby in his early days). All of his children inherited a love of fishing, horses and hunting. He is an outstanding example of a charming family man and expert surgeon who has lived life to the full in every aspect.

O'NEILL, Patrick (Paddy)

Consultant ENT Surgeon

b. 1903

LRCP & SI, LM, RCS, 1927

Consultant ENT surgeon, Altnagelvin Hospital (preceded Ronald Harvey [q.v.]).

O'REILLY, James Alphonsus (Seamus)

Consultant ENT Surgeon

MB, NUI, 1948; FRCS Eng, 1960; FRCS Ed, 1960

Consultant ENT surgeon, Dungannon and Magherafelt Hospitals.

PEARSE, Patrick S.

Ophthalmic and Aural Surgeon

LRCP, LRCS Edin., LFDS Glas, 1897

House surgeon, Royal Victoria Eye and Ear Hospital, Dublin.
Civil surgeon in charge of troops.
Ophthalmic and aural surgeon, St John's Hospital, Limerick.
Member, BMA.

PEDLOW, Margaret Ethel

ENT Surgeon

Educ. Trinity College, Dublin

MB, TCD, 1925

ENT surgeon, Royal Victoria Eye and Ear Hospital, Dublin.

Margaret Pedlow was an affable northerner who worked in the ENT Outpatient Department at Eye and Ear Hospital. Her consulting rooms were at 31 Upper Fitzwilliam Street. She insisted that an ashtray should be always available for her during the clinic.

She liked to socialise over a cup of coffee mid-morning with her ophthalmic colleagues in the library. She left some non-specified funds to the hospital in her Will and Eric Fenelon [q.v.], then Chairman of the Medical Board, felt that she would best appreciate funding a new carpet for the library, which was duly purchased.

PIEL, Paul Douglas

ENT Surgeon

Educ. Trinity College, Dublin

MB, TCD, 1924

ENT surgeon, Royal Victoria Eye and Ear Hospital, Dublin.

Paul Piel worked in the ENT outpatient clinic in the Eye and Ear Hospital and had consulting rooms in 35 Fitzwilliam Place. He was a cautious individual and non-committal in inscribing patients' notes. He was said to have been amused that his surname, Piel, was the same as that of the Little Flower, St Thérèse of Lisieux, though he was of a different religious persuasion. His photographic portrait in the library of the Eye and Ear Hospital shows a slightly portly individual with a small moustache and a steady gaze.

ROBERTS, Michael (Mickey)

Consultant ENT Surgeon

b. 1911
Educ. Trinity College, Dublin
m. Eithne (a champion golfer; she was later non-playing captain of the Curtis Cup Irish and UK women's team in America); 6 children (sadly two died in childhood, a girl at 5 and a boy at 9)
d. 1993

MB, BCh, TCD, 1925; MCh, 1928

Postgraduate training in Birmingham and Vienna.
Consultant ENT surgeon, Barrington's Hospital, Limerick, where he remained on staff for forty-nine years.

Mickey Roberts was an excellent surgeon, precise and efficient. He did major head and neck surgery, parotids and thyroids, long before ENT training caught up with these areas. Peadar Keogh [q.v.] recalls offering, in latter years, to help Mickey with a laryngectomy the following day. Mickey thanked him and asked him to come to theatre around ten o'clock. When Peadar duly arrived, the larynx was already in the tray — an unmistakable message.

Mickey Roberts was dapper, genial and well dressed, with a full head of hair, and energy that belied his years. He spoke softly and quickly, with an unmistakable accent. Once, following an ample dinner hosted by the IOS Travel Club in Florence,

Mickey stood up and volubly thanked his Italian colleagues 'for the surgical demonstrations' the group had seen. One of the Italians asked a Northern Ireland colleague sitting beside him what Dr Roberts had said; he just shrugged his shoulders and replied, 'Who knows?'

An old-school gentleman, he was a man of character, intelligence and good humour. Altogether a memorable colleague.

ROBINSON, Peter John

Consultant ENT Surgeon

Educ. Trinity College, Dublin

MB, TCD, 1958; FRCS

Postgraduate training in Birmingham.
Consultant ENT surgeon, Galway Regional Hospital.

Peter Robinson retired early and went to live in Cornwall.

RODDY, Patrick J.

ENT Surgeon

CSI, LRCPI, LM, 1920

ENT surgeon, Jervis Street Hospital, Dublin; Royal Victoria Eye and Ear Hospital, Dublin (mainly in the Outpatient Department); St Michael's Hospital.

Paddy Roddy had a quiet, retiring personality. He was a strong supporter of Fianna Fáil and his brother was a TD.

SANDFORD, Arthur W.

Ophthalmic and Aural Surgeon

Educ. Queen's College, Cork

MD, MCh, LM, RUI, 1882 (QCC)

Surgeon, Cork Ophthalmic and Aural Hospital.
Ophthalmic surgeon, Cork District Lunatic Asylum.
Ophthalmic and aural surgeon, Hospital for Incurables, Cork.

Author of 'Reports of an outbreak of ophthalmia' in Cork Workhouse and in Baltimore Fishery School. Monograph on 'Importance of physical voice training for public speakers and others in connection with throat troubles'. 'Tubercular iritis' (read before Ophthalmic Society London) and 'Importance of early attention to infections of the special senses in children'.

SHAW, Cecil Edward

Consultant Oculist

Educ. Queen's College, Belfast

MA, MD, MCh, RUI, 1887 (QCB, London, Marburg, Vienna, Paris)

Clinical assistant, Moorfield's Ophthalmic Hospital; Golden Square Throat, Nose and Ear Hospital, London.
Honorary laryngological surgeon, Hospital for Consumption and Diseases of the Chest, Belfast. Consultant oculist, Alexandra Hospital, Ballymena; County Antrim Infirmary, Lisburn; Mater Infirmorum Hospital, Belfast.
Lecturer in ophthalmology, QUB.

Published papers include 'Sympathetic ophthalmia and the case of associated movement of eyelid and jaw'. Author of *Diseases of the Eyes*, 1895.

SHEPPERD, Harold Walter Henry

Consultant ENT Surgeon

Educ. Queen's University, Belfast

MB, QUB, 1947; FRCS Eng, 1954; DLO Eng, 1952

Postgraduate posts as senior registrar, ENT, Middlesex Hospital, London; ENT registrar, RVH, Belfast.
Consultant ENT surgeon, North Down and Downpatrick Hospitals, 1959; RVH, Belfast; Lagan Valley Hospital, Lisburn.
Member, Court of Examiners, RCS England; examiner, FRCSI.
Fellow, Royal Society of Medicine; President, IOS.

Harold Shepperd practised general ENT with a special interest in head and neck surgery. He had an attachment with the Royal Navy Reserve for nearly thirty years. A tall, urbane amiable and charming individual, with a full head of hair and handsome appearance, he retired in 1986. He is very good company and his quiet demeanour is complemented by his lively and vivacious wife, June. They like to travel and frequently visit their several children who are living in Canada.

SINGH, Kulunder Paul (Paul)

Consultant ENT Surgeon

Educ. Parjat, India

MB, BS, Parjat, India, 1965; FRCS Ed, 1972, DLO

Postgraduate training in Northern Ireland.
Consultant ENT surgeon, Craigavon Area Hospital.

Widely experienced in all aspects of his specialty, Paul Singh was decisive, with a meticulous surgical technique. He was quite intense when working, and drove his juniors hard like himself. A very pleasant, energetic person with a good sense of humour, he was relaxed on holiday. He retired in 2005 and returned to India with his family.

SIMPSON, Noreen

Audiologist

m. David Craig [q.v.] after he was widowed
d. 1975

Audiologist, Royal Belfast Hospital for Sick Children.

Noreen Simpson was appointed to the Royal Belfast Hospital for Sick Children in 1950 to aid in the development of the Audiology Department, to ease the burden of David Craig's work. The department, which was primitive, was moved twice until adequate facilities were eventually provided in 1970. Noreen Simpson made a major contribution to the welfare of deaf children in Northern Ireland. She helped to establish audiology clinics in Ballymena, Larne, Downpatrick, Omagh, Dungannon, Enniskillen and Londonderry. She also organised the training of health visitors to recognise the early signs of deafness in newborn children.

Having visited the major centres of electrophysiological investigation of young children with hearing problems, in Bordeaux and Oxford, she laid the groundwork for evoked response audiometry services in Northern Ireland. The first equipment for carrying out these tests arrived in 1975, the year of Noreen Simpson's premature death. Her work was continued and further developed by Bob McCrea [q.v.].

SIRIPURAPU, Ankaiah ('Mr Siri')

Consultant ENT Surgeon

b. 1943, India, sixth in a family of 7
Educ. primary and secondary school in India; Andhra Medical College, Visakhapatnam
m. Kasteri (a gynaecologist)

MB, Andhra Medical College, Visakhapatnam, India, 1965; DLO, 1972; MS (ORL), 1974; FRCS Ed (ORL), 1979

Postgraduate ENT training in India; Mount Vernon Hospital, Northwood, Glasgow; Belfast and Derry.
Senior registrar, Royal Victoria and Belfast City Hospitals.
Consultant in ENT surgery, Altnagelvin Area Hospital, 1984–95.
Member, BAO; HNS; IOLS.

Influenced in his work by Prof. O. P. Gupta, T. J. Wilmot [q.v.], I. P. Munro, G. D. L. Smith and A. J. Kerr.
His main interests were general ENT and head and neck surgery.

Mr Siri, as he was known, and his wife enjoy gardening, bird watching and photography.

He describes himself as 'tallish, long fine-fingered, quiet, loves teaching, firmly combative with loathed managers'. He introduced individual outpatient appointments in his clinics in 1985. He modestly describes his sporting interest as 'golf (failed)'.

SMYTH, Gordon Dill Long

Consultant ENT Surgeon

b. 1929, son of Dr Jack Smyth (physician and biochemist, RVH, Belfast)
Educ. Queen's University Belfast
d. 1992

MB, QUB, 1953; FRCS Eng, 1959; DLO Eng, 1957; DSC, 1971; MCh, 1976; MD, Belfast, 1961
Trained as an otologist in Memphis, Tennessee (with John Shea who popularised stapedectomy for deafness), and in Belfast.
Consultant ENT surgeon, Eye and Ear Clinic, RVH, Belfast, 1964.

Gordon Smyth was one of the major medical figures in Britain and Northern Ireland in the twentieth century, with an internationally recognised reputation. As a consultant, he devoted himself to all aspects of ear surgery, in particular to the treatment of middle ear disease, including cholesteatoma. He built up a huge series of personally performed tympanoplasty procedures, which he critically and honestly analysed in meticulous detail. Because the incidence of middle ear disease was high in Northern Ireland and the population at that time was static, with emigration rare, the size and detail of his follow-up was unique in the world.

His precision surgery, tailored for each individual patient, with indefinite critical follow-up, seven days a week, resulted in the publication of nearly 200 papers on his work. He enthusiastically taught all who came to visit him in Belfast, as well as lecturing all over the world. His lectures were models of clarity and conviction, delivered in a forthright inimitable style.

His long-term follow-up and critical assessment led him to limit the indications for combined approach tympanoplasty, which he had enthusiastically supported in his early career. He co-operated in many papers with Alan Kerr [q.v.].

Apart from middle ear surgery, which was his main focus, Gordon Smyth was a keen gardener, cultivating superb rhododendrons at his home. A man of personal courage, when he was being treated for the carcinoid tumour that eventually led to his demise, he organised the follow-up and treatment of each individual patient in his care, so that they would be properly looked after as he would wish.

Gordon Smyth was a great loss, not only to his family and friends but to the medical profession as a whole. He showed that dedication, enthusiasm, hard work and unbiased reporting could produce world-beating results, even in a relatively small community. His work significantly advanced our understanding and management of the complex processes in middle ear disease.

STEWART, Terence James (Terry)

Consultant ENT Surgeon

b. 1941, third child of James and Florence Stewart
Educ. Down High School, Downpatrick; Carrickmallon Primary School, Ballygowan; Royal Belfast Academical Institution; Queen's University Belfast
m. Carole (physiotherapy and amateur drama); 3 d (Nicola, an artist; Tara, a production manager, BBC; Heidi, a broadcast journalist and champion 3-day eventer)

MB, QUB, 1964; FRCS 1970

Postgraduate training: Royal Victoria Hospital; senior registrar in ENT, Belfast City Hospital, 1971–72; Massachusetts Eye and Ear Infirmary; Harvard Medical School, Boston (clinical Research Fellow, 1972–74, then staff member and clinical instructor).
ENT Consultant, Ulster, Ards and Downe Hospitals, 1974; Belfast City Hospital, 1986.
Founder member, Otopathology Society (in honour of Prof. Schuknecht).
Member, IOS; BAO; HNS.

Significant influences in his career were Gordon Smyth [q.v.], Kennedy Hunter [q.v.] and Professor Harold Schuknecht.

His special interests were in ear surgery: in particular, combined approach tympanoplasty and stapes surgery.

Terry Stewart particularly enjoyed paediatric otology septoplasty. Pharyngeal pouch surgery and glossopharyngeal nerve section were also particular interests. An enthusiastic teacher and perfectionist, he was keen on smartly turned out doctors, and insisted on white coats being worn. He officially retired in 2002, but continues to do locum NHS work and private practice.

Tall, athletic, dressed to perfection and always cheerful and friendly, Terry is great company. He was a distinguished rugby player in school and a member of the team that won the medallion shield and schools cup. He was also the winner of the Mike Hawthorn Memorial Trophy for motor racing, Kirkistown, in 1962.

A keen family man, he also had a high standard in motor cars.

THOMSON, Matthew P.

Consultant ENT Surgeon

Educ. Kerala, India

MB, BS, Kerala, India, 1958; FRCS Ed, 1977; DLO Eng, 1967.

Consultant ENT surgeon, Craigavon Hospital.

TOBIN, Kieran Edward

Consultant ENT Surgeon

b. 1943

Educ. University College Galway

m. Ann (MA, Honorary Vice-Consul for Spain in the west of Ireland); 2 s (one in Galway; one in California)

MB, UCG, 1966; FRCS Eng, 1972; FRCSI, 1973; DLO, London, 1971

Postgraduate training: Liverpool ENT Infirmary; Alder Hey Children's Hospital; St Mary Abbot's Hospital, Kensington, London; University College Hospital, Galway.
Consultant ENT surgeon, Worcester Royal Infirmary, 1977; University College Hospital, Galway, 1978–2003.
Lecturer and head of ENT Department, UCG, 1988–2003.

President, IOS.

Member, European Academy of Facial Plastic Surgery.

His career was influenced by major ENT figures, Philip Stell and Robert Pracy in Liverpool, Tony Bull in London, and Alec Blayney [q.v.] in Galway.

Kieran Tobin practised general ENT, with special interests in head and neck surgery, children's airway problems and rhinoplasty. An alert, friendly, upright figure, who sports a well-trimmed beard and always a bow tie, he took early retirement in 2004, following a period of ill-health from which he made a full recovery, to devote himself to a second successful career. He is a superb landscape artist. His pictures, which show his capacity for detailed observation, are done in pastel and, as with the work of other notable artists, his paintings do not need a signature to be instantly recognisable as his work. His exhibitions are always completely sold out.

WILMOT, Thomas James (Tom)

ENT Surgeon

b. 1920, eldest son in a family of four of Thomas and Bessie Wilmot
Educ. Lydgate House Preparatory School, Hunstanton, Norfolk; Epsom College, Surrey; Middlesex Hospital Medical School

MB, Middlesex Hospital Medical School, 1943; DLO, 1948; FRCS, 1950; MS, 1950; FRCSI
Postgraduate training in Inverness, Scotland; Mount Vernon Hospital; Middlesex Hospital; Gray's Inn Road Royal National Throat, Nose and Ear Hospital.
ENT surgeon, Tyrone County Hospital, Omagh, 1951–81.
Member, Royal Society of Medicine, London; later president, section of otology.
Member (and past president), IOS.

He was influenced in his career by C. P. Wilson, FRCS, Middlesex Hospital.
Author of *Ménière's and its Management*, 1984. Also remarkably published at least one peer-reviewed paper for every year as a consultant in Omagh (thirty years). This was a huge achievement and a beacon to all.

Tom Wilmot had a particular interest in vestibular problems and their investigation. As well as running a first-class ENT department and service, he also avidly pursued his interests in fishing. It was alleged at interview for his job in Omagh that good local fishing was a motive for his moving to Northern Ireland. Though initially apparently sceptical of the possible success of the Irish Otolaryngological Society, Tom was, in due course, elected president of this thriving association.

Tom did things with style, and was often seen motoring through the Fermanagh countryside in his chauffeur-driven Bentley, on his way to and from the ENT clinic he also held at the Erne Hospital, Enniskillen. Shortish, bespectacled, quizzical and sometimes peppery, he had great enthusiasm for ENT, fishing and life in general. With his alert intelligence and individualistic viewpoint and sense of humour, he is a great companion in the Travel Club. He is currently focusing his attention on painting.

WILSON, T. G. D. (Tom, 'TG') PRCSI 1958–1960

Dublin ENT Surgeon

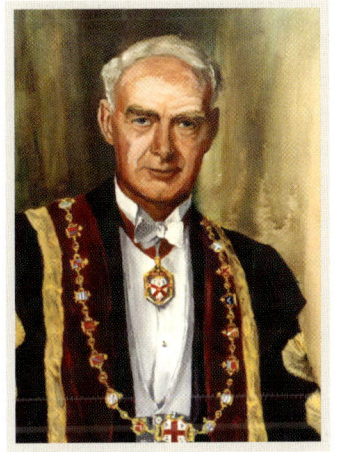

b. 1901, Belfast
Educ. Trinity College, Dublin
m. 1928, Mary Babington, daughter of Sir Anthony Babington KC; 2 s, (Thomas [q.v.], who followed the family tradition into ENT and painting; and Anthony), 2 d (Lucinda and Prudence)
d. 1969

MB, TCD, 1923; FRCSI, 1927; DLitt (*hon. causa*), TCD; FRCS Eng (Hon.); FRCS Ed (Hon.); FACS (Hon.)

Consultant ENT surgeon, Dr Steevens' Hospital, Dublin; Drumcondra Hospital; Mercer's Hospital; National Children's Hospital, Harcourt Street.
Member, collegium, ORLAS.

Member of Council, RCSI; President, 1958–60.
Professor of Anatomy, Royal Hibernian Academy; honorary member.
Commissioner of the Irish Lights.

Published and illustrated the first book on paediatric ENT surgery that demanded a second edition. Also wrote biographies of Dean Swift and Sir William Wilde.

TG Wilson famously assisted some British servicemen who had been interned in the Republic during the Second World War to escape to Belfast. He was put on trial and was fined and sentenced to twelve months' imprisonment but this was suspended. He had a larger-than-life, flamboyant and intimidating personality but he could also be charming and congenial. He was a gifted artist, writer and surgeon, and maintained international contacts. He was very competitive both at work and as a sailor (his yacht was called Fenestra).

Presidents of the RCSI have their portrait painted, which then hangs in the College. It says much of Tom Wilson that his is an excellent self-portrait. Tall, handsome, really distinguished and well built, with a military bearing, he cared little for others' opinion of him. On retirement, he enjoyed his many and varied interests and remained creative all his life.

WILSON, Thomas

Consultant ENT Surgeon

b. 1934, son of T. G. Wilson [q.v.] (ENT surgeon) and Mary Wilson (*née* Babington)
Educ. Eton College; Trinity College, Dublin
m. Biddy; 3 children

MB, TCD, 1958; FRCS Ed

Postgraduate training in Edinburgh (with Simpson Hall); London (with Sir Terence Cawthorne); Memphis, Tennessee (studied otology with John Shea); Los Angeles (Howard House).
Senior registrar, St George's Hospital, London, 1962–67; attended National Hospital for Nervous Diseases, Queen's Square, for otoneurology.
Consultant ENT surgeon, St George's Hospital, 1969; City of Dublin Hospital, Baggot Street, 1970; Sir Patrick Dun's Hospital (later St James's Hospital); Monkstown Hospital.
Resigned Dublin hospital appointments in 1982, and worked in Irish-managed and Irish-staffed PARC Hospital, Baghdad. Later worked for some years in Our Lady's Hospital for Sick Children, Crumlin.

Tom Wilson, like his father TG, is talented at music and art. He achieved full voice training as a singer. While working in Baghdad, he continued to develop his special interests as consultant on voice problems to many leading actors and singers. Though retired now from ENT surgery, he is an active artist and vocal consultant. In addition, he is a prolific painter, mostly in watercolours.

Tall, warm, handsome, friendly and gregarious, with a distinctive personality and notable sense of humour, he is a wonderfully entertaining companion.

WOODS, Robert Rowan (Bobbie)

ENT Surgeon and Consultant Laryngologist

b. a son of Sir Robert Woods [q.v.] (former PRCSI) and Margaret Woods (*née* Shaw)
m. twice married

BA, Dub, 1925; MB, BCh, BAO, TCD, 1927; FRCSI, 1929

Postgraduate training in Vienna, and Salford Royal Infirmary, Manchester.
ENT surgeon, Sir Patrick Dun's Hospital; St Luke's Hospital, Dublin.
Consultant laryngologist, Rotunda Hospital, Dublin; Drogheda Cottage Hospital; Dublin Dental Hospital.
Fellow, RAMI; Royal Society of Medicine in London.

An original thinker, Robert Woods designed and made some of his own instruments. A fine ear surgeon, he went to see John Shea in Memphis. He worked with the Leitz Microscope and performed head and neck cancer surgery of quality in St Luke's Hospital. Tall, darkly handsome with a forthright personality, he was quite chatty at times, but an occasional brusqueness of manner could be misunderstood. He was probably the best operator in ENT surgery of his era.

WOODS, Sir Robert Henry PRCSI 1910–1912

Dublin Otologist and ENT Surgeon

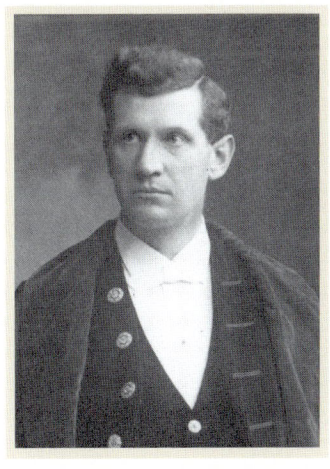

b. 1865
Educ. Wesley College; Trinity College, Dublin
m. Margaret Shaw of Belfast; 5 children (eldest son, Lieutenant Thornley Woods, killed in action in October 1916; Bobbie Woods [q.v.] was another son)
d. 1938

BA, MB, TCD, 1889; FRCSI, 1893; FACS (Hon.), 1921

Studied in Vienna.
Surgeon, Department of Throat, Nose and Ear, Sir Patrick Dun's Hospital, Dublin.
Member of Council and President, RCSI.
Surgical Travelling Prize, TCD, 1891.
President, IMA; British Laryngological Society.
Professor of ENT, TCD.

MP, University of Dublin, 1919
KB, 1913.

Author of papers on 'Restoration of nose by modified Indian operation', 'Excision of half the larynx', 'Ear disease with intractable complications' and 'Chronic laryngitis', (trans) RAMI, 1895–99.

Robert Woods took his duties as an MP seriously and spoke eloquently many times in the House of Commons. He said he was not an apologist for Sinn Féin but pleaded for an understanding of their point of view — brave words from a knight of the realm in Westminster in 1921.

With an imposing presence, bright and eagle eyed, he had a ready tongue (perhaps too ready at times) and could be abrupt and dismissive, but he was a superb surgeon and one of the few Irish medical men of the time who was truly an international figure.

19
THE EVOLUTION OF PAEDIATRIC SURGERY

Prof. E. J. Guiney

THE EVOLUTION OF PAEDIATRIC SURGERY

The evolution of paediatric surgery as a defined specialty within the spectrum of surgical skills was an inevitable development following the spectacular advances in all branches of medical practice in the latter half of the twentieth century. There was a greater appreciation that up to 2 per cent of all infants born alive have a life-threatening congenital anomaly such as congenital heart disease, a great variety of intestinal obstructions, urinary tract anomalies and spina bifida. Many of these need early specialised surgery and this led to the development of neonatal surgery. The care of most childhood ailments in specialised children's hospitals became the accepted norm in the developed world.

Historically, specialised children's hospitals were established in many cities where their foundation was provoked by social and charitable needs. In Dublin, the National Children's Hospital eventually settled in Harcourt Street. It is now incorporated with the Meath/Adelaide complex at Tallaght. St Joseph's/the Children's Hospital at Temple Street, now called the Children's University Hospital, led the way in providing specialised care by trained paediatricians. With one notable exception, surgical care was provided very much on a part-time basis by surgeons whose main commitment was to adult surgery. The exception was John Shanley [q.v.] who, at Temple Street Children's Hospital, was a pioneer paediatric surgeon in Europe, dedicated to providing his considerable surgical skills exclusively to infants and children.

From the mid-twentieth century, the momentum for the development of specialised neonatal and child surgery gathered momentum. There was inevitable resistance, memorably countered by Sir Denis Browne (1892–1967) with the mission statement, 'We seek not to create a monopoly, but to set a standard.'

In Dublin, the opening in 1956 of Our Lady's Hospital significantly advanced the movement towards the provision, in Crumlin, of full-time paediatric surgery for sick children. This hospital had 320 beds and cots. It had a full staff of paediatricians, neonatologists and, with the appointment of Barry O'Donnell [q.v.], a fully trained children's surgeon. In 1965, a Children's Research Centre was established there, and this had a major impact on all branches of paediatrics in the country. The three hospitals all had academic affiliations. The National Children's Hospital, Harcourt Street, was affiliated to Trinity College, Dublin, and the other two gave undergraduate and graduate teaching and training to students from UCD and the RCSI. Under the guidance of Barry O'Donnell, and with the unstinting support of AB Clery [q.v.], Surgical Director, paediatric surgery prospered at Our Lady's. At Temple Street, James O'Neill [q.v.], Kevin Maughan [q.v.] and Frank Duff [q.v.] were the active surgeons. Stanley McCollum [q.v.] provided services to the National Children's Hospital. In 1966, after a year's specialised training as a senior registrar at the Alder Hey Hospital, Liverpool, Eddie Guiney [q.v.] was appointed to Our Lady's and shortly afterwards to Temple Street and Harcourt Street hospitals. Barry O'Donnell provided a back-up service to these latter two. Thus a service was provided for Dublin and the rest of the country, even though it was thinly spread. Ray Fitzgerald [q.v.] was appointed in 1978, Prem Puri in 1991 and Martin Corbally in 1993. Barry O'Donnell retired in 1993, after thirty-seven years as a consultant, and Eddie Guiney in 1996. Fergal Quinn had done an eight-year locum before he was appointed to the now four-man team, which covers the entire republic.

There has been considerable discussion regarding the ideal number of paediatric surgeons to cover a population. The British Association of Paediatric Surgeons recommends that there should be one surgeon for each 500,000 of the population, preferably located in one major centre. The units should have four surgeons of whom one should be a paediatric urologist. The present population of 4.4 million would need eight or nine surgeons, two of whom would be primarily paediatric urologists. Paediatric urology resembles paediatric surgery rather more closely than it resembles adult urology. The successful repair of oesophageal atresia, which has a predictable incidence of one in 5000 births, which comes out at about fourteen per annum in the Republic, best represents the acme of paediatric surgery. Success in this problem requires high-level anaesthetic and nursing skills. The ability to provide such a service is a status symbol reflecting the high quality of care to be found in that institution. Inevitably hospital staffs compete to acquire this 'seal of approval', but centralisation has not been achieved in Dublin.

Much more importantly, the failure of efforts to amalgamate the National Children's Hospital and Our Lady's Hospital, which came tantalising close to success in the late 1970s and early 1980s, and which had the whole-hearted support of the medical staff of both institutions, was a grave disappointment. The benefits which would have resulted from such a union in economic, educational, research and day-to-day service to the community would have had a major impact and avoided the present imbroglio about the siting of a new children's hospital.

There is a cross-border Society of Irish Paediatric Surgeons with the euphonious and promising acronym of SIPS. It was founded in the mid-1980s with Brian Smyth [q.v.] of Belfast as first President. Meetings are held alternately in Belfast and Dublin. 'Informal' would be at the upper end of the register of adjectives to describe these enjoyable get togethers.

Paediatric Surgeons

SHANLEY, John

Dublin Paediatric Surgeon

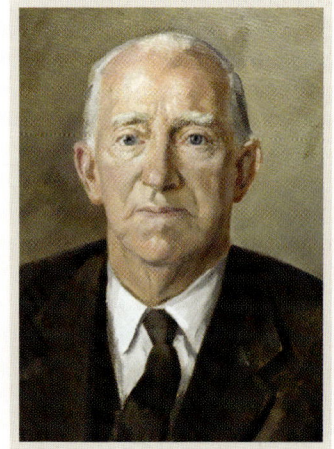

b. 1895, first child of Peter W. and Mary M. Shanley
Educ. O'Connell School, Dublin; University College Dublin
m. 1932: Una O'Mara, daughter of James O'Mara, MP & TD
d. 1995

MB, UCD; DPH; MD; BSc; FRAM

Surgeon, St Joseph's Hospital (Children's Hospital), Temple Street, 1923–70.
Surgeon, Orthopaedic Hospital, Cappagh, Dublin.
President, IMA, 1940.
Chairman, Irish Red Cross Society, 1948; Hospitals Commission, 1970; Government commission on the salaries of President, Taoiseach and Cabinet Ministers, 1936.

Founder member, Irish Orthopaedic Club and Irish Paediatric Association.
Honorary member, British Association of Paediatric Surgeons.
Examiner in surgery of children, UCD.

Numerous publications on medical, nursing and social issues.

John Shanley was Ireland's first dedicated paediatric surgeon. A man of total integrity who gave his life to the Children's Hospital, Temple Street, but also gave generously of his time to scores of voluntary organisations and groups, he was a tireless defender of professional independence and was in demand as a scrupulously fair chairman even when his own pet interests were threatened. He was particularly expert on paediatric orthopaedics and had a huge experience in talipes (club foot). He had a special welcome for new members of the paediatric community.

John had few interests outside medicine and it is a tribute to his character that he attended medical board meetings in total silence, long after he had retired from the staff, well into his nineties.

Of middle height and unsmiling, he walked everywhere and had a distinctive moist, carrying voice. Serious, hugely respected and much loved, with trademark unkempt hair, he did not have an enemy in the world when he died in his one hundred and first year.

MAUGHAN, Kevin Matthew

Dublin Paediatric Surgeon

b. 1903, elder son of Dr Mathew Maughan and Margaret Maughan (*née* Masterson)
Educ. Castleknock College; University College Dublin
m. 1934: Avice (a stunning society beauty who still looked wonderful at 92), daughter of P. A. Hearne and Josephine Hearne (*née* Spillane); 5 s (two deceased), 1 d (deceased)
d. 1975

MB, UCD, 1928

Postgraduate work included house surgeon, Mater Hospital (under Robert Farnan); casualty officer, Royal Sussex County Hospital, Brighton; house officer, King George V Hospital, Ilford; St Michael's Hospital, Dún Laoghaire; resident medical officer, New End Hospital, Hampstead, London.
Senior surgeon, Children's Hospital, Temple Street, Dublin; St Ann's, Northbrook Road; St Anthony's Clinic, Merrion Road.
Visiting consultant surgeon, Cappagh.
Founder member and president, Irish Paediatric Association.

After graduation, Kevin Maughan spent seven years in all, in various London hospitals where he assisted many famous 'stars'. He had learned tonsil dissection from Denis Browne at Great Ormond Street, and he pioneered this (guillotine tonsillectomy was still practised in Dublin in the 1960s) and pharyngoplasty in Dublin. Dapper, well groomed and courteous, he was a neat, tidy surgeon, with interests ranging from cleft lip to Hirschprung's disease. He and his family had lived and he consulted at 10 Merrion Square and later at 12 Fitzwilliam Square. He also maintained a discreet private adult surgical practice at the Bon Secours Hospital, Glasnevin. His wardrobe was filled with pinstripe suits and tailored shirts, and he looked like a transplanted Harley Street specialist, with an immaculate, self-maintained Daimler to match. He played golf at Milltown Golf Club.

A family member remembers, 'Kevin had enormous self confidence in his own ability and talents and he was an outstanding diagnostician. He was not an easy colleague as he was certain that nobody was more medically knowledgeable than himself. However, when it came to nurses and patients, his popularity soared, as witnessed by the Valentine cards he received from the nurses in Temple Street just three months before his death.' A classic twentieth century-Dublin surgeon.

O'NEILL, James Patrick (Jimmy)

Dublin Paediatric Surgeon

b. 1916, eldest son of James W. O'Neill and Christine O'Neill (*née* Murphy)
Educ. University College Dublin
m. 1950: Martha Tohall (LRCP & SI); 7 s, 2 d (6 doctors, including Prof. Desmond O'Neill, Prof. Geriatrics, TCD. A wondrous legacy!)
d. 1999

MA, BComm, NUI, 1937; LRCP & SI, 1944; MB, UCD, NUI, 1946; FRCSI, 1950; MCh, NUI, 1950.

Postgraduate posts at Jervis Street Hospital; National Children's Hospital, Dublin. Surgical registrar, Jervis Street; civilian surgical specialist, British Military Hospital, Trieste, Italy. Periods of study in Vienna and Bologna.
Surgeon, Temple Street Children's Hospital, 1952–86; St Ultan's Hospital, 1952–82; Bon Secours Hospital, 1952–86.
Occupational physician to Unidare and Cement Roadstone.
Registrar, deputy governor and governor, Apothecaries Hall, Dublin.
President, Irish Society of Occupational Medicine; Medical Union.
Founder member, Medical Union. Played a major part in negotiation of Consultants' Common Contract.

Jimmy O'Neill loved history and travel and visited many countries worldwide. He spoke French, German and Italian. Not tall, aldermanic, balding, tenacious, humorous, he was a dedicated family man with a huge fund of general knowledge. His passion was medical politics.

O'DONNELL, Barry PRCSI 1998–2000

Dublin Paediatric Surgeon

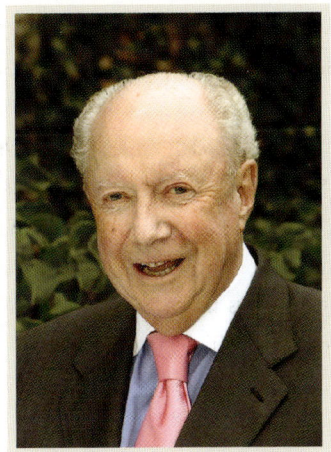

b. 1926, Cork, eldest son of Michael O'Donnell and Kitty O'Donnell (*née* Barry)
Educ. Christian Brothers College, Cork; Castleknock College, Dublin; University College Cork
m. 1959: Mary Leydon (BA, BComm, BL), only child of John Leydon (KC St Gregory, DLitt, the senior civil servant of his day, described by Seán Lemass (Taoiseach 1959–66) as 'the ablest man I ever knew') and Nan Leydon (*née* Layden); 3 s (John, barrister and poet; Michael, financial services; Nicholas, corporate real estate and international yachtsman), 1 d (Catherine, financial services)

MB (hons), UCC, 1949; MCh, NUI, 1954; FRCSI, 1953; FRCS Eng, 1953; FRCS Ed (*ad hom.*) 1993; FRCP & S (Glas qua chir), 1999; FACS (Hon.), 1999; FRCS Eng (Hon.) 2007

Postgraduate posts in Winchester, Brighton, Leicester; Hospital for Sick Children, Great Ormond Street, London.
Registrar, Royal Northern Hospital, London; Whittington Hospital, London.
Senior Registrar, Hospital for Sick Children, Great Ormond Street (Sir Denis Browne, Sir D. I. Williams).
Ainsworth Travelling Scholarship from UCC to Lahey Clinic, Boston (Drs Richard B. Cattell, Herbert Adams, Samuel Marshall, Ken Warren), and Boston Floating Hospital for Infants and Children (Dr Orvar Swenson).
Consultant surgeon, Our Lady's Hospital for Sick Children, 1957–93; Children's Hospital, Temple Street, 1977–88; National Children's Hospital, Harcourt Street, 1965–80.
Professor of Paediatric Surgery, RCSI, 1986–93.
Honorary Fellow, Singapore Academy of Medicine and Surgery, 1999; Malaysian Academy of Medicine and Surgery, 2000; College of Surgeons, South Africa, 2001; section of surgery, American Academy of Pediatrics; American Pediatric Surgical Association; American Surgical Association; New England Surgical Association; Boston Surgical Association.
President, British, Canadian and Irish Medical Associations, 1976–77; British Association of Paediatric Surgeons, 1981–82; surgical section, RAMI, 1990–92.
Chairman, Journal Committee, BMA (including BMJ), 1982–88.

National People of the Year award jointly with Prof. Prem Puri, 1984.
Hunterian Professorship, RCS Eng, 1986.
Denis Browne gold medal, British Association of Paediatric Surgeons, 1989; urology medal, American Academy of Pediatrics, 2003; Distinguished Alumni Award, UCC, 2004.
Eponymous addresses in Australia, US and UK.
Visiting professor to six US universities, including twice to Harvard.
Director, Standard Chartered Bank (Ireland), 1977–88; West Deutsche LandesBank (Ireland), 1988–96.

Sixty-four peer-reviewed publications. Four books (two co-authored) including *Terence Millin: a Remarkable Irish Surgeon*.

A sound, compassionate, listening clinician and a first-rate operating surgeon, Barry O'Donnell describes himself as 'a second-class brain with a world-class training'. In his prime years he was greatly influenced by his close friend and contemporary, Hardy Hendren of Boston, who was the leading paediatric surgeon in the world at the time.

Barry's proudest achievement was being the mainspring of the Children's Research Centre (founded 1965) at Our Lady's Hospital for Sick Children. The Centre, which was his idea, became a small part of the national fabric, and funds were raised for it in every corner of every county in Ireland and abroad. The innovation of endoscopic correction of vesicoureteric reflux (1984), which was developed jointly with Professor Prem Puri, changed the management of the commonest major condition in paediatric urology.

Before he became president of the IMA, he had been for about ten years one of the principal negotiators for the consultants in their relations with the government. As president of the RCSI, he oversaw major property expansions, introduced the highly successful Mini-Med School for the lay public, changed many of the ways the Council did its business but also conceived the full-time post of Director of Surgical Affairs, an appointment of a surgeon which allowed focus and action on 'events' (crises), and created a closer and sounder symbiotic relationship with the Department of Health.

Recreations include rugby football (Colours, UCC, 1946–48 'hooker'), sailing offshore with mutinous family and consenting adults (includes Fastnet Race, 1979 and 1981), really incompetent golf.

On his honeymoon in Rome in June 1959, Pope John XXIII blessed his hands, and then said (in Italian), 'I'd better bless his head as well because that's where the decisions are made.' The biggest and best decision (Mary) had already been made. She was able to say 'Don't be silly' to BO'D on the frequent occasions when nobody else could say it.

Barry is 5'7", stocky, combative and energetic. He loves gossip and talks all the time. (Reality check: 'humble, yes: modest, no' , 'not quite as vain as he appears', 'just a little bit too pleased with himself', 'when playing rugby for UCC it seems likely that his was the last name on the team sheet. He was nine stone nine pounds of naked aggression, could not catch, kick or run but was a lucky hooker and a reckless tackler', 'as an offshore sailor he could hardly steer and he was a real liability as he could get seasick in the bath', 'he probably made more after dinner speeches than any recent Irish surgeon', 'never mind the quality feel the width', it was said that he had 'nineteen jokes in all but this was disputed; it could have been twelve' (favourite saying 'never ask an Irishman where he is from: if he is from Cork he will tell you and if he is not you will only embarrass him') and 'never claimed that anything came easy to him but a Rolls Royce training with the best in the world at the time built up a surgical capital and a confidence which he depleted over the years'. 'About the two, much vaunted, visiting professorships to Harvard it should be remembered that the second visit was to apologise for what he said on the first'… 'All the posts he occupied were an education for him and a great education for the people who elected and appointed him'. It is alleged that after a talk in the US when someone asked him 'Who are you anyway?' he replied, 'It would take me too long to tell you.' It was said, 'he exceeded his mother's expectations.' Not many Cork boys do that.)

GUINEY, Edward J. (Eddie)

Dublin Paediatric Surgeon

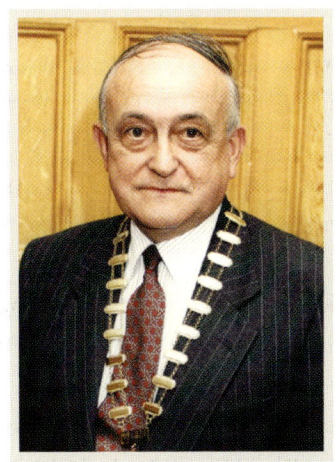

b. 1931, Dublin

Educ. Belvedere College SJ; University College Dublin

m. 1962: Dr Sheila McNamara (consultant anaesthetist; d. 2006); 2 s (Michael is consultant radiologist, Dublin; Edward produces award-wining films), 1 d

MB (first place with hons), UCD, 1955; MCh, NUI, 1961; FRCSI, 1960; FRCS Eng, 1962

Postgraduate years at St Vincent's Hospital Dublin (with the professors of surgery and medicine); senior house officer and registrar, Regional (Teaching) Hospital, Galway, 1957–58; senior registrar and tutor in surgery, St Vincent's Hospital, Dublin, 1958–62.

Two-year travelling Fellowship in surgery awarded by NUI.

Lecturer in surgery, St Thomas's Hospital, London, 1960–61.

Research Fellow, Massachusetts General Hospital and Harvard Medical School.

Senior resident, Massachusetts General Hospital, 1961–63.

Lecturer in surgery, UCD, 1963–65.

Senior surgical registrar, Alder Hey Children's Hospital, Liverpool (with Peter Paul Rickham), 1965–66.

Consultant paediatric surgeon, Our Lady's Hospital for Sick Children, Crumlin; Children's Hospital, Temple Street, 1966–97; National Children's Hospital, Harcourt Street, 1970–86; MANCH Hospital, Tallaght, 1986–97.

Professor of Paediatric Research, NUI, and director (the first director), Children's Research Centre at Our Lady's Hospital for Sick Children, 1976–1991 (resigned).

Professor of Paediatric Surgery, RCSI, 1991–97; now Emeritus Professor.

Director of Intercollegiate Basic Skills Course for seven years, 1997–2004. President, UCD (Students) Medical Society; UCD Medical Graduates Association; Society for Research into Spina Bifida and Hydrocephalus; Irish Paediatric Association; British Association of Paediatric Surgeons, 1995–96.

RCSI gold medal from RCSI for postgraduate teaching.

Wide range of publications on research and clinical topics in peer-reviewed journals and book chapters.

Particular interest was in the ethical problems of severe congenital abnormalities.

Eddie Guiney has been actively involved in research during his entire career, culminating in his appointment as Director of Research at the Children's Research Centre, in 1976. At St Thomas's he was involved in work on the lymphatic system. At the Massachusetts General, it was transplantation biology. In Dublin, the main thrust was in biliary atresia and other liver problems of the newborn and older child. He is an authority on xanthogranulomatous pyelonephritis. Experimental liver transplant surgery at the UCD Research Centre in Woodview resulted in the survival of a number of pigs, one of which gave birth to fourteen piglets. In 1972, this was a world first and led to his involvement in the national liver transplant programme at St Vincent's Hospital, Dublin.

Following a brilliant undergraduate career, Eddie had a first-rate, enviable training in London and Boston, as well as Dublin. It showed. He was a quick, superb technical surgeon and was easy to assist. The trainees really enjoyed working with him and quickly forgave the odd irritability due to overwork. He developed the biggest practice in the country because the paediatricians liked and trusted him. He eagerly undertook the care of the spina bifida patients and showed great humanity in dealing with patients and parents. A prodigious worker, often working a one-on-one rota in his three hospital appointments, he was an admirable, hugely supportive colleague. His election as president of the British Association of Paediatric Surgeons against a strong London candidate was a tremendous personal achievement and mirrored the esteem in which he is held.

He used to play golf but now really enjoys himself yarning with his wide circle of friends.

FITZGERALD, Raymond James (Ray, 'RJF')

Dublin Paediatric Surgeon

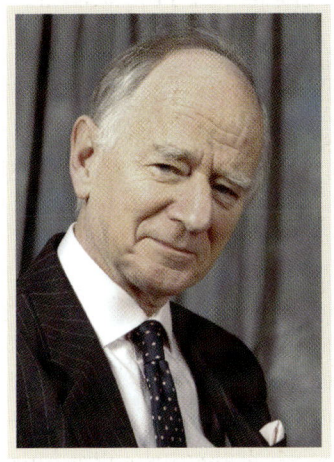

b. 1941, only son of Thomas Fitzgerald and Eleanor Fitzgerald (*née* Rickerby)
Educ. Caludon Castle School, Walsgrave, near Coventry; Trinity College, Dublin
m. 1968: Joy Carson (SRN, Adelaide Hospital), daughter of William and Mary Carson; 2 s, 1 d

MB, TCD, 1967; MA, TCD, 1968; FRCSI, 1973; FRCS Eng, 1973; FRACS (paediatric surgery), 1977; European Board of Paediatric Surgery, 1997; FRCS Ed (*ad hom.*)

Junior posts at the Adelaide Hospital (with Prof. Nigel Kinnear [q.v.]).
Surgeon Lieutenant, Royal Navy, 1968–73; served in Fleet Air Arm Base, HMS Osprey, Naval Hospitals and Broadgreen Hospital, Liverpool.
Junior post at the Hospital for Sick Children, Great Ormond Street (with Harold Nixon and Herbie Eckstein); registrar, paediatric surgery, Our Lady's Hospital for Sick Children (with Barry O'Donnell [q.v.] and Eddie Guiney [q.v.]); senior registrar, Royal Children's Hospital, Melbourne, 1977–78 (with E. Durham Smith, Nate Meyers, Peter Jones, Justin Kelly and Bob Fowler).
Consultant paediatric surgeon, Children's University Hospital and Our Lady's Hospital for Sick Children, 1979–2005.
Associate Professor of Paediatric Surgery, TCD, 1996.
President, British Association of Paediatric Surgeons; Member, Council of RCS England, 2006–08.
President, Society for Research into Hydrocephalus and Spina Bifida, 2006–09; European Association of Paediatric Surgical Associations; Irish Paediatric Association; Association for the Welfare of Children in Hospital
Chairman, National Advanced Trauma Life Support Committee at RCSI.

Influenced by Surgeon Commanders Richardson, Drinkwater and Fulford and John Shepherd of 'Acute Abdomen' fame. Prof. Stanley McCollum influenced him to do paediatric surgery.
Special interests in paediatric surgical oncology; hydrocephalus and spina bifida.

All his presidencies are a tribute to Ray Fitzgerald's outstanding characteristic — his integrity. In addition, he was hardworking, collegial, accommodating and public-spirited. He was highly organised (perhaps a naval input) in a centripetal sort of way and a really good organiser. The paediatricians loved him. He encouraged residents to 'write' and helped them to do so.

Of average height, 5'9", which makes him by some distance the tallest paediatric surgeon in the jurisdiction, he is erect and sartorially conservative. Half-moon gold-rimmed spectacles are a parapet over which bushy eyebrows can bristle threateningly at theatre nurses and somnolent assistants. He sports bow ties.

His interests include holding a private pilot's licence since 1982, gardening with a chainsaw, and studies in German and French. Previously a sailor, wild-fowl hunter and coarse rugby player, he now enjoys woodwork and is an armchair follower of rugby and cricket.

Sources close to the Throne write: 'An average day in the hospital means everyone is on edge, registrars checking their notes, theatre staff checking their instruments, anaesthetists checking their watches. Rounds are conducted at top speed; residents are breathless; parents are reassured. He was relentlessly honest, and one was never in doubt as to where one stood with him (even though it was often in the doghouse). Always to the fore in helping to organise the Christmas concert and lately the butt of many sketches and jokes at these events, he received a surprise send-off from his colleagues with an evening of *This is Your Life* entertainment, much more suitable for the man than a formal Festschrift.' An admirable professional and good companion.

20
PLASTIC SURGEONS IN THE REPUBLIC OF IRELAND

PLASTIC SURGEONS IN THE REPUBLIC OF IRELAND

CONDON, Kevin Callaghan ('Cal')

Cork Accident and Emergency and Plastic Surgeon

b. 1927, younger son of Justin C. ('The Boss') and Anne Condon, Youghal, Co. Cork
Educ. Christian Brothers School, Youghal; Castleknock College, Dublin; University College Cork
m. 1956: Dr Margaret (Peg) O'Donoghue, daughter of Dr Patrick and Catherine O'Donoghue, Killarney; 3 s (Cal is a Dublin dermatologist)

MB, UCC, 1950; MCh, NUI, 1954; FRCS Ed, 1956; FRCSI (*ad eundem*), 1980

Postgraduate training in Irish and English regional hospitals: St Mary's, Portsmouth; Bury General; resident surgical officer (two years), St Catherine's, Tralee. Study and courses at Guy's Hospital, Westminster Hospital and St Thomas's Hospital, London.
Training in plastic surgery: senior house officer, Rookstown House, Basingstoke, Hampshire (Sir Harold Gillies and Charles McCash); registrar, St Lawrence's Hospital, Chepstow (Welsh National Plastic Surgery Unit; with Emlyn Lewis); registrar Rookstown House, 1956–58; senior registrar, Queen Elizabeth Hospital Birmingham, 1958–60, and registrar, plastic surgical unit.
General surgeon, Bon Secours (private) Hospital, Tralee, 1960–71.
Consultant A&E and plastic surgeon, Southern Health Board, Cork, 1971–94.
Representative of plastic surgery, Irish Postgraduate Training Committee.
Chairman, Irish branch, British Association Plastic Surgeons.
Surgical Advisory Board in Plastic Surgery.

Although Cal Condon was a fully trained plastic surgeon, there were no vacancies in Ireland, in the 'lost decade' of the 1950s, and he spent eleven years in Tralee as general surgeon, with some plastic surgery sessions, firstly in Mallow, Co. Cork, and then in Cork. St John O'Connell [q.v.] (orthopaedic surgeon) and Maurice

Hickey [q.v.] (cardiothoracic surgeon), two powerful figures of the time, got him formal sessions in Cork. In 1969, a post of consultant plastic surgeon was created and, as it was thought that he would not have enough to do, the post of consultant in A&E services was added to the job. By the time of his retirement, there were three plastic surgeons and three A&E consultants.

A progressive Captain of Tralee Golf Club, Cal became a highly successful offshore sailor and did a hairy transatlantic passage in a 35' engineless sailboat. He is the kind of man you would want in your lifeboat. Genial, genuine, really smart, with a thin self-deprecating veneer ('an honorary Kerryman'), he was a fine technical surgeon and made a big difference to many aspects of the Cork surgical scene.

EDWARDS, Gerald Ernest (Gerry)

Dublin Plastic Surgeon

b. 1933, Dublin, younger son of Percy Edwards and Florence Edwards (*née* Von Ackermann)
Educ. Catholic University School; St Fintan's School; Royal College of Surgeons in Ireland
m. 1966: Ita McGowan, younger daughter of John McGowan and Mary McGowan
(*née* Gallagher); 2 s, 2 d
d. 1999

LRCP & SI, RCSI, 1956 (gold medal in surgery), FRCSI, 1961

Postgraduate plastic and reconstructive surgery training at St Mary's, Roehampton, London, 1961–65.
A&E consultant, Jervis Street Hospital, early 1970s.
Consultant plastic surgeon, Dr Steevens' Hospital; Our Lady's Hospital for Sick Children, Crumlin; St Anne's Skin and Cancer Hospital; St James's Hospital.
Member, Irish/British burns specialist team who visited Chelyabinsk, USSR, following gas explosion.

An excellent technical surgeon, Gerry Edwards was an expert in handling 'revision' operations where the first had not been totally successful. He had a gentle, soothing way of dealing with anxious patients and parents. He did a lot of charity work, particularly for the Children's Research Centre at Our Lady's Hospital for Sick Children, Crumlin, where he was responsible for raising large sums over many years. He was in great demand as a medico-legal witness.

Passionate about sport, he became Captain of his beloved Portmarnock Golf Club. Earlier he had sailed competitively. He earned his private pilot's licence at 60.

He was a big man in every way — in body, heart and mind — with a huge capacity for friendship. Opera singing was in the family and his party pieces were traditional — 'Jerusalem' and 'Bless This House' sung in a deep bass baritone. Gregarious, he loved informal gatherings with family and friends. He is much missed.

HOGAN, Niall James

Dublin Maxillofacial Surgeon

Educ. Trinity College, Dublin

MB, Dublin, 1939; BDentSc, 1947; FFD, RCSI, 1963 (TCD)

Postgraduate posts as dental surgeon, Westminster Hospital, London; senior registrar, Plastic and Jaw Unit, Hill End Hospital, St Albans; Captain, Royal Army Medical Corps.
Surgeon, Maxillofacial Department, Dr Steevens' Hospital, Dublin.
Dental surgeon, Sir Patrick Dun's Hospital; St Luke's Hospital; Royal Victoria Eye and Ear Hospital.
Oral surgeon, Incorporated Dental Hospital, Ireland; Dr Steevens' Hospital, Dublin.
Dental surgeon and oral surgeon, St Laurence's (Richmond) Hospital, Dublin.
Lecturer in oral surgery, TCD.

McHUGH, Matt

Dublin Plastic Surgeon

b. 1939, younger son of Thomas and Ann McHugh
Educ. St Patrick's College, Cavan; University College Dublin
m. 1970: Eileen Quirke; 1 s, 3 d

MB, UCD, 1963; BSc, 1965; FRCSI, 1969

Postgraduate posts as intern, St Vincent's Hospital, Dublin; lecturer in anatomy, UCD 1964–66; registrar, general surgery, Regional Hospital, Galway, 1966–70; senior registrar, Dr Steevens' Hospital, Dublin, 1970–71; registrar, hand surgery, Derby Royal Infirmary, 1970–72; registrar, plastic surgery, Canniesburn Hospital, Glasgow.
Senior registrar, Dr Steevens' Hospital, 1973–76; St Thomas's Hospital and Hospital for Sick Children, Great Ormond Street, London, 1976–77; senior registrar, plastic surgery, Dr Steevens' Hospital, 1977–79.
Consultant plastic surgeon, Dr Steevens' Hospital; St James's Hospital; Our Lady's Hospital for Sick Children, Crumlin, Dublin, 1979–2003.
Director, National Burns Unit, St James's Hospital, Dublin.

Matt McHugh had a superb training in four centres of excellence, and it showed. He was quick, deft and accurate, rarely having to put in a suture a second time. He had been at the hand surgery unit in Derby, when it was one of the best in the world, and tendon repairs were his forte, but he cut freehand skin grafts with great skill. The operating list was over, and Matt was gone before anyone realised it.

Goalkeeper for the Co. Cavan Gaelic football team, he was memorably photographed for a local newspaper making a brilliant save for the county while he was registrar 'on call' some miles away; this led to some questions which would have been embarrassing had they not won. He was devoted to vintage cars, which he changed all the time, and this sometimes made it difficult for the 'trainees' to know whether or not he was in the building.

Above medium height, sharp-featured, with thinning fair hair and a gangling walk, which was almost a trot, he kept his shape and was in great demand as a medico-legal witness in the courts outside Dublin, where he imparted sincerity and integrity.

Ó RIAIN, Séamus Morgan

Dublin Plastic Surgeon

b. 1930, Dublin, son of Dr James (Jim) and Mairin Ryan (*née* Cregan). Dr Ryan was an Irish patriot who, as a qualified doctor, was in gaol three times for his republican activities. He was an Irish Cabinet Minister almost continuously from 1932 to 1959 and was the first Minister for Health, in 1949. His mother, who was also jailed, wrote award-winning children's books.
Educ. Holy Faith nuns, Greystones; Christian Brothers School, Blacklion, Co. Cavan; Catholic University School, Dublin; Glenstal Priory, Co. Limerick, University College Dublin
m. Married with 5 children (daughter Fiona is a nurse)

MB, UCD, 1954; FRCSI, 1963; FRCS Eng, 1963; MCh, NUI, 1964

Postgraduate posts at St Vincent's and Meath Hospitals, Dublin.
Ship's surgeon, P&O Line to Australia.
Four years' general surgery and four years' plastic surgery, mainly in the UK mentored by Frank Duff [q.v.] (past PRCSI) and John Barron, plastic surgeon, Oddstock Hospital, Salisbury and the Hammersmith Hospital
Consultant plastic surgeon, Children's Hospital, Temple Street, 1968–77; St Vincent's Hospital, 1969; Dr Steevens' Hospital. 1972.
Plastic surgeon, PARC Ibn Al-Bitar Hospital, Baghdad, 1989–91.

Séamus Ó Riain's main interest was in cleft lip and palate surgery, a subject to which he made a number of durable contributions. He was also an expert on hand surgery and successfully re-implanted an amputated forearm, which was functional twenty years later.

The PARC Ibn Al Bitar Hospital in Baghdad was built by the Iraqi government opposite Saddam Hussein's principal palace, and functioned from 1978 to 1991. It was administered and staffed by Irish nurses and doctors and, principally because of the superb nursing services, was at the time one of the best hospitals in the Middle East. Séamus spent two years there and encountered lots of burns from the open fires.

He has made a number of family cruises to France, and later enjoyed sailing, wind surfing and scuba diving. At 5'6", he was a bustling scrum half with Greystones Rugby Club at various grades for eighteen years. He is still full of energy at 77.

PRENDIVILLE, Joseph Brendan (Brendan, 'BP')

Dublin-Based Founder of Plastic Surgery in Ireland

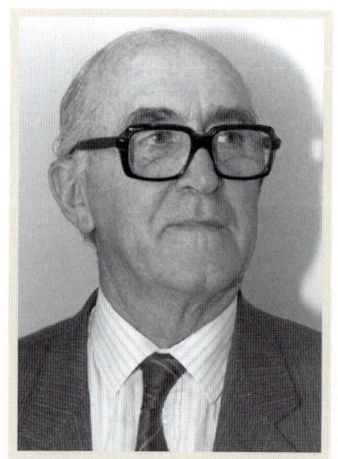

b. 1922, son of Dr Joseph Prendiville (Killorglin, Co. Kerry) and Kathleen Prendiville (*née* Evans)
Educ. Clongowes Wood College, Kildare; Royal College of Surgeons in Ireland
m. 1951: Teresa O'Neill, daughter of Edward and Brigid O'Neill (d. 2007); 1 s (Edmond, FRCSI); 2 d (Anne, a public health consultant; Julie, a consultant dermatologist)

LRCP & SI, 1946 (Stoney Memorial gold medal, 1942; gold medal in operative surgery, 1946: in each case a remarkable second generation award); FRCSI, 1949

Postgraduate posts as resident surgical officer, Manchester Northern Hospital, 1950; senior registrar, plastic surgery, Manchester Region Hospital Board, 1951; senior registrar, plastic surgery, Cardiff United Hospitals and Welsh Regional Board including Chepstow, 1952–54.
Surgeon, Dr Steevens' Hospital, 1957–90.
Member of Council, British Association of Plastic Surgeons.

BP was the first plastic surgeon in Ireland, but the prophet of a new specialty is not always welcome. His appointment to Dr Steevens' as a general surgeon was to become a problem much later when plastic surgery training posts had to be accredited as such, without a general surgery component. Every one of that generation of Dublin plastic surgeons trained with Brendan Prendiville.

In his early years, he travelled around to other hospitals and pressed for further appointments in the specialty. He had a particular interest in burns and campaigned successfully against flammable children's nightwear. He established a maxillofacial surgery unit with Niall Hogan [q.v.], and it has grown to five plastic surgeons, with two oral surgeons and appropriate supporting staff. A great legacy.

BP was a methodical operator who got admirable results. In later years, he was in demand as an expert court witness, an area he greatly enjoyed. He is an acknowledged expert in flora and fauna and wrote a chapter on the subjects for his beloved Portmarnock Golf Club's centenary book. He had a real interest in antiquarian bookbinding and was Keeper of the Worth Library at Dr Steevens' Hospital for a while. He also restored vintage cars.

Tall, ascetic, monklike and balding, he works hard to conceal a proven first-rate brain. Careful in his choice of words, he never loses his Kerry cadences, and is remembered by his patients as someone for whom no minutiae of care were too much trouble.

O'CONNOR, Thomas Paul Fawcett (Tom)

Cork Plastic Surgeon

b. 1943, Cork, younger son of Dr T.P. O'Connor and Pauline O'Connor (*née* Fawcett)
Educ. Christian Brothers College, Cork; University College Cork
m. 1970: Claire Ryan, daughter of Josephine and William ('The Doc') Ryan, Glengariff, Co. Cork; 2 s, 2 d

MB, UCC,1966; FRCSI, 1972; FRCS Eng, 1973; Certificate of Specialist Training in Plastic Surgery, RCS Eng, 1977

Postgraduate posts in South Infirmary Hospital, Cork; general surgery, Bantry Hospital; St Finbarr's Hospital, Cork; Our Lady's Hospital for Sick Children, Crumlin, Dublin, 1969–70. Surgical Research Fellow, Our Lady's Hospital for Sick Children, Crumlin, Dublin; senior house officer, plastic surgery, Hospital for Sick Children, Great Ormond Street, London; senior house officer, A&E Department, University College Hospital, London, 1970–71; surgical registrar, rotation, University College Hospital, London. 1971–73; plastic surgery registrar, Frenchay Hospital, Bristol, 1973–74; senior registrar, plastic surgery, Frenchay Hospital, Bristol, 1974–79; surgical Fellow (head and neck surgery), Rigas Hospitalet, Copenhagen, 1976.
Consultant plastic surgeon, Cork University Hospital.
Clinical lecturer in surgery, UCC, 1979–2004.
Chairman, Intercollegiate Board in Plastic Surgery, 1995–97; Irish Association of Plastic Surgeons, 1995–2000.
Director, Plastic Surgical Department, Cork University Hospital, 1992–2001.
Ainsworth Travelling Scholarship, UCC, 1976.

Following hard on the heels of Cal Condon [q.v.], Tom O'Connor drove the unit at Cork University to new heights, and he did this while remaining extremely popular with his colleagues and all members of the extended medical profession.

Part of his training had been spent with one of the great twentieth-century masters of plastic surgery, David Matthews of London, with whom he had a warm friendship to the end. Tom was a superb technical surgeon, regarded by many as the best in Ireland in his time. He had been trained by the best and it showed.

A fearless scrum half for UCC, he later took up fishing, shooting (a passion), golf and boating. He is currently involved in bridge, Spanish and learning to play the guitar. Of medium height, he has a dark, youthful, handsome appearance, is quiet and sensitive by nature, and has a great sense of humour, especially when relaxed. He is even tempered but known to have 'a black look' when angry. He has been known to sing a song or two when encouraged. A warm generous colleague. A milestone man.

21
UROLOGISTS IN THE REPUBLIC OF IRELAND

BUTLER, Michael Raymond (Mick) PRCSI 2002–2004

Dublin Urologist

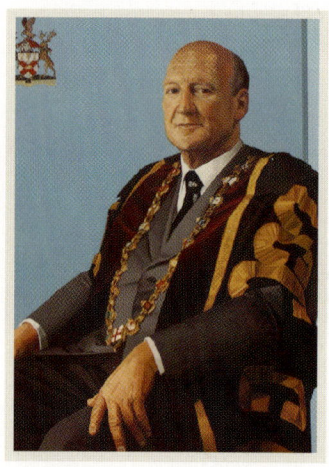

b. 1941, Dublin, son of Andy [q.v.] (Mater Hospital surgeon) and Ethna Butler: one of 5 sons and 3 daughters

Educ. St Michael's College, Ailesbury Road, Dublin; Rockwell College, Co. Tipperary; University College Dublin

m. 1967: Joan Connolly; 4 s

MB, UCD, 1965 (hons and first place in a particularly brilliant class); BSc Anatomy (hons), 1966, UCD; FRCSI, 1969; FRCS, 1970; FRCS Ed (Hon.), 2004.

Postgraduate training at Mater Hospital, Dublin (with Prof. Eoin O'Malley [q.v.], S. Heffernan [q.v.], FX O'Connell [q.v.], W. Hederman [q.v.], Patrick MacAuley [q.v.]); Meath Hospital urological unit (with Dermot O'Flynn [q.v.] and Victor Lane [q.v.]); University of Pennsylvania and Penn Hospital, Philadelphia (with John Murphy and Terry Molloy, two really big names in the specialty). Staff, Penn Hospital, 1973–74.

Consultant, Meath Hospital; St James's Hospital; St Anne's Hospital; National Rehabilitation Centre, 1974–04.

Member, Council, RCSI; President, 2002–04.

Interested in general urology and reconstructive surgery, particularly urethral reconstruction, a technically demanding area.

A really first-class brain, allied to superb operative skills and a charming, easy manner, put Mick Butler straight into the front rank. He was hardworking, quick and careful, and gave assiduous postoperative care. He had a large and appreciative 'carriage trade', spread through word of mouth by the great and the good. He wrote little on the basis that anything worth saying had already been said, and he rarely spoke at major specialty meetings.

He served on the Council of the RCSI for over 20 years and chaired several important committees before becoming President. He has a lightning intelligence, and a speedy appreciation of the real issues involved, and one of his most endearing characteristics is that he never loses his cool with the 'slow learners' on whatever group he is chairing.

A great family man, Mick is passionate about golf and played to a handicap of four for twenty-three years. It is alleged that he changes his clubs every nine months ('wear and tear', particularly 'tear'). He is a keen practising pianist and flies model aircraft. He was scrum half and captain of the invincible Rockwell College rugby team of 1959 and captained the Munster Schools rugby team. Above average height, with hunched shoulders, thinning reddish hair and a permanent grin, his trademark twinkle has been even brighter since his premature retirement.

DUFF, Francis Arthur Mary (Frank) PRCSI 1972–1974

Dublin Urologist

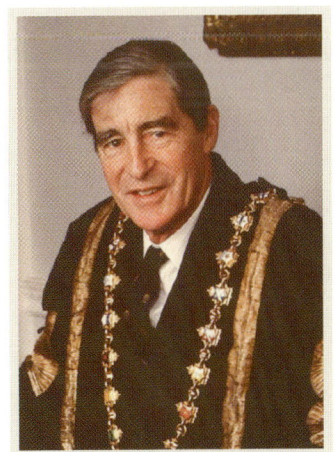

b. 1916, Dublin, son of Arthur Joseph Duff and Sheila Duff (*née* Kirwan); grew up in Goresbridge, Co. Kilkenny
Educ. St Dominick's School, Cabra; Clongowes Wood College; University College Dublin
m. 1950: Joan Devane (founder, Irish Museums Trust; President, Board of Visitors of the National Museum), daughter of John Devane (Limerick's most distinguished surgeon); 6 d, 1 s
d. 1997

MB, UCD, 1939 (first class hons and McArdle surgical prize); DPH, BSc, UCD, 1941; FRCSI, 1943; MCh, NUI, 1944; FRACS (Hon.); FCS&P South Africa (Hon.)

Postgraduate posts at St Vincent's Hospital and Mayo Clinic on travelling scholarship to study urology.
Surgeon/urologist, St Vincent's Hospital; Children's Hospital, Temple Street; Coombe Lying-in Hospital; National Maternity Hospital; St Luke's Hospital.
Lecturer in clinical urology, UCD; Acting Professor of Surgery, UCD, 1978–79.
Member, Council, RCSI; President, 1972–74.

Frank Duff was an absolutely superb operating surgeon who made everything look easy and obvious. He was a first-class diagnostician. Although he was a 'bloodless' operator, he was at his best when a big bleed did occur. He always maintained that this was the real test of a surgeon, and he certainly gave a master class on how to do it. He was easy to assist.

In 1973, he presided over an international meeting to commemorate the bicentenary of the birth of Abraham Colles. He expertly chaired the vital College Council meeting which gave the go-ahead to a building that would more than double the size of the College. He did this as an act of faith in the future, at a time when inflation was running at almost 20 per cent and national economic prospects were bleak. He served the Council for over twenty-five years and was chairman of the College Bicentenary Committee and the Finance Committee.

In his Doolin Lecture on 'The Making of a Doctor' (IMA, 1976), he made a plea that medical students be selected from a cross-section of those with adequate rather than just top grades in entry examinations. Perceptively he argued for a graduate, mature-student entry as well as the mainstream.

No account of Frank could omit his legendary courtesy. He never, ever, said a harsh word about anyone, even about those who richly deserved it. The most he would say was, 'It was a pity that he did/said that.' If he had a fault, it was that it was difficult for him to say 'no'. Tall, 6'1", he had the appearance of a film star or the scion of a thousand-year-old family of the French aristocracy, and a beautiful speaking voice.

Frank was hugely admired as a surgeon and as a professional. He was a much-loved presence who lit up any event in which he took part. His death from prostatic cancer was an irony, as this gentle man, who cared so much about patients, was himself long in considerable distress.

HANSON, John Senan (Seán)

Dublin Urologist

b. 1939, Clare, younger of two sons of John Hanson, Kilrush, Co. Clare
Educ. Christian Brothers Schools, Kilrush; University College Dublin
m. Anne McHugh; 2 s (one radiologist; one plastic surgeon), 2 d (one nurse; one psychologist)
d. 3 October 2006

MB, UCD, 1963; BSc Anatomy (hons), UCD, 1965; FRCSI 1971

Postgraduate post as anatomy demonstrator, UCD, 1964.
Junior training positions at Jervis Street Hospital (with Prof. P. G. Collins [q.v.], A. Walsh [q.v.], P. G. Brady [q.v.], D. A. Ryan [q.v.]) , 1963–68; registrar, City Hospital, Belfast (with J. Kennedy [q.v.] and Prof. M. McGeown), 1968–71; registrar and senior registrar, Institute of Urology, London (with J. D. Ferguson, R. Turner Warwick, J. Wickham), 1971–73; Department of Urology, Meath Hospital (with Dermot O'Flynn and Victor Lane [q.v.]), 1973.

Consultant urologist and renal transplant surgeon, Jervis Street Hospital, 1974–86.
UN travelling scholarship to US, to UCLA in San Francisco and Los Angeles.
Surgeon Prosector, Department of Anatomy, RCSI, 1986.

Developed and perfected a surgical technique for creation of arterio-venous shunt for vascular access in dialysis patients, which was published in the *British Medical Journal*, accompanied by an editorial.

Seán Hanson had been trained by the best people in the best places and was a gifted technical surgeon. He cheerfully undertook the heavy burden of a kidney transplant surgeon. Responsible for the introduction of HLA tissue typing to Dublin, he retired prematurely following surgery for a large pituitary adenoma which had not gone completely according to plan, but he never complained.

A gifted teacher, he was appreciated by all his classes for his kindness and extensive knowledge of anatomy. For twenty years he taught undergraduates clinical anatomy with good humour — he always had a smile on his face — and infinite patience, and undertook excellent dissections. He died prematurely of a ruptured aortic aneurysm. In 2007, the anatomy prize for the best student in the graduate entry programme was named in honour of Seán and his colleague Kamal Sayed — the Sayed-Hanson Memorial Medal. In the same year, the renal transplant unit in Beaumont Hospital was named in his honour.

KELLY, Daniel G. (Dan)

Dublin Urologist

b. 1934, Ballinahinch, Co. Tipperary, eighth and youngest child of Denis and Mary Kelly
Educ. Dominican College, Newbridge; University College Dublin
m. Geraldine Kelly [q.v.] (FRCSI, consultant ophthalmologist); 3 s (one deceased; Robert cardiologist, Dublin), 1 d (trainee ophthalmologist)

MB, UCD, 1957; FRCSI, 1960; MCh, NUI, 1961

Postgraduate training at St Vincent's Hospital, St Stephen's Green Dublin; Cornell Medical School, New York City (with Victor Marshall, who was at the height of his powers); Albany University, New York State.
Consultant urologist, St Vincent's Hospital, Dublin, 1966–2000; St Michael's Hospital, Dún Laoghaire; Children's Hospital, Temple Street; National Maternity Hospital, Holles Street; Coombe Women's Hospital.
European Board of Urology, 1992.
Greatly influenced by Frank Duff [q.v.], a superb operator with silky social skills to match.
Prof. Patrick Fitzgerald [q.v.] instilled his love of surgery.

A rapid, tireless surgeon who built a massive practice based on his surgical skills and attractive personality, Dan Kelly was a role model for junior staff ('Great with the patients,' said a trainee) and for his colleagues ('Great with staff' said a matron). Now well into his seventies, he continues to operate. He just loves his work. He was also a peerless chairman of Medical Boards who appreciated his conciliatory skills and his ability to get things done.

A huge man, 6'1", and 16 stone, he has been a successful farmer and horse trainer. He also enjoys golf and entertaining. A warm generous spirit who can light up a room.

KIELY, Matthew David (David)

Cork Urologist

b. 1935, Cork, second eldest of four sons of John Kiely ('K John') [q.v.] and Helen Kiely (*née* Goggin), BDS; three brothers surgeons (Roger, FRCS Eng, deceased)
Educ. Christian Brothers College, Cork; University College, Cork
m. 1965: Rosalie Dyer, eldest daughter of Dr Arthur Dyer (family doctor), Co. Kilkenny; 5 children (Paul is trainee orthopaedic surgeon)

MB, UCC, 1958; FRCS Eng

Postgraduate posts as registrar, Bradford Royal Infirmary (with Charles Macalister who had been Millin's [q.v.] assistant, and, after Millin himself, was probably the greatest exponent of the Millin prostatectomy).
Surgeon, Mercy Hospital, Cork.
President, Irish Society of Urology.

An outstanding technical operating surgeon, David Kiely was a selfless professional and, as a consultant, he assisted other surgeons in the hospital with complex procedures before it had a full quota of trainees. Not many have done that. Decisive, practical and methodical, he was an expert at getting the best out of his staff and never failed to distribute praise when praise was due.

Handsome, jovial and attractive (the nurses couldn't do enough for him), David was capped five times for Ireland as a rugby 'wing-forward', as it was then. A marvellous companion on continental cycling tours (and elsewhere), he is universally popular in his home 'town' where he was a competitive golfer until the legacies of rugby, that ultimate contact sport, caught up with him.

LANE, Thomas Joseph Daniel (Tom, if you dared)

Founder of Irish Urology

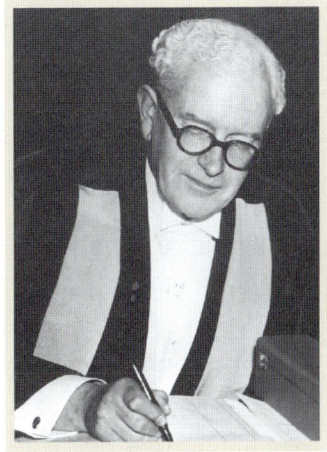

b. 1893, Ferozepore, Pakistan (then British India), son of Colonel D. T. Lane (doctor in Indian Medical Service, which had a long tradition of having a TCD graduate at, or near, the top)
Educ. Our Lady's Bower, Athlone; Clongowes Wood College; Trinity College, Dublin
m. Agnes McLoughlin; son, Victor Lane [q.v.], a urologist
d. 1967

MB, TCD, 1916 (first in class; Fitzpatrick scholarship); Dip. Tropical Medicine & Health, Lond, 1920; MA, TCD, 1921; MCh (*hon. causa*) TCD, 1951; FRCSI (Hon.), 1957

GP, Co. Limerick.
Pathologist; radiologist; urological surgeon, Meath Hospital.
Consultant, Meath Hospital, 1928–67.

Tom Lane worked in the Meath Hospital first as a pathologist, then as radiologist and finally as a urological surgeon, all without a major degree in surgery. He quickly realised that the results of surgery in Ireland lagged far behind those in Britain and particularly those in the United States. A visit to the Mayo Clinic in 1939 convinced him of the necessity of specialisation and the need for a national unit for urology. He began a crusade and pursued it doggedly and single-mindedly. He had pointed out that in the 1930s the mortality for prostatectomy, then 70 per cent of urology, was 20 per cent in Dublin and general hospitals in London, 10 per cent in London specialist units and down to almost 7 per cent in the best American centres. He was convinced and convincing that focus would improve results. And it did. He prevailed on two distinguished British urologists to write to the Irish government, and this, combined with Lane's international reputation, won the day. After delays, to some extent resulting from the ongoing religious 'wars' of the time, the Meath Hospital urological unit was opened in 1954 and prospered from the beginning.

Lane had also been imbued with the passion for good medical records, which was part of the Mayo Clinic culture, and those in the new unit were second to none. Follow-up was rigorous and there followed a long series of world-class clinical research papers, with Dermot O'Flynn, then his 'first assistant', reporting 3,000 prostatectomies with a mortality of less than 3 per cent. Ironically the preferred method of prostatectomy was transurethral, though another Irish surgeon working in London, Terence Millin, had perfected an open operation, which was in worldwide use in the late 1940s and 1950s. There was a constant stream of 'pilgrims' and the unit in the Meath attracted first-rate trainees, particularly from Australia; for many years, it was probably the most visited surgical unit in Ireland.

The man himself could be a charmless martinet with Victorian ideas of 'keeping people in their place'. When he got a substantial sailboat, he found it difficult to get and keep crew. In this, he was the complete opposite of his son, Victor, who joined him on the unit and was so much loved.

Somewhat below middle height, with urologist's stoop and piercing eyes behind thick spectacles, he gave specialist advice readily, usually tinged with overtones that the patient would be better off in his unit. One man can make a difference, and he certainly did. The undisputed Father of Irish Urology, he set the highest possible standards.

LANE, Victor PRCSI 1984–1986

Dublin Urologist

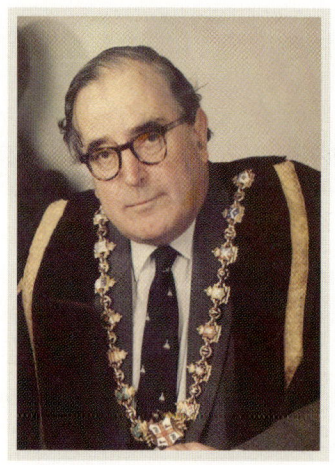

b. 1924, son of T. J. D. Lane [q.v.] (founder of modern Irish urology) and Dr Agnes Lane (*née* McLoughlin)
Educ. Belvedere College; Clongowes Wood College; Trinity College, Dublin
m. 1955: Nuala McGilligan, daughter of Dr Joseph McGilligan, Dundalk; 4 children
d. 1992

BA, TCD, 1946; MB, TCD, 1948 (Purser Medal, EH Bennett Medal and Surgical Travelling Prize); FRCSI, 1950; MCh, TCD, 1954

Postgraduate posts at Meath Hospital; Ancoats Hospital, Manchester; Addenbrooke's Hospital, Cambridge; Northern Hospital, Liverpool.
Surgical registrar, General Hospital, Nottingham; Radcliffe Infirmary; Churchill Hospital, Oxford. Postgraduate Medical School, Hammersmith, London.
Urological surgeon, Meath Hospital; St Kevin's Hospital; Rotunda; National Children's Hospital.
Lecturer in urology, TCD.
President, Irish Society of Urology, 1982–83.
Council, RCSI, 1966–98; President, 1984–86.

There was a certain inevitability that Victor Lane would follow his father into urology, but it was there that the resemblance ended. Tom Lane, an outstanding organiser and surgeon, had few friends and practised the 'fine art of making enemies'. Victor, on the other hand, had a talent for friendships which he raised to an art form, and he kept them in good repair. He was a great joiner and participator and it was said that he never refused membership of an organisation. He was invited to join many exclusive American and European urological societies because of his excellence as an urologist but also because he was an old-fashioned, all-round, good fellow.

He loved tradition: Trinity, the Royal St George Yacht Club, the Irish Cruising Club, and high on the list, the Band of the Irish Guards, or indeed any brass band, were all part of his warm enthusiasms. Others were Kinsale, Dublin, Manhattan and Nantucket Island. He had a great sense of humour and a broad outlook.

A perfect gentleman, as PRCSI he defended the primacy of the office and the Council in the affairs of the College. He was capable of 'storm force ten' interventions when he thought these were in danger but, as with summer storms, they quickly blew through. Everyone remembers Victor with affection.

McLEAN, Peter PRCSI 1996–1998

Dublin Urologist

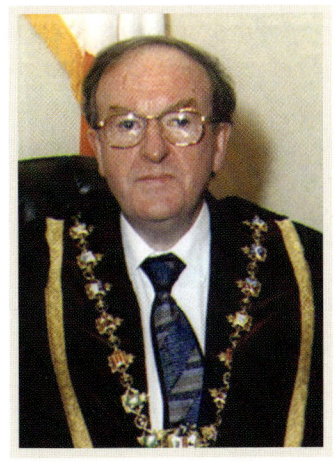

b. 1934, Donegal, younger son of John and Bridget McLean, Dunfanaghy, Co. Donegal
Educ. St Eunan's College, Letterkenny, Co. Donegal; Royal College of Surgeons in Ireland
m. 1962: Dr Nuala Kilcoyne (RCSI graduate); 1 s, 1 d

LRCP & SI (hons), 1958; FRCSI, 1962; FRCS Eng, 1964; FRCS Ed, 1964; MS (urology), University of Minnesota, 1968; FACS, 1974; FRCP & S Glasgow (Hon. *qua surg.*); FCS SA

Postgraduate internship in Ohio, USA. General surgical training in Charitable Infirmary, Jervis Street, Dublin; Hammersmith Hospital, London. Urology residency, Mayo Clinic, Rochester, Minnesota, 1965–68. Edward John Noble Foundation Award at Mayo Clinic.
Consultant surgeon in urology and transplantation, Charitable Infirmary, Jervis Street, subsequently Beaumont Hospital, 1968–99.
Council, RCSI 1984–98; President, 1996–98; President, Biological Society and Association of Graduates

Honorary Fellowship, Academy of Medicine, Malaysia and Singapore.
Donegal Person of the Year, 1986.
Bartholomew Mosse Oration, Rotunda Hospital, 1998.
Vice-President, International Federation of Surgical Colleges, 2004.
Chairman, Voluntary Hospital Consultants Group, IMA.
Medical Staff Ombudsman, Beaumont Hospital Board (a unique appointment in Ireland).
Founder, Kidney Transplant Foundation of Ireland.

Peter McLean returned to Ireland from the Mayo Clinic as a completely trained, highly skilled urologist of international standard. His foremost achievement was to co-ordinate and establish the infrastructure for a kidney transplant programme in the Republic. He harvested the first kidney for transplantation, which he and Tony Walsh [q.v.] put in place, in the Charitable Infirmary. This achievement put the hospital right in the front rank and it remained there. He was a talented technician and had a huge practice, public and private, from other urologists around the country as well the city of Dublin.

Peter had deep tribal loyalties to the RCSI, where he won scholarships; the Mayo Clinic, to which he was invited back many times; and the Charitable Infirmary, known to the rest of Dublin as the 'Jerv'. He wears his heart on his sleeve in the politics of the day (probably his most famous patient was Charles Haughey) and perhaps his proudest moment was conferring the Honorary Fellowship of the RCSI on President Mary McAleese (1998). He had obtained the anchor contribution for the building of the RCSI Smurfit Clinical Science Building at Beaumont and his intimate relationship with the Charitable Infirmary Trust ensured many bequests to the RCSI, including the magnificent stained-glass windows in the Albert Theatre.

Peter claims to enjoy life now on his 'small' farm in Donegal, complete with thatched-roof cottage, where he has Connemara ponies and Jacob sheep, with a bit of horse riding as a distraction, but the reality is that his life is his profession, his patients and his institutions, all of which he served with complete dedication. Short, with slight urologist's stoop, and reddish thinning hair, he has great reserves of energy and determination.

MILLIN, Terence John PRCSI 1963–1966

London Urologist

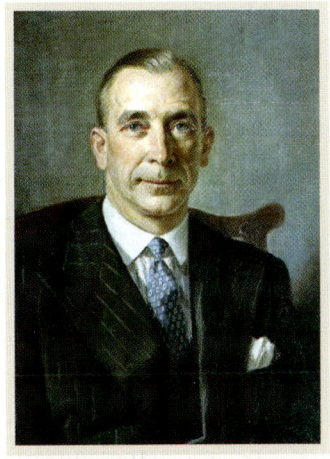

b. 1903, Helen's Bay, Co. Down, only son of Samuel Shannon Millin (barrister) and Ella Catherine Millin (*née* Morton, of Stirling, Scotland)
Educ. St Andrew's School, Dublin; The Abbey School, Tipperary town (scholarship); Trinity College, Dublin
m. 1939: Alice ('Molly') Neville of Guernsey; 2 d
d. 1980

MB (hons), TCD, 1927; MRCS, London, 1928; FRCSI, 1928; FRCS Eng, 1930; MA, TCD, 1931; MCh, TCD, 1931; FRACS (Hon.), 1968; FACS (Hon.)

Training posts in Northampton and Sir Patrick Dun's, Dublin; travelling scholarship to Guy's Hospital and the Middlesex Hospital, London; Royal National Orthopaedic Hospital, Great Portland Street, London.
Urologist, All Saint's Hospital, Pimlico; Southall Hospital; Royal Masonic Hospital; Chelsea Hospital for Women; Mitcham Hospital; St Helier Hospital, Carshalton.
President, British Association of Urological Surgeons, 1954.
Council RCSI, 1960–75; President, 1963–66 (an unprecedented three years).

Although Terence Millin never practised in Ireland, no account of Irish surgery in the twentieth century could omit him. He had a brilliant academic undergraduate career but he was also an outstanding rugby footballer (centre three quarter or five eighth), captained the invincible Trinity teams and played and scored for Ireland against Wales in 1925. A travelling scholarship allowed him to go to London and, with examinations out of the way, he became assistant to Canny Ryall, a Trinity graduate who had set up urological practice in his own hospital in London (All Saints in Vauxhall Bridge Road and subsequently Austral Street, Southwark, 'a slum hospital in a slum area', where they saw a lot of venereal disease). Canny Ryall died suddenly in 1934 and the 31-year-old Millin inherited a thriving Harley Street practice. He prospered.

In 1945, Millin published 'Retro-pubic prostatectomy: a new extravesical technique', in the *Lancet*, and became world famous almost overnight. The new operation for removal of the enlarged obstructing prostate gland was a huge advance on existing methods. He was in demand everywhere as a superb operating surgeon with this innovative procedure, which reduced death from open prostatectomy from perhaps 15 per cent to 3 per cent. He was tall, dark, handsome, utterly charming and a polished, amusing public speaker. He had it all. For five years, he was the biggest surgical earner in London. Taxation rose to a peak rate of 98 per cent in the UK and, in 1950, Millin decided to work part-time in London and spend the remainder of his time on an estate he had purchased in Doneraile, Co. Cork. The practice declined though he formally retired from surgery only in 1963.

Millin operated overseas on many famous patients. He gave operative demonstrations in Dublin either as principal surgeon or assisting an overwhelmed tyro. He moved to Co. Wicklow and was elected to the RCSI Council. He was hugely effective as PRCSI and gave all around him great confidence in the institution, which was going through a lean spell. He travelled widely, raising funds, and his name opened doors everywhere.

His fortunes declined dramatically during the hyperinflation of the 1970s and he moved twice to progressively more modest accommodation. In 1977, he developed a rare tumour of the vocal cords, had radiotherapy but declined radical surgery. He had a tracheotomy and was in great distress at his death in 1980.

The operation he described lost favour in the 1970s but paradoxically the retropubic (Millin) approach is the standard access for the now common operation of radical prostatectomy for carcinoma of the prostate. He lives on in the RCSI through Millin House, a student residence for which he had obtained the funds, and an annual Millin scientific meeting, the highlight being an eponymous lecture by a senior trainee. He lives on also in the memory of those who knew him as a remarkable, warm, lovable Irishman and a superb surgeon.

O'Flynn, James Dermot (Dermot) PRCSI 1992–1994

Dublin Urologist

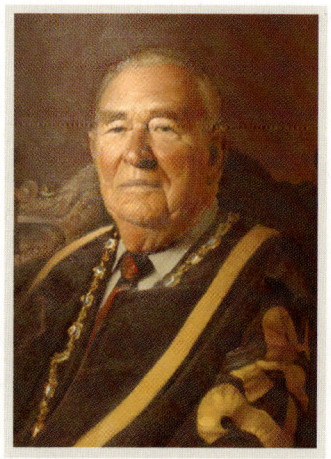

b. January 1920, Cork, eldest child of John and Margaret O'Flynn of Cobh, Co. Cork; brother Maurice, an anaesthetist; sister Mary, a scientist

Educ. Presentation College, Cobh; Cork Technical School (physics and chemistry); University College Cork, 1937–42

m. Monica Kelleher (MB, UCC, 1950; d. 1984); 4 s (Kieran is consultant urologist, Manchester); 1 d

MB (hons and second place in surgery); FRCS Ed, 1948; MCh, NUI, 1949; FRCSI (*ad eundem*), 1968; FRCS Eng (Hon.), 1993; FRCP & S Glasgow (Hon.), 1993.

Trainee posts at Mansfield General Hospital; Lincoln County Hospital.

Captain, Royal Army Medical Corps at Westminster Hospital, London, 1945–47.
Registrar and clinical tutor, Western General Hospital, Edinburgh (with David Band and Selby Tulloch); visiting trainee, Urology Department, Mayo Clinic, on Ainsworth Scholarship from UCC, 1952.
Senior surgeon, Meath Hospital Urological Unit; National Medical Rehabilitation Centre (succeeded Tom Lane [q.v.])
Surgeon, St Luke's (cancer) Hospital; St Kevin's (later St James's) Hospital.
Elected or government appointed as Board Member or Chairman of all his hospitals.
Lecturer in urology, TCD.
Elected member, Medical Council of Ireland, 1983–93.
First *ad eundem* FRCSI to be elected President and first President from Cork.
Presidential gold medal, RCS Ed.
Chairman, surgical section RAMI.
President, Irish Society of Urology.
Guest professor and lecturer, New York; Stanford; Ann Arbor; St Peter's Hospital, London; Urological Society of Australasia.

Dermot O'Flynn set the standards in the surgery of benign prostatic enlargement and the management of the neuropathic bladder, in many parts of the world outside Ireland. His published review of 3,000 prostatectomies (1967) was a milestone of great technical surgery and relentless follow-up. It was widely quoted, as was his paper in the *Journal of Urology* on the bladder in spinal injury. The Meath unit always had excellent medical records, long before computerisation, but Dermot devised and supervised a much-improved punch-card system. At the peak of his powers, scientific papers poured out of the Meath Hospital Urology Department, and he is one of Ireland's best-known, and best-liked surgeons at home and abroad. He built up the unit, emphasising the invincibility of teamwork and by shrewd choice of personnel, and he attracted many overseas trainees, especially from Australia, to the unit.

Calm, kindly, warm and non-confrontational, Dermot retired in July 1987. Of middle height and really strong, with big hands (a former rugby centre three quarter with safe hands and a big tackle), he walks for 18 holes of golf at 85. Dermot generated tremendous loyalties amongst friends, colleagues, nursing staff and trainees. A role model.

O'SULLIVAN, Denis Christopher ('Denis P')

Cork Urologist

Educ. University College Cork

m. Dr Marie Gould; son, Denis, is consultant urologist, Hermitage Clinic, Dublin

MB, UCC, 1953; FRCSI, 1958; FRCS Eng, 1958; FACS

Postgraduate posts included four years at the Mayo Clinic, Rochester, Minnesota, when it was at its zenith.
Consultant urologist, St Finbarr's Hospital and subsequently Cork University Hospital; Bon Secours Hospital.

A brilliant student, Denis O'Sullivan was the first trained, committed urologist south of Dublin, and he built up a huge practice as an extremely hard worker and a state-of-the-art technician. There were two doctors Denis O'Sullivan in Cork, the other being 'Denis J', the hugely popular, iconic Professor of Medicine. To distinguish them, the urologist involuntarily became 'Denis Pee'.

A dedicated fisherman and accomplished shot, he is also an astute art collector with an eye for rising stars. In Cork iconoclasm is a major, participatory blood sport. When a Cork doctor eventually wins a Nobel Prize there will be a pause for reflection and then the considered comment: 'He's not the worst of them.' That's Cork.

SMITH, James Michael (Séamus)

Dublin Urologist

b. 1940, Kells, Co. Meath, younger son of Matthew Smith and Mary Ann Smith (*née* Duffy)
Educ. Blackrock College; University College, Dublin
m. 1970: Patricia Ann Webster, daughter of Jim and Nora Webster, Bridlington, Yorkshire, England; 2 s (James, MRCS, is with Médecins Sans Frontières in Africa), 3 d (eldest is radiologist, Memorial Sloan Kettering, New York)

MB, UCD, 1963; FRCSI, 1967; FRCS Eng, 1968; FRCS Urol, 1976

Postgraduate work at Bradford Royal Infirmary (with 'Tiny' Martin, a large man who had been the last house surgeon to the great Lord Moynihan [1865–1936]); Leicester Royal Infirmary (with Paul Hickinbottom and John Leslie); Addenbrooke's Hospital, Cambridge (with John Withycombe); Meath Hospital, Dublin (with Dermot O'Flynn [q.v.] and Victor Lane [q.v.]. At the Meath, he also operated with and for Terence Millin [q.v.]).
Consultant urologist, Mater Misericordiae Hospital; Children's University Hospital, 1979–2005.
President, Medical Society, UCD, 1994 (the students' choice is a token of their affection); Irish Society of Urology, 2000–02.
First Millin Lecturer, RCSI, 1978.

A brilliant, gifted operating surgeon, Séamus Smith trained with the best, and it showed. He was particularly interested in prostate and bladder cancer and carried out large numbers of successful radical retro-pubic prostatectomies. He worked at great pace and crammed as much as possible into the day. He was an inspiring teacher and his ward rounds drew large attendances. He was also a good storyteller, with a weakness for delicious, spicy gossip. The operating room was calm, fun and even hilarious at times. He was very dedicated to his patients and loved by the nurses and secretaries.

To say that Séamus is a keen golfer is to understate the matter by an order of magnitude. He is a fanatic who has played to between 1 and 6 handicap for over forty-five years, and has won many prizes and representative honours, as well as captaincies and presidencies of golf clubs and societies.

Tall, slim, dark, very good-humoured, highly organised and punctual, he worked hard at all facets of the profession but perhaps it is as a popular figure and superb technician that he will be best remembered.

WALSH, Anthony (Tony, 'Narky')

Dublin Urologist

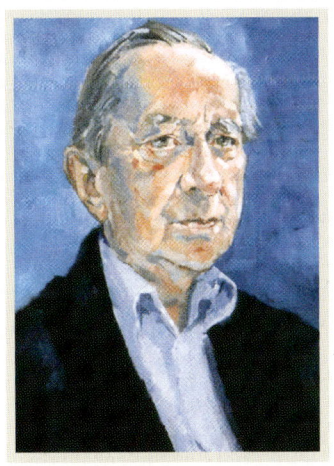

b. 1922, Sligo, only son of James J. Walsh (barrister, d. 1938) and Dora Heartsease Byrne
Educ. Belvedere College, Dublin; Ampleforth College (Benedictine), Yorkshire; Trinity College, Dublin
m. 1954: Josephine (Jossy) Schulte ('a saint'), daughter of Hans and Leonie Schulte of the Netherlands, her family are connected with the retail giants C&A; 3 s, 2 d (2 nurses and a doctor).
d. 1997

MB, TCD (first class hons; Bennett Medallist, 1944; Dublin University Surgical Prize, 1945); Primary and Final exams, FRCSI, 1947; DSc (Hon.), TCD, 1992; MA, TCD, 1993; FACS

Postgraduate posts at Cheltenham General Hospital, 1944–45. Resident surgical officer, Sefton General Hospital, Liverpool; Dreadnought Seaman's Hospital, Greenwich, London. Clinical assistant in Urology, St John's Hospital, Lewisham (with Mr Winsbury White); senior surgical registrar, Royal Southern Hospital, Liverpool (with J. Cosbie Ross).
Senior consultant urologist, Jervis Street Hospital, Dublin, 1953–87; founder and head of department.
Urologist, James Connolly Memorial Hospital, Blanchardstown, 1974–87.
Lecturer in urology, RCSI; examiner undergraduate and Fellowship.

President, International Society of Urology; European Dialysis and Transplantation Society; Irish Society of Urology; Irish Biomedical Engineering Society.
Honorary member, American, Australasian, British and Japanese Urological Associations.
Visiting Professor at more than ten university medical schools and gave scores of invited lectures.

Author of 83 articles in various publications; three books, four book translations and ten chapters in books.

J. Cosbie Ross, an international authority on genitourinary tuberculosis, and Mr Winsbury White were career influences.

A really first-rate urologist, who read omnivorously and was certainly the best informed in the specialty in the city of Dublin, Tony Walsh had had a very sad childhood. His mother walked out of the family home when he was two and his father died of tuberculosis when Tony was 16. It is widely believed that some of his years in Ampleforth College owed something to the generosity of orthopaedic surgeon Arthur Chance [q.v.], who was unmarried at the time. He got into Trinity on a scholarship and was constantly short of money for such basics as the examination fee, which on one occasion was paid by his tutor. As a student, he acted with the Gate Theatre Company, on the stage with Micheál Mac Liammóir, Hilton Edwards and Orson Welles, to augment his income. He also had to give 'grinds', which cut into his study time but did not influence his brilliant results.

Tony Walsh wrote articles all the time, which was unusual in those days for someone who did not have a major academic appointment, and he was an expert on the history of the specialty. His biggest achievement was getting dialysis and renal transplant started at Jervis Street which, at that time, was regarded as being well behind the Lane Urological Unit at the Meath Hospital. He was leader of the team that performed the first kidney transplant in Ireland. He had little interest in private practice. It never bothered him that his nickname was 'Narky'; he just knew that he was right.

Tony was a fine teacher and, even though he was hard on the students, most of them knew that he had their interests at heart. Overseas trainees were sometimes treated poorly, however, and he could be patronising beyond belief. Nevertheless, he generated great loyalties amongst the nursing staff and many of his trainees. He was hospitable and generous, and each year at Christmas his splendid home in Herbert Park was 'open house' all day and well into the night, but there was also much hospitality through the year. He had a beautiful speaking voice, which resonated regularly through his local church. He was a good friend to the local clergy.

Tony Walsh's fame overseas was never reflected in Ireland, and cynics said that those who elected him to high international office in sunnier climes saw him for only a few days a year. Despite numerous attempts, he never came close to being elected to the RCSI Council. This unpopularity did not upset him even when his junior colleague, Peter McLean, was elected PRCSI. 'He was his own worst enemy but he was several other people's as well.' He was a complete urological snob with a negligible sense of humour.

Above middle height, with dark good looks, he had a figure that was a tailor's joy and he was always beautifully turned out, with trademark dark quiff over his forehead. He had the languid manner of an intellectual, which he certainly was. He also had many trophies for rowing. His family loved him and the urological community missed him. There is an appropriate memorial of a sponsored travelling Fellowship in his name. He richly deserves it. An icon who was not a role model. Only Tom Lane [q.v.] is ahead of him in the Irish urology pantheon.

22
ANAESTHESIA

Prof. Richard Clarke

ANAESTHESIA

THE END OF THE NINETEENTH CENTURY

Anaesthesia was initiated in Ireland by John MacDonnell, who gave ether in the Richmond Hospital on 1 January 1847. Its acceptance in London and Dublin a few weeks after its first use in Boston indicates that the world was eagerly awaiting such a humanitarian development. Chloroform, introduced by James Young Simpson in Edinburgh, was first used in Dublin in November 1847, and from this time both agents were used for anaesthesia throughout Ireland. Chloroform was preferred for its ease of administration, with little coughing, but its dangers were known from the outset and it was avoided in patients with 'weak hearts'. Ether was regarded as safer than chloroform, but the coughing, salivation and vomiting that it caused gave poorer operating conditions and it was considered undesirable for use in patients with chest problems. The rules for the use of both agents are marshalled by George Foy and it is clear that towards the end of the nineteenth century Foy and his colleagues had a preference. He actually states that 'The death rate from chloroform is high; it is calculated as one in 525 administrations...' but he does not accept this figure and quotes series of 15,000 and 30,000 without a fatality, so that overall he attributes many of the deaths to the patient's poor health or to bad administration.

Nitrous oxide, though its anaesthetic properties were known in the 1840s, was much less used in the nineteenth century. This was largely because of the difficulties of storing the gas and administering it safely with air. However, cylinders of nitrous oxide were available, and Foy describes its use as sole agent for dentistry, or combined with ether for general surgery.

The apparatus used for the majority of ether and chloroform anaesthetics was of the simplest — a wire cage covered with thick cloth or Gamgee, onto which the liquid was dropped from a drop bottle. This type of mask was introduced soon after 1850 and remained in use, particularly for children, until the 1950s. Ormsby's ether inhaler, used in the Meath Hospital, Dublin, consisted simply of a sponge onto which ether was poured, attached to a face mask. Clover's portable ether inhaler was more elaborate, with a chamber filled with ether, surrounded by a jacket filled with warm water and attached to a bag, so that higher and more predictable concentrations of ether could be given. In various forms it was used well into the twentieth century. The advantages of giving oxygen, particularly with chloroform anaesthesia, were realised in the nineteenth century but, as with nitrous oxide, the difficulties of supplying a gas limited its general acceptance.

Developments in the Twentieth Century

The first major development in anaesthesia during the twentieth century was the introduction of tracheal intubation. This had been practised earlier for resuscitation and to avoid a tracheostomy for obstruction of the larynx. However, it was after the trauma of the First World War that it came into its own, as used by anaesthetists working with Sir Harold Gillies in Kent. The two main figures were Ivan Whiteside Magill (1888–1986) and Edgar Stanley Rowbotham (1890–1979). Ivan Magill was born in Larne, Co. Antrim, and graduated from Queen's University Belfast, in 1913. Having served with the Royal Army Medical Corps during the First World War, he was appointed assistant to the Queen's Hospital for Facial and Jaw Injuries, in Sidcup, Kent, in 1919. There he developed the technique of blind nasal intubation and also designed his endotracheal tubes and laryngoscope. He never practised in Ireland, being on the staff of the Brompton Chest Hospital in London from 1923 and of the Westminster Hospital from 1924. Queen's University has the unfortunate distinction of having turned down his MD thesis, though it later made up for this by awarding him a DSc (*hon. causa*) in 1945. Equally important for the development of the specialty was his role in establishing the Association of Anaesthetists of Great Britain and Ireland (1932), the Diploma of Anaesthetics (DA) examination (1935) and finally the Faculty of Anaesthetists of the Royal College of Surgeons of England (1947).

The next landmark in anaesthesia was the development of intravenous drugs to induce sleep, since a small needle-prick is regarded by most adults as preferable to having the face-mask applied while conscious. After trials of other barbiturates, thiopentone was synthesised in 1932 in Germany and slowly introduced into clinical practice, though the longer-acting pentobarbitone continued in use through the 1930s. The dangerous aspect was that when intravenous anaesthetics were introduced it seemed appropriate to use them as sole agents or with only nitrous oxide and oxygen. This required large doses, caused prolonged sedation and, since no analgesic was usually given, was followed by much restlessness — a situation well described by O. J. Murphy (of St Vincent's Hospital, Dublin) in his article of 1946. On the other hand, the anaesthetic appeared smooth for the surgeon and avoided the postoperative vomiting associated with ether. Only after the work of Professor Cecil Gray of Liverpool and the studies of their clinical pharmacology by John Dundee in Belfast did these drugs become truly safe and satisfactory. This eventually led to the introduction of their shorter-acting successors, methohexitone and althesin, which were also pioneered by John Dundee.

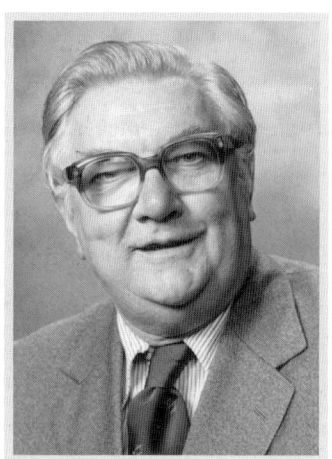

Dr John Dundee

The introduction of muscle relaxants to clinical practice began in 1942 with Griffith and Johnston in Canada and probably had an even bigger influence on surgery than intravenous anaesthesia. By relaxing the abdominal muscles, curare removed the need for deep anaesthesia while giving better operating conditions. Similarly, by paralysing the respiratory muscles in thoracic and cardiac surgery, it provided, if not a motionless operating field, a degree of quiet and predictable movement, which facilitated delicate surgery.

Other twentieth-century developments in anaesthetic pharmacology have been less conspicuous — but there has been a steady improvement in the safety of inhalational anaesthetics, resulting in the elimination of cardiac and hepatic toxicity, as we have moved from chloroform and ether, through cyclopropane, trichloroethylene and halothane, to sevoflurane and desflurane. These changes, together with improvements in anaesthetic monitoring and equipment, have gradually made anaesthesia safer throughout the twentieth century.

The advent of intensive care, on the other hand, has involved much greater and more extensive changes within every hospital. The widespread epidemic of poliomyelitis in Copenhagen in 1952 stretched resources to the limit and it became clear that the best solution was to set up a new type of ward, heavily staffed with nurses, and under the care of anaesthetists, for only they had the expertise to ventilate patients for prolonged periods. In Ireland, this development began around 1960, with a unit in the Mater Misericordiae Hospital, Dublin, for the postoperative ventilation and monitoring of cardiac surgical patients. The respiratory failure unit in the Royal Victoria Hospital, Belfast (1961), was at first concerned mainly with ventilatory support for victims of poliomyelitis, tetanus (after suppression of spasms with muscle relaxants) and other causes of respiratory weakness. The intensive care unit of 1965 in the Adelaide Hospital, Dublin, had a mixed medical and surgical background. However, it gradually became apparent that the anaesthetists and their colleagues had the skills to manage nutrition, renal function, blood volume, electrolyte disturbance and cerebral protection, as well as supporting the cardiovascular system with inotropic drugs and aortic balloon pumps, if required. With this went the development of equipment for measuring blood gases and electrolytes, and this often required the setting up of a new laboratory, since at that time no hospital laboratory could provide a sufficiently rapid service. In addition, new skills of arterial and central venous cannulation had to be learned as the monitoring equipment gradually improved. The growth of the intensive care unit has inevitably meant a concentration of medical and nursing expertise, and now the adequacy of intensive care provision is often the limiting factor in the volume of cardiac, neuro- and other major surgery that can be carried out.

The other field of expansion of the anaesthetist's role has been that of pain management. The first pain clinics were started in the early 1960s to treat chronic pain, usually post-traumatic or resulting from malignancy. The methods of pain relief included oral opioids with appropriate antiemetics, but the more specialist field involved some unusual nerve blocks (trigeminal, cervical, coeliac, etc). Gradual specialisation has led to the reduction in the number of anaesthetists involved, with only a few clinics in the major cities.

A separate development in acute pain relief services in many hospitals followed from the realisation that many postoperative patients were not receiving analgesia when they most needed it. In fact, its administration was related more to the availability of a doctor or nurse than to the severity of the pain. This led to the adoption of patient-controlled intravenous infusions of morphine. In parallel came the increased use of postoperative epidural analgesia, following its growing use in obstetrics. Both these methods carry a high risk of accidental overdosage, and safety has been ensured only by having pain management teams of a doctor and several nurses, with responsibilities spread widely through a hospital.

THE FACULTY OF ANAESTHETISTS

The formation of the Association of Anaesthetists of Great Britain and Ireland in 1932 had given all career anaesthetists in these islands some corporate identity, and many anaesthetists from Ireland subsequently took the Diploma of Anaesthetists examination of the Royal Colleges of Physicians and Surgeons in London (e.g. Dr Olive Anderson, Dr Stafford Geddes and Dr Patrick Nagle in 1936; Dr John Dorman in 1941; Dr Maurice Brown in 1945; Dr Edmund Delaney in 1955; Dr Joseph Galvin in 1959). The logical next move was to develop a Diploma of the Irish Colleges of Physicians and Surgeons, which came about in 1943 and was taken by, among others, Dr John Boyd [q.v.], Dr Thomas Gilmartin and Dr George Hamilton in 1943, Dr Frank Whyte (1947), Dr Alexander Blayney (1950), Dr John Goodbody (1951) and Dr John McCarthy (1953).

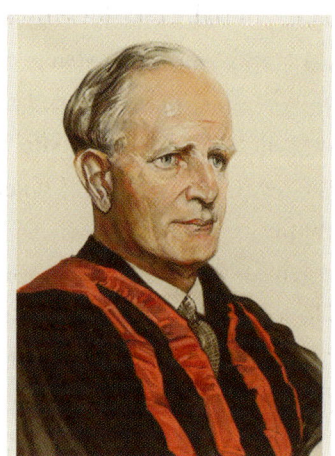

Dr Thomas Gilmartin

This undoubtedly proved a satisfactory level of competence, though it was not defined as a 'Fellowship' or 'membership', and most Irish anaesthetists did not sit the DA in the 1940s or 1950s. The position of anaesthetists in 1946 is well described by Richard W. Shaw. The Irish anaesthetists, compared with the surgeon, had no definite training, no equivalent qualification, no Royal College, no university professorship, no position on a hospital board, could usually work only in the morning since most operating was carried out then, and were paid by the surgeon rather than by the patient. The challenge for the specialty was to set about correcting these deficiencies, and the Faculty of Anaesthetists of the Royal College of Surgeons (London), founded in 1948, seemed the obvious model. In the United Kingdom in the 1950s, the Fellowship of the Faculty of Anaesthetists was emerging as the normal qualification for consultants, indicating a satisfactory level of training, and was considered comparable to the FRCS and MRCP. A steering committee of the Royal College of Surgeons in Ireland was formed with Thomas Gilmartin as chairman, and the first meeting of the new Board of the Faculty of Anaesthetists took place on 15 December 1959. The members were Dr Thomas Gilmartin as Dean, Dr Victor McCormick as Vice-Dean, Dr Drury Byrne, Dr Ray Davys, Dr John Dundee, Dr Sheila Kenny, Dr Harold Love, Dr Paul Murray, Dr Patrick Nagle and Dr Joseph Woodcock, with Mr Desmond Riordan FRCS as representative of the College Council. The initial considerations were largely concerned with Fellowship of the new Faculty — who should be awarded the Fellowship (on payment of a fee) and who should have to sit the new examination (which started with a primary examination in 1961). The Faculty celebrated its inauguration by granting Honorary Fellowships to Dr Ivan Magill, Dr John Gillies and Dr Geoffrey Organe, and Ivan Magill reciprocated by presenting the Dean with a ceremonial medal and chain of office.

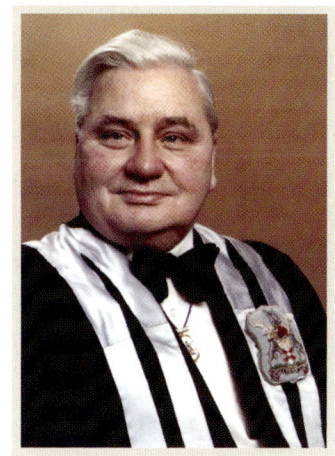

Dr Joseph Woodcock

From the outset, education was prominent, with the first Irish national meeting in 1960, soon followed by courses for the examinations. Once the final clinical exam (part II) was established and the Fellowship became the standard qualification, members of the Board felt that the DA should be abolished. The anaesthetists were particularly concerned that county hospitals would accept it as an adequate qualification for a consultant appointment and delay the recognition of the FFA as the national standard. However, it brought in revenue to the Colleges of Physicians and Surgeons and continued to be taken by many from outside Ireland, so that the argument between the surgeons' and the anaesthetists' points of view continued at almost every Board meeting into the late 1970s.

It was now clear that an approved period of clinical training was an essential preliminary to the Fellowship, and the question of where the training had taken place became relevant. This evolved in the 1960s into a programme of hospital inspections, which could be used as a threat to both anaesthetists and administrators to ensure the highest standards of training and supervision of junior doctors.

The concept of a Faculty of Anaesthetists as a part of the College of Surgeons was bound to have many areas of disagreement. Initially the College Council felt that choice of examiners and conferring of Fellowships was a College matter, and the College had a representative on the Board of the Faculty. However, one by one, these areas of involvement in Faculty affairs (as they were seen by anaesthetists) were removed. In the mid-1970s the possibility of having a Faculty representative on the College Council was explored but found to be legally almost impossible. Another intermediate phase of development was consideration in the early 1990s of amalgamation of the Irish Faculty with the newly established Royal College of Anaesthetists in London. However, this would inevitably have resulted in the loss of the Irish Faculty's identity, and the idea was abandoned.

The most serious arguments with the College of Surgeons were over finances, with some degree of financial separation requested as early as 1964, and a Faculty honorary treasurer appointed in 1967. Naturally this became more urgent as the Faculty's capital and income increased, coming from new Fellows, courses and meetings, and annual subscriptions. The examinations remained a College function until the end of the century, since the College gave them their status and essentially the College maintained that they were non-profit-making. This description might suggest that there was a constant battle between Faculty and College, but this would be quite untrue and these issues came out only occasionally at Board meetings, while day-to-day co-operation, particularly with the examinations, was complete.

The next important step forward, though it was a move by the College of Surgeons rather than the Faculty, was the creation of a Chair of Anaesthetics in 1965, with Professor T. J. Gilmartin as first occupant. It must be said that the Chair did not come with a Department of Anaesthetics or any facilities for teaching or research, and this was the situation during the tenure of Professor Gilmartin. However, when Dr Tony Cunningham succeeded him in 1986 it was as head of a complete academic department. The new chair was followed in 1967 by the inauguration by the Faculty of a lecture in memory of Dr T. P. C. Kirkpatrick, though, after the first ten years, the lecture has rarely been given. A few years later, a medal fund was announced in memory of Dr Edmund

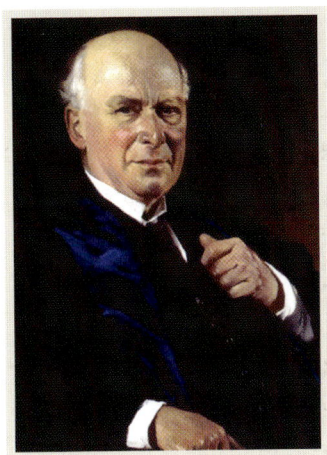

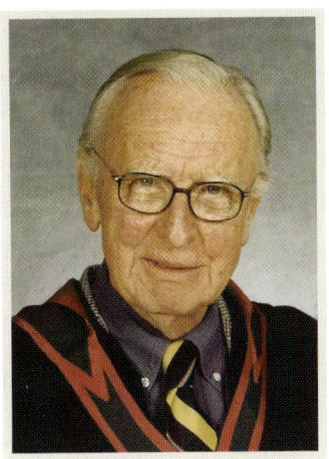

Dr T. P. C. Kirkpatrick   *Dr W. S. Wren*

Delaney, an energetic early member of the Board, who died in 1979. Trainees in the presentation of a prize essay compete for this annually. The third honour created by the Faculty was in 1984, with the first Gilmartin Lecture, to be given on a non-anaesthetic topic at the Annual Scientific Meeting.

The creation of a national training programme for senior registrars, though not strictly a Faculty enterprise, was the idea of Dr Bill Wren, and meetings with the Department of Health began in 1970; a structured programme had been achieved by 1975 while Dr Wren was Dean. It ensured that trainees throughout the Republic could achieve a full experience in all fields of anaesthetic practice and were fully prepared for consultant posts.

Progress of the Faculty to an independent College was probably inevitable, though it was completed only on 23 September 1998 with the inauguration ceremony, and an Honorary Fellowship for the President of Ireland, Mary McAleese. In 2003, 22 Merrion Square North was bought and it was opened in the following year as the College of Anaesthetists' new home.

Deans of the Faculty of Anaesthetists, from 1959

1959–64	Professor T. J. Gilmartin (Dublin)
1964–67	Dr J. A. Woodcock (Dublin)
1967–70	Dr G. R. Davys (Dublin)
1970–73	Professor J. W. Dundee (Belfast)
1973–76	Dr W. S. Wren (Dublin)
1976–79	Dr S. H. S. Love (Belfast)
1979–82	Dr J. R. McCarthy (Dublin)
1982–85	Dr G. W. Black (Belfast)
1985–88	Professor P. W. A. Keane (Galway)
1988–91	Professor D. C. Moriarty (Dublin)
1991–94	Professor R. S. J. Clarke (Belfast)
1994–97	Dr J. Cooper (Belfast)

Presidents of the College of Anaesthetists, from 1997

1997–2000	Dr W. Blunnie (Dublin)
2000–03	Professor A. J. A Cunningham
2003–06	Professor J. P. H. Fee
2006–09	Dr J. McAdoo (Cork)

The Practice of Anaesthesia

Around 1890–1910, doctors specifically described as anaesthetists began to be appointed to the main Irish hospitals, but outside the major centres, as late as the 1950s, large numbers of anaesthetics were still being administered by medical students, house officers, junior surgeons and general practitioners. In London, there had been some specialisation from the outset and the pioneering work of John Snow (1813–58) and Joseph Clover (1825–82) is well known. In Ireland, there were specialists such as George Foy, FRCS (1845–1934), of the Whitworth Hospital, Dublin, who wrote extensively on the history and practice of anaesthesia, though his main specialty was surgery, and Charles O'Neill (1861–1924) of Belfast, who wrote up a series of 600 anaesthetics in 1896. The general pattern in the early twentieth century was of appointing young doctors, usually budding surgeons, to serve as anaesthetists for a short time, before they moved on to a settled career. The effect of having surgeon-anaesthetists and non-specialist anaesthetists was that the choice of anaesthetic and technique remained very much in the surgeons' hands. It was also normal practice for surgeons to give their own spinal anaesthetics since they often had no adequate anaesthetic help.

Anaesthetic practice did not develop in a uniform way everywhere but in accordance with the needs and resources of particular hospitals. In Northern Ireland, the advent of the National Health Service in 1948, with parity of salaries for all consultants, made it possible for anaesthetists to devote themselves exclusively to anaesthetic practice, though a few continued to combine it with general practice. However, in many cities in the Republic, the transition was delayed for many years by financial uncertainties. The names of only some of the earlier anaesthetists have survived but it is worth highlighting a few figures from the first half of the century in the various hospitals. After technical and organisational developments in the 1950s and 1960s, it is possible to mention only some of those who made a wider contribution to the national scene.

Anaesthesia in Dublin

The Charitable Infirmary, Jervis Street — This hospital was not only the first voluntary hospital in Ireland, founded in Cook Street, Dublin, in 1718, but also the first hospital where chloroform was given, in December 1847. The hospital was, however, slow to appoint a visiting anaesthetist, an idea taken up only in 1910. Dr Joseph Daniel (LRCPI, LRCSI, 1906) was appointed to work on two mornings a week, from ten o'clock, but received no payment or fees from medical students. It is recorded that the hospital spent 23 shillings in 1911 for purchase of a new Clover inhaler, but clearly anaesthesia was neither expensive nor highly valued. Dr Daniel resigned after two years and, after a number of short-term appointments, the post lapsed. The next appointment was Dr Frank O'Grady (MB, 1921) in 1926. He was appointed on a yearly basis, at a salary of £100 per annum, and he also was followed by a number of short appointments.

Eventually, in 1946, Dr Joseph Woodcock (LRCPI, LRCSI, 1944; DA, Irel, 1946; d. 1997) was appointed as assistant anaesthetist and he was to dominate life in the Anaesthetic Department of the hospital for nearly forty years. He fostered the growth of the intensive care unit, the surgical day-care centre and the dialysis unit, being Director of the last for many years. He was approached by the Department of Health in 1966 to set up a National Poisons Information Service and was a key figure in its success. Beyond the hospital he was one of the main figures in setting up the Faculty of Anaesthetics and was its second Dean 1964–7, after Dr Thomas Gilmartin. After this campaign was successful, he lobbied, along with his colleague Dr Desmond Riordan, for a Chair of Anaesthetics within the College and, on his retirement in 1986, was succeeded in his clinical appointment by Dr Anthony Cunningham (MB, 1972), who became the first *full-time* Professor of Anaesthetics in the Republic of Ireland.

Mercer's Hospital — Mercer's Hospital was opened in 1734 and the old building now houses the library of the Royal College of Surgeons. The first anaesthetist to be appointed, in 1913, was Dr James Beckett (MB, 1911), uncle of the future playwright and Nobel prize winner. He moved to the Adelaide Hospital in 1919 and was replaced by Dr Joseph Brennan (LRCP, LRCS, 1917) followed by Dr Patrick Gaffney (LRCPI, LRCSI, 1921), soon to become Dublin's coroner for forty years. In 1932, Dr Thomas J. Gilmartin (1905–1986; LRCPI, LRCSI, 1929) was appointed assistant anaesthetist and, in his long life, made the most outstanding contribution to Irish anaesthesia. As well as Mercer's he was consultant to the City of Dublin Skin and Cancer Hospital, Hume Street, and the Dublin Dental Hospital and Peamount Sanatorium. He was the first anaesthetist in Ireland to use curare, but his great contribution was a belief in sound training and in the corporate identity of anaesthetists. He was a founder member of the Association of Anaesthetists of Great Britain and Ireland and was given the DA of the RCPSI in 1943. Later he was to be chairman of the steering committee which created the Faculty of Anaesthetists of the Royal College of Surgeons in Ireland (1959) and its first Dean, and he was appointed Professor of Anaesthesia, on a part-time basis, by the College in 1965. In 1965, he was also awarded the John Snow Medal by the Association of Anaesthetists, and the Faculty of Anaesthetists in his honour created the Gilmartin Lecture in 1984.

The Richmond, Whitworth and Hardwicke Hospitals — This group, known collectively as the House of Industry Hospitals or St Lawrence's Hospital, dates its foundation to the years 1803–17 and can claim the distinction of having given birth to anaesthesia in Ireland, on 1 January 1847, Dr John MacDonnell giving the anaesthetic. The first anaesthetists appointed as such were Dr John Meyler (LRCPI, LRCSI, 1899) and Dr Alfred Boyd (MB, 1896), both appointed in 1905. Dr Meyler resigned in 1911 but Dr Boyd continued until 1925, writing papers on 'oil-ether colonic anaesthesia'. Thereafter there was a succession of anaesthetists, with Dr Paul Murray (LRCPI, LRCSI, 1929; d. 1981), who was on the staff c.1936–73, taking a special interest in neurosurgical anaesthesia and leading the anaesthetic team in 1968 for the pioneering attempt to separate conjoined twins. Dr John Conroy (LRCP, LRCS, 1947; DA, Dub, 1951; d. 2004) came in 1955 and was first Director of Anaesthetics from 1961, and Dr Hugh Raftery (MB, 1950; DA, Dub, 1952), came in 1977 and established the hospital's pain-relief clinic. Dr Thomas Breen (LRCPI, LRCSI, 1951; DA, Dub, 1954) was consultant anaesthetist 1969–87 and laid the foundations of thoracic anaesthesia, introducing the first ventilator to the hospital — a Radcliffe. The group was amalgamated with the Charitable Infirmary, Jervis Street, and Mercer's Hospital in the new Beaumont Hospital in 1987.

Dr Steevens' Hospital — This hospital was founded in 1720 in association with Trinity College, Dublin. The first anaesthetist was appointed in 1899, the celebrated Dr Thomas Percy Claude Kirkpatrick (1869–1954; MB, 1895). Although he resigned in the following year to become a physician, he continued to practise as an anaesthetist, in both Dr Steevens' and the Dental Hospital, for the rest of his career. In addition, he was lecturer in anaesthetics at Trinity College. He was Registrar of the Royal College of Physicians for the extraordinary period of 1903–53, and in this role became a distinguished medical historian. As well as his accounts of *Medical Teaching in Trinity College* (1912) and *Dr Steevens' Hospital* (1924), he wrote innumerable articles and compiled an extensive biographical archive, now housed in the Royal College of Physicians. Later anaesthetists have included Dr Richard Shaw (MB 1919) and Dr Edmund Delaney (MB 1949). The latter became a member of the Board of the Faculty in 1965, and was later Vice-Dean. A prize medal given by the Faculty commemorated his early death in 1979.

The Meath Hospital — Founded in 1753, this hospital is unusual in having an early and detailed history by Lambert Ormsby, FRCS, published in 1888. However, it inevitably has little record of anaesthesia and it is only in 1945 that names of anaesthetists begin to appear on the hospital staff lists: Dr Charles Wilson (MB, 1926; DA, Dub, 1943), Dr Silver Dean-Oliver (MB, 1926; DA, Lond, 1943) and Dr Maureen Murphy (MB, 1938; DA, Dub, 1944). They were later followed by Dr Patricia Delany (MB, 1939; DA, Dub, 1951), Dr Kevin O'Sullivan (MB, 1945; DA, Dub, 1952), Dr Margaret Una Comer (MB, 1952;

DA, Dub, 1954; m. Dr Brendan Callaghan) and Dr Joseph Galvin (LRCPI, LRCSI, 1955; DA, Lond, 1959).

Sir Patrick Dun's Hospital — This hospital opened in 1802 and was from the outset closely associated with Trinity College. The first recorded anaesthetist was Dr Richard Kennan (MB, 1892), appointed in 1898, prior to his becoming a surgeon and joining the Colonial Medical Service. He was followed by a succession of anaesthetists on the surgical ladder. The first appointment of a visiting anaesthetist in the hospital was Dr William Smyly (MB, 1909), who was in post *c.*1911–50, followed by Dr Victor McCormick (MB, 1923; d. 1970), who was in post *c.*1925 until he retired *c.*1967. He belonged to the generation before the Diplomas of Anaesthetics were set up and instead took the MRCPI exam in 1928 and became FRCPI in 1930. Nevertheless, he was early in the use of curare for abdominal surgery (1946) at a time when 'supplies are still very limited' and 0.5 to 1.0 gram of thiopentone was regarded as a moderate dose. He was awarded the FFA RCSE in 1948 and was Vice-Dean of the first Board of the Faculty in 1959. He was joined about 1952 by Dr Frank Whyte (MB, 1939; d. 1976) and Dr John Goodbody (MB, 1951).

The Adelaide Hospital — The Adelaide opened in 1839, and the first anaesthetist, Dr Paul Piel (LRCSI, 1884), was appointed in 1886 to work two half-days per week. He appears to have used mainly ether given by Clover's inhaler, but occasionally chloroform or nitrous oxide was given for a pleasanter and smoother induction. However, when in 1906 he asked for the hospital board's permission to use a gas-oxygen apparatus he was told, 'gas alone would be less complicated for ordinary hospital purposes and much less expensive'. Dr Piel was never appointed to the honorary medical staff, but was graded as anaesthetist and lecturer in anaesthetics. When he retired in 1919, he was followed by Dr Isabella Webb (MB, 1904), Dr James Beckett (MB, 1911), Dr Robert Jackson (MB, 1923) and Dr John Stephens (MB, 1927), who from the outset were members of the honorary medical staff. The next event in terms of personalities was the appointment of Dr Sheila Kenny (*née* Wilson, MB 1933; d. 1990) in 1934 as the first full-time anaesthetist in the hospital. She had trained in England and took the London DA in 1946. The formation of the intensive care unit in 1965 was driven by Mr Nigel Kinnear [q.v.], and Sheila Kenny created its scientific basis with her blood-gas laboratory. The Adelaide

Ventilator (designed by Dr Michael Lewis, who later moved to Belfast) also belongs to the early period of the intensive care unit. She was on the first Board of the Faculty of Anaesthetists in 1959 and was later its Vice-Dean. Another Adelaide anaesthetist widely involved in the Faculty of Anaesthetists and academic life in Dublin was Dr John Goodbody (MB, 1951). He was also on the staff of Sir Patrick Dun's Hospital and was consultant anaesthetist in the Adelaide Hospital from about 1962 to 1986.

St Vincent's Hospital — Founded in 1834 in St Stephen's Green, this hospital moved to its present site in Ballsbridge in 1970. We know of only one visiting anaesthetist in the 1920s, Dr Oswald Murphy (MB, 1914), who returned from the post of colonial surgeon in St Helena with a strong interest in anaesthesia and seems to have combined that with the post of deputy coroner of the city of Dublin. He was joined in 1946 by Dr Ray Davys (MB, 1942; DA, Dub, 1947), followed by Dr Michael Nash (MB, 1944; DA, Lond, 1946), Dr Denis O'Leary (MB, 1951; DA, Dub, 1953), Dr Richard Nolan (MB, 1961; DA, Lond, 1963) and Dr Marian Rice (MB, 1956; DA, Eng, 1959) in 1972, and the staff continued to expand. Dr Ray Davys was a member of the first board of the Irish Faculty of Anaesthetists and became the third Dean 1967–70. Dr Richard (Dick) Nolan sadly died in 1983 at the peak of his career, following major surgery. Other anaesthetists prominent on the board of the Faculty included Dr Edmund Gallagher and Dr Vincent Hannon, both appointed to the hospital staff in 1989.

The Mater Misericordiae Hospital — The hospital dates from 1861 and the first visiting anaesthetist appointed to the hospital was Dr Patrick Joseph O'Farrell (LRCP, LRCS, 1903) in about 1906, who continued to work in the hospital and in private practice until about 1937. He was joined in about 1922 by Dr Hugh Kelly (MB, 1915) and about 1932 by Dr Patrick Drury Byrne (MB, 1926; d. 1978). No further anaesthetists were appointed to the staff until around 1947, when Dr Patrick Nagle (MB, 1929; d. 1980) joined. He had already been in anaesthetic and general practice in London, where he had taken the Diploma of Anaesthetics in 1936 and had worked for some years in Jervis Street Hospital. During the 1950s and 1960s the staff slowly expanded to include Dr Alexander Blayney (MB, 1947; d. 1974) and Dr John McCarthy (MB, 1951). The appointment of the latter as assistant anaesthetist in 1961 and full consultant in

1969 coincided with the development of open-heart surgery, and this remained his major interest throughout his career. As the Mater became the principal centre for open-heart surgery in the Republic, he pioneered the technique of using an epidural block as the main means of analgesia for these patients. Having taken the DA Dub in 1953, he was made one of the early Fellows of the new Faculty of Anaesthetists in 1962. Subsequently he joined the Board of the Faculty and was Dean 1979–82.

The next appointments in the 1970s were Dr John Magner (MB, 1960), Dr Declan Tyrrell (MB, 1960; d. 2007) and Dr Denis Moriarty (MB, 1968). Dr Moriarty also had a special involvement in cardiac anaesthesia, having trained in London and worked as consultant in the National Heart and Brompton Hospitals. After his appointment to the staff of the Mater Hospital in 1976, he became lecturer in anaesthetics at University College, Dublin, and its first Professor of Anaesthetics in 1991. He joined the Board of the Faculty in 1980 and was chairman of its examination committee from 1986 through the formation of the new College of Anaesthetists until 2001, apart from his term as Dean of the Faculty 1988–91. He thus had an enormous influence on the shape of the Faculty's examinations, particularly the Final/Part III over this long period. This period saw the expansion of the Faculty and College in overseas teaching and examinations from Singapore and Kuala Lumpur in the East to the USA and Caribbean in the West.

The Dublin Children's Hospitals — During the first half of the twentieth century, specialist treatment for children was concentrated in the National Children's Hospital, Harcourt Street, and the Children's Hospital, Temple Street. In Harcourt Street, Dr Dorothea Bennett (MB, 1925; DA, Dub, 1943) and Dr Silver Dean-Oliver (MB, 1926; DA, Dub, 1943) were the main specialist anaesthetists, later joined by Dr Sheila Kenny and Dr Ray Davys of the Adelaide and Vincent's Hospitals. In Temple Street, the anaesthetists in the same period were Dr Ita Brady 1931–36 and Dr Patrick Nagle, also of the Mater Hospital, 1941–57. During the second half of the century, Our Lady's Hospital for Sick Children, Crumlin, became the main specialist centre for paediatric surgery and anaesthesia. Development of the specialty there was led by Dr William (Bill) Wren (MB, 1952; DA, Lond, 1954; d. 2006), who had trained at the Hammersmith and London Hospitals. He was Dean of the Faculty of Anaesthetists 1973–76 and was closely associated with the development of the

National Training Scheme. He it was who established the first purpose-built intensive care unit for infants and children. He was joined by Dr Kevin Moore (MB, 1961), who overcame severe problems of ill-health to play a large part in the Faculty and in organising higher training.

ANAESTHESIA IN BELFAST

The Royal Victoria Hospital and Group — It is clear from newspaper reports that Dr Alexander Gordon and Dr Horatio Stewart were using anaesthesia in the General Hospital in January 1847. Alexander Gordon became the first Professor of Surgery of Queen's College, and Horatio Stewart, who was later the first Professor of Materia Medica, may be regarded as the first anaesthetist of the hospital. Thereafter there were no official anaesthetists until 1900, when Dr Victor Felden and Mr Robert Johnstone were appointed to part-time honorary posts in the re-named Royal Victoria Hospital. By 1902, Robert Johnstone had moved to gynaecology (later to become professor) but Victor Felden remained the pillar of anaesthesia in the hospital for the rest of his working life.

Dr Victor Felden (1867–1946) was born in Plymouth but the family moved to Belfast when he was 15. He obtained the licentiate of the Pharmaceutical Society of Ireland (first place) in 1890 and graduated in medicine at Queen's College, Belfast, in 1892. After this, he was a demonstrator in pharmacy at Queen's College and retained a broad interest in the subject, helping Professor William Whitla for many years with his highly successful *Materia Medica* and *Dictionary of Treatment*. He was appointed to the honorary attending staff of the Royal Victoria Hospital in 1911 and obtained the MD of Queen's University in 1912 for a thesis on 'Ethyl chloride'. Subsequently he served in the Royal Army Medical Corps during the First World War and worked in the hospital until 1932. He also carried on a private practice in anaesthesia in the afternoons and was certainly the doyen of anaesthesia in this era. He is remembered as having favoured chloroform given with the semi-accurate Vernon Harcourt machine, throughout his career.

Two assistant anaesthetists were appointed to the hospital in 1923, Dr Olive Anderson (1894–1985), who worked from 1923 to 1944, and who obtained the MD by thesis in 1932, and Dr Stafford Geddes (*c.*1892–1969), who worked from 1923 to 1956. Both obtained the DA, Lond, in 1936. Neither was appointed to replace Victor Felden on the visiting staff, partly because anaesthetists had no equivalent to the FRCS (though not all surgeons had this), but mainly because it was thought inappropriate by the established surgeons and physicians. In fact, no women were appointed until the advent of the National Health Service in 1948 when Dr Stafford Geddes was also 'elevated'. Dr George Hamilton (1887–1967) combined general practice with anaesthesia in the hospital in 1935–52, taking the DA in Dublin in 1943. Probably the most notable of these pre-war anaesthetists was Dr John Boyd (1902–81), who was assistant anaesthetist at the Belfast Hospital for Sick Children from 1928 and at the Royal Victoria Hospital from 1937. He was given visiting status in the Sick Children's Hospital in 1945 and consultant status in both hospitals in 1948. He had obtained an MD for a thesis on 'Rectal avertin' in 1933, and the Dublin DA in 1943. He was a master of the blind nasal intubation in children, but had the eccentric belief that no patient should have ventilatory assistance after suxamethonium, on the grounds that this delayed the return of spontaneous respiration.

The real change in anaesthesia in the hospital came with the appointment of Dr Maurice Brown (1912–93; MB, 1931; DA, Lond, 1945) in 1946. He had served in the Royal Navy during the war and took up anaesthesia following disfigurement by severe facial burns. He trained in London under Dr Ivan Magill and worked mainly in thoracic anaesthesia. He was also the first Queen's University lecturer in anaesthesia, though this involved very little teaching, and that only of undergraduates. Other specialists in the 1950s were Dr James ('Minty') Bereen (1913–87; MB, 1937; DA, Lond, 1940), who, having trained in the Royal Army Medical Corps during the war, worked exclusively in neurosurgery from 1950 to 1977, and Dr James Elliott (1915–83; MB, 1938; DA, Lond, 1942), who was early in thoracic anaesthesia, managing some of the first thoracoplasties in Whiteabbey Hospital with Mr 'Barney' Purse [q.v.], at a time when blood transfusion was not available. He was on the staff of the Royal Victoria Hospital in 1954–80.

In 1958, a joint consultant/senior lecturer post in anaesthetics was created and Dr John Wharry Dundee (1921–91) was appointed. He had graduated at Queen's University and trained at Liverpool under the legendary Professor T. Cecil Gray, taking the MD in 1951 and the relatively new Fellowship of the Faculty of Anaesthetists of the Royal College of Surgeons (of England) in 1953. He consolidated his research experience in Philadelphia with the Liverpool PhD in 1957. In Belfast, he immediately created a vigorous programme of training and rotation for anaesthetists, which became a model for his own and most other specialties. He also began a programme of clinical research, at first continuing his own work on thiopentone, but gradually, in over 400 published papers, covering the whole range of pharmacology as it impinged on anaesthesia. He was appointed professor in 1964 and remained a prolific author and international lecturer even after he retired in 1986. He was a member of the first Board of the Faculty of Anaesthetics of the Royal College of Surgeons in Ireland in 1959, and was its fourth dean, 1969–73.

Dr Richard Clarke (MB, 1954) joined Professor Dundee in 1965 and combined a long-term involvement in intensive care and cardiac surgical anaesthesia with a steady output of human pharmacological research. Like John Dundee he was an examiner in the Irish Faculty for most of his career and was Dean of the Faculty from 1991 to 1994. He held a personal chair in the university from 1980 and was Professor and head of the department from 1988 until his retirement in 1994. His successor in the Chair, Dr Howard Fee (MB, 1972), was President of the College of Anaesthetists 2003–6.

Professor Dundee's other contribution to the hospital was the initiation of a Research Fellowship in intensive care from 1959 to 1961, which was filled by Dr Robert (Bob) Gray (MB, 1949; DA, Dub, 1953). His combination of perseverance and tact gradually overcame all resistance as the unit moved from a two-bedded room in the neurology ward, via an eleven-bed purpose-built unit in 1970 to the present twenty-five-bed unit in the 'new' (2001) Royal Victoria Hospital. Dr Gray remained senior consultant (later Director) of the unit until 1987. The work of the unit began with a high percentage of tetanus, poliomyelitis, polyneuritis and self-poisoning, but trauma took over in the worst period of 'the Troubles', and no one will forget the casualties from the Abercorn Restaurant bombing in 1972. However, even in this period, road traffic accidents (often alcohol-related) occupied as much bed space in the unit.

Apart from the pioneering career of Dr John Boyd already mentioned, few anaesthetists had more than a part-time and brief involvement in the Belfast Children's Hospital. Dr Harold Love (MB, 1945) was the first to make paediatric anaesthesia a life interest, being appointed to the Royal Victoria and Belfast Children's Hospitals in 1954. He had taken the Dublin DA in 1949, followed by the MD of Queen's University in 1952 and was Dean of the Irish Faculty 1976–79. Dr Gerald Black, who also became Dean of the Faculty of Anaesthetists of the RCSI 1982–85 and retired in 1990, joined Harold Love in 1962 in the Royal Victoria and Children's Hospitals. When Dr Samuel Keilty took up the post of consultant anaesthetist in the Children's Hospital in 1970, he became the first anaesthetist in Belfast to work exclusively in paediatrics.

Thoracic surgery was carried out in the Royal Victoria Hospital as well as a number of chest hospitals in the greater Belfast area, from the 1930s. Closed cardiac surgery (mainly mitral valvotomy) began in Belfast in 1950 and later, in the 1950s, closure of atrial septal defect under hypothermia was practised. Anaesthesia for these procedures involved Dr James Elliott during the 1940s and later Dr Maurice Brown and most of the senior anaesthetists. Progress was slow with open-heart surgery and was not really satisfactory until Mr Pat Molloy was appointed in 1968, with Dr Morrell Lyons (MB, 1960) providing full-time anaesthetic cover. This growing unit covered all forms of cardiac surgery, in adults and children, for the whole of Northern Ireland and had its own cardiac recovery unit (later Cardiac Surgical Intensive Care Unit). Morrell Lyons also found time to serve on the Board of the Faculty in Dublin and the Council of the Association of Anaesthetists of Great Britain and Ireland, becoming President of the latter 1994–96, the only anaesthetist practising in Ireland to do so.

The Belfast City Hospital — This hospital is derived from the old Belfast workhouse infirmary and fever hospital which existed on the site from 1838 to 1948 and seems to have had little need for anaesthetists for most of that period, though Dr James Lynass (MB, 1892) was appointed in the role in 1899. Surgery was certainly carried out in the pre-National Health Service era by Dr Joseph Fulton but it was probably on a small scale and under very poor conditions. The first professional anaesthetist was Dr John Dorman (MB, 1940; DA, Lond, 1941), who had trained with the Royal Army Medical Corps and in the Royal Berkshire Hospital and was appointed in 1948. The staff was slowly built up, with Dr James McNeilly (MB, 1947; DA, Dub, 1951; retired 1977) and Dr Thomas McErvel (MB, 1937; DA, Lond, 1949), who had served and trained, 1938–53, with the regular army, being appointed consultants in 1953. As well as a steady expansion in general surgery, the first renal transplants in Northern Ireland were carried out in 1968, involving a heavy anaesthetic workload for Dr John Cecil Hewitt (MB, 1938; DA, Lond, 1949) and Dr John P. Alexander (MB, 1954).

The Mater Infirmorum Hospital — This hospital dates from 1883, and remained an independent voluntary hospital until 1972 in spite of the advent of the

National Health Service. Unusually, as early as 1924, it appointed a full-time anaesthetist, Dr Claire McGuckin (MB, 1923), who had attended a course at the Hammersmith Hospital, run by Dr Ivan Magill. She relinquished the post when she married in 1928 and was followed by many short-term appointments before Dr John A. Macaulay (MB, 1937; DA, Irel, 1945; d. 1971) joined about 1941. Dr John Cooper (MB, 1954) was appointed consultant in 1965, joined the Board of the Faculty of Anaesthetists in 1984 and was Dean 1994–97.

The Ulster Hospital for Children and Women — This was founded in 1872 as a voluntary hospital for children, and only later became a general hospital. Until 1941, it was situated in Belfast on the east side of the river, but during the German air raids suffered a direct hit and was rebuilt in 1957 on a new site outside the city. Anaesthesia during the earlier period was conducted largely by the same anaesthetists as in the Royal Victoria Hospital, Dr Victor Felden and Dr Stafford Geddes. The first consultant anaesthetist appointed to the new hospital was Dr James Camac (Mac) Clarke (MB, 1949; DA, Dub, 1951). He planned the department from the outset and had a special skill with the engineering problems of anaesthesia. He was joined in 1962 by Dr William Bingham (MB, 1941; DA, Dub, 1947), who moved from Lurgan and later became the first treasurer of the Faculty of Anaesthetists.

ANAESTHESIA IN CORK

The first anaesthetist recorded is Dr Denis Donovan (O'Donovan) (LRCP, LRCS Edin, 1870), who combined anaesthesia in the North Infirmary with general practice. He was followed in the 1920s by Dr Denis Fennell (MB, 1919) and he by Dr John Finbarr O'Sullivan (MB, 1936), who also practised in the Cork Dental Hospital and was known as 'Jackie Gas'. Anaesthetists recorded in the South Infirmary include Dr Timothy Stanislaus (Stan) Reynolds (MB, 1918), Dr Edmund Donovan (MB, 1922), and Dr H. G. Birkhan, the last becoming Professor of Anaesthesia in the University of Haifa, Israel. Dr Walter Rahilly (O'Rahilly) (LRCPI, LRCSI, 1911) was anaesthetist and later surgeon at the Mercy Hospital, but gave up surgery when he won the Irish Sweepstake. Dr Victor Joseph Dillon (MB, 1934) was anaesthetist in the Bon Secours Hospital in the 1930s.

The first trained anaesthetist to practise in Cork was Dr Brendan Vincent Lyne (MB, 1944; DA, Dub, 1947), who had trained at the Royal Victoria

Hospital, Belfast, University College and Hammersmith Hospitals, London, and the Radcliffe Infirmary, Oxford, learning the use of thiopentone and blind and laryngoscopic intubation. He was anaesthetist to the Bon Secours Hospital 1947–49, but then emigrated to Auckland, New Zealand, where he took the Australasian FFA (1956) and the Irish FFA (1960). He was followed as visiting anaesthetist in the Bon Secours Hospital by Dr James Daniel Bourke (MB, 1943; DA, Lond, 1946), who had trained at the Edinburgh Royal Infirmary and introduced into Cork curare and 'total spinal block' for sympathectomy. He went on to Kilkenny and became a Freeman of that city. From there he moved away to become consultant in the Dudley Road and other hospitals in Birmingham.

Dr Eugene (Owen) Thomas (MB, 1941; DA, Lond, 1947) was appointed as anaesthetist in 1948 to the Regional Thoracic Surgical Unit, which was then the Mallow Chest Hospital, with Mr Maurice Hickey [q.v.] as surgeon. He had trained in the Central Middlesex Hospital and Sheffield Royal Infirmary and employed all the techniques of thoracic anaesthesia in use at the time, including intravenous anaesthesia and muscle relaxation, endotracheal and endobronchial intubation and endobronchial blocking. He was also involved with the team caring for patients needing ventilation during the major polio epidemic in Cork in 1956. He was elected first President of the newly formed South of Ireland Society of Anaesthetists (now Association of Anaesthetists) in 1955. The unit moved in that year to the newly opened Sarsfield Court Hospital and Dr Thomas moved to Birmingham in 1957 to be replaced, 1957–58, by Dr Arthur Moore before he settled in Galway. Both were using standard hypothermia for cardiac surgery in this period. Dr Maureen (Maura) O'Driscoll (MB, 1941; DA, Lond, 1950) was also consultant anaesthetist in this sub-specialty (made permanent in 1955).

Dr John Desmond Gaffney (LRCPI, LRCSI, 1944; DA, Dub, 1949) was appointed to the unit in 1960 and the next phase was to introduce profound hypothermia by the Drew technique, resulting in a paper to the Dublin meeting of the Association of Anaesthetists in 1961. He later became anaesthetist in administrative charge of the new Department of Anaesthesia, based first at St Finbarr's Hospital and then at the Cork Regional Hospital (now Cork University Hospital).

Dr Daniel (Don) Gerard Coleman (MB, 1946; DA, Dub, 1949) trained in Oxford and Liverpool and was appointed to the Mercy Hospital in 1950 and subsequently to the South Infirmary in 1955. He used spinal anaesthesia, which he had learned in Oxford, on a regular basis. Epidural anaesthesia for caesarean section was introduced by Dr Maurice (Mossie) Flynn (MB, 1948; DA, Dub, 1952), who was appointed to the Bon Secours Hospital in 1952. When he was joined by Dr John Gerard Casey (MB, 1954; DA, Lond, 1960) as a consultant anaesthetist in 1960, they established an epidural service for pain relief in labour.

The first purpose-built intensive care unit in Cork was opened with four beds at St Finbarr's Hospital in 1969. It was planned and operated by Mr Michael Patrick Brady [q.v.], Professor of Surgery, with the anaesthetists, Dr Talbot David Seigne (appointed in 1968) and Dr John Desmond Gaffney. Another two-bedded intensive care unit was opened in Bantry General Hospital in 1972 by Dr Derek McCoy, consultant physician.

What subsequently became a national service for the definitive diagnosis of malignant hyperthermia in patients and the identification of susceptible relatives was set up in 1979 by Dr James Heffron (later Professor) of the Biochemistry Department of University College, Cork, and Dr John Curran (MB, 1967), who was at that time consultant anaesthetist at the Cork Regional Hospital. Patients and relatives travelled to Cork from all over Ireland for muscle biopsy under general anaesthesia, and standardised halothane and caffeine contracture tests were carried out on the live muscle fibres in UCC.

In 1997, Professor George Shorten was appointed to a new Chair of Anaesthesia and Intensive Care Medicine at University College, Cork.

Anaesthesia in Galway

The first anaesthetist appointed officially to the old Central Hospital was Dr Sarah (Sally) O'Malley (*née* Joyce; MB, 1923) in 1943. Her husband was Dr Conor O'Malley [q.v.], an eye, ear, nose and throat surgeon also of the Central Hospital, and Sarah covered anaesthesia for these specialties in particular. She was followed by Dr James Thomas Bolger (MB, 1940), Dr Kevin Bernard Glynn (MB, 1943) and Dr Arthur Moore (MB, 1938; DA, Lond, 1948). Dr Moore, who had trained in Liverpool generally and in Broad Green Hospital for chest surgery, and had worked for a time with Dr Joseph Woodcock in Jervis Street, Dublin, was appointed to the Central Hospital in 1949. These were all on a voluntary appointment basis, working as general practitioners in the afternoons, but around this time sessional rates of payment were agreed and full-time practice of anaesthesia became possible. The first Boyle machines were also becoming available but it was still the practice to dilute the Novocaine tablets for spinal anaesthesia from water sterilised and held in a Winchester bottle from the beginning of the week. Dr Moore also worked in Castlerea Hospital, Co. Roscommon, where chest and mitral valve surgery were being carried out around 1950 by Mr Maurice Hickey [q.v.] and Mr Keith Shaw [q.v.].

In 1970, Dr Padraic Keane was appointed as the first full-time consultant anaesthetist to the Regional Hospital (which had replaced the Central Hospital) and Merlin Park (the medical and surgical chest unit), and lecturer in anaesthetics to University College, Galway. He had graduated at Galway in 1960, taken the Irish DA in 1964 and FFA RCS in 1967, followed by a year in Boston as Research Fellow and an MD of Galway University in 1970 for a thesis on 'The effects of Ketamine on the contractile element of isolated heart muscle'. He was thus well qualified to set up a new department involving both training and research. Subsequently he set up a six-month exchange programme between Galway and the Milwaukee Medical Centre, under Professor John Kampine, which gave three senior resident trainees a valuable introduction into research.

An intensive care unit was opened in 1972 in the Regional Hospital but it remained inadequate in size and staffing until 1978, when it was enlarged to seven beds. A hyperbaric oxygen unit was also set up in 1976 under the care of Dr Peter O'Beirn (d. c.1990), who had a special interest in underwater medicine. It was used not just for diving accidents, but also for patients with badly traumatised limbs, multiple sclerosis and other medical conditions, and members of the Galway Sub-aqua Club contributed to the care of patients needing the chamber. The same year (1976) also saw the foundation of the Western Anaesthetic Society and its Annual Symposium, a key event not only for the west of Ireland but for the whole island. Dr Keane played an important role as Treasurer of the Faculty of Anaesthetists in establishing its financial independence and was Dean of the Faculty 1985–88. In 1989, Dr Keane was appointed as the first Professor of Anaesthesia in the National University, Galway, a post which he held until his retirement in 2001. Dr John Laffey succeeded him in the Chair.

Note: I am grateful to Dr John Cooper, Dr Seamus Hart, Professor Padraic Keane, Dr Morrell Lyons, Professor Denis Moriarty and Ms Mary O'Doherty for their help with material.

CLARKE, Richard Samuel Jessop (Richard)

Belfast Anaesthetist

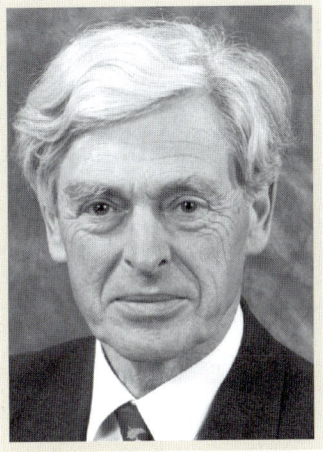

b. 1929, Elder son of Dr Brice R. Clarke (consultant chest physician) and Doreen Clarke (*née* Cassidy)
Educ. Royal Belfast Academical Institution; Queen's University Belfast
m. 1958, Elizabeth Kyle ('Kyleen') Colhoun, daughter of John Gordon Colhoun of Londonderry and Elsie Colhoun (*née* Roden); 1 s ; 2 d (Daughter Dr Anne Haigh of Livingston Scotland)

BSc (Hons) 1951, MB, QUB, 1954; MD 1958, FFA RCS Eng 1961; PhD Belfast 1969; FFA RCSI 1971

Postgraduate posts at Royal Victoria Hosp and St Bartholomew's Hospital, London (lecturer in physiology); member of scientific staff, Medical Research Council. Department of Human Anatomy, Oxford 1955–58, successively tutor, senior lecturer, reader, Professor of Clinical Anaesthetics and then Professor of Anaesthetics and Head of Department QUB 1988–94.
Consultant anaesthetist, Eastern Health Board, DHSS, NI. Special interest in cardiac and thoracic anaesthesia and in intensive care.
Dean of Faculty of Anaesthetics RCSI 1991–94. President, Section of Anaesthetics, Royal Society of Medicine, 1995–96.

Distinguished clinical and research anaesthetist with scores of publications. In retirement he became a polished medical historian. Honorary Archivist to the Royal Victoria Hospital, he produced a major work, *The Royal Victoria Hospital*, which was a master class of its kind. His affectionate biography of Sir Ian Fraser was exactly what the great man deserved.

He is keen naturalist and is a Trustee of the Ulster Historical Foundation. Author/editor of 31 volumes of 'Gravestone inscriptions', Down, Antrim and Belfast. He collects Irish maps, Worcester porcelain, and enjoys opera, gardening and walking. A man of culture and a cultured man, he is erudite over a wide range of subjects. A doting grandfather and a generous host.

Five foot seven, distinguished appearance with mane of white hair intact, he has admirable obsessions with getting things 'right' without descending into nit picking. A real scholar and a delightful companion.

23
RADIOLOGY

Prof. David McInerney

RADIOLOGY

The Dawn of Radiology

Radiology was born on the afternoon of Friday, 8 November 1895. Professor Wilhelm Conrad Röntgen was studying the effect of cathode rays, alone in his laboratory. In the darkened room, he noticed a faint glow from an object placed some distance away. This was a greenish light that varied with the discharges of an induction coil which he was using to produce cathode rays. He deduced that some radiation was coming from the tube and striking the barium platinocyanide screen, producing this light. For the next two months, Röntgen, alone in his laboratory, studied this radiation intensively. He produced the first radiograph of his wife's left hand with her wedding ring. By the end of 1895, Röntgen published a very comprehensive analysis of the properties of these new rays. In the proceedings of the Würzburg Physical Medical Society they were called X-rays because their nature was unknown.

Uniquely among medical specialties, radiology came into existence almost fully formed from the beginning. All over the world, in the year following Röntgen's discovery, there was an explosion of activity in radiologic imaging. No major medical discovery ever had so rapid an adoption as that of X-rays. In January 1896, the *Lancet* and *British Medical Journal* wrote of it. and it is also mentioned in the *Freeman's Journal* in Dublin in mid-January as 'newly-discovered light'. Over a thousand medical articles were published on the 'new rays' in 1896.

Early Radiology in Ireland

The physical instruments for generating X-rays were widely available in laboratories, and many scientists and doctors immediately set about duplicating

Röntgen's findings. The late Professor James Murray of UCG suggested that the first X-ray in Ireland was taken in Clongowes Wood College by Rev. Henry Gill, SJ. Medical radiographs are recorded in Ireland from several sources in 1896. These include Professor Barrett of the RCSI in Dublin, Dr Cecil Shaw [q.v.] in Belfast, Dr John O'Donnell in the Mater and W. S. Haughton [q.v.] in Sir Patrick Dun's and Dr Steevens' Hospital. In Dr Steevens' Hospital, Professor Barrett located a broken needle which had been in a girl's hand for over two years; Surgeon McCausland successfully removed it. This case was published in the *British Medical Journal* in March 1896. In this month also, W. S. Haughton in Sir Patrick Dun's had acquired his own X-ray equipment, becoming the first Irish radiologist.

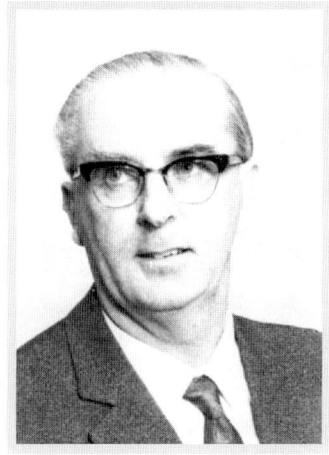

Professor James Murray

In the beginning, hospitals thought X-rays of no great importance, assigning the process little space or equipment. Physicians who wished to practise radiology often had to purchase the equipment and operate it themselves. Nevertheless, within a year or two, there were many hospitals utilising X-rays regularly, both on hospital patients and on patients referred by outside doctors. In the Mater in Dublin, the first X-ray department was established under the cupola of the roof of the hospital, uniquely as most other departments were in the basement of hospitals.

The clinical utilisation of radiology in Ireland was led by W. S. Haughton, who lectured and published extensively. He developed the use of dental radiology. One of his students, a Major Battersby, utilised his equipment in treating casualties in the course of the war in Sudan in 1898. While practising radiology, Haughton continued as a surgeon throughout his life. His great achievements were recognised by his election as first President of the Radiological Society of Ireland, in 1932, and by the international annual award of the Haughton medal by the Faculty of Radiologists invited radiologists who have achieved an international reputation. Haughton's student, Dr E. J. M. Watson, practised radiology at Sir Patrick Dun's Hospital in 1900 and subsequently also in the Richmond and Adelaide Hospitals.

In the Meath Hospital, Richard Lane Joynt commenced radiology in 1896 and, like Haughton, continued also as a surgeon until his death in 1928. In St Vincent's Hospital, J. S. McArdle [q.v.] obtained X-ray equipment in 1896. In a court case in 1904, he observed that he had been performing domiciliary consultations outside Dublin and taking radiographs. J. N. Meenan was appointed in 1905 to St Vincent's Hospital to direct a purpose-built X-ray department. He had an interest in the radiology of gunshot wounds.

In Dr Steevens' Hospital, Walter Clegg Stephenson was appointed X-ray officer in 1904, but continued also as a surgeon. Although most of the early radiologists were surgeons, the Adelaide Hospital appointed Geoffrey Harvey, a physician, in 1905. He had an interest in radiology of the chest and the use of contrast media for gastrointestinal examination. He was 'to undertake the duties of Surgical Pathologist and to take entire charge of the X-ray Department at an annual salary of 26 guineas per annum'. This was unusual because at that time radiologists were generally unpaid and indeed often had to provide their own equipment. In Jervis Street Hospital, Dr Henry W. Mason was appointed in 1909, on condition that he provide his own apparatus and supply it gratis to the department. In 1912, Dr Garret Hardman was appointed to the Richmond, Adelaide and Baggot Street Hospitals, and in 1913 Dr O'Hea was appointed to St Vincent's.

In Cork, the first radiographs were taken in Queen's College in 1896. A surgeon in the North Infirmary, C. Y. Pearson [q.v.] directed an X-ray department and also opened a second department in the Victoria Hospital.

The first full-time radiologist was Dr Maurice Hayes, appointed as 'Medical Electrician' to the Mater Hospital in 1907. He is recorded in the minute book of 1907 as 'to be Medical Electrician Dr Maurice Hayes'. Hayes was interested in localising foreign bodies in the orbits because of a childhood injury which left him with monocular vision. He was appointed in 1922 as Director General of the Irish Army Medical Corps and, within nine months, had organised a medical service for the National Army, after which he returned to his practice. Dr John Geraghty succeeded Dr Hayes. Geraghty was the first radiologist with a formal qualification in radiology, appointed to the Mater in 1926 with the DMRE of Cambridge University, a qualification which had been established in 1920. In Galway, Dr Conor O'Malley was appointed to the Central Hospital in 1928 and was succeeded in 1932 by Dr W. J. McHugh who had obtained a diploma in radiology in Newcastle, around 1928.

In the early days, X-ray exposures were quite prolonged. It is recorded that for a kidney examination, Dr Watson in the Adelaide Hospital would switch on, say the Eton Grace, and switch off, the results being reasonable for those days and capable of demonstrating calculi.

In Belfast, Dr John Rankin was appointed to the Royal Victoria Hospital in 1903 and was publishing scientific articles on radiology in 1906. In 1919, Dr Maitland Beath was appointed to the RVH.

The Development of Radiology in Ireland

Steady incremental development took place in radiology in the decade following Röntgen's discovery. Gradually the features of a modern X-ray department emerged. Radiology moved away from medical photography and the hospital electrician and came under medical direction. It ceased to be the hobby of a small group of enthusiastic doctors and became the full-time professional occupation of specially trained physicians. It ceased also to be one of the minor duties of the harassed surgical registrar. No longer were radiologists expected to work gratis and supply their own equipment. Hospitals moved to invest in premises and equipment. Substantial budgets were allocated. Instead of X-ray apparatus being built ad hoc from generic electromagnetic items, great international companies set about the design and provision of X-ray equipment of increasing capacity.

It took a long time for radiology to be fully recognised as a separate and distinct discipline. Until mid-century many doctors, particularly chest physicians and orthopaedic surgeons, would have their own X-ray equipment in their rooms. In due course, speed and quality issues and the wish to avail of specialist expertise persuaded them to locate all imaging facilities under the umbrella of the Radiology Department.

Dr Thomas Eustace was appointed to the Mater Hospital in 1934. He was the first Irish radiologist to obtain the Fellowship in London, in 1935.

An X-ray examination from that time is described by an Adelaide nurse from the 1930s: 'alarming stories of the crowds of staff and students packing into that small area to see a barium meal examination in the darkened room — sparks flying everywhere'.

Records in Jervis Street describe the building and equipment by Dr Mason of the X-ray Department in 1927, all taking place within one year and costing less than £2,500. Not content with this achievement, Dr Mason raised the money by running a successful dance during Horse Show Week in 1928.

Dr Maitland Beath was appointed in 1919 to the Royal Victoria Hospital and later to the Belfast Union Infirmary, which became the City Hospital. He subsequently became President of the British Association of Radiologists and was associated with the formation of the Faculty of Radiologists in the UK. His partner, Dr (later Sir) Frank T. Montgomery, succeeded him. At the Mater Hospital in Belfast, Dr Colm Kelly was appointed in 1946. Dr James Owen Cole was appointed to the Royal Victoria Hospital in 1958 and was elected Dean of the Faculty of Radiologists, 1977–79. Colonel Desmond Whyte had had a distinguished military career in the Far East when he was appointed to Altnagelvin Hospital in 1954. He had a strong influence on the graduates of the School of Radiography established there in 1958, whose training under his direction was considered of the highest quality.

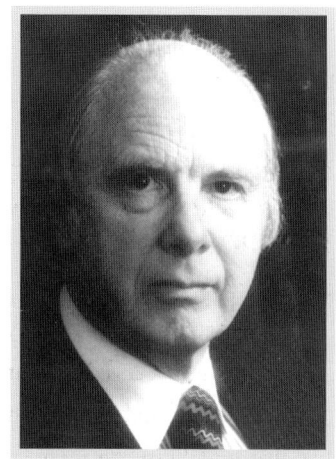

Dr James Owen Cole

Until mid-century specialist services in radiology were limited outside the teaching centres of Dublin, Cork and Galway. In Galway, the Regional Hospital was opened in 1956 and major radiology upgrading took place there and in Merlin Park Hospital and Portiuncula. In 1948, in Limerick, Kevin McMahon became radiologist at Barrington's Hospital, and John Wallace practised in Tralee in 1954.

In 1951, a group of regional radiologists was appointed, initially for the South Eastern and North Eastern regions. Seven posts were filled, including Dr J. J. O Connell and Dr Ken Reynolds in the south, Dr Mervin Clarke in the northwest, Dr Michael Loughlin in the midlands, Dr James McLoughlin in the midwest and Dr Jack Hurley in the northeast, which indeed also included north Donegal. These newly appointed radiologists had very heavy workloads, onerous travelling obligations and had to upgrade and even establish new radiology departments, all this at a time of scarce resources and economic depression. It is to their credit that all the radiologists appointed at that time remained in their posts until retirement, despite the difficulties.

The Radiological Society of Ireland

The Radiological Society of Ireland was established in 1932. It was the precursor of the Faculty of Radiologists. W. S. Haughton was elected President and Dr M. O'Hea was elected Honorary Secretary and Honorary Treasurer. The society was registered legally with memorandum and articles of association. The society sent a delegation to the fourth International Congress of Radiology, at Zürich, in 1934. A joint annual meeting was conducted with the British Faculty of Radiologists in Dublin in 1955, under the presidency of Dr Peter Kerley, a graduate of UCD. Dr Kerley was editor of the major radiology textbook of that time, *A Textbook of Radiology by British Authors*. The Society established a section of radiology at the Royal Academy of Medicine in 1955. Over time, the membership of the society increased from the original sixteen to thirty-eight in 1967. The society prepared reports on many areas of radiology, submitting them to the government.

The Radiological Society held joint meetings with the Ulster Radiological Society in 1965 and 1970, and with the Scottish Radiological Society in 1967. Most of the functions of the society over time became the province of the Faculty until, by the end of the century, the society survived solely as a negotiating body for radiologists in discussion with the authorities on financial and contractual matters

Past Presidents, Radiological Society of Ireland

1932	Professor W. Haughton	1976	Dr McCarthy
1952	Dr M. O'Hea	1979	Dr J. C. Carr
1954	Dr W. McHugh	1983	Dr B. Hourihane
1956	Sir Frank Montgomery	1986	Dr N. Blake
1958	Dr J. S. Boland	1988	Dr J. Daly
1960	Dr O'Farrell	1990	Dr J. Masterson
1962	Dr W. McHugh	1993	Dr E. Breathnach
1964	Dr D. O'Sullivan	1998	Dr D. McInerney
1967	Dr O. Cole	2002	Dr F. McGrath
1970	Dr Henderson	2005	Dr D. O'Keeffe
1972	Dr S. Douglas	2007	Dr M. O'Driscoll
1974	Dr P. McCann		

The Faculty of Radiologists

A committee of the Radiological Society of Ireland, chaired in 1960 by Dr Desmond Riordan, proposed that the society should form a Faculty of Radiologists in association with the Royal College of Surgeons. The standing orders of the Faculty of Radiologists state that the objectives of the Faculty are (1) to advance the science, art and practice of radiology and of allied sciences and (2) to promote education, study and research in radiology. Dr Desmond Riordan was appointed first Dean. A radiotherapist, he was director of St Anne's Hospital, Dublin, and a Council member of the College of Surgeons. Dr S. J. Boland of St Vincent's Hospital was appointed Vice-Dean and Dr Finbar Cross, a radiotherapist at St Luke's Hospital, was appointed Honorary Secretary.

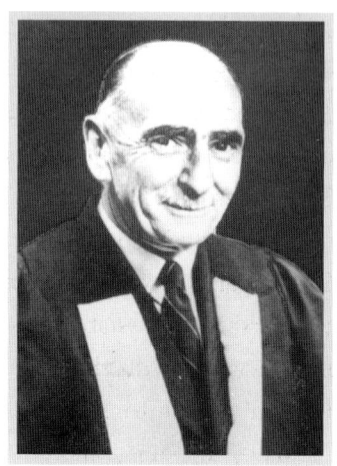

Dr Desmond Riordan

The Faculty commenced its academic programme with undergraduate lectures in radiology at the College of Surgeons. A training programme in radiology was set up and the first examinations held in 1966. Details of the training scheme were negotiated with the Department of Health, and Dr Malachy Powell chaired the co-ordinating committee. The course for Fellowship was four years, with the candidate taking the DMRD examination of the conjoint board in London after two years. Physics teaching was provided by Dr John O'Connor of St Luke's Hospital. Following negotiations with the London College, reciprocal recognition was achieved with London for the Primary Fellowship Examination and it was also agreed that part II of the Fellowship examination should be *ex-aequo* with the London Fellowship. These negotiations were conducted by the then Dean, Dr Dermot Cantwell, with the Warden of the London College, Professor Robert Steiner, who was a graduate of UCD from the 1940s. At the time, this recognition gave strong support to the development of radiology training in Ireland. In subsequent years, the Faculty training programme has become the training programme of choice of Irish medical graduates, as radiology itself has become one of the most sought-after sub-speciality training positions.

There has been a substantial and increasing contribution by Fellows of the Faculty at national and international meetings. Fellows have been elected or appointed to major positions in many international associations. A programme of radiology training in developing countries has been conducted since the later 1970s. At the present time, a complete programme of radiology training is conducted in Kuwait, in association with the Kuwait Institute of Medical Specialisation. This involves Faculty members being invited to Kuwait to teach and to hold the part I and part II examinations in Kuwait. A Third World Scholarship, in memory of the late Dr Dara O'Halpin, The O'Halpin-Linders Scholarship, was established in 2005. At present, this programme is conducted in association with the University of Nairobi in Kenya and involves funding a Kenyan doctor to Ireland every year to carry on a full training course in radiology for four years.

Radiology has now become an integral part of medical teaching both for medical students and in postgraduate courses. Radiologists participate as teachers of anatomy and pathology. There are professorial Chairs in Dublin, Cork, and Galway.

In addition to undergraduate, postgraduate and sub-specialty training, the Faculty conducts scientific meetings and invites international figures to lecture to its Fellows. The Faculty's major scientific meeting is held at the end of September and consists of original scientific research by Faculty members and trainees, presentation of review papers and invited lectures from international figures. Honorary Fellowships are conferred on invited radiologists of distinction. In 1962, the Faculty conferred Honorary Fellowships on Dr Peter Kerley, Dr Rohan Williams, and Sir Frank Montgomery. In 2006, Honorary Fellowship was conferred on the President of Ireland, Mrs Mary McAleese. A further meeting is held outside Dublin in spring each year. Sub-specialty groups associated with the Faculty in nuclear medicine, paediatrics, breast radiology and interventional radiology conduct their meetings in association with the Faculty also. A management meeting is held in February each year and there is a further meeting in association with radiographers, physicists and other associated professional groups.

Past Deans of the Faculty of Radiologists

1961–64	Dr D. Riordan
1964–67	Dr S. Boland
1967–70	Dr O. Chance
1970–73	Dr W. MacHugh
1973–75	Dr D. O'Sullivan
1975–77	Dr D. Cantwell
1977–79	Dr O. Cole
1979–81	Dr M. Ryan
1981–83	Dr P. McCann
1983–85	Dr N. O'Connell
1985–87	Dr J. Carr
1987–89	Professor M. O'Halloran
1989–92	Dr M. Daly
1992–94	Dr G. Hurley
1994–96	Professor D. MacErlaine
1996–98	Dr A. O Dwyer
1998–2000	Dr J. Masterson
2000–02	Dr L. Johnston
2002–04	Dr D. Mc Inerney
2004–06	Dr E. Breatnach
2006–08	Professor P. McCarthy

Academic Work of the Faculty

Library and study facilities are provided in the Mercer's Unit of the College of Surgeons and they are regularly upgraded, together with the purchase of audiovisual aids, film, museums, textbooks and journals. The Faculty training programme in radiology is conducted over five years. Candidates are selected after public advertisement and interview. About fourteen places are available each year. These places are in the teaching hospitals in Dublin, Cork and Galway, associated with the university medical schools. Following an intensive course, including physics, radiography and techniques, the part I Fellowship examination is taken at the end of the first year. After a further two and a quarter years, the Fellowship examination is taken. A programme of sub-specialty training for a fifth year is then provided in the teaching hospitals.

Research occupies a central role in radiology. A casual perusal of the medical literature confirms the importance of radiological imaging in medical science. Radiology trainees are expected to participate from the beginning in research, and to publish. The research committee of the Faculty of Radiologists invites applications for funding from trainees and advises on research methods. John Henry of the Physics Department of Queen's College, Galway, was awarded a grant for two years by Eastman Kodak in 1896 for research into X-ray photography. What appears to be the first Research Fellowship in Ireland, if not in the UK, was awarded in 1896 in Galway.

The Faculty recognised the importance of formal evaluation of continuing medical education, with the establishment of a CME committee in 1994. A voluntary programme of CME recording and regulation was set up to assess Faculty and other meetings for CME. Together with the other postgraduate faculties, ongoing discussion continues with the Medical Council and the Department of Health in relation to a national CME programme.

In Europe, the Faculty officers have been involved for many years with the European Association of Radiology (EAR), now subsumed into the European Society of Radiology, (ESR). A former Dean, Dr Gerard Hurley, was President of the EAR in 2005. Many faculty officers hold or have held significant posts in radiology associations in Europe.

Regulation of Imaging with Ionising Radiation

Many of the pioneers of radiology in the early days suffered severe burns to exposed areas, particularly their hands. The potential dangers of radiation burns first came to notice in Ireland with a court case in February 1904. A young boy who had frequent examinations to locate a needle, which was thought to be in his knee, subsequently developed an ulcer with scarring at the site of radiation. The danger of radiation was soon recognised and, in due course, statutory regulations were established.

Conscious of the hazards of radiation, the Radiological Society in Ireland, in 1957, set up a sub-committee under Dr John Geraghty to prepare recommendations for the protection of patients and staff. In Ireland, St Luke's Hospital in the 1950s commenced a personal dosimetry programme. In 1970, the National Radiation Monitoring Service was formally established. Its functions were assumed in 1992 by the Radiological Protection Institute of Ireland (RPII), which replaced the Nuclear Energy Board.

Radiology and Technology

The discipline of radiology has always been dependent on technological advances. This pace of change quickened noticeably in the 1960s and has accelerated to a remarkable degree since then. From the 1960s onwards, there has been a series of major organisational and technical changes, which have completely altered the face of radiology.

To begin with, in the 1960s, the image intensifier replaced the dark-room fluoroscope. From the earliest days of radiology, fluoroscopy was carried out by direct examination of a fluoroscopic screen in a dark room, the radiologist having adapted his eyes to the dark by wearing red plastic goggles throughout the day. Electronic enhancement of the fluoroscopic image, with projection onto a television screen, now allowed fluoroscopy to be carried out in daylight. This made it easier to use instrumentation in the course of intervention procedures directed by fluoroscopy. Automatic film processing replaced the older hand-operated photographic methods. This led to a great increase in the speed of radiographic throughput.

Hounsfield's discovery of computerised tomographic (CT) scanning was in 1973. Commencing in the late 1970s, magnetic resonance imaging had developed greatly by the late 1980s. Positron emission tomographic (PET) scanning and the development of molecular imaging came late in the 1990s. All these technological advances were underpinned by the information revolution brought about by computer technology. There is constant striving for the ideal of specialist diagnosis occurring in real time, thereby having the greatest impact on patient care.

A combination of flexible catheters and instruments, together with the use of contrast medium, led over time to the sub-specialty of intervention radiology, in which procedures of increasing complexity are carried out. In recent years, great advances have been made in therapeutic procedures where minimally invasive procedures have replaced what previously were complex operations.

From the beginning, researchers sought to improve their images by using chemical agents to enhance photographic contrast. The earliest intravenous contrast medium was unmodified iodide salt. Administered intravenously in small quantities, these were very hazardous and gave only faint opacification of the renal tract. By mid-century, complex organic iodides became available, with a much greater capacity to opacify, though these still had some significant hazard. Later, the development of non-ionic and isotonic contrast media has made parenteral administration safer. These are not completely hazard-free, however, and administration in very large volumes may still be attended by occasional mortality. The traditional bismuth and then barium contrast media used for gastrointestinal opacification reached their apex in the 1970s and 1980s but are now much less used, as endoscopy has taken over many of these studies. Similarly biliary tract contrast medium, always more troublesome than angiographic contrast, has been replaced by other methods of biliary evaluation. More exotic procedures which used air or other gases as contrast media up to the 1970s (such as retro-peritoneal air insufflation and air encephalography) now belong to history.

Ultrasound was the first of the major new imaging technologies, appearing in the 1970s, inspired by wartime localisation of hostile vessels, using sonar. The early ultrasound apparatus required the same type of electronic support as the early computers but the equipment has become perfected and miniaturised with the progress of technology. Moderate portable ultrasound is now available to be brought to the patient's bedside. Because of its low cost, ease of use and absence of ionising radiation or other hazards, ultrasound will become more and more widely used as a primary diagnostic tool.

Following Hounsfield's invention of CT in 1973, the first CT scanner in Ireland was installed in the old Richmond Hospital (now relocated to Beaumont Hospital), where national neurological services were then located. There was huge demand for the service. As time passed, it became obvious that much more extensive CT provision was required, and eventually CT equipment was provided in virtually every acute hospital in the country. Higher resolution and greater speed have extended the scope of this technique and now CT coronary angiography is moving to replace traditional catheter studies.

As with CT, magnetic resonance imaging started with a single national installation, and considerable time elapsed before there was wider provision. There was such great demand for MR that a sub-committee of radiologists was established in the late 1970s, with staff of the Richmond and some outside hospitals, to monitor requests for examinations from all over the country. By the end of the century, MR services were available in most acute hospitals in the country, in many places provided by a mobile service. MR imaging has had a major impact throughout medicine but in particular on neurological and musculoskeletal practice.

The provision of PET scanning requires proximity to a cyclotron to generate the isotope, and the first cyclotron was located in the Blackrock Clinic. PET scanners are now established or planned in several major teaching hospitals and it is clear that this technique will be the frontier of imaging in the early decades of the twenty-first century.

The traditional X-ray department was located in the basement and characterised by huge filing rooms for films and a pervasive odour from the thiosulphate and other chemicals used for processing. Digital technology has done away with all of this. The entire archive of a major teaching hospital can now be stored electronically in a small cabinet and retrieved instantly through picture archiving and communications systems (PACS). These systems are linked through the hospital information system and with the radiology information system and there is progress towards a completely electronic patient record (EPR). The first completely filmless PACS installation was in Tallaght Hospital, opened in 1998.

Radiology Staffing

The Faculty of Radiologists has worked tirelessly to ensure that radiology posts are properly structured, that the value of radiology is recognised and that appointees are properly trained. Since its inception, the Faculty has constantly reminded the health authorities of the relatively low numbers of radiologists in post in Ireland, by international standards, and has published several manpower surveys. The Faculty has encouraged the establishment of many extra posts. Through the Postgraduate Medical and Dental Board (PGMDB), the Faculty has obtained funds and official support to increase the numbers in training in Ireland in radiology. Comhairle and the PGMDB have now been absorbed into the Health Services Executive (HSE), which is proposing to take a much more active part in postgraduate training than heretofore. It is to be hoped that future structures will continue to give the Faculty the central role in radiology training that it has had up to the present.

Appointment to the public service of a radiologist in Ireland requires possession of the Fellowship of the Faculty or equivalent specialist qualification, possession of a recognised basic medical degree, and a minimum of five years of accredited training in radiology. Radiologists who have trained abroad and who wish to work in Ireland apply to the Medical Council, which seeks the advice of the Faculty in relation to accreditation of training.

Radiology has travelled quite a distance since earlier times when clinicians were expected to be able to do their own radiology. Competence in radiology was required as a qualification for clinical posts both in surgery and medicine even as late at 1962. Only the difficult cases might be referred to the radiologists.

The institution of the Health Boards and the setting up of Comhairle na nOspidéal in the 1970s led to a more planned development of radiology staffing on a national basis. Each of the health boards had a major regional hospital in which a cadre of experienced radiologists was built up, allowing the development of specialty interests. The closure of many small hospitals in the 1980s, particularly in Dublin, led to a similar process through centralisation.

The Future of Radiology

What of the future of radiology? The traditional radiologist was a generalist and a diagnostician who examined patients referred by medical colleagues. Now the field of radiology is far too wide to be comprehended by one person. Staging of disease and assessment of response to treatment are required in addition to diagnosis. Finally, in some interventional areas, radiologists are becoming primary treating physicians, having beds allocated, and doing their own ward rounds. Traditional radiology has become the victim of its own success.

For much of the twentieth century, radiologists strove to bring all medical imaging under one roof. Surgeons and physicians came to recognise the advantages of centralising the location of complex equipment and encouraging the development of specialist expertise in imaging. The process of sub-specialisation continues, yet a countertide of differentiation and separation of the imaging sub-specialties also exists. In addition, the boundary with interventional radiology and image-assisted surgery is very fluid. In the past, radiotherapy was separated from radiology. At present, some radiology sub-specialties are differentiating to a greater or lesser extent both in Europe and in the United States. This is occurring with interventional radiology and neuroradiology. In Ireland, while the great majority of radiologists remain generalists, most now have sub-specialty interests, and these are becoming more pronounced with the passage of time.

The wide availability of radiological equipment, particularly where non-ionising radiation is involved, has encouraged clinical disciplines to learn to use them. This has occurred particularly with ultrasound. Some clinical disciplines such as cardiology now have major diagnostic imaging involvement. Nuclear medicine and imaging is practised as a separate discipline in many countries.

The development of teleradiology means that sub-specialty evaluation of images can be made promptly available from distant centres. Teleradiology reduces the necessity for on-site availability of the radiologist. The demand for immediate radiology reporting has led in America to the situation where, in large hospitals, radiologist staff may rotate to offices on the opposite side of the globe so that overnight radiology reporting can be provided in real time by a radiologist working in daytime, for example, in Australia. Teleradiology also allows overseas radiology reporting in countries where there is unclear and perhaps less supervision of standards, and this is a matter of concern at a time when there is a tide of commercialisation in medicine. The maintenance of traditional professional structures in radiology and medicine generally becomes more difficult in these circumstances. There is a movement also for non-medically trained specialists, chiefly radiographers and physicists, to carry out direct reporting of medical images.

What is certain is that radiology will be in the forefront of scientific and medical advances and that its practitioners will have an exciting and fulfilling professional career.

McINERNEY, David Patrick (David)

A Dublin Radiologist

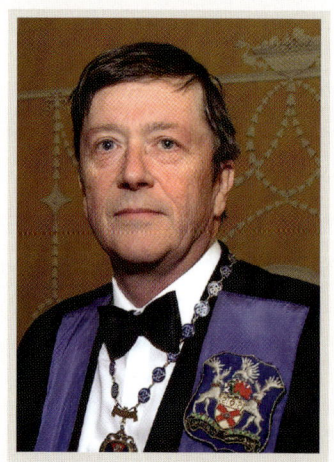

b. 1946, second son of Michael and Bernadette (*née* McGrath) McInerney.
Educ. Christian Brothers Schools, Synge Street, Dublin; University College Dublin
m. 1969: Maire McNeill, daughter of Patrick and Catherine McNeill. 3 s (two engineers and one lawyer)

MB, UCD, 1969; MRCPI, 1972; MRCP, UK, 1973; FRCR, 1976; MD, 1978; FFRCSI, 1981; FRCPI, 1982.

Postgraduate general medical training St Vincent's Hospital and St James's Hospitals, Dublin 1969–73. Commenced radiology training course in Dublin 1973 and moved to Bristol 1974–77.
Lecturer in radiology, Flinders Medical Centre, Adelaide, South Australia 1977–78. Influenced at Bristol by Howard Middlemiss (a towering figure in the specialty) and Rhys Davis. Consultant radiologist, Federated Dublin Voluntary Hospitals and St James's 1978. Attended Dr Steevens's Hospital, Meath and Adelaide Hospitals prior to move to Tallaght Hospital 1998.

Special interests in skeletal and spinal radiology, mammography and computerised applications of radiology.
Dean, Faculty of Radiologists RCSI 2002–04.

Formerly UCD oarsman. Coarse golf and tennis. Enjoys Brahms, Beethoven and Dvorak as well as modern history. David is understated on first impression, but the RCSI firmly advised the editor: 'If you want to get something done get David McInerney.' (They were right.) He enjoys teaching and feels fortunate to have worked through a 'golden age of radiology'. A dedicated family man, he and his charming wife tramp the hills of the west of Ireland when they get a chance. He dislikes clutter and is on record as suggesting that if Santa Claus came to his home he would be delighted if he would remove a couple of sackfuls. An amiable, admirable professional.

AFTERWORDS

It is difficult to summarise this book. It is the story of surgery in a small island with little in the way of natural resources. For most of the century the whole island was poor. In 1900 the gross national product per head of population was less than two-thirds of that of Great Britain. The northeast, centred on Belfast, prospered until about 1930, but the remainder remained poor by all measurable standards until the 1990s. It was said that Ireland was a failed Scotland. This relative poverty was reflected in the quality of the health services. As a measure it has been said that the infant mortality in Dublin (the Dublin of James Joyce's *Ulysses* in 1904) was worse than that of Calcutta.

There were six medical schools but in the first seventy-five or eighty years perhaps 75 per cent of graduates emigrated permanently. They could not make a living in such a depressed country. Up to 1948 there were two kinds of hospitals in Northern Ireland, Voluntary Hospitals and Local Authority Hospitals. The well-to-do went to nursing homes for surgery. The Royal Victoria Hospital, Belfast was by some distance the largest and best hospital in the island. Dublin had three medical schools but surgery was spread over at least nine voluntary institutions with a deep sectarian divide and absolutely no attempt at co-operation on any issue.

Hospitals are expensive to run. Presently (2008) an acute hospital needs five employees for every in-patient. This is one reason why they are more expensive than hotels, which run on a ratio of less than one employee per resident. Public hospitals are still being designed and built without en suite bathroom facilities, which is one of the principal reasons patients go into private accommodation. The much praised, entirely governmental, Canadian Health

Service does not allow any competing private insurance scheme except for issues such as private hospital accommodation. The health services in Great Britain and Ireland do not allow choice of surgeon, place of surgery or a choice of timing for the intervention. In most of Europe and North America the reverse is true. Here most areas and specialties have only about one-third of the specialists required to give around-the-clock, around-the-year service with adequate time for teaching and some research, as well as managerial responsibilities. Surgeons overwhelmed by the sheer numbers of patients for whom they have responsibility cannot be expected to fill other roles.

Patients who benefit from hospital treatment, particularly life-saving treatment, will return again with the same or other complaints until they die. As more and more can be done for patients they are living longer and longer, receiving further forms of treatment, often using high-cost technology. 'Old age does not come alone.' This is part of the reason why there are crowded Emergency Medicine departments with many patients on trolleys waiting for admission and cure. And then the cycle starts again. 'Everybody wants to go to Heaven but nobody wants to die.' Nobody wants to hear of it but even Lazarus died in the end.

In the second half of the twentieth century both parts of the island of Ireland had inherited a system of surgical staffing based on the British model. There was a multiplication of junior 'trainee' posts, which were initially filled by local British and Irish graduates. As the number of consultant surgeons more than trebled in those fifty years each one looked for a 'team' of trainees. There simply weren't enough doctors to fill the posts but on the other hand there were thousands of English-speaking doctors – eligible for British and Irish Medical Registration – from the Indian subcontinent anxious to get some training and avail of the much higher salaries. Their courtesy and industry were bywords even if sometimes there were communication and cultural divides. In the last years of the century trainees' payment for overtime sometimes exceeded the salary. Many were simply economic migrants seeking a better life for themselves and their families. The editor was one such when he went to England in 1949 with no prospect of returning to Ireland.

The 'entitlement' to a 'team' of assistants now appears enshrined in new consultants' expectations. It can only continue if we go on welcoming 'international' (the new politically correct word) graduates. India, Pakistan and

Bangladesh have a combined population of over 1.5 billion and they also need doctors. As President of the British, Canadian and Irish Medical Associations the editor visited New Delhi in 1977 for a meeting of the Commonwealth Medical Association (don't ask). When he was introduced to the Oxford-educated Prime Minister Mrs Indira Ghandi, she said directly and loudly, 'We don't want *you* here. You are taking all our best people.' It is impossible to forget this remark and its implications.

As long as we have a ratio of more than two 'trainees' to one consultant, more than half of the surgery, even on patients with private insurance in a public hospital bed, will be performed by these 'trainees'. Close supervision is often impossible and it would be naïve to believe that all the results are no different from those of a consultant. There has been little effort to train operative assistants who are not medically qualified and new 'infill' grades are resisted by the medical and nursing professions.

The government is reluctant to increase consultant numbers because the teams they need are so expensive, but increased numbers are what the public wants. A retired secretary of the Department of Health told the editor that within two years a new hospital surgeon generates costs of ten times his/her salary. Intensive care is expensive care.

Despite the free labour market in Europe the language barrier is often bigger than the hurdle of medical registration. There are almost no international doctors in mainland Europe and Scandinavia. Consequently there are many more specialists. The USA, after many years of raising the bar against 'international graduates', is now largely dependant on them for care outside the most elite of teaching institutions. As an example, more than half the doctors in the local medical society in Fort Worth, Texas (population over 650,000) are international graduates. So the doctor shortage problem is no longer just a rural phenomenon.

The next issue is subspecialisation. This is happening all the time and affects even commonly performed intermediate-level operations. Foot surgeons get better results with hallux valgus (which the public see as a small operation on a big toe) than general orthopaedic surgeons because they do more. Collective reviews of recurrence following repair of inguinal hernia remains anchored at about ten per cent, with specialist clinics reporting figures of just over one per cent. Patients want perfection all the time. The dilemma of urgent major surgery on a potentially lethal condition, such as a leaking aortic aneurysm, in the hands of someone who hasn't seen one for a year, does not bear thinking about. More specialists and subspecialists per capita provide better health care. It's as linear as that.

An important and increasing cultural issue is the ever-higher numbers of surgeons who marry other doctors or have doctors as partners. Both want full- or part-time posts within a reasonable radius of one another. If the locality cannot provide these posts they simply won't go to that locality. With a combined income of, at the very least, €350,000 further incentives are difficult to provide. Lifestyle, duty hours, as well as career paths, are increasing considerations.

BETTER LEFT UNSAID

The Brief Biographies do not provide a complete picture of the subjects. No biography does. There is no finality. Remember that was an all-male world. These men were dealing with life and death all the time. And in the early years there was much more death and despair because of how little could be done. Between themselves there was, then as now, a certain irreverence, some of it resembling locker room banter. Competition for practice was much more acute and mild backbiting even more common.

In the present book there are various constraints on the Brief Biographies, mainly involving issues of taste rather than legal grounds. Halos are tilted, sometimes quite askew. The phrases, if attached to an appropriate name, are all defensible, and in the case of those living, witnesses could be called to testify to the accuracy. But it would be messy. Indeed they are not all 'hanging offences' but are examples of the traits and foibles of the almost infinite variety of people who become surgeons.

Below is a partial list of phrases expunged. Be it noted that there are many more Brief Biographies than there are expunged phrases and that some subjects might have more than one phrase expunged. It might also have been necessary to use the same phrase for a number of subjects.

All feared him and many but not all idolised him

A poor listener

Genial, unpopular

A somewhat autistic bedside manner

A disagreement with the Revenue about what might rightly be called declared
 income

A deplorably colourful life

A question of interpretation of the exchange controls regulations involved the impounding on the airport tarmac of a 'carry-on' (appropriate) containing £25,000 in banknotes

A man who cared nothing for public opinion, which was just as well

An appalling male chauvinist

Bullied nurses and trainees, regularly reduced nurses to tears

Difficult to get nurses to scrub up (assist him) in theatre

A known skinflint and tightwad

Constantly at war with the administration

Had a bulging, overflowing patient complaints file

Always late, rarely apologised

Total disregard of other people's commitments

Inconsiderate

Professor on the Richter scale of charismatic leadership, the needle barely moved

More respected than admired

He realised his potential

Rarely operated on 'public', 'entitled', 'charity' patients

Regularly dashed away, leaving an unfinished list for an unsupervised trainee

Recidivist racist

His masterly inactivity was really a total lack of concern

Chronic fatigue syndrome

Avoided outpatient sessions as far as possible

Would be late on a Sunday

Brusque and rude…with patients and relatives

A surgical black hole

A strong supporter of the grievance industry

A top seed in any competition for least liked

Liked as much as disliked, often by the same people

A lifetime achievement award for the courting of controversy

Confrontational in negotiation

Little time for teaching students, trainees or nurses…'pays badly' 'interferes with practice'

A collapsible accent

His retirement was early rather than premature

Taciturn…humourless…two separate issues

Little time for hair-splitting theology (atheist)

Affably apathetic

He was always able to sink to the occasion

He brings out the worst in people

Motivational deficiency disorder

Never put a foot right

X was his own worst enemy. And several other people's too.

Was a little too pleased with himself

Liver made of brass

Less vain than he appeared

On the issue of misbehaviour in theatre, he wrote the book

Attractive women students were importuned

Never missed an opportunity of missing an opportunity

The mention of research sent him into a state of resentful coma

Saying that he had a drink problem is like saying that Willie Sutton the bank robber made unauthorised withdrawals

The most overrated in a crowded field

Abused his access to the hospital pharmacy

Socially retarded

No sense of humour whatever

Saw jokes only by appointment

Despite a certain predictability about the event and the widespread and welcome adoption of the Gregorian calendar, his sixty-fifth birthday seems to have taken him by surprise and there were no home-grown candidates for his important post

Regardless of the length and complexity of the operating list he left the operating theatre at 12.40 p.m.

Little was given in the way of advice

Responded well to a short term of rehabilitation

He enjoyed family life so much that he had more than one family

You always knew where you were with X…he would *always* let you down

Despite his high office many candidates refused to be examined by him

A unique talent for attracting personal animosity

His farewell party was a really low-key affair

For many years the administration knew the date of his retirement to the day and he was not allowed to do his own locum

Nothing, absolutely nothing, in the hospital's experience had prepared it for what lay ahead
Provided a benchmark in operating theatre bad behavior
Sometimes a dram or two short of his best
He made sturdy cars appear fragile
His eye for the ladies remained bright
No nonsense (disruptive committee man); disliked committees (ditto)
Choleric (easily and often angered…bad tempered)
Not only collected grievances but nurtured and fed them by repetition
A modern day Robin Hood: he took from the rich and he took from the poor.

In another jurisdiction the surgeon himself was not invited to his vast, joyous, retirement party.

One of the above phrases was made up by the editor and therefore does not apply to anyone. At least two others apply to the editor himself.

To surgeons active and retired may we just say, 'You are in there somewhere?' Readers who have played the children's blindfold game of 'pinning the tail on the donkey' may see some parallels.

Enjoy.

NOTES

9 PROFESSORS OF SURGERY IN THE REPUBLIC OF IRELAND

Biography of Sir Frederick Conway Dwyer

Lyons JB. An Assembly of Irish Surgeons. Glendale Press; 1984, pp. 43–45.

Widdess JDH. The Richmond Whitworth and Hardwicke Hospitals, 1772–1972. Bacon Printing Co.; 1972, 143–7.

Biography of Jack Henry

Personal communication, Dr George Henry.

Coakley Davis. Baggot Street. Board of Governors, Royal City of Dublin Hospital; 1995.

Werner LE. Obituary. BMJ 1970.

Biography of Coley Byrnes

Obituary. BMJ: 9 April 1966.

Obituary. Journal of the Irish Medical Association. 1966; LVIII, 344: 55.

Biography of Johnny McArdle

White RJ. chapter in A Century of Service. Published for the Centenary of St Vincent's Hospital. Browne & Nolan; 1934.

Meenan FOC. St Vincent's Hospital 1834–1994: A Historical and Social Portrait. Gill and Macmillan; 1995.

21 Urologists in the Republic of Ireland

Biography of Terence Millin

O'Donnell Barry. Terence Millin. A Remarkable Irish Surgeon. A&A Farmar: 2003.

22 Anaesthesia

Boes JB, Zorab JSM. Sir Ivan Magill contribution to anaesthesia. In: Ruprecht J, van Lieburg MJ, Lee JA and Erdman W. Anaesthesia; Essays in its History. London; 1985, pp. 13–7.

Centenary: Mater Misericordiae Hospital, Dublin, 1861–1961. Dublin; 1961.

Foy G. Anaesthetics, Ancient and Modern. London; 1889, pp. 128–9.

Haslett WHK. Ne obliviscaris — lest we forget. Presidential Address to the Northern Ireland Society of Anaesthetists, 1999.

Hewitt JC, Dundee JW. Development of anaesthesia in Northern Ireland. Ulster Medical Journal 1970; 39: 97–107.

McCormick VO. Anaesthesia in abdominal surgery. Irish Journal of Medical Science 1946; 256: 665–71.

Meenan FOC, editor. The Children's Hospital, Temple Street, Dublin, 1872 — Centenary — 1972. Dublin; 1972.

Meenan FOC. St Vincent's Hospital 1834–1994. Dublin; 1995.

Mitchell D. A Peculiar Place: The Adelaide Hospital, Dublin, 1839–1989. Dublin; 1989.

Murphy, OJ. Intravenous anaesthesia. Irish Journal of Medical Science 1946, 256: 696–703.

Murray JP. Galway: A Medico-Social History. Galway; 1992.

O'Brien E, Brown L, O'Malley K. The House of Industry Hospitals, 1772–1987. The Richmond, Whitworth and Hardwicke (St Laurence's Hospital). A Closing Memoir. Dublin; 1988.

Shaw RW. Irish Journal of Medical Science 1946; 256: 662–4.

The Medical Directory. London, published annually.

Tracey J. The Department of Anaesthesia. In: O'Brien E., The Charitable Infirmary, Jervis Street, 1718–1987. Dublin; 1987, pp. 127–36.

Widdess JDH. The introduction of ether and chloroform to Dublin. Irish Journal of Medical Science 1946; 256: 649–55.

INDEX

Académie Royale de Chirurgie, 14
Acheson, Howard, 209
The Active Management of Labour, 403–4
Adair, Ian, 141
Adelaide Hospital, 266–8, 390, 540
    anaesthesia, 581, 590–1
    radiology, 605, 606, 607
Agarwala, Rasewar Prasad, 478
Ahern, Tom, 369
Aitken, Henry, 478–9
Alexander, John P., 596
Allen, Patrick, 109
Altnagelvin Hospital, 608
American Surgical Association, 39
anaesthesia, ix, 3, 5, 367, 477, 578–601
    Belfast, 593–7, 601
    Cork, 597–9
    Dublin, 587–93
    Faculty of Anaesthetists, 582–6
    Galway, 599–600
Anderson, Olive, 582, 593–4
Anderson, William, 416
antibiotics, 5
Antrim, 98–103
apprenticeship model, 14–15, 16
Archer, Desmond, 417
Ardkeen, 365
Ards, 105–6
Armagh, 104–5, 408, 419
Armstrong, Gordon, 141

Arnott, Eric, 409
Arnott, Lady, 408
Ashe, Matthew (Peter), 322–3
assistant surgeons, 17, 25, 26
Association of Anaesthetists of Great Britain and Ireland, 579, 582
Association of Surgeons of Great Britain and Ireland, 39
Atkins, C.M. (Murphy), 427
Atkins, Thomas, 334
audiology, 477, 530
Augustine, Sr, 368

Baggot Street (City of Dublin Hospital), 166, 275, 365, 366, 374, 390, 606
    surgeons, 276–8
Bailey, Ian, 134–5
Bailie, Hugh, 116
Baird, David St Clair, 142
Baird, Robert, 418
Baker, George, 141–2
Baker, Seán, 213–14
Ball, Sir Charles Arthur Kinehan, 169–70
Ball, Sir Charles Bent, 166–7
Ballinasloe, 218
Ballymena, 98–9
Ballymoney, 99–100
Ballyshannon, 215
Balmer, John (Jack), 104

629

Banbridge, 106, 109
Bannigan, Charles, 215
Bantry, 213–14, 599
Barnard, Christiaan, 7, 39
Barniville, Henry (Barney), 199–200
Barrett, Connor, 230
Barrett, John (Jack), 334–5
Barrington's Hospital, Limerick, 355, 608
Barros D'sa, Aires, 64–6
Barry, Arthur, 392, 398, 399
Barry, Geraldine, 444–5
Barry, Patrick, 389, 390, 393
Barter, George, 426
Bassett, William, 105
Beath, Maitland, 607, 608
Beaumont Hospital, 21, 589, 615
Beckett, James, 588, 590
Beesley, William, 266
Belfast, xiii, 23–4, 620
    anaesthesia, 580, 593–7, 601
    obstetricians and gynaecologists, 399–402
    ophthalmic surgeons, 408, 410–23
    professors of surgery (Queen's), 51–62
    radiology, 607, 608
    surgeons, 63–96
    surgeons, specialist, 127–62
Belfast City Hospital, 86–8, 419, 596, 608
Belfast Hospital for Sick Children, 594
Belfast Ophthalmic Hospital, 408, 410, 413–15
Belfast Royal Hospital, 408, 410–12
Bell, David Millar, 86
Benn, Edward, 408
Benn Ulster Hospital, 408, 410, 415–16
Bennett, Dorothea, 592
Bennett, Edward, 176–7
Bennett, Harry Milne, 120–1
Benson, Arthur, 479
Benson, Arthur Hy, 430–1

Bereen, James ('Minty'), 594
Bevan, Aneurin, 33
Bicknell, Michael, 479–80
Biggart, Hugh, 480
Bingham, John, 128–9
Bingham, William, 597
Birkhan, H.G., 597
Black, Gerald, 586, 595
Black, Sir James, 11–12
Black, John (Ian), 481
Blackrock Clinic, 34, 368, 472, 615
Blair, Paul, 65
Blake, John, 439
Blake, N., 609
Blakeney, Edward, 243
Blayney, Alexander, 582, 591
Blayney, Alexander John Edward (Alec), 482
Blayney, Alex Joseph McAuley, 280
Blayney, John, 240
Blundell, James, 110–11
Blunnie, W., 586
Boland, Charles, 322
Boland, Denis, 245
Boland, J.S., 609
Boland, S.J., 610, 612
Bolger, James, 599
Bonnar, James, 405
Bonney, Victor, 391
Bon Secours Hospital, 544, 597, 598, 599
Boston, Victor ('Slick Vic'), 157–8
Bouchier-Hayes, David, 186–7
Bouchier-Hayes, Thomas, 296–8, 311
Bourke, James, 598
Bowell, Roger, 444
Boyd, Alfred, 588
Boyd, John, 582, 594
Boyd, John Craig, 215
Boyd, John Stewart, 108
Boyle, Hilary, 388–9
Bradshaw, R., 227
Bradshaw, R. Jnr, 227

Brady, Ita, 592
Brady, Michael P., 192–3, 599
Brady, Patrick (Gerry), 452
Braidwood, Walter, 105
Breathnach, E., 609, 612
Breen, Thomas, 589
Brenan, Richard, 266–7
Brennan, Joseph, 588
Brennan, Wilfred, 121
Brereton, William Westropp, 351
Bresnihan, Patrick (Paddy), 234–5
British Association of Paediatric Surgeons, 39
British Association of Plastic, Reconstructive and Aesthetic Surgery, 39
British Association of Urological Surgeons, 39
British Orthopaedic Association, 39
broncho-oesophagology, 476, 477
Broomfield, Humphrey, 208
Brown, James, 483
Brown, Maurice, 582, 594, 596
Browne, Alan, 404–5
Browne, Denis, 540, 544
Browne, Harold, 303–4
Browne, Hyacinth, 305
Browne, James M., 424–5
Browne, Sir John Walton, 413
Browne, Michael ('Bomber'), 449–50
Browne, Noël, 370
Browne, Samuel, 408
Brunnell, Sterling, 476
BST (Basic Surgical Training), 23
Buckley, Timothy ('Ted'), 380–1
BUPA, 33
Burke, Michael Plunkett, 306
Burke, Thomas, 335–6
Burns, Hugh, 483–4
Butler, Andrew, 281
Butler, Michael, 560–1
Byrne, John A., 389
Byrne, John Edward Thomas, 484

Byrne, Louis, 268
Byrne, Patrick Drury, 583, 591
Byrnes, Colman K. (Coley), 183–4
    Irish Surgical Travellers' Club, 42
Byrnes, Dermot, 135–6

Cahill, Joseph, 336
Cairns, Hugh, 136, 137
Calder, Alexander Mackay, 105
Calderwood, James, 142–3
Calman, Sir Kenneth, 23
Calvert, Cecil, 136–7
Cameron, Sir Charles, vii, xiii
Campbell, Brian, 422
Campbell, Robert, 66–7
Cannon, Dominick, 221–2
Cantillon, Charles, 427
Cantwell, Dermot, 610, 612
Cappagh Orthopaedic Hospital, 463
cardiac surgery, 7, 275, 364–77, 596
    surgeons, Northern Ireland, 128–34
    surgeons, Republic of Ireland, 370–7
Carey, Patrick (Paddy), 381–2
Carlow, 208–9
Carr, J.C., 609, 612
Carrick-on-Shannon, 227
Casey, John, 599
Cashel, 247–8
Cassidy, Hugh, 442
Castlebar, 232–6
Castlerea, 365, 600
Catell, Richard B., viii, 4
Catholic University of Ireland, 166
Cavan, 209–11
Central Remedial Clinic (CRC), 455
Certificate of Specialty Training, 22–3
Chance, Arthur, 181–2
Chance, Sir Arthur, 282, 302
Chance, O., 612
Charitable Infirmary (Jervis Street), 41, 568, 587
    anaesthesia, 587–8
    radiology, 606, 607–8

surgeons, 268–75
Chater, Eric, 452–3
Cherry, John (Jack), 278–9
Children's Hospital, Temple Street, 540, 541, 592
Children's Research Centre, 541, 546, 553
Children's University Hospital, 540
chloroform, 578, 579, 587
Cinnamond, Michael, 485
City of Dublin Hospital (Baggot Street), 166, 275, 365, 366, 374, 390, 606
    surgeons, 276–8
City of Dublin Skin and Cancer Hospital, 588
City of Limerick Infirmary, 355
Clare, 211–13
Clarke, James Camac ('Mac'), 597
Clarke, James Joseph, 230
Clarke, Mervin, 608
Clarke, Richard, 595, 601
    operated on by Purse, 81
    publications, 31, 69, 601
Clarke, R.S.J., 586
Clarke, Stewart, 67
Cleland, John (Jack), 129
Clery, Anthony Burton ('AB'), 307–8
Clery, Anthony Patrick Tully, 308–9
Clover, Joseph, 586
Coady, Edward, 221
Coffey, William, 253
Cole, Graham, 108
Cole, James Owen, 608, 609, 612
Cole, Warren, 86
Coleman, Daniel (Don), 598–9
Coleraine, 116–17, 420
Colles, Abraham, vii, 297
Collins, Patrick G. (Paddy), 269–70, 274
Collum, Louis, 441
Colohan, Nicholas, 350
Colville, James, 453–4
Colville, John, 160
Comer, Margaret Una, 589

Comhairle na nOspidéal, 20, 617
common contract, 19, 34
Condon, Kevin ('Cal'), 552–3
Condon, Patrick, 449
Condon, Richard, 448
Connolly, Mary, 434
Conroy, John, 589
consent, informed, 11–12
Coolican, John Edward Francis (Jack), 298–9
Coolican, John Henry (Jack), 299
Coombe Hospital, 388–9, 390, 392, 398, 405
Cooper, John, 586, 597
Coppinger, Charles, 283
Corbally, Martin, 541
Corbett, Cornelius ('Curly'), 485
Corcoran, John, 283–4
    RCSI dinner photo, 8
Cork, 165, 188, 369
    anaesthesia, 597–9
    cardiothoracic surgeons, 370–1
    neurosurgeons, 380–1
    ophthalmic surgeons, 408–9, 423–8
    orthopaedic surgeons, 464–5, 466, 467–8
    otolaryngologist, 490
    plastic surgeons, 552–3, 557–8
    professors of surgery, 188–93
    radiology, 606, 611, 612
    surgeons, 334–50
    urologists, 564, 572
Cork, County, 213–14, 598, 599
Cork Eye, Ear and Throat Hospital, 31, 408–9, 423–8
Cork Eye Infirmary, 408
Cork University Hospital, 423, 557, 598, 599
Corkery, J. Allison, 417
Corrigan, Thomas, 284
county hospitals, 44–7
County Infirmary, Limerick, 355, 358
county surgeons, 47–50

Cowan, Eric, 412, 418
Craig, David H., 486
Craig, James, 411, 486
Craigavon, 104–5
Crawley, Frank, 433
Creedon, Francis, 337
Creighton, Patrick, 122
Croly, Henry, 276
Cronin, Jeremiah (Jerry), 487
Crookes, Gearóid P., 438
Croom, 228
Cross, Finbar, 610
Crymble, Barry Templeton, 143
Crymble, Percival Templeton, 55
CT scanning, 477, 614, 615
Cummins, Joseph, 433
Cunningham, A.J.A., 586, 588
Cunningham, Herbert, 413–14, 487
Cunningham, John F., 397
Cunningham, Tony, 584
Curran, John, 599
Curry, Rodney, 87
Curtin, John Michael McAuliffe ('Mac'), 488–9
Curtin, Laurence (Larry), 489

d'Abreau, Abundius, 254
Daly, J., 609
Daly, M., 612
Daniel, Joseph, 587
Davidson, Isaac, 416
Davys, G.R., 586
Davys, Ray, 583, 591, 592
Dawson, Cliff, 367
Dean, H.C.C., 104
Dean-Oliver, Silver, 589, 592
Delaney, Edmund, 582, 584–5, 589
Delaney, Peter, 361–2
Delany, Patricia, 589
Delap, John (Cyril), 490
Dempsey, Sir Alexander, 401
Dempsey, Alexander Joseph, 402
Dempsey, Patrick, 491

Dennis, Augustine, 491
Derry see Londonderry
de Valera, Éamon, 392, 397, 405
Devane, Dermod ('Derry'), 357–8
Devane, John Francis, 355–6
De Wytt, William, 454–5
Dickie, William (Wilbert), 159–60
Dickson, Ronald, 102–3
Dillon, Victor, 597
Dilworth, George (Ray), 144
Donegal, 215–18, 608
Donovan, Denis, 597
Donovan, Edmond (Ned, 'Dongo'), 337–8
Donovan, Edmund, 597
Donovan, Patrick (Feargus), 382–3
Doolin, William, 323–4
Doran, James, 401
Dorman, John, 582, 596
Douglas, D.H., 437
Douglas, Shalto, 384–5, 609
Down, 105–11
Downpatrick, 107–8
Doyle-Kelly, Walter, 505–6
dress of surgeons, 18, 35
Drogheda, 231–2
Dr Steevens' Hospital, 278–9, 390, 589, 605, 606
Drumm, John, 405
Dublin
	anaesthesia, 587–93
	cardiothoracic surgeons, 370–7
	hospitals see individual hospitals
	neurosurgeons, 381–6
	obstetricians and gynaecologists, 392–8, 404–5, 406
	ophthalmic surgeons, 409, 429–45
	orthopaedic surgeons, 452–63, 465–7, 471–3
	paediatric surgeons, 542–50
	plastic surgeons, 553–7
	professors of surgery, 166–87, 196–206

633

radiology, 605–8, 615–20
surgeons, 265–332
urologists, 560–8, 570–5
Dublin Dental Hospital, 588, 589
Dublin Obstetric Society, 393
'Dublin School', vii
Dublin Surgical Committee, 19
Duff, Francis, 561–2
Dundalk, 230–1
Dundee, John, 134, 580, 583, 586, 594–6
Dundon, John, 189–90
on fees, 32
Dundon, John Conor, 338
Dungannon, 122–4
Dún Laoghaire, 322–3
Dunlop, John (Boyd), 455
Durkin, Francis, 227
Dwyer, Sir Frederick Conway, 180
Dwyer-Joyce, Patrick Jnr, 443
Dwyer-Joyce, Patrick Snr ('Robert'), 442
on fees, 32

ear, nose and throat surgery, 476–538
Eaton, Arthur, 125
Edwards, Gerald, 553–4
Egan, Thomas (Joe), 360–1
Ekin, William, 87
El-Kordi, Fatah, 492
Elliott, James, 594, 596
emigration, 26, 46, 164, 620
Ennis, 211–13
Enniskillen, 111–16
ENT *see* ear, nose and throat surgery
ether, 578, 579
Eustace, Peter, 443
Eustace, Thomas, 607
exchange programmes, 21
eye surgery *see* ophthalmic surgeons, 408–50

Fagan, Albert, 492–3
Fagan, Patrick, 324
Fannin, Thomas, 137
Faris, George, 211
Farnan, Robert, 389
Fee, J.P.H., 586, 595
Feeney, J.K., 392
fees, 31–4, 519–20
Fegan, George, 178–9
Felden, Victor, 593, 597
Fenelon, Robert (Eric), 493
Fennell, Denis, 597
Fennell, Francis, 494
Fenton, George, 144
Fenton, Maurice, 440
Fermanagh, 111–16
Finnegan, Laurence, 237
Fitzgerald, Charles, 431
Fitzgerald, Colman, 495
Fitzgerald, Patrick ('Paddy Fitz'), 201–2, 332
Fitzgerald report, 45, 202
Fitzgerald, Raymond, 549–50
Fitzgibbon, Henry, 276
FitzPatrick, David, 456–7
Fitzsimons, John Joseph, 310–11
Flanagan, Sean, 45
Flemming, Horace, 112–13
Flood, Fr John (JC), 270–1
Flynn, Mark, 457
Flynn, Maurice (Mossie), 599
Fogerty, William A., 357
Foley, J.H., 426
Foley, Michael, 405
Fothergill, William, 391
Foy, George, 578, 586
Fraser, Sir Ian, 67–9, 74, 132
knighthood, 38
work with Fullerton, 54, 68
FRCS, 17–23
Friel, Robert, 250
Fullerton, Andrew, 54–5, 68
Fulton, Joseph, 596
Furlong, Sidney, 495
Furlong, Stanislaus, 261

634

Gabriel, William Bashall, 267
Gaffney, Desmond, 371
Gaffney, John, 598, 599
Gaffney, Patrick, 588
Gaffney, Peter, 214
Gallagher, Edmund, 591
Gallagher, Herbert, 106
Gallagher, Joseph, 458
Galvin, Colm, 353
Galvin, Joseph, 582, 590
Galway, 165, 350, 369, 409, 445
    anaesthesia, 599–600
    ophthalmologists, 445–9
    orthopaedic surgeons, 452–3, 460, 461
    professors of surgery (UCG), 193–6
    radiology, 606, 608, 611, 612, 613
    surgeons, 350–5
Galway, County, 218
Galway County Hospital, 350
Geddes, Stafford, 582, 593–4, 597
George VI, King, 9–10, 134, 202
Geraghty, John, 606, 613
Gibbon, John, 365
Gibbons, John, 130
Gibson, Jack, 222–3
Gibson, Roy, 495–6
Gill, Frederick, 316–17, 318
Gill, Rev. Henry, 605
Gillies, Sir Harold, 579
Gillies, John, 583
Gilligan, Conor, 91
Gilmartin, Thomas, 582, 583, 584, 586, 588
Given, Frederick, 195–6
Gleadhill, Colin, 138
Glynn, Kevin, 599
Gogarty, Oliver St John, 496–7
    on Keogh, 508
    Purefoy and, 268
    on Shipsey, 252
Golden, James, 218
Goodbody, John, 582, 590, 591

Gordon, Alexander, 593
Gordon, Derek, 139–40
Gordon, Thomas Eagleston, 177
Gormley, Peter, 421
Goulding, H.B., 434
Goulding, Lady Valerie, 455
Graham, Patrick F., 356
Graham, Thomas ('Togo'), 497–8
Graham, William, 104–5
Grant, William, 498–9, 520
Gray, Robert, 595
Gray, T. Cecil, 580, 594
Greer, Ian, 116–17
Greig, George William Vause (Bill), 101–2
Guild of St Mary Magdalene, 14
Guinan, Philomena, 437
Guiney, Edward, 547–9
gynaecologists and obstetricians, 388–405
    Northern Ireland, 399–402
    surgeons, 392–406

Hackett, Edward (Bill), 499
Hackett, Hawksworth, 426
Hadden, David, 260
Hadden, David Jnr, 261
Hall, Henry Potter, 118
Hall, James Campbell, 239
Halsted, William, 22
Hamilton, George, 582, 594
Hanley, Joseph, 217
Hanlon, James, 499–500
Hanna, Boulos, 211
Hanna, Henry, 411
Hanna, Mary, 420
Hanna, William Alexander (Will), 87–8
Hanna, William Swanston (Bill), 98–9
Hannon, Vincent, 591
Hanson, John (Séan), 562–3
Harcourt Street (Children's Hospital), 540, 541, 542, 592
Hardman, Garret, 606

Hardwicke Hospital, 588–9
Hargrove, Martin, 367, 369
Harley, J.M.G., 401
Hart, Patricia, 419
Harvey, Geoffrey, 606
Harvey, Ronald, 500–1
Haughton, William Steele ('Baldy'), 459, 605, 606, 609
Hayden, Patrick, 271
Hayes, Maurice, 606
Hayes, Patrick, 196–7
Hayes, W.B., 219
Heatley, Seymour, 317–18
Hederman, William, 285–6
Heffernan, Daniel, 502
Heffernan, Seán, 286
Heffron, James, 599
Hegarty, Daniel, 339
Hegarty, George, 339–40
Hendren, Hardy, 546
Henley, Andrew (Finbarr), 220–1
Hennessy, Thomas, 174–5
Henry, A.K., 384
Henry, Harold, 502
Henry, John, 613
Henry, Robert (Jack), 182–3
Heuston, Francis, 267
Hewitt, John Cecil, 596
Hewson, George, 446
Hickey, John (Jack), 249
Hickey, Maurice, 370–1, 598, 600
Higher Surgical Training Programmes, 19–20
Hingorani, Ram Kumar, 502
historical developments, 1–50
    anaesthesia, ix, 3, 5, 367, 477, 578–601
    cardiac surgery, 7, 275, 364–77, 596
    county surgeons, 47–50
    ear, nose and throat surgery, 476–8
    medical schools, 164–6, 620
    obstetrics and gynaecology, 388–405
    ophthalmic surgery, 408–10, 455

    paediatric surgery, 7, 540–2
    radiology, ix, 10, 477, 604–19
    training, 13–28
Hobart, Nathaniel Henry, 424
Hobart, Nathaniel Joseph, 424
Hogan, David, 366, 367
Hogan, John Joseph, 251
Hogan, Mary (Gay), 309–10
Hogan, Niall, 554
Hogan, Patrick, 247
Holles Street Hospital, 389, 390, 392, 393, 394, 397, 404, 405
Horgan, John Bowering (JB), 503
Horne, Sir Andrew, 392–4
Hospital Council, 20
hospitals, 30–1, 620–1
    county hospitals, 44–7
    see also individual hospitals
Hourihane, B., 609
house surgeons, 17
Houston, John, 275
Hughes, Joseph, 226
Hughes, Norman Campbell, 158–9
Hunter, Kennedy, 503–4
Hunter, W.B., 118
Hurley, Gerard, 612, 613
Hurley, Jack, 608
Hyland, Gabriel (Gay), 239
hysterectomy, 390, 391

Illingworth, Charles, 60
infirmaries and county hospitals, 44–7
informed consent, 11–12
Institute of Clinical Science, 57
Irish Medical Organisation (IMO), 336
Irish Surgical Postgraduate Training Committee, 20
Irish Surgical Travellers' Club, 42
Irwin, John (Sinclair), 69–70
Irwin, Sir Samuel, 70–1
Irwin, Terence, 70

Jackson, Chevalier, 476

Jackson, Robert, 590
Jacob, Arthur, 275
Jacob, William Gardiner, 240
James, Charles, 223
James, William (Jimmy), 145
Jefferson, Fred, 412
Jellett, James, 251
Jervis Street Charitable Infirmary, 41, 568, 587
    anaesthesia, 587–8
    radiology, 606, 607–8
surgeons, 268–75
Johnson, Stewart, 419
Johnston, George Jameson, 180–1
Johnston, George Weir, 71–2
    work with Rodgers, 57, 72
Johnston, Joseph, 236
Johnston, L., 612
Johnston, R.J., 400
Johnston, Stafford, 504
Johnstone, Robert, 593
Joynt, Richard Lane, 606

Kampine, John, 600
Keane, Anthony, 405
Keane, Padraic, 600
Keane, P.W.A., 586
Keane, Thomas, 504–5
Kearney, Anthony, 257
Kearney, John Joseph (JJ), 340–2
Kearney, Kevin, 342–3
Keartland, Paul, 367
Keaveny, Thomas (Vincent, TVK), 326
Keegan, John, 271–2
Keelan, Patrick, 257–8
Keenan, Richard, 590
Keilty, Samuel, 595–6
Kelly, Colm, 608
Kelly, Daniel, 563–4
Kelly, Geraldine, 444–5
Kelly, Hugh, 591
Kelly, John, 343–4
Kelly, Joseph M., 460

Kelly, Vivian, 505
Kemp, Richard (Ernie), 103
Kenefick, Cyril, 506–7
Kennedy, Denis ('The Doc'), 327
Kennedy, Dermot Patrick (DP), 358–9
Kennedy, Desmond, 507
Kennedy, Evory, 393
Kennedy, Frank, 402
Kennedy, Joseph, 161
Kennedy, Terence Leslie (TLK), 73–4
Kenny, Francis ('Fred'), 460
Kenny, Sheila, 583, 590–1, 592
Keogh, Peadar, 508, 527
Keogh, P.J., 508
    on fees, 32
Kerley, Peter, 609, 611
Kerr, Alan, 509
Kerry, 219–21, 608
keyhole surgery, 9, 477
Kidd, Leonard, 111–12
Kiely, John ('K John'), 345–6
    on fees, 33
    Irish Surgical Travellers' Club, 42
Kiely, Matthew (David), 564
Kiely, Patrick (Paddy, 'PK'), 190–2
    RCSI dinner photo, 8
Kiely, Patrick Bartholomew ('PB'), 346
Kiely, Patrick Edward (Paddy, 'PE'), 346–7
Kildare, 221–3
Kilkenny, 223–5
Killen, James Wallace, 510
Killen, William Marcus, 415, 420, 510
Kinkead, Richard, 351
Kinnear, Nigel, 172–3, 590
Kirk, Thomas ('Surgeon Kirk'), 74
Kirklin, John, 365
Kirkpatrick, Thomas Percy Claude, 584, 585, 589
Kneafsey, Desmond, 372
knighthoods, 38
Knott, Middleton O'Malley, 232–3
Kocher, Theodor, 459

Laffey, John, 600
Laird, Robert, 103
Lamki, Harith, 401
Lane, Arbuthnot, 9
Lane, Brian, 272
Lane, David, 319
Lane, Thomas, 565–6, 567
Lane, Victor, 566–7
Lanigan, John, 383
    RCSI dinner photo, 8
Laois, 240–2
Larne, 101
Lavelle, Edward, 287
Lavelle, Eoghan, 461
Lavelle, James ('Ruaire'), 238–9
Laverty, Thomas, 229, 258
Lavery, Frank J., 436
Lavery, Frank Linton, 450
Lavery, Maurice, 92
Law, Kathleen, 510
Law, Samuel, 511
Leahy, Edward (Gerry), 235
Lee, George (Angus), 262
legal work, 49
Leitrim, 227
Lempert, Julius, 476, 519
Lentaigne, Sir John, 287
Letterkenny, 216–18
Lewis, John, 365
Lewis, Michael, 591
lifestyles of surgeons, 35–6, 48, 623
Lifford, 215
Lillehei, C. Walton, 365
Limavady, 117
Limerick, 355, 409, 608
    eye surgeon, 447
    surgeons, 228, 355–62
Limerick County Hospital, 228
Limerick Regional Hospital, 358–62, 447
Linehan, Gerard ('Gus'), 347
Lisburn, 101–3
Little, Martin, 461

Livingston, Reginald, 75
Loane, Robert (Ronnie), 122–3
Local Appointments Commission, 24–5, 33
Logan, Hume, 88–9
Logan, Patrick (Paddy), 372–3
Logan, William Caskey, 419
Londonderry City, 118–21, 408
    specialist surgeons, 142, 144, 151
Londonderry, County, 116–21
Longford, 229–30
Longmire, William, 58
Loughlin, Michael, 608
Loughridge, James, 75–6
    RVH photo, 6
Loughridge, William (Gordon), 162
    RVH photo, 6
Louth, 230–2
Love, Harold, 583, 586, 595
Love, Harold, 31
Love, R.J. McNeill, 267
Lowery, C.S., 400
Lowry, John Barbour, 123
Lowry, John Henry, 145
Luke, David, 369
Lurgan, 105, 109
Lynass, James, 596
Lynch, Gearóid, 311–12
Lynch, Vincent, 373–4
Lyndon, Thomas, 264
Lyne, Brendan, 597–8
Lynn, Beatrice, 415
Lyons, George, 219–20
Lyons, J.B., xiii
Lyons, Morrell, 596

McAdoo, J., 586
Macafee, Alastair, 146
Macafee, C.H.G., 392, 400–1
McArdle, John, 197–8, 393, 606
MacArevey, J.B., 434
McAuley, Catherine, 442
MacAuley, Charles, 288

638

McAuley, Francis, 439
MacAuley, Henry (Harry), 461–2
Macauley, John A., 597
MacAuley, Patrick (Paddy), 462–3
McBride, Anthony ('Daddy'), 233–4
McCalister, Alexander, 89–90
McCann, P., 609, 612
McCarthy, Annette, 367
McCarthy, Charles, 244–5
MacCarthy, Hugh, 312–13
McCarthy, John, 582, 591–2
McCarthy, John R., 367, 586
McCarthy, P., 612
McCaughan, Daniel, 513
McCaughan, David, 421
MacClancy, John, 212
McCollum, Stanley, 173–4
McConnell, Adams A., 170, 384–5
    Gleadhill and, 138
McCormack, Charles, 242
McCormack, Michael, 218
McCormick, Victor, 583, 590
McCoy, Derek, 599
McCrea, Robert, 514
McCrea, W.B., 437
McCready, Wyclif, 414
McCullen, Patrick (Oliver), 515
McDermott, Edward Neale (Neil), 352
McDermott, Patrick, 227
McDevitt, Joseph (Brendan), 246
MacDonald, Dermot, 405
McDonnell, H., 230
MacDonnell, John, 578, 588
MacDougald, T.J., 437
McDowell, Cecil, 463–4
MacDowell, Effingham Carroll, 244
McEnri, Seaghain, 445
MacErlaine, D., 612
McErvel, Thomas, 596
MacFetridge, W.C., 434
McGarry, Philip, 92
McGeown, Mollie, 86
McGinley, J.P., 216

McGovern, Eilis, 369
MacGowan, William, 184–6
McGrath, F., 609
McGrath, Joseph, 464
McGuckin, Claire, 597
McHugh, Matt, 554–5
McHugh, Thomas, 351
McHugh, W.J., 606, 609, 612
McIndoe, Sir Archibald, 159
McInerney, David, 618–19
McKee, Frederick, 313–14
McKelvey, Samuel, 77
Macken, Arthur P., 392
MacKenzie, Sir Morrell, 476
McKeown, William, 415
McKernan, R.L., 437
McKibbon, Alistair (Andy), 115–16
Mackillip, Neil, 348
McLaren, Hugh, 406
McLaughlin, Francis, 511
McLean, Peter, 567–8, 575
McLeod, Norman, 146
McLoughlin, James, 608
McLoughlin, James Neill, 118
McMahon, Kevin, 608
McMechan, Eric, 77, 84
    RVH photo, 6
McMullin, Joseph Columba, 209–10
McMullin, Joseph Patrick O'Byrne
    ('Shos', 'Joe Mac'), 329
McNaughten Jones, H., 423
McNeilly, James, 596
Madden, Jack, 428
Madden, Thomas Moore, 389
Magee, Reginald, 76
Magherafelt, 121
Magill, Ivan Whiteside, 579, 583, 594, 597
Magner, John, 367, 592
Maguire, Andrew, 512–13
Maguire, Charles, 418
Maher, James, 328
Mahon, Ralph, 351

Makesy, George, 250
Mallow, 214, 598
Maltby, Alfred (Cecil), 125–6
Manning, Kevin, 513
Martin, Norman, 147
Martin, Victor, 418
Martin, William, 99
Mason, Henry W., 606, 607–8
Mastership system, 388
Masterton, J., 609, 612
Mater Infirmorum, Belfast, 3, 4, 24, 420, 596, 608
   anaesthesia, 596–7
   obstetricians and gynaecologists, 401–2
   ophthalmic surgery, 408, 410, 420–2
   surgeons, 91–6
Mater Misericordiae Hospital, 19, 442
   anaesthesia, 581, 591–2
cardiac surgeons, 275, 365, 366–7, 368
obstetricians, 389, 392
ophthalmic surgeons, 442–5
radiology, 605, 606, 607
   surgeons, 280–91
Mater Private Hospital, 368
Mathews, Richard Hy, 515
Mathews, William, 516
Matthews, David, 558
Matthews, Joseph, 300
Matthews, Richard, 433
Maughan, Kevin, 543–4
Maunsell, Charles, 300
Maxwell, Euphan, 433
Maxwell, Patrick W., 431, 516
Mayne, Nathaniel, 229
Mayo, 232–6
Mayo Clinic, 15, 42, 565
Meade, Henry (Harry), 200–1
   on fees, 31, 32
   on visiting clinics abroad, 16
Meagher, Declan, 403, 404
Meagher, Timothy, 226
Meath, County, 237–9

Meath Hospital, 292–6, 390, 540, 565–6, 571, 574, 589
   anaesthesia, 579, 589–90
medical schools, 164–6, 620
Meenan, J.N., 606
Megaw, John, 88
Mehigan, John (Gussie), 325
Meigs, Joe, 391
Mennell, Zebulon, 3
Mercer's Hospital, 166, 365, 390, 588
   surgeons, 296–303
Merlin Park, Galway, 365, 600, 608
Meyler, John, 588
microsurgery, 477
Middleton, William, 257
Miller, Anthony, 517
Miller, Joseph Ewing, 118
Miller, Sir W., 118
Millikin, James, 320
Millin, Terence, 569–70
   pioneering work, 38, 566, 569
Mina, Amal ('Mike'), 260
Mitchell, Arthur, 77–8
Mitchell, Oswald, 106
Mitchiner, Philip, 74
Mollan, Raymond (Rab), 147–8
Molloy, Patrick, 130–1, 596
Moloney, Michael, 240
Moloney, Patrick ('PD'), 210–11
Monaghan, 239–40
Montgomery, Douglas, 292
Montgomery, Sir Frank T., 608, 609, 611
Montgomery, Robert J., 432, 517
Mooney, Alan, 435
Mooney, David, 441
Mooney, Herbert, 432
Mooney, Robert, 222
Moore, Arthur, 599, 600
Moore, F.D., x
Moore, Frederick, 464–5
Moore, Henry, 277
Moore, Hy Francis, 237

Moore, James ('Barney'), 93
Moore, Kevin, 593
Moriarty, D.C., 586
Moriarty, Denis, 367, 368, 592
Moriarty, James, 93–4
Morissey, Joseph, 251
Morrin, Francis ('Pops'), 330
Morris, William, 250
Morrison, Ernest, 78–9
Morton, William, ix
Mosse, Bartholomew, 388
Moynihan, Lord, 456
MRI scans, 8, 477, 615
Mulcahy, Ursula, 231
Mulholland, Patrick, 420
Mullingar, 257–60
Mulvihill, Cornelius ('Niall'), 465
Murphy, Bernard, 354
Murphy (Atkins), C.M. (Nuala), 427
Murphy, John F., 406
Murphy, Maureen, 589
Murphy, Michael, 359–60
Murphy, Michael Kevin, 466
Murphy, O.J., 580
Murphy, Oswald, 591
Murphy, William, 518
Murray, Desmond, 273
Murray, James, 605
Murray, Paul, 583, 589
Myles, Sir Thomas, 314–16

Nadaraja, Thiaga, 518
Nagle, Patrick, 582, 583, 591, 592
Nash, David, 109–10
Nash, Michael, 591
National Cardiac Surgical Centre, 366, 368, 369–70
National Children's Hospital (Harcourt Street), 540, 541, 542, 592
National Eye and Ear Hospital, 409
National Health Service, 17, 23, 26, 33, 476
National Maternity Hospital (Holles Street), 389, 390, 392, 393, 394, 397, 404, 405
National Radiation Monitoring Service, 613
National University of Ireland (NUI), 165
National University of Ireland Galway (NUIG), 165
Navan, 237–9, 463–4, 470
NCHD (non-consultant hospital doctors), 18, 27
Neligan, Maurice, 374–5
Nelson, Joseph, 410
Nenagh, 249
neurosurgeons, 8
    Northern Ireland, 134–40
    Republic of Ireland, 380–6
Newry, 109–11
Newtownabbey, 103
nitrous oxide, 578, 579
Nixon, James, 149
Nolan, John, 446–7
Nolan, Richard, 591
Nolke, Lars, 368
Noonan, Timothy, 248
Northern Ireland, xii, xiii, 620
    anaesthesia, 587, 593–7, 601
    income and fees, 33
    neurosurgeons, 134–40
    obstetricians and gynaecologists, 399–402
    ophthalmic surgeons, 408, 410–23
    orthopaedic surgeons, 141–55
    paediatric surgeons, 156–8
    plastic surgeons, 158–60
    professors of surgery (Queen's), 51–62
    radiology, 607, 608
    surgeons, 63–126
    surgeons, specialist, 127–62
    training developments, 23–4, 27

O'Beirn, Peter, 600

O'Beirn, Seán, 194–5
obituaries, xv–xvi
O'Brien, Brian, 518–20
O'Brien, Michael, 520
O'Brien, Timothy, 466–7
obstetricians and gynaecologists,
    388–405
    Northern Ireland, 399–402
    surgeons, 392–406
O'Connell, Cornelius (Con), 521
O'Connell, Francis Xavier (FX), 290
O'Connell, James, 259
O'Connell, J.J., 608
O'Connell, Michael John, 241–2
O'Connell, N., 612
O'Connell, Sir Peter, 94–5
O'Connell, Richard, 468–9
O'Connell, St John Gerard, 467–8
O'Connell, Thomas Columba James
    (Bob), 331–2, 365
O'Connor, Ina, 427
O'Connor, John, 610
O'Connor, John ('Surgeon O'Connor'),
    228
O'Connor, Maurice, 521–2
O'Connor, Thomas, 557–8
Odevaine, Ferdinand, 431, 522
Odling-Smee, George, 80
O'Doherty, Edward, 523
O'Doherty, John, 95
O'Domhnaill, Seamus, 249
O'Donnel Browne, T.D., 394, 398, 399
O'Donnell, Barry, vii–viii, 545–7
O'Donnell, John, 605
O'Donnell, Joseph, 348–9
O'Donoghue, Hugh, 444
O'Driscoll, Kieran, 403–4
O'Driscoll, M., 609
O'Driscoll, Maureen (Maura), 598
O'Driscoll, Robert, 469
O'Dwyer, A., 612
O'Farrell, Patrick Joseph, 591
Offaly, 226–7

O'Flynn, James (Dermot), 570–1
O'Grady, Frank, 587
O'Grady, Seán, 225
O'Hagan, J.V., 230
O'Halloran, M., 612
O'Halloran, Sylvester, 14
O'Halpin, Dara, 611
O'Hanrahan, John ('Jock'), 243
O'Hara, Mary, 367
O'Hea, Mick, 327, 606, 609
O'Hea Cussen, Vernon, 425
O'Higgins, Niall, 205–6
O'Kane, Hugh, 131–2
O'Keeffe, D., 609
O'Leary, Denis, 591
O'Loughran, Francis, 523–4
Omagh, 124–6
O'Mahony, John J., 524
O'Malley, Charles, 445–6
O'Malley, Conor (professor), 524
O'Malley, Conor (radiologist), 606
O'Malley, Eoin, 203–4, 366, 369, 375,
    377
O'Malley, Michael, 193–4
O'Malley, Sarah (Sally), 599
O'Meara, Patrick (Paddy), 525
O'Meara, William, 208
O'Neill, Brendan, 376
O'Neill, Charles, 586
O'Neill, Henry, 79
O'Neill, James, 544–5
O'Neill, Patrick (Paddy), 525
O'Neill, Tom, 321
ophthalmic surgeons, 408–50
    Northern Ireland, 408, 410–23
    private, 449–50
    Republic of Ireland, 408–9, 423–50
O'Rahilly, Walter, 597
O'Reilly, Sir Anthony, x
O'Reilly, James (Seamus), 526
O'Reilly, John (Jack), 255
Organe, Frank, 583
Ó Riain, Séamus, 555–6

Ormsby, Sir Lambert, 293, 589
O'Rourke, Kathleen, 455
orthopaedic surgeons, 6–7, 18
    Northern Ireland, 141–55
    Republic of Ireland, 452–73
O'Shea, John, 229–30
Osterberg, Paul, 150
O'Sullivan, D., 609, 612
O'Sullivan, Denis ('Denis J'), 572
O'Sullivan, Denis ('Denis P'), 572
O'Sullivan, John Finbarr ('Jackie Gas'), 597
O'Sullivan, John Frederick (Jacko), 289
O'Sullivan, John Phillip Brennan, 263
O'Sullivan, Kevin, 589
otolaryngology, 477
    surgeons, 484–5, 488–90, 503, 509
otology, 477
    surgeons, 509, 520, 523, 537
Our Lady's Hospital for Sick Children, Crumlin, 365, 366, 367, 368, 541, 542, 546, 553
    anaesthesia, 592–3

PACS, 616
paediatric surgery, 7, 540–50
    anaesthesia, 592–3, 594, 597
    surgeons, Northern Ireland, 156–8
    surgeons, Republic of Ireland, 542–50
pain management, 581–2
Parks, Thomas (George), 61–2, 88
Pate, Alexander ('Sandy'), 385
patronage, 25
Peamount Sanatorium, 588
Pearse, Patrick S., 526
Pearson, Charles Yelverton, 188–9, 606
Pearson, William, 177–8
Pedlow, Margaret, 526
penicillin, 476
PET scanning, 614, 615–16
Phelan, William, 224
Piel, Paul, 527, 590

Piggott, James, 151
Pinto, Domingos, 126
plastic surgeons, 7
    Northern Ireland, 158–60
    Republic of Ireland, 552–8
Portadown, 105
Portiuncula, 608
Portlaoise, 240–2
Powell, Malachy, 610
Power, William (Liam), 256
Prenderville, Joseph (Brendan, BP), 556–7
Prenderville, Walter, 405
Price, Gavin, 151
Price Thomas, Sir Clement, 134
Primary Fellowship Examination, 19
Pringle, John, 171
Pringle, Seton, 301–2
private eye surgeons, 449–50
private health insurance, 33–4, 472
professors of surgery
    Queen's University Belfast, 51–62
    Republic of Ireland, 166–206
public perception of surgeons, x, 35
Purefoy, Robert Dancer, 268
Puri, Prem, 541, 546
Purse, George ('Barney'), 80–1, 84, 594
Pye, Joseph, 350
Pyper, James (Jay), 152
Pyper, John (Graham), 119

Queen's University Belfast, 24, 52
    professors of surgery, 51–62
Quill, Denis, 209
Quinn, Fergal, 541

Radiological Society of Ireland, 609, 610
radiology, ix, 10, 477, 604–19
    Faculty of Radiologists, 610–13, 616
radiotherapy, 5
Raftery, Hugh, 589
Rahilly, Walter, 597

643

Rankin, John, 607
RAS (resident assistant surgeon), 17, 25, 26
RCSI *see* Royal College of Surgeons in Ireland
Redmond, Mark, 368
registrars, 17, 20, 22, 26
Regius Chair of Surgery, 166–75
Reiter, Fritz, 367
Relihan, Michael, 243–4
resident assistant surgeon (RAS), 17, 25, 26
resident surgical officer (RSO), 17, 19, 22, 26–7
Reynolds, Ken, 608
Reynolds, Timothy (Stan), 597
Rice, Marian, 591
Richmond Hospital, 19, 21, 385
  anaesthesia, 578, 588–9
  radiology, 605, 606, 615
  surgeons, 303–16
Riordan, Desmond, 583, 588, 610, 612
Robb, John, 100
Robb, John C., 107
Roberts, James, 357
Roberts, Michael, 527–8
Robinson, Derek, 294
Robinson, Peter, 528
Roche, T.F., 438
Roddy, Patrick, 528
Rodgers, Harold, 56–7, 72
  training development, 24
Roemmele, Peter, 116
Röntgen, Wilhelm Conrad, ix, 604
Roscommon, 243–4, 365, 600
Rosen, Samuel, 476
Ross, Charles, 237
Rotunda, 388, 389, 392, 394, 396, 404
Rowbotham, Edgar Stanley, 579
Roy, Arthur (Douglas), 59–60
  training development, 24
Royal Academy of Medicine in Ireland, 39, 40

Royal Belfast Hospital for Sick Children, 530
Royal City of Dublin (Baggot Street) Hospital, 166, 275, 365, 366, 374, 390, 606
  surgeons, 276–8
Royal College of Physicians in Ireland, 165
Royal College of Surgeons in Ireland (RCSI), vii, 14, 28, 164–5, 185, 541, 583, 584
  professors of surgery, 180–7
Royal Maternity Hospital, Belfast, 399–401
Royal University of Ireland (RUI), 165
Royal Victoria Eye and Ear Hospital, Dublin, 409, 429–42
Royal Victoria Hospital, Belfast, 6, 23, 24, 408, 581, 620
  anaesthesia, 593–6, 601
  ophthalmic surgeons, 417–19
  radiology, 607, 608
  surgeons, 64–85
RSO (resident surgical officer), 17, 19, 22, 26–7
Russell, George Hy, 247
Rutherford, Sir Ernest, xi, 2
Ryall, Isaac, 409
Ryan, Daniel, 273–4
Ryan, John (Louis), 448
Ryan, M., 612

St Anne's Hospital, 610
St Finbarr's Hospital, 344, 365, 371, 598, 599
St James's Hospital, 166, 275, 369, 389, 392
  surgeons, 322
St John's Hospital, 355, 358
St Joseph's (Temple Street Children's Hospital), 540, 541
St Kevin's Hospital, 365
St Laurence's Hospital *see* Richmond Hospital

St Luke's Hospital, 610, 613
St Mark's Hospital, 409
St Michael's Hospital, Dún Laoghaire, 322–3
St Stephen's Hospital, 365
St Vincent's Hospital, 365, 367, 382, 389, 392, 458, 519, 548, 591
    anaesthesia, 591
    surgeons, 323–32, 382–3, 458
Salter, Robert, 141
Sandford, Arthur Wellesley, 423, 528–9
Sarsfield Court Hospital, 598
Savage, John, 96
Sayed, Kamaludeen, 386, 563
Scannell, Timothy, 470
Scarisbrick, Joseph, 225
Seigne, Talbot, 599
Senate of Surgery of Great Britain and Ireland, 18
Shanahan, Edward (Ted), 238
Shanahan, Michael, 219
Shanley, John, 542–3
    pioneering work, 540
Shaw, Cecil, 413, 529, 605
Shaw, Cyril, 422
Shaw, Joseph (Terry), 90–1
Shaw, Keith Meares, 376–7, 600
    pioneering work, 275, 366, 370, 377
Shaw, Richard W., 582, 589
Shea, John, 477
Sheehan, James, 471–2
Sheehan, Michael (Vincent), 231–2
Shepperd, Harold, 529
Shiggins, Richard, 261
Shipsey, Maurice, 252
Shorten, Donal, 447
Shorten, George, 599
Simpson, Noreen, 530
Sinclair, Samuel, 412
Sinclair, Thomas, 52–3
Singh, Kulunder (Paul), 530
Siripurapu, Ankaiah ('Mr Siri'), 531

Sir Patrick Dun's Hospital, 166, 365, 390, 590, 590, 605
    surgeons, 316–21
Sisters of Charity, 30–1
Sisters of Mercy, 30–1, 442
Slater, Ronald MacCollum, 160
Sligo, 244–6, 409, 447
Smiley, Thomas, 132–3
Smiley, William, 393, 394
Smith, Alfred, 389
Smith, James (Séamus), 572–3
Smith, Robert, 176
Smyly, William, 590
Smyth, Brian, 156–7
Smyth, Gordon, 531–2
Smyth, Patrick ('Parkey'), 291
Smyth, William, 125
Snow, John, 586
Society for Cardiothoracic Surgeons, 39
Society of British Neurological Surgeons, 39
Society of Irish Paediatric Surgeons (SIPS), 542
Society of Perfusionists of Great Britain and Ireland, 367
Solomons, Bethel, 395–7
Somerville-Large, L.B. ('Beecher'), 436–7
Spain, Alex, 392, 398, 399
Spillane, Dermot, 221
Stanley, Anthony, 229, 258
Staunton, Edward, 212–13
Staunton, Frederick, 251
Steiner, Robert, 610
Stephens, Brandon, 294–5
Stephens, John, 590
Stephenson, Walter Clegg, 606
Stevenson, Alex. Berchmans, 224
Stevenson, Howard, 82
Stevenson, Howard (Morris), 133–4
Stewart, Horatio, 593
Stewart, Terence, 532–3
Stinson, Robert (Roy), 99
Stokes, Henry, 295–6

Stoney, Richard Atkinson, 277–8
Storey, Sir John Benjamin, 430
Strahan, Jack, 114
Stuart, Joseph, 398, 399, 405
subspecialisation, 622–3
Sugars, John, 472–3
Sullivan, Jack V., 427–8
surgery and surgeons, vii, ix–xiii, 1–50, 620–3
    county surgeons, 47–50
    dress of surgeons, 18, 35
    future of, 620–3
    historical developments, 1–50
    anaesthesia, ix, 3, 5, 367, 477, 578–601
    cardiac surgery, 7, 275, 364–77, 596
    ENT, 476–8
    obstetrics/gynaecology, 388–405
    ophthalmic surgery, 408–10, 455
    paediatric surgery, 7, 540–2
    radiology, ix, 10, 477, 604–19
    honours and awards, 38–9
    income and fees, 31–4, 519–20
    international graduates, 621–2
    life expectancy, 35–6
    lifestyles, 35–6, 48, 623
    marriage and family, 36–7, 48, 623
    medical schools, 164–6, 620
    medico-legal work, 49
    public perception, x, 35
    qualities of surgeons, x–xi
    scientific papers and research, 40
    subspecialisation, 622–3
    training developments, 13–28
    travelling clubs, 40–2
    women surgeons, xi
    working day of surgeons, 37–8
Swan, Thurloc, 245–6
Swanzy, Sir Henry Rosborough, 429–30
Swenson, Orvar, viii, 15

Tait, Lawson, 390
Tallaght Hospital, 389, 540, 616
Tanner, Arthur, xii
Tanner, Norman, xvii, 287
Tate, Thomas, 107
Taylor, Alexander, 140
Taylor, Edward, 167–8
Taylor, Trevor Childs, 152
Taylor, Sir William, 168–9
Temple Street Children's Hospital, 540, 541, 592
Templeton, John, 153
Thomas, Eugene (Owen), 598
Thompson, Edward, 124
Thompson, E.W.L., 398, 399
Thomson, Matthew, 533
Timmon, W.P., 237
Tipperary, 247–9
Tobin, Kieran, 533–4
Tobin, Richard ('Daddy'), 332
Tompkin, Alex, 440
Tompkin, Harris, 435
Townsend, Henry, 424
training development, 13–28
    medical schools, 164–6
    trainees' lives, 25–7
Tralee, 219–21, 608
travelling clubs, 40–2
Trinity College Dublin (TCD), 30, 164, 166, 541
    professors of surgery, 166–79
Tullamore, 226–7
Tweedy, Ernest Hastings, 394–5
Tyrell, Declan, 592
Tyrone, 122–6

Ulster Hospital, 88–91
Ulster Hospital for Children and Women, 597
Ulster Radiological Society, 609
Ulster Surgical Club, 42, 110
ultrasound, 7, 615
University College Cork (UCC), 165, 188
    professors of surgery, 188–93

University College Dublin (UCD), 165, 389, 541
    professors of surgery, 196–206
University College Galway (UCG), 165, 445
    ophthalmologists, 445–9
    professors of surgery, 193–6
University of Dublin, 164
    Regius Chair of Surgery, 166–75
urologists, 7
    Northern Ireland, 161–2
    paediatric, 541–2
    Republic of Ireland, 560–75

vascular surgery, 7
Vella, Leonardo, 274–5
VHI, 34, 472
Vincent, Samuel, 83
voluntary hospitals, 19, 30, 33–4

Wallace, John, 608
Walsh, Anthony ('Narky'), 573–5
Walsh, Joseph, 440
Walsh, Martin, 473
Ward, John Turner, 123–4
Ward, O.C., 368
Ward, Pauline, 368
Ware, Charles, 419
Waterford, 250, 365, 409
    cardiothoracic surgeons, 372
    ENT surgeon, 485
    ophthalmic surgeons, 448–9
    orthopaedic surgeons, 457, 468–9
    surgeons, 250–6
Waterford County and City Infirmary, 250
Waterford Regional Hospital, 448–9
Watson, E.J.M., 605, 607
Watson, John, 124
Webb, Isabella, 590
Webb-Johnson, Sir Alfred, 316
Welbourn, Richard, 58–9
Wells, Spencer, 390, 395

Werner, Louis J. Jnr, 434
Werner, Louis J. Snr, 432, 442
Wertheim, Ernest, 391
Western Anaesthetic Society, 600
Westmeath, 257–60
Wexford, 260–3
Wheeler, James, 412
Wheeler, Thomas, 83
Wheeler, Sir William Ireland de Courcy, 302–3, 396
Whelton, William (Frank), 349–50
White, Vincent, 254
Whitla, William, 593
Whitworth Hospital, 588–9
Whyte, Col. Desmond, 608
Whyte, Frank, 582, 590
Wicklow, 264
Widdess, J.D.H., vii
Wilde, Sir William, 409, 429, 437
Williams, Rohan, 611
Wilmot, Thomas, 534–5
Wilson, Charles, 589
Wilson, Denis, 428
Wilson, H., 101
Wilson, Robert Irvine, 153–4
Wilson, T.G. (Tom, 'TG'), 535–6
Wilson, Thomas, 536
Wilson, Willoughby, 84–5
Withers, Robert (Jimmy), 155
Wood, Freddie, 368
Woodcock, Joseph, 583, 586, 587–8, 599
Woods, Sir Robert Henry, 537–8
Woods, Robert Rowan, 537
Woodside, Cecil ('Cocky'), 85
working day of surgeons, 37–8
Wren, W.S. (Bill), 368, 585, 586, 592–3
Wright, Peter Paul, 96

X-rays *see* radiology

Young, George, 102

Zaheer, Syed, 101